Endovascular Surgery and Devices

Zaiping Jing • Huajuan Mao • Weihui Dai
Editors

Endovascular Surgery and Devices

SSTP

Springer

Editors
Zaiping Jing
Department of Vascular Surgery
Changhai Hospital
Second Military Medical University
Shanghai
China

Huajuan Mao
Department of Vascular Surgery
Changhai Hospital
Second Military Medical University
Shanghai
China

Weihui Dai
School of Management
Fudan University
Shanghai
China

ISBN 978-981-10-8269-6 ISBN 978-981-10-8270-2 (eBook)
https://doi.org/10.1007/978-981-10-8270-2

Library of Congress Control Number: 2018944593

Printed on acid-free paper

This Springer imprint is published by the registered company Springer Nature Singapore Pte Ltd.
The registered company address is: 152 Beach Road, #21-01/04 Gateway East, Singapore 189721, Singapore

Foreword 1

This book is a much-needed and excellent addition to the fields of endovascular treatments, vascular surgery, and vascular interventions. In many ways, it is a treasure.

Since the world's first and well-recognized description of mini-invasive endovascular treatment of an abdominal aortic aneurysm in 1991, the endovascular treatment of most vascular diseases have made explosive progress, becoming an overriding trend in vascular surgery and other disciplines. The combination of creativity, ingenious technology, and wonderful manufacturing skills have given birth to the innovative endovascular devices that serve as the basis of developing endovascular procedures to benefit patients.

This book is an important part of the theoretical system of endovascology, which was first proposed by the prominent and well-known Chinese vascular surgeon Zaiping Jing in 1997. This volume expands on this system and introduces for the first time the new term of "endovasdevicology." It also provides excellent guidance and important information about endovascular devices and their clinical application in the treatment of vascular diseases.

China has an old saying: "Spend 10 years grinding a sword." This means that outstanding achievements come from diligent persistence. This book provides a clear and excellent classification of numerous endovascular devices and gives precise information about their optimal clinical usage. It also provides a rich source of clear and artful illustrations. Many of these illustrate the application of these endovascular devices in the treatment of particularly difficult cases. This book could not have been conceived and written without the authors' decades of rich experience focusing on the progressive development of these endovascular devices, or without their systematic and creative contributions as this experience accumulated. Professor Jing and all the authors deserve to be congratulated on the great and successful effort that went into this important volume.

This book represents the combined effort of expert vascular surgeons and leaders in nursing and management. Their cooperation reflects their multidisciplinary knowledge and participation in the efficient clinical application of these endovascular devices. This volume also analyzes the characteristics and requirements of the various devices during different endovascular procedures. It introduces the use of an agile supply-chain management system, autonomous intelligence technology, and other advanced information techniques to assure the availability of the devices when they are needed. These systems assure that device supply will automatically be adjusted to endovascular procedural needs. Finally, this device supply model will integrate with external supply-chain resources to provide the "best supply strategy" and assure that vascular surgeons will have the endovascular devices they need, even in urgent circumstances. This supply-chain model will also make the selection of endovascular devices more scientific and economical. In addition, it will provide data-mining technology to facilitate analysis and reporting of results with appropriate statistical aids. In this way, early warning of poorly-chosen devices will be provided and clinical outcomes optimized.

As the first description of endovasodevicology (Endovascular Surgery and Devices), this book will provide a knowledge system and scientific research method for the optimal clinical application of endovascular devices. As such, it should prove useful to individuals around the world who are interested in improving outcomes of endovascular procedures in the future. It should also further advance the field of endovascology (first proposed by Professor Jing)—a field that continues to evolve and grow exponentially. As it does, this originally surgical discipline must merge with and incorporate the skills of device management and information technology. This merger and cross-disciplinary integration is begun by this book, which should prove beneficial to all the vascular patients that we serve globally.

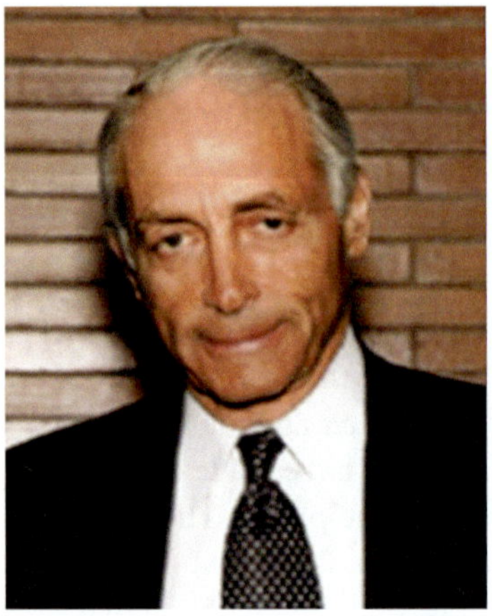

New York, USA
May 2018

Frank J. Veith

Frank J. Veith is Professor of Surgery, New York University, and the William J. von Liebig Chair in vascular surgery at the Cleveland Clinic. He graduated from Cornell University Medical School with honors before completing an internship at Columbia–P&S and his surgical residency training at Peter Bent Brigham Hospital and Harvard Medical School. Thereafter, he achieved success with his pioneering work in experimental and clinical lung transplantation. In the 1970s and 1980s, his attention turned toward vascular surgery with an emphasis on lower extremity revascularization procedures, many of which he innovated. He and his colleagues were the first to advocate an aggressive approach to saving limbs threatened by arteriosclerosis and gangrene when most patients with this problem were being treated by major amputation. His group were recognized as world leaders in this field and had more than 300 published articles related to it. In the early 1990s, Dr. Veith, long an advocate of endovascular treatments, became involved with endovascular grafts, using them to treat a variety of vascular lesions. Many of these procedures he and his associates performed were "firsts." He and his group were the first to perform an endovascular graft repair of an abdominal aortic aneurysm, or EVAR, in the USA. They were also the first in the world to perform an EVAR for a ruptured abdominal aneurysm. In 1995, he was elected President of the Society for Vascular Surgery (SVS) and had a major role in promoting the endovascular treatment of many vascular diseases. He was a driving force behind the endovascular revolution. Dr. Veith held positions as Chief of Vascular Surgery and Chairman of Surgery at Montefiore Medical Center—Albert Einstein College of Medicine for many years. He was also the William J. von Liebig Chair in vascular surgery at these institutions. In 2006, he was appointed to his present positions at New York University and the Cleveland Clinic. Over the years, he has received numerous awards and honors as a leader, outstanding teacher and innovator in vascular surgery. He chairs the largest vascular meeting, the VEITH symposium, held annually in New York City. In 2018, the meeting will celebrate its 45th year. In 2010, Dr. Veith received the SVS Distinguished Lifetime Achievement Award. In 2013, an endowed chair, the Frank J. Veith Chair in Vascular and Endovascular Surgery, was established at Langone New York University Medical Center to honor him. Dr. Veith received the Lifetime Achievement Award at the Houston Aortic Symposium in 2013, the ISET Lifetime Achievement Award in 2016, and the Charing Cross Lifetime Achievement Award in 2018.

Foreword 2

This book focuses on the endovascular devices field, including not only arterial procedures but also the entire venous area. Today, the modern heart and vascular surgeon is faced with challenges not only in the endovascular treatment of thoracic and abdominal aneurysms, but also in minimally invasive heart valve repair.

Prof. Jing is one of China's leading vascular surgeons. I first got to know him on my visit to China in March 1997. I was accompanied by Prof. Müller-Wiefel (Duisburg) and Mrs. Agatha-Lindenthal, representing BsC. Professor Jing, along with his team, and I were first to introduce the EVAR procedure to China at Changhai Hospital (affiliated with the Second Military Medical University, Shanghai). Since then, I have visited Shanghai several times a year to perform an EVAR surgery with Prof. Jing. Over this time, Prof. Jing and his team have proven to be highly qualified. In fact, Prof. Jing and his team not only helped to improve the surgical techniques of EVAR surgery, but they also offered valuable contributions for improving pre- and postoperative care.

Prof. Jing was ahead of the times by realizing the value and importance of vascular treatment for arterial and venous diseases. He had already opened a vascular surgery department at Changhai Hospital in 1989. Then, in 1998, Prof. Jing completed the first domestic thoracic endovascular aneurysm repair case in a patient with aortic dissection. Prof. Jing's department has grown famous for treatment focusing on the thoracic aorta and its branches, including the aortic arch and the ascending aorta. As a logical consequence, Prof. Jing and his team also specialize in minimal invasive transcatheter heart valve surgery.

Numerous presentations, publications, and frequent visits from different vascular surgeons at his clinic have greatly contributed to the growth of vascular surgeons all over China. Since 1997, the Endovascology congress has taken place in Shanghai annually in October. This congress has continued to grow, with a steadily increasing number of attendees from China and especially from overseas. Prof. Jing's work has been honored with numerous awards, including one from President Jinping Xi in 2017 and his induction into the Hall of the People in Beijing.

Besides the supraaortic trunk, this book also covers endovascular therapy of the extra- and intracranial carotid artery. Additional chapters cover the intestinal arteries, obliterations of the lower extremity, and the management of venous occlusive disease, including malformations. Unfortunately, these procedures have never been sufficiently recognized in Western cultures. I am pleased that this important book is now also offered in English thanks to Springer Verlag/ Heidelberg. This will contribute to further recognition all over the world.

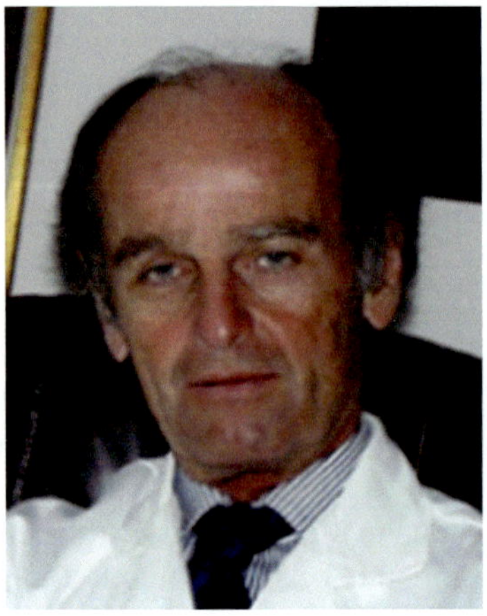

Erlangen, Germany
May 2018

Dieter Raithel

Professor Dr Dieter.Raithel is foremer Head of the Germany Society for Vascular Surgery (1999–2000), former Director director and Head of the Department of Vascular Surgery from (1984–2010) at the University of Erlangen-Nuremberg School of Medcine, and honorary professor at the Second Military Medical University, Shanghai, China. He is also honorary doctor at the University of Cluj-Napoca, Romania. Prof Raithel is an expert in the diagnosis and surgical treatment of difficult and complex carotid artery diseases, and has done more than 40000 carotid endarterectomies. Because of the short time and low complication rate of carotid endarterectomy, he is known as "the European fast shooter" and used to be awarded a medal from the German President (Bundesverdienstkreuz) and was honored with the medal of Bavaria (Bayerischer Verdienstorden).

Preface 1

Devices integrated with technology and art.

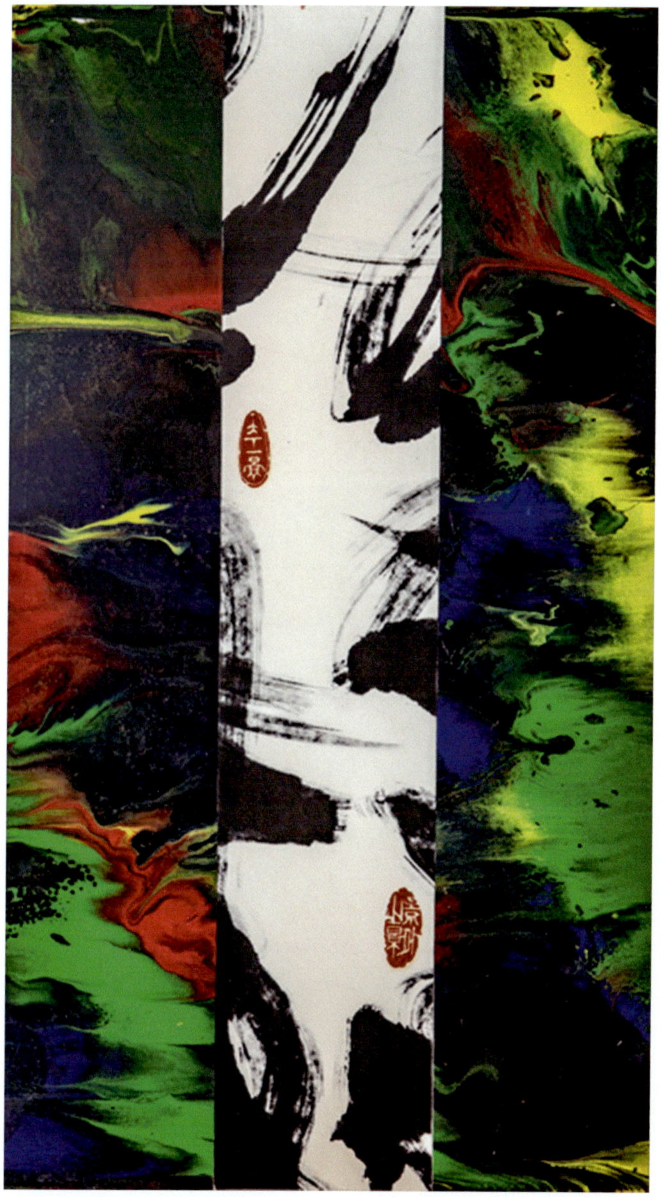

Shanghai, China
July 2018

Zaiping Jing

Zaiping Jing

Preface 2

Having engaged in research on translational medicine and medical information management for more than 20 years, I have always been focusing on the clinical application and information-based management of endovascular devices. Modern endovascular devices are the combined efforts of various high and new technologies and advanced techniques, which not only promote the translation of technological developments in minimally invasive endovascular treatment to clinical applications, but also refuel the technological innovation of the endovascular device itself. These two aspects acting together give rise to a sustainable and innovative eco-chain. Medical information is evolving from information-based management toward big data-driven intelligent decision-making, from rational machine intelligence to smart healthcare integrated with emotional intelligence and from in-hospital management to patient-centered ubiquitous service integration, triggering in-depth reform to traditional medical management patterns.

Ever-changing multifarious endovascular devices have become the most extensive and most sophisticated invasive devices for human bodies. However, they have complex requirements and peculiarities in terms of research, development, design, production, storage, selection, use, and surgical skills. In particular, in distribution coordination for clinical procedures, we must not only take into account the dynamically changing requirements and the use habits of doctors, but also build an agile supply-chain system centered on personalized scale demands in relation to its stocking pattern and emergency distribution patterns, where decision-making involves the multi-sided benefits to patients, doctors, suppliers, and hospitals. Information-based management of endovascular devices is a field of clinical application that requires the widest coverage, the highest intelligence level, and the most sophisticated decision factors. Therefore, professional study and talent development for the above-mentioned devices and their management are urgently required for the disciplinary development and clinical application of medical devices.

Endovascodevicology, as proposed in this book, constitutes an important part of the endovascology founded by Professor Zaiping Jing, China's well-reputed expert in vascular surgery. It is a subdiscipline following the cross-development of modern medical devices and related disciplines with the clinical application of endovascology. The unique contents, knowledge structure, theoretical system, research direction and fields, and other issues regarding the above-mentioned discipline need to be further investigated and discussed. However, its research and development will inevitably provide richer contents for endovascology, create an organic eco-chain between scientific innovation and application translation of endovascular devices, and produce a far-reaching influence on the close integration between medical device disciplines and clinical applications, as well as the development of relevant professional talents.

Weihui Dai

Shanghai, China
July 2018

Preface 3

As China steps into an aging society, various vascular diseases with fast-growing mortality rates have become a common problem that seriously threatens national health in China. Since the first minimally invasive endovascular aortic aneurysm repair (EVAR) surgery succeeded in 1991, minimally invasive endovascular surgery has become the first choice for many patients, especially elderly high-risk patients, and represents a development trend for the surgical treatment of relevant diseases. The success of EVAR depends largely on the innovative development of endovascular devices. Meanwhile, device management and their distribution coordination during clinical operation are not only fundamental for surgical success, but also exert a direct influence on the satisfaction of the patients, physicians, and suppliers, as well as the quality of medical service and economic benefits of hospitals.

Endovascular devices are of multifarious types and specifications, so their storage and indication selections are very complicated. Various accidents may happen at any time during clinical operations; thus, there exist different requirements for distribution coordination of devices. This book has been written with the knowledge of doctors, nurses, and suppliers involved in minimally invasive endovascular surgery; it is China's first professional publication in the field of endovascular devices. Based on many years of clinical experiences in the Vascular Surgery of Changhai Hospital (affiliated with the Second Military Medical University) and written from a fundamental, practical, technical, pioneering and standardized management perspective, this book provides a systematic description of the existing management of endovascular devices in the vascular surgical suite. It consolidates relevant new theories, new technologies, new experiences, and special cases, while vividly expounding the structures, functional characteristics, use conditions, and management essentials of various devices with rich texts and illustrations.

This book was conceived and written under the personal guidance of Professor Zaiping Jing from the Vascular Surgery of Changhai Hospital (affiliated with the Second Military Medical University) and under the auspices of our affiliated hospitals and device suppliers. It is a great achievement after 4 years of painstaking efforts by the editorial group of clinical specialists and medical workers of the Vascular Surgery of Changhai Hospital (affiliated with the Second Military Medical University) and particularly, my tutor, Professor Weihui Dai from the School of Management, Fudan University. The achievements in this book have yielded excellent results in practical use; for example, the Distribution Coordination and Management System Based on Agile Supply China was honored with second prize for the Science and Technology Progress Award of Shanghai Municipal Government in 2015, significantly fueling advancements in management innovation and technological progress. For this, I am very grateful for the support and help from our affiliated hospitals and suppliers. My thanks go to all the editorial members for their wisdom and hard work! In particular, special thanks must be given to my assistants Meiqing Shi and Fuxiang Wang, who contributed greatly to compiling this book by data collection and sorting. I also thank my family because their support and concern contributed to the success of the book.

Because innovations in endovascular devices develop very quickly, many clinical experiences from other hospitals have not been incorporated and there is still much imperfection in this book. Thus, corrections and advice from readers and experts are appreciated.

Shanghai, China
July 2018

Huajuan Mao

Contents

List of Contributors and Editors

Contributors

Junmin Bao Department of Vascular Surgery, Changhai Hospital, Second Military Medical University, Shanghai, China

Zhiyong Chen Department of Vascular Surgery, The First Hospital, Anhui Medical University, Anhui, China

Weihui Dai School of Management, Fudan University, Shanghai, China

Jian Dong Department of Vascular Surgery, Changhai Hospital, Second Military Medical University, Shanghai, China

Jiaxuan Feng Department of Vascular Surgery, Changhai Hospital, Second Military Medical University, Shanghai, China

Rui Feng Department of Vascular Surgery, Changhai Hospital, Second Military Medical University, Shanghai, China

Xiang Feng Department of Vascular Surgery, Changhai Hospital, Second Military Medical University, Shanghai, China

Wenping Hu Department of Vascular Surgery, Changhai Hospital, Second Military Medical University, Shanghai, China

Zaiping Jing Department of Vascular Surgery, Changhai Hospital, Second Military Medical University, Shanghai, China

Haiyan Li Department of Vascular Surgery, Changhai Hospital, Second Military Medical University, Shanghai, China

Guangqin Liu Department of Vascular Surgery, Changhai Hospital, Second Military Medical University, Shanghai, China

Qingsheng Lu Department of Vascular Surgery, Changhai Hospital, Second Military Medical University, Shanghai, China

Ye Lu Department of Vascular Surgery, Changhai Hospital, Second Military Medical University, Shanghai, China

Huajuan Mao Department of Vascular Surgery, Changhai Hospital, Second Military Medical University, Shanghai, China

Zhijun Mei Department of Vascular Surgery, Changhai Hospital, Second Military Medical University, Shanghai, China

Yifei Pei Department of Vascular Surgery, Changhai Hospital, Second Military Medical University, Shanghai, China

Meiqin Shi Department of Vascular Surgery, Changhai Hospital, Second Military Medical University, Shanghai, China

Chao Song Department of Vascular Surgery, Changhai Hospital, Second Military Medical University, Shanghai, China

Wen Tian Department of Vascular Surgery, Changhai Hospital, Second Military Medical University, Shanghai, China

Fuxiang Wang Department of Vascular Surgery, Changhai Hospital, Second Military Medical University, Shanghai, China

Hongfei Wang Department of Vascular Surgery, Changhai Hospital, Second Military Medical University, Shanghai, China

Xiaolong Wei Department of Vascular Surgery, Changhai Hospital, Second Military Medical University, Shanghai, China

Yu Xiao Department of Vascular Surgery, Changhai Hospital, Second Military Medical University, Shanghai, China

Liangxi Yuan Department of Vascular Surgery, Changhai Hospital, Second Military Medical University, Shanghai, China

Lei Zhang Department of Vascular Surgery, Changhai Hospital, Second Military Medical University, Shanghai, China

Zhiqing Zhao Department of Vascular Surgery, Changhai Hospital, Second Military Medical University, Shanghai, China

Jian Zhou Department of Vascular Surgery, Changhai Hospital, Second Military Medical University, Shanghai, China

Yufeng Zhuang Department of Vascular Surgery, Changhai Hospital, Second Military Medical University, Shanghai, China

Lei Zhang Department of Vascular Surgery, Changhai Hospital, Second Military Medical University, Shanghai, China

About the Editors

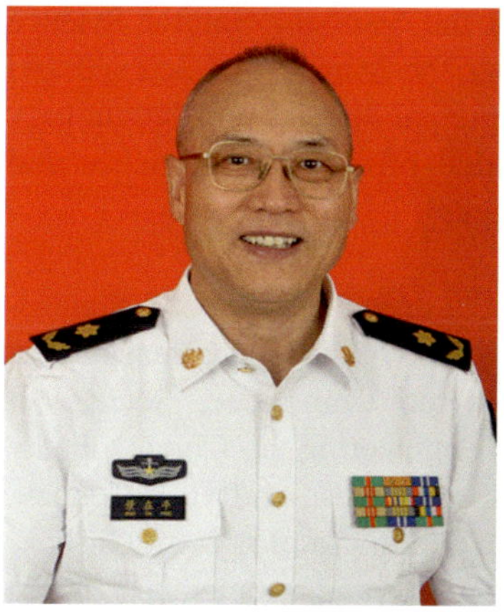

Zaiping Jing is a professor, chief physician, doctoral tutor, well-reputed expert on vascular surgery, and the founder of endovascology. He is currently serving as the director of Vascular Surgery at Changhai Hospital Affiliated with the Second Military Medical University, director of the Shanghai Clinical Medical Center of Vascular Diseases, director of the Military Research Institute of Vascular Surgery, leader of the Military Vascular Surgery Group, director of Society of Endovascology (secondary commission) of the Chinese Doctor Association, council member of Asian Vascular Surgery Association, and a member of European Society for Vascular Surgery and International Society for Endovascular Specialists. Dr. Jing is a certified expert of the Central Healthcare Office and Central Military Commission Healthcare Office and received the Special Allowance of the State Council. He has made breakthroughs in clinical development, such as the pioneering practice of minimally invasive therapies for abdominal aortic aneurysm, aortic dissection and aortic valve in China. The minimally invasive treatment and device research in the aortic arch and ascending aortic dissection has also reached internationally advanced level. He has received grants for nearly 40 state-level invention patents and utility models, with related achievements published in the *Journal of the American College of Cardiology* (impact factor 19.9), as well as more than 500 papers in various Chinese core journals. Dr. Jing has published more than 10 monographs and obtained more than 10 provincial, ministerial, and state-level awards for his major achievements, including second prize in the National Science and Technology Progress Award, first prize in the Science and Technology Progress Award of the Ministry of Education, first prize in the Chinese Medical Science, State-Level Award of Teaching Achievement, Award of Military Science and Technology Progress, Award of Military Medical Achievement, Shanghai Medical Science and Technology Award, Award of Shanghai Outstanding Scientific Achievement, and Award of Shanghai Medical Achievement. He has been engaged in medical service for nearly 40 years. Dr. Jing was named as one of the Top 10 People Moving Shanghai in 2014 and a Moral Model of the PLA General Logistics Department in 2015 for his painstaking innovation and enthusiasm for charity.

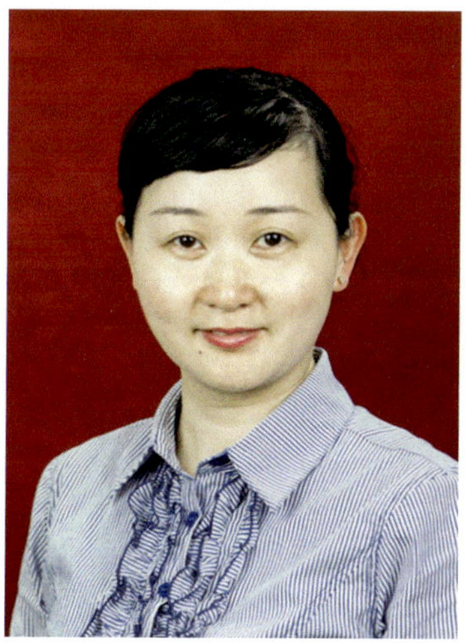

Huajuan Mao M.A., is a senior nurse in charge of vascular surgery devices at Changhai Hospital (affiliated with the Second Military Medical University), with 20 years of clinical experience in vascular surgery. She received a master's degree in software engineering from Fudan University in 2010. Huajuan Mao is mainly responsible for the management of research on endovascular devices, as well as the coordination of nursing for endovascular minimally invasive surgeries. She is currently the deputy director of the Research and Transformation Expert Council, Specialized Committee of Endovascology of Chinese Medical Doctor Association; deputy director of the Specialized Committee of Nursing, Chinese Chapter Congress of International Union of Angiology; and a council member of the Neuromanagement and Neuroengineering Research Committee, Society of Management Science and Engineering of China. She has applied for and obtained more than 10 national patents for invention, has more than 10 publications on utility model and design as the first author, has published indexed articles in a number of academic journals, and participated in compiling five monographs. As a key member of various project teams, she has participated in and completed five major scientific and technological research programs, including the major research program of the National Natural Science Foundation of China, the international cooperation program of the Ministry of Science and Technology of China, and research programs of Shanghai Municipal Science and Technology Commission, China, in addition to being honored with second prize for the Science and Technology Progress Award of Shanghai Municipal Government.

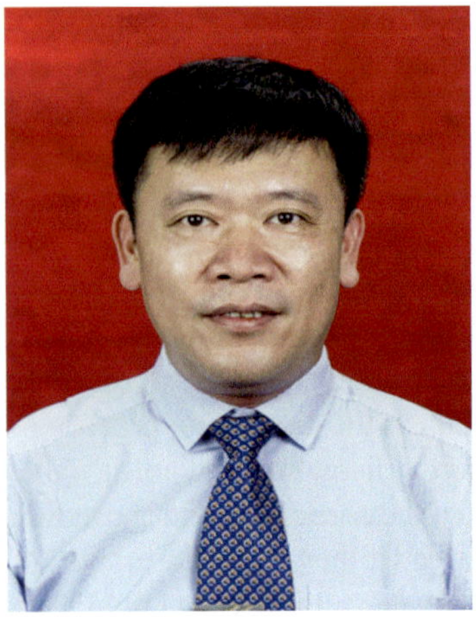

Weihui Dai Ph.D., is a professor in the School of Management, Fudan University; chairman of the Neuromanagement and Neuroengineering Research Committee, Society of Management Science and Engineering of China; deputy director of the Research and Transformation Expert Council, Specialized Committee of Endovascology of Chinese Medical Doctor Association; a standing member of the Neuroeconomics and Management Committee, China Society of Technology Economics; a council member of the Technical Committee on Collaborative Computing of China Computer Federation; a committee member of the Shanghai Charter, China Computer Federation; and a committee member of the Chinese Cultural Industries Management Committee. He received his Ph.D. in Biomedical Engineering from Zhejiang University in 1996. He was engaged in postdoctoral research work on management science and engineering at the School of Management, Fudan University from 1997 to 1999, where he served as the president of the Postdoctoral Fellowship of Fudan University and the executive vice president of Shanghai Postdoctoral Fellowship. Dr. Dai was a visiting scholar at the Massachusetts Institute of Technology Sloan School of Management, United States, in 2000; a volunteer professor at Yunnan University to support education in border areas appointed by the Ministry of Education of China in 2002; a visiting professor at Chonnam National University, Korea, in 2002; and a visiting professor at the Columbia University Medical School, United States, in 2014. He also previously worked as a chief technology officer, senior investment analyst, and advisory director of the listed companies. Dr. Dai has completed more than 22 key scientific and technological research projects as the principal investigator, including projects with the National High-Tech R&D Project (863 Program) of China, the National Natural Science Foundation of China, the National Social Science Foundation of China, an international collaborative project with the Ministry of Science and Technology of China, and key scientific and technological projects with the Shanghai Municipal Science and Technology Commission. In addition, he has completed more than 30 large-scale planning, design, and consultancy projects, including designing the information management system of China's first-batch pilot cities for social medical insurance, planning China's first digital community, and designing the Western Medicine Valley in China. He has published more than 180 academic papers and 6 books, as well as drafted China's Standard for Digital Community Management and Service Classifications and Codes and the Development Strategy for China's Transformation Medicine: Prospective Medical Information Technology. Dr. Dai has received 11 awards and honorary titles, including the first prize of National Commerce Science and Technology Progress Award, the second prize of Science and Technology Progress Award of Shanghai Municipal Governments, the second prize of Shanghai Excellent Teaching Achievement Award, and the National Fine Course Award of China.

Introduction

Endovascular devices are the various instruments and devices used for endovascular lesion exploration and surgical treatment, including puncture needles, vascular sheaths, wires, catheters, balloons, stents, Y valves, filters, embolizations, snares, connectors, inflation devices, vascular closure devices, embolic protection devices, liquid embolic systems, thrombus aspiration and thrombectomy devices, plaque excision systems, endovascular grafts, vascular prostheses, and others, which comprise multifarious and sophisticated types, specifications, shapes, and functions. These devices have become the most sophisticated and extensively applied invasive devices for human bodies. At present, there are no uniform standards for the classification of the above-mentioned devices. Therefore, they are roughly classified in clinical use based on their common applications, procedures, and locations in the body. Among them, consumable devices are classified into two categories of high-value and low-value consumables, according to their value.

Endovascular devices are combined efforts of high and new material, mechanical, electronic, and biological technologies and advanced techniques. Because relevant technologies and technique levels have developed rapidly in recent years, endovascular devices have experienced ever-changing innovative developments, providing advanced technological support and developments in minimally invasive endovascular surgery. Endovascular devices must be designed and produced by taking into account the vascular shapes, structures, and lesions in different parts of the human body, as well as surgical operability, influence on hemodynamics, and possible occurrence of various complications. In practical use, the preferred combination of devices must be selected according to different states of illness and surgical targets, which are closely related to a clinician's familiarity with using these devices. In storage, advanced professional requirements are necessary for the management of environments, containers, labels, and expiry dates, as well as personnel management.

Devices and consumables involved in clinical procedures are multifarious, with high stock costs and management difficulties. Therefore, common stocks are generally available to clinical departments; devices and consumables required during actual operations are directly delivered by the suppliers to the surgical suite. Consequently, distribution management involves a series of links from delivery by the suppliers, logistics distribution, and hospital stock warehousing to stock removal, which are related to the multisided benefits to patients, doctors, suppliers, and hospitals. Information-based management of endovascular devices is a field of clinical application that requires extensive coverage, a high level of intelligence, and sophisticated decision-making. Therefore, professional research and talent development for the previously mentioned devices and their management are urgently required for the discipline development and clinical practice of medical devices.

In 1997, Professor Zaiping Jing, a well-known Chinese expert in vascular surgery, proposed the new concept of endovascology and presided over the first international endovascology meeting. In 2014, the Specialized Commission of Endovascology of Chinese Doctor Association was officially established. With developments spanning nearly two decades, endovascology is becoming a new clinical discipline linked to other disciplines and directed at minimally invasive endovascular therapy.

The concept of endovascodevicology proposed in this book constitutes an important part of endovascology. It is a subdiscipline that formed after the cross-development of modern medical devices and relevant disciplines in the clinical applications of endovascology, involving research, development, production, application, management, talent development and related theoretical and application knowledge of endovascular devices. Major research coverage in the field includes the following: (1) the materials, structures, shapes, and functions of endovascular devices; (2) the process design of endovascular devices; (3) the influence of endovascular devices on human physiology; (4) the clinical application of endovascular devices; (5) research and development innovation in endovascular devices; (6) the production of endovascular devices; (7) coordination management of endovascular devices and their distribution; and (8) the development of professional talents for endovascular devices.

As the first book on endovascodevicology in internation, this book provides systematic descriptions of the basic knowledge, clinical applications, management theories, and methods of endovascular devices. The book is divided into 3 parts and 22 chapters, as follows.

Part One, Basics of Endovascodevicology (Chaps.1–10): From the perspective of percutaneous transluminal angioplasty (PTA), endovascular stent technique, endovascular stent graft technique, embolization of abnormal vessels, and revascularization (indwelling catheter thrombolysis, thrombus or plaque aspiration or excision) of occluded blood vessels, these chapters illustrate the developmental history of endovascular devices and summarize the characteristics, specifications, models, functions, and indications of the various endovascular devices currently used in clinical procedures.

Part Two, Applications of Endovascodevicology (Chaps. 11–19): From the viewpoint of frontier clinical technologies, these chapters introduce the major endovascular surgical procedures, endovascular devices to be produced, operation procedures, and keys for intraoperative observation. These chapters also analyze and illustrate surgical essentials, the use of special devices, and relevant experiences for special and complicated cases by way of actual applications.

Part Three, Management of Endovascodevicology (Chaps. 20–22): Starting from the characteristics of dynamic demands and requirements for distribution coordination of endovascular devices, these chapters illustrate the management theories, methods, and autonomous intelligent management technology of agile supply chains for the above-mentioned endovascular devices. The chapters also analyze the storage and use of devices in clinical departments, the construction of device platforms and personnel management, and the methods for the neuromanagement and smart medical service of patients.

Part I

Basics of Endovascular Surgery and Devices

Development History of Endovascular Surgery and Devices

1

Jiaxuan Feng and Zaiping Jing

Abstract

There are six major techniques for endovascular treatment, i.e., percutaneous endovascular balloon angioplasty, endovascular stent angioplasty, endovascular graft exclusion for artery dilatations, endovascular thrombolysis, endovascular embolectomy, and minimally invasive endovascular replacement of cardiac valves, none of which can do without continuous improvement and innovation of endovascular devices. While Seldinger percutaneous vascular puncture has opened the first chapter of endovascular treatment, percutaneous endovascular balloon angioplasty is the first step of endovascular treatment. It has experienced the stages of catheter dilatation, classical balloon dilation, special drug-eluting balloon, and so forth, having laid the foundation of endovascular treatment. Similarly, stent, a representative of endovascular implants, has also undergone continuous innovations of bare stent, drug-eluting stent, and absorbable stent. However, when it comes to comparing the long-term advantages and disadvantages of stents of different configurations and materials after having been applied at different sites of the human body, more clinical researches are required for further confirmation. Besides progress in peripheral arterial devices, fast-changing innovations are also being carried out on devices used for the endovascular treatment of aortic diseases. As for endovascular devices applied to aortic dilatations, from the coating materials at the beginning, through the small-caliber delivery systems, to the innovations in the overall configurations of stent grafts, more and more aortic diseases which could not handle minimally invasive endovascular treatment in the past can now be cured through endovascular treatment. In short, endovascular devices adopt further minimally invasive treatment, higher disease adaptability and better long-term effectiveness as their development directions, and the endless emergence of new design concepts (such as individualized customization), new materials and new manufacturing processes forecasts the accelerated arrival of an era in which all vascular diseases can be cured through minimally invasive endovascular treatment.

Keywords

Endovascular treatment · Development history of endovascular devices

The development of endovascular therapy cannot be separated from the continuous improvement of endovascular devices. Endovascular therapy relates roughly to six major techniques: percutaneous endovascular balloon angioplasty, endovascular stent angioplasty, endovascular graft exclusion for artery dilatations, endovascular thrombolysis, endovascular embolectomy, and minimally invasive endovascular replacement of cardiac valves. The six therapies alone or in combination continually improve the effect of endovascular treatment, and the scope of treatment enlarges gradually. Because percutaneous endovascular balloon angioplasty, endovascular stent angioplasty, and endovascular graft exclusion for artery dilatations represent the major development trend for endovascular treatment, the following will focus on three techniques to introduce the development history of related endovascular devices, and in particular, taking abdominal aortic aneurysm (AAA) [1], the emblematic endovascular aortic surgery, as the example, expound the improvement history of aortic stent grafts, and analyze the development direction and trend of endovascular devices.

J. Feng · Z. Jing (✉)
Department of Vascular Surgery, Changhai Hospital,
Second Military Medical University, Shanghai, China
e-mail: jingzp@xueguan.net

Z. Jing et al. (eds.), *Endovascular Surgery and Devices*, https://doi.org/10.1007/978-981-10-8270-2_1

1.1 Percutaneous Endovascular Balloon Angioplasty

In 1953, Seldinger invented the percutaneous vascular puncture technique which is currently recognized as the beginning of modern endovascular treatment. By virtue of this pathway, percutaneous coronary intervention (PCI) and endovascular therapy for structural heart diseases have seen their fast development, among which, the representative percutaneous endovascular balloon angioplasty is the most extensively used time-honored technique in the history of endovascular surgery.

In 1964, the American physician Dotter first passed a catheter through a stenosis, then used a 2.54 mm (0.1in) taper-tipped catheter to insert into the first catheter to dilate the stenosis, and finally used a 5.1 mm (0.2 in) catheter to re-dilate the stenosis, thus pulling off the first PTA in the world. In 1974, Dotter invented the basket balloon catheter and used it for the treatment of iliac artery stenosis, reaching a success rate of over 90%. In the 1970s, Gruentzig of Sweden invented the one- and two-cavity balloon dilation catheter and subsequently used it successfully for percutaneous transluminal coronary angioplasty (PTCA). Two-cavity balloon dilatation catheter expands the scope of PTA treatment and gradually replaces Dotter's coaxial catheter technique, which is still the most commonly used dilatation catheter. Till now, the balloon can be divided into three kinds according to their use characteristics: over the wire (OTW), rapid exchange system (RX), and balloon on wire, among which, balloon on wire is basically no longer for clinical practice, while OTW and RX are currently the mainstream balloons in clinical practice.

With the advancement of bioengineering and pharmaceutical engineering, some specially designed balloons such as perfusion balloon, cutting balloon, dual-wire balloon, drug-coated balloon (DCB), frozen balloon, and others are gradually playing an important role in treating various difficult lesions, resulting in a miraculous effect [2]. For example, DCB, a drug-coated balloon, is a balloon developed to reduce the incidence of restenosis after PTA and stenting, which is subject to plasma sputtering etching (PSE) on the surface of the balloon so as to form a nanoscale microporous structure on the surface, on which the drug-coating is prepared. In 2001, the German scholar Scheller completed the preliminary design of DCB, Germany B. Braun company first introduced DCB, and first applied it to the treatment of coronary artery diseases. At present, the application value of DCB in coronary artery diseases has been confirmed, but its application in peripheral vascular disease is still in the clinical trial stage, and its initial clinical results prove worth waiting.

1.2 Endovascular Stent Angioplasty

Endovascular stent is used to prevent post-PTA stenosis or local dissection after PTA treatment and other complications and improve the long-term patency rate of vascular lesions. In 1983, embolization-type endovascular stents wound with Ni-Ti memory alloy wire were produced by Dotter and Crag, respectively, and implanted in dog's lower extremity and abdominal aorta for laboratory purpose. In 1984, Mass et al. produced a spring-type artery stent wound with duo-helix flat memory alloy sheet and used it to carry out 70 cases of thoracic and abdominal aortic and inferior vena cava implantation tests for dogs and cattle. In 1985, Palmaz reported a balloon-expandable wire mesh braided endovascular stent and carried out animal experiments with it. And later, to pursue for a larger circumferential tension, he improved the structure of the stent, where he first hollowed out many longitudinal notches on the seamless stainless steel pipe by laser and then introduced it into bodies by balloon dilation, by which the metal pipe could no longer retract after exceeding the modulus of elasticity and thus formed a diamond mesh-type tubular stent with a larger diameter [3]. Fairly satisfactory results were achieved after researches with implantation into dog's aorta, pulmonary artery, coronary artery, renal artery, and vena cava, and this is the earliest US FDA-approved Palmaz stent. In the same period, Gianturco developed a "Z"-shaped foldable stainless steel stent with a larger expansion compression ratio, the Gianturco stent. In 1985, Volodos first reported the clinical application of stents in iliac arteries and aorta. In 1987, Sigwart et al. first reported the clinical application of metal stents in human coronary arteries. Palmaz and Schatz reported in the same year the use of Palmaz stent in human body, symbolizing that endovascular metal stents officially entered into clinical application. Since then, metal stents have developed into multifarious shapes, specifications, and varieties, and their placement extends from coronary artery to abdominal aorta and from artery to veins, almost covering all large and medium blood vessels of human bodies. Commonly used stents at present include balloon dilation stents represented by Palmaz stent and self-expanding ones represented by Wallstent stent. The combination of PTA with endovascular stenting significantly improves the long-term patency rate after vascular surgery.

In 2003, Cordis introduced the first drug-eluting stent, followed by Boston Scientific, which immediately launched a drug-eluting stent for coronary angioplasty, marking the advent of the drug-eluting stent era. Drug-eluting stent (DES) is coated with drugs that are slowly released to inhibit intimal hyperplasia, where the drugs on the coating selectively inhibit hyperplasia and migration of the intima and smooth muscle cells and effectively avoid vascular restenosis while supporting the blood vessels. Its design and production involve materials science, biomedical science, and other interdisciplinary sciences, requiring for extremely complex process technology, and at present, the technology is available with such foreign companies as Cordis and Boston Scientific. China's domestic drug-eluting stent was launched into market in 2004 and then rapidly promoted for application in coronary atherosclerotic stenosis with a market share far-exceeding the bare stent, marking the DES era for coronary interventive treatment. Currently the drugs carried with DES mainly include three kinds: rapamycin (sirolimus), rapamycin derivatives, and paclitaxel, whose anti-intimal hyperplasia effect has no significant difference at present. Domestic manufacturers such as Shanghai MicroPort, Beijing Lepu, and Shandong Jiwei have launched their own DES. But for peripheral arteries, drug-eluting stent is mainly used in the treatment of low-profile arterial diseases such as infra-popliteal artery disease and vertebral artery stenosis, mainly because the diameter of peripheral arteries is significantly larger than that of coronary artery, and the economic benefit ratio for bare stent and DES is not as significantly different as that of coronary arteries. The self-expanding DES currently available to international market includes Cook Zilver PTX stent and Boston Scientific Eluvia stent.

However, the drug-eluting stent means not all roses. In 2006, the side effects of intra-stent thrombosis (IST) were disclosed, the reason for which was that the drug inhibited the proliferation of normal endothelial cells and delayed the healing of the intimal vessels. If the metal beam of the stent is not covered by the endothelium, it is easy for platelets to adhere to the blood vessel wall, thus giving rise to thrombosis. The polymer coating on DES plays a role in controlling the slow release of drugs, but the polymer coating will also lead to vascular inflammatory response, resulting in the formation of late thrombosis. Although the overall incidence is only 1% at present, it might be of catastrophic consequences once it happens to coronary DES, with a mortality rate of up to 40% [4]. Therefore, the patient with stent graft, especially DES, must strictly take two antiplatelet drugs.

In order to enhance the safety of endovascular stents, biodegradable stents evolve gradually, such as stenting development with soluble polymer, zero polymer, and improved biocompatible polymer [5]. Research and development of this bio-resorbable vascular scaffold (BVS) have been started by Duke University of the USA as early as in the 1980s. When bioengineering characteristics of materials, skeleton design of scaffold, coating carrier controlling drug release, and other sophisticated scientific difficulties were solved one after another, this kind of stent was launched into the market after repeated tests of 30 years [6]. BVS has all the advantages of metal drug stents, including excellent delivery capacity and vascular wall support strength, and effectively inhibits the drug release pattern on the surface of the vascular intimal hyperplasia. Recent clinical reports suggest that BVS has the same effect as the drug scaffolds currently available to the market, with a stent restenosis rate of only 4% [7]. The development of BVS basically compensates for some shortcomings and deficiencies in drug scaffolds. It is not like the metal materials that are permanently retained in the blood vessels and thus can restore the original anatomical morphology of blood vessels. Furthermore, blood vessels can restore the physiological shortening and diastolic function, and the coronary artery will be more reasonably adjusted to meet the blood supply required for myocardial metabolism. BVS stents start their own dissolution 3 months after implantation into human bodies and disappear completely in 2 years on average. The polylactide material in the stent will be degraded into lactic acid and ultimately metabolized to carbon dioxide and water.

Although BVS stent is another milestone in the history of endovascular stent, it is, after all, a new product with a history of only 5 years, and we need more clinical information to assure its long-term safety and effectiveness. The next study, published at the annual conference of American College of Cardiology (ACC) Annual Conference in 2014, is currently the largest prospective, multicentered, random, and open test for comparing the biolimus bio-resorbable eluting scaffold (BES) with the everolimus-eluting scaffold (EES) [8]. With 1-year follow-up, there was no significant difference in the rate of revascularization, cumulative incidence rate of intra-stent thrombosis, and cumulative mortality for target lesions between the two groups. In the BASKET-PROVE II and EVOLVE II studies released on AHA (American Heart Association) Annual Conference in 2014, a comparative study was conducted between the first generation and second one of biodegradable polymer drug-eluting stents and the second-generation everolimus-eluting stents. With a 1-year follow-up, there was no significant difference in the rate of revascularization and cumulative incidence rate of intra-stent thrombosis between the two groups, suggesting that the two biodegradable polymer scaffolds were not inferior to the permanent polymer drug-eluting stents. EVOLVE study compared the second generation of BES and the first generation of BES, both having non-inferiority, but the former has thinner stent that can be absorbed in 3–4 months, superior to the latter of 9 months [9].

BVS has been reported recently in the early clinical application of infra-popliteal artery lesions of the lower extremity, but the international community has been dedicating to the development of degradable stents exclusively used for peripheral vascular diseases, and till now, no such products have been launched for use; the reason for this is that the peripheral vascular stents and the coronary stents have different requirements for the material, profile, and length of the biodegradable stents: the coronary stent is small in diameter, short in length, and free from external mechanical compression and, comparatively speaking, requires relatively low fatigue resistance, while the peripheral vascular stent requires a diameter of at least 5–6 mm, larger than that of 2–3 mm of the coronary one, and a length much longer than 1–2 mm of the coronary stent [10].

1.3 Endovascular Graft Exclusion for Artery Dilatations

The earliest report of endovascular grafts (endografts) was seen in 1969. Dotter reported researches of transluminal placement of vascular grafts into canine femoral and popliteal arteries, and the grafts used were of plastic materials. In 1985, the physician Nichok Volodos et al. of the former Soviet Union succeeded in using endovascular graft to treat iliac artery stenosis, with the test results published in Russian version. In the late 1980s, research reports on arteriectasia-specific endovascular devices were seen. In 1986, surgeon Balko et al. of Medical Center of Brown University in the USA first reported the application of straight self-expanding full "Z"-shaped stent made of stainless steel and nickel-titanium alloy fabric and covered with polyurethane film in the treatment of canine abdominal aortic aneurysm. In fact, Argentine vascular surgeon Parodi began to conceive for arteriectasia-specific endovascular graft as early as in 1979, and in 1988 Parodi sutured Palmaz stent and Dacron-woven vascular prosthesis together to produce the proximal or both-end supported straight graft system. On September 6, 1990, he carried out the first case of treatment of abdominal aortic aneurysm with aneurysm repair in the world. In 1991, Parodi first reported five cases of clinical application of stent grafts in the treatment of abdominal aortic aneurysm, a milestone event in the history of endovascular treatment. The successful experience of Parodi has led to the rapid promotion of aneurysm repair in aortic aneurysm treatment in the international context. In 1998, Dake M and Nienaber C, respectively, reported on the New England Journal of Medicine in the same period the early clinical results of ANEURYSM REPAIR treatment of aortic dissection proximal rupture, marking the beginning of endovascular treatment era for aortic dissection. At present, endovascular graft exclusion has become the preferred treatment for Stanford type B aortic dissection [11]. Abdominal aortic aneurysm (AAA) is the earliest aortic lesion using stent grafts. Therefore, we make use of the development and evolution of the AAA endovascular devices to reflect the entire progress of ANEURYSM REPAIR.

The first generation of abdominal aortic aneurysm stent grafts, represented by Medtronic AneuRx, Guidant Ancure, Gore Original Excluder, and Cook Zenith, is marked by relatively rigid skeleton, suitable for lesions with aneurysmal neck twist angle of less than 60°and neck length greater than 15 mm [12]. It has ordinary release performance, and clinical failure in release was reported. Moreover, interim and long-term clinical results showed a high rate of conversion to open surgery, an internal leakage rate, an endovascular reoperation rate, and a graft rupture rate. According to clinical evaluation, it is not indicated for patients with poor aneurysmal neck, and its long-term efficacy still needs to be improved [13].

The progress of the new generation of abdominal aortic aneurysm stent grafts is mainly reflected in the following aspects: (1) The outer diameter of the delivery system gradually reduces from the 27F Ancure delivery system launched in 1999 down to only 14F Ovation system launched in 2013 [14]. The delivery system with a small outer diameter can more easily pass through the twisted, narrow, and calcified iliofemoral artery and avoid arterial injury, which is more suitable for female patients and results in less puncture point complications [15]. Different stent grafts have different ways to reduce the diameter of the delivery system. Gore's new Excluder uses thinner, more robust fabrics to reduce the outer diameter. Cook Zenith LP uses a nickel-titanium alloy stent to replace the stainless steel stent, reducing the delivery system from 18~22F to 16F. (2) Stent grafts have more diversified sizes to suit for different aneurysmal neck diameters from 16 to 32 mm. (3) The release system is improved, making proximal landing more accurate, with Gore C3 stent graft as a representative, whose rear release and foldable retrieval design facilitates the positioning and release of the stent graft. (4) Windowing and other modifications can be made with the existing stent grafts, making the stent grafts available to lesions with an extremely short or even no aneurysmal neck. (5) Reform in the landing patterns of proximal aneurysmal neck leads to such ring-shaped stents as Ovation and Aorfix for proximal landing, featuring excellent flexibility of its proximal landing zone, suitable for lesions with an extremely twisted aneurysmal neck. At the same time, Heli-FX endostapler can assist with proximal neck landing [16]. (6) Cook and Gore designed a variety of iliac or stent grafts for the retention of internal iliac artery, making the patients suffer less risk of postoperative pelvic ischemia and improve their postoperative quality of life. In general, the new generation of abdominal aortic stents is much more suitable for patients with complex neck conditions, having better anchoring adhesion, less internal leakage rate, and more reliable long-term efficacy, so that many AAA patients who are formerly unsuitable for endovascular treatment can now be treated with minimally invasive endovascular therapy.

In addition, the Nellix system put into initial clinical use in the USA in recent years uses Endobag for endovascular sealing, transforming the traditional EVAR (endovascular aneurysm repair) concept to EVAS (endovascular aneurysm sealing), aimed at solving such problems as difficult and complex aneurysmal neck conditions and dislocation of long-term grafts, which is expected to become a new generation of AAA endovascular treatment device [17, 18]. However, it has not yet entered the Chinese market, and its interim and long-term efficacy remains to be observed.

1.4 Summary

Today, endovascular surgical treatment has been extended to various fields, like arteriectasia, artery occlusive disease, veno-occlusive disease, venous reflux disorder, congenital vascular malformations, vascular trauma, and many other areas. Meanwhile, the emerging new devices promote the everlasting improvement of the endovascular surgical procedures, with the treatment spectrum enlarging gradually and treatment effect improving continually, which reflects the close integration with material science, bioengineering, and clinical medicine and the accelerated transformation from basic research to clinical application [19]. Endovascular devices develop toward more minimally invasive therapy, better pathological adaptation, and higher long-term efficacy. New design concepts, materials, and production techniques come out thick and fast, indicating the accelerated advent of an era of complete minimally invasive endovascular treatment.

References

1. White GH, Yu W, May J, et al. Endoleak as a complication of endoluminal grafting of abdominal aortic aneurysms: classification, incidence, diagnosis and management. J Endovasc Surg. 1997;4(2):152–68.
2. Naghi J, Yalvac EA, Pourdjabbar A, et al. New developments in the clinical use of drug-coated balloon catheters in peripheral arterial disease. Med Devices (Auckl). 2016;9:161–74.
3. Chaikof EL, Blankensteijn JD, Harris PL, et al. Reporting standards for endovascular aortic aneurysm repair. J Vasc Surg. 2002;35:1048–60.
4. Veith FJ, Baum BA, Ohki T, et al. Nature and significance of endoleaks and endotension: summary of opinions expressed at an international conference. J Vasc Surg. 2002;35:1029–35.
5. Baxendale BR, Baker DM, Hutchinson A, et al. Haemodynamic and metabolic response to endovascular repair of infrarenal aortic aneurysms. Br J Anaesthesia. 1996;77:581–5.
6. Baum RA, Carpenter JP, Cope C, et al. Aneurysm sac pressure measurements after endovascular repair of abdominal aortic aneurysms. J Vasc Surg. 2001;33:32–41.
7. Mehta M, Veith FJ, Ohki T, et al. Significance of endotension, endoleak and aneurysm pulsatility after endovascular repair. J Vasc Surg. 2003;37:842–6.
8. Hagan PG, Nienaber CA, Isselbacher EM, et al. The international registry of acute aortic dissection (IRAD): new insight into an old disease. JAMA. 2000;283:897–903.
9. Zimpfer D, Schima H, Czerny M, et al. Experimental stent-graft treatment of ascending aortic dissection. Ann Thorac Surg. 2008;85:470–3.
10. Wang Z, Massimo C, Li M, et al. Deployment of endograft in the ascending aorta to reverse type A aortic dissection. Asian J Surg. 2003;26:117–9.
11. Feng R, Zhao Z, Bao J, et al. Double-chimney technology for treating secondary type I endoleak after endovascular repair for complicated thoracic aortic dissection. J Vasc Surg. 2011;54:212–5.
12. Yuan L, Feng X, Jing Z. Endovascular repair of a thoracic arch aneurysm with a fenestrated stent-graft. J Endovasc Ther. 2008;15:539–43.
13. Lu Q, Jing Z, Zhao Z, et al. Endovascular stent graft repair of aortic dissection type B extending to the aortic arch. Eur J Vasc Endovasc Surg. 2011;42:456–63.
14. Lin C, Lu Q, Liao M, et al. Endovascular repair of the half aortic arch in pigs with an improved, single-branched stent graft system for the brachiocephalic trunk. Vascular. 2011;19:242–9.
15. Hayashida K, Lefevre T, Chevalier B, et al. Transfemoral aortic valve implantation new criteria to predict vascular complications. JACC Cardiovasc Interv. 2011;4:851–8.
16. David HD, Manish M, Karthik K, et al. The phase I multicenter trial (STAPLE-1) of the Aptus endovascular repair system: results at 6 months and 1 year. J Vasc Surg. 2009;49:851–7; discussion 857–858.
17. Leon MB, Smith CR, Mack M, et al. Transcatheter aortic- valve implantation for aortic stenosis in patients who cannot undergo surgery. N Engl J Med. 2010;363:1597–607.
18. Reijnen MM, de Bruin JL, Mathijssen EG, et al. Global experience with the nellix endosystem for ruptured and symptomatic abdominal aortic aneurysms. J Endovasc Ther. 2016;23:21–8.
19. Stone GW. Bioresorbable vascular scaffolds: more different than alike? JACC Cardiovasc Interv. 2016;9:575–7.

2 Conventional Endovascular Devices

Huajuan Mao, Fuxiang Wang, Junmin Bao, and Zhiyong Chen

Abstract

Conventional endovascular devices provide a basic guarantee for endovascular treatment. They include puncture needle, sheath, wire, Y-type valve, connecting pipe, inflation pump, vascular closure device, etc. This chapter gives a detailed introduction to the structures, features, models, brands, and other information of the abovementioned devices and offers a conclusion and summary about the operation steps of vascular closure devices from the perspective of clinical application.

Keywords

Conventional endovascular devices · Structure and features · Model · Usage in operation

2.1 The Puncture Needle

2.1.1 Product Structure

The puncture needle is the basic device for percutaneous vascular puncture, mostly trocar, composed of an outer cannula and a needle core, where, in use, the protrusion at the rear end of the needle core is inserted into the groove at the rear end of the outer cannula so that the slope direction of the needle tip is in the same direction as the slope direction of the cannula tip. To facilitate holding the needle and identifying the slope direction of the needle tip, some puncture needles are equipped with a tail flap at the end. Puncture needles are mostly made of stainless steel, with their outer cannula being plastic.

As the tips of the puncture needles are different, there are two kinds of trocars:

- Seldinger needle, with blunt outer cannula and needle of pointed tip and sharp surface
- Bailey needle, with sharp-faced outer cannula and needle core with blunt tip not protruding out of the outer cannula

Apart from the two kinds of trocars, another commonly used puncture needle is the front-wall puncture needle, or single-wall needle, without outer cannula, usually made of metal, where, in use, the front-wall needle needs not to pass through the back wall of the vessels, with easy operation and popularity in clinical practice.

2.1.2 Models and Specifications

The diameter size of the puncture needle is usually expressed in G (gauge) internationally, where the gauge number goes up and the diameter size goes down. But in China, it is mostly expressed in number, where the bigger the number is, the larger the size will be. For example, we use Nos. 8, 9, and 12 to express 0.8, 0.9, and 1.2 mm outer diameter of the puncture needle, respectively. G relates to number roughly like this: 14G = No. 20, 16G = No. 16, 18G = No. 12, 20G = No. 9, 21G = No. 8, and 22G = No. 7. For adults, usually 16–19G puncture needles are used, but for children, 18–19G, and wire with a maximum inserted diameter of 0.97 mm (0.038in) can be used for endovascular treatment. At present, there are various puncture needle brands, and this section mainly introduces Cook and Terumo puncture needle.

H. Mao (✉) · F. Wang · J. Bao
Department of Vascular Surgery, Changhai Hospital, Second Military Medical University, Shanghai, China
e-mail: czymm8@163.com

Z. Chen
Department of Vascular Surgery, The First Hospital, Anhui Medical University, Hefei, China

Z. Jing et al. (eds.), *Endovascular Surgery and Devices*, https://doi.org/10.1007/978-981-10-8270-2_2

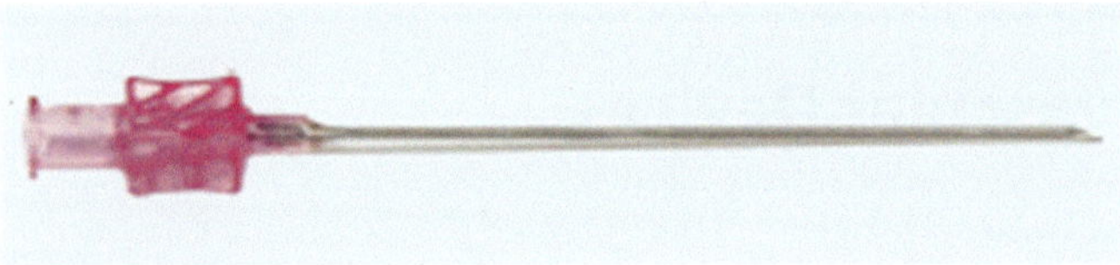

Fig. 2.1 Cook puncture needle

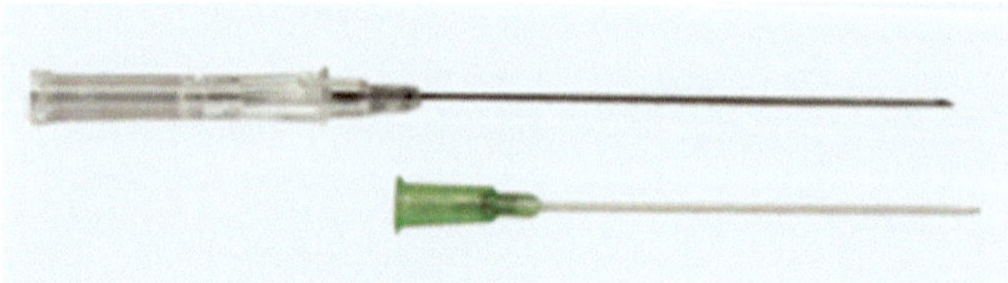

Fig. 2.2 Terumo puncture needle

2.1.3 Brand Information

2.1.3.1 Cook Puncture Needle

The US Cook-produced puncture needle (Fig. 2.1) is a front-wall puncture needle, with its tube made of stainless steel, its tube base of plastics, without outer cannula, at a diameter of 18G (21G for micropuncture needle used for 4F micropuncture sheath) and a length of 7 cm.

2.1.3.2 Terumo Puncture Needle

The Japanese Terumo-produced puncture needle (Fig. 2.2) is a Seldinger trocar, composed of plastic cannula and metal puncture needle, a supportive product with Terumo vascular sheath, having 18G needle core and 8.5-cm-long inner core. Its outer cannula is 7.5 cm long and slightly shorter than the puncture needle, where, in use, the puncture needle is withdrawn after puncture into the vessels, with the outer cannula left inside to insert the wire. Compared with metal puncture needle, the plastic trocar features sound flexibility and soft tip, which can be bent into the vessels with the wire, not liable of damage to vessels or wire. Usually, the trocar first penetrates through the vascular back wall and then withdraws into the vascular cavity.

2.2 Vascular Sheath

2.2.1 Product Structure

The vascular sheath kit is composed of a vascular sheath and a dilator. The vascular sheath is a cannula sheath made of plastics, which is placed outside the dilator and inserted into the vessels together with the dilator. When the dilator is pulled out, the catheter is inserted, and thereafter, all operations can be performed via the vascular sheath. The vascular sheath can not only facilitate intraoperative operation, support and guide the catheter and wire, but also reduce the bleeding at the puncture and the pain of patients.

2.2.1.1 Vascular Sheath

At the proximal end of the sheath, there is a sidearm and a short connector, the end of which connects a three-way valve. Through this connector diluted heparin can be injected to avoid the formation of blood clots among the intrathecal catheter gaps. There is a rubber sheet at the joint of the sheath, with a gap in the middle, where the catheter can be inserted. As the rubber sheet is closely attached to the catheter, the blood within the blood vessels is not easy to leak. Therefore, this kind of vascular sheath is often referred to as the leak-proof sheath.

2.2.1.2 The Dilator

The dilator head gradually shrinks to expand the passage of the skin to the vascular wall for subsequent placement of the catheter. When the wire enters into the blood vessels through the puncture needle, pull the wire through the dilator and insert the dilator into the vessel together with the wire. Please note that the dilator used should be slightly smaller than the subsequently used catheter, preferably 0.5F, and should not be larger than the subsequently used catheter. Otherwise, with the catheter inserted into the blood vessels, blood may leak around the catheter, seriously affecting the operation. If this happens, replace it with a larger catheter or insert the vascular sheath immediately.

2.2.2 Models and Specifications

The diameter unit of the vascular sheath, the guide catheter, the catheter, the balloon catheter, and the stent is expressed in Fr., or abbreviated as F. Fr. was originally a unit measuring the circumference, invented by a French physician, and an abbreviation of the English word French. Fr. system is based on π (pi), where the French size of the catheter or cannula is divided by π or 3 so as to obtain the catheter or cannula diameter.

The vascular sheath can be divided into a short vascular sheath (short sheath) and a long vascular sheath (a long sheath or an introducer sheath) in terms of its length:

- The short sheath is indicated for common vascular access, angiography, as well as vascular anterograde or retrograde puncture of the lower extremity. The short sheath's inner diameter (ID) is 4–14F, of which 5 F and 6 F short sheaths are the most commonly used. The length of the short sheath is generally 10–20 cm.
- The long sheath is indicated for puncturing distant vessels at a long distance, such as the carotid artery, vertebral artery, subclavian artery, renal artery, and other blood vessels, and different vascular sheaths can be selected according to different positions of lesions. The inner diameter of the long sheath is 4–26 F. The length of the long sheath can be determined according to the length of

the lesion to access, for example, 45–55-cm-long sheath can be used for accessing renal artery stenosis from femoral artery and 70–90 cm sheath if being accessed from brachial artery. It is noteworthy that, in choosing the long sheath with a longer length, a catheter about 10 cm longer than the long sheath shall be selected to coordinate with the use. In addition, the long sheath has straight and curved tips for selection to suit for vessels of different lesions and different positions.

At present, vascular sheath brands mainly include Terumo, St. Jude, Cook, Cordis, Arrow, Gore, Merit, LifeTech, and others. In this section, we focus on introducing Terumo, St. Jude, Cook, Cordis, Arrow, Gore, and LifeTech vascular sheaths.

2.2.3 Brand Information

2.2.3.1 Terumo Vascular Sheath

The Japan Terumo-produced short sheath (Fig. 2.3) has inner diameter of 5–9F, sheath body being hydrophilic coating, indicated for various angiography and endovascular treatment and most commonly in clinical use.

- The Japan Terumo-produced long sheath (Fig. 2.4) has inner diameter of 6–8F, with the sheath body being hydrophilic coating, sheath tip being straight and curved, at a length of 45–90 cm, suitable for endovascular treatment of visceral artery, carotid artery, vertebral artery, and subclavian artery.

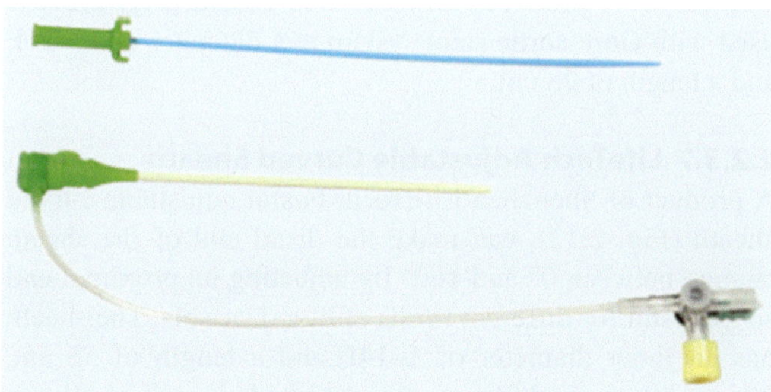

Fig. 2.3 The short sheath (Terumo)

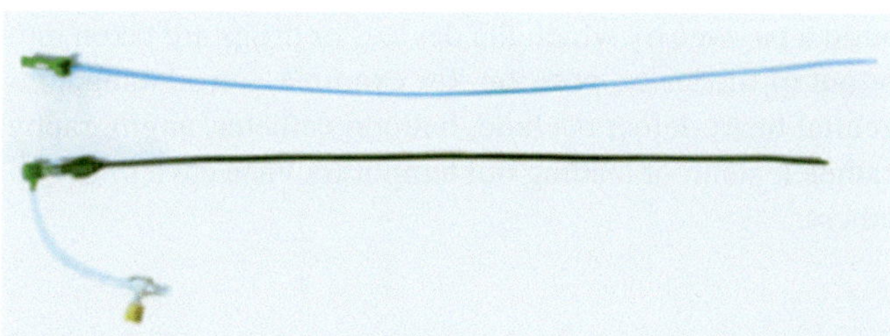

Fig. 2.4 The long sheath (Terumo)

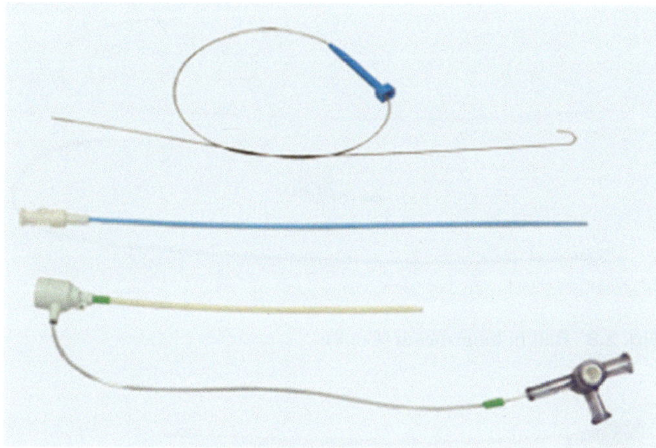

Fig. 2.5 The short sheath (St. Jude)

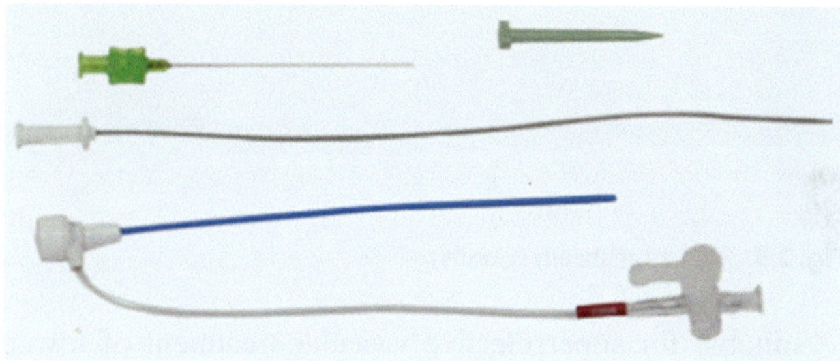

Fig. 2.6 The short sheath (Cook)

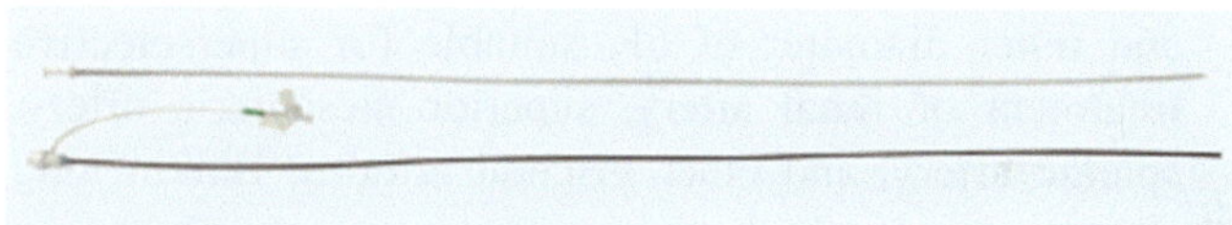

Fig. 2.7 Raabe long sheath (Cook)

2.2.3.2 St. Jude Vascular Sheath

The US St. Jude-produced short sheath (Fig. 2.5) has an inner diameter of 5–10F, indicated for the anterograde puncture of lower extremity, angiography, and other kinds of endovascular treatment.

2.2.3.3 Cook Vascular Sheath

- The US Cook-produced short sheath (Fig. 2.6) has an inner diameter of 4–14F, among which 4F short sheath is micropuncture sheath used with 21G micropuncture needle and 0.46 mm (0.018in) wire, indicated for the retrograde puncture of arterioles of lower extremities. 12F and 14F short sheaths are equipped with 8F and 10F dilators, respectively.
- The US Cook-produced long sheath is classified as Raabe long sheath (Fig. 2.7), Ansel long sheath, Balkin long sheath (Fig. 2.8), and others. Raabe long sheath has a straight tip at a length of 55 cm, 70 cm, 80 cm, and 90 cm, respectively, and has an inner diameter of 4–10F,

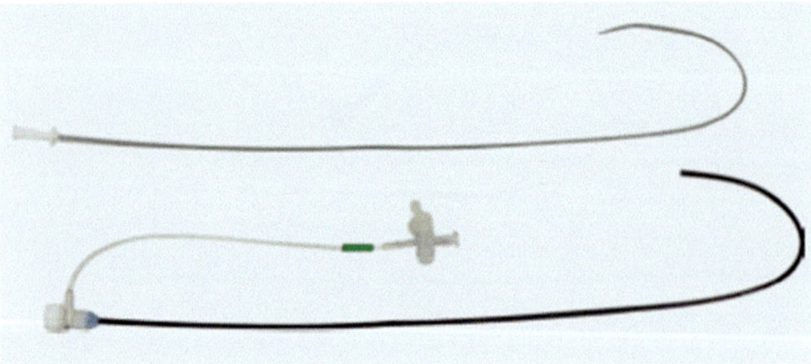

Fig. 2.8 Balkin long sheath (Cook)

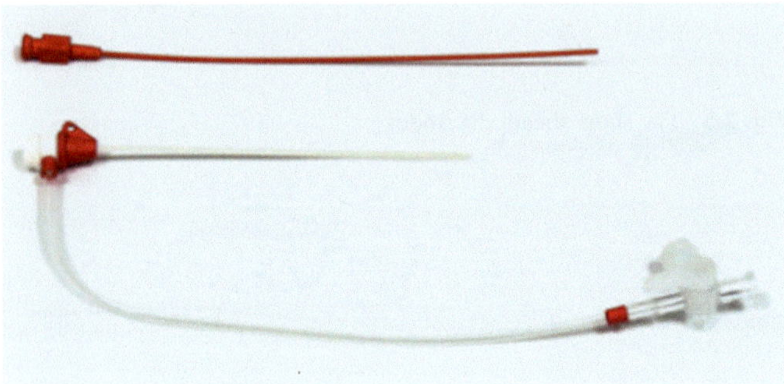

Fig. 2.9 The short sheath (Cordis)

suitable for superselective vascular treatment of lower extremity arteries, carotid artery, vertebral artery, and subclavian artery. Ansel long sheath has a curved tip specially designed for renal arteries at a length of 45 cm and inner diameter of 6F, suitable for superselective treatment of renal artery, superior mesenteric artery, splenic artery, and other visceral arteries. Balkin long sheath, commonly known as crossover sheath, has a curved tip specially designed for crossover treatment of lower extremity arteries, with a length of 40 cm and an inner diameter of 6–8F, suitable for crossover treatment of lower extremities.

2.2.3.4 Cordis Vascular Sheath

The US Cordis-produced short sheath has an inner diameter of 4–8F, among which 4F short sheath (Fig. 2.9) is indicated for the retrograde puncture of lower extremities and also for the puncture treatment of children or thinner blood vessels, available to accessing through 0.89 mm (0.035in) wire.

2.2.3.5 Arrow Vascular Sheath

The US Arrow-produced long sheath (Fig. 2.10) has a cannula made of metal coil. Compared with other long sheaths, Arrow long sheath is softer and has easy access through twisted blood vessels but with poor supportive force. The long sheath has an inner diameter of 6–10F and a length of 35–90 cm.

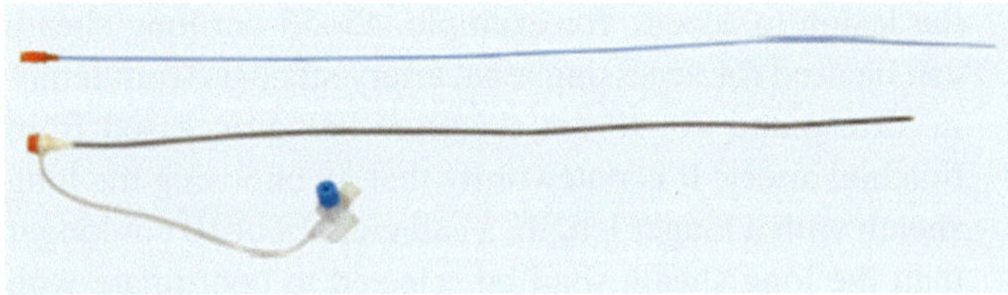

Fig. 2.10 The long sheath (Arrow)

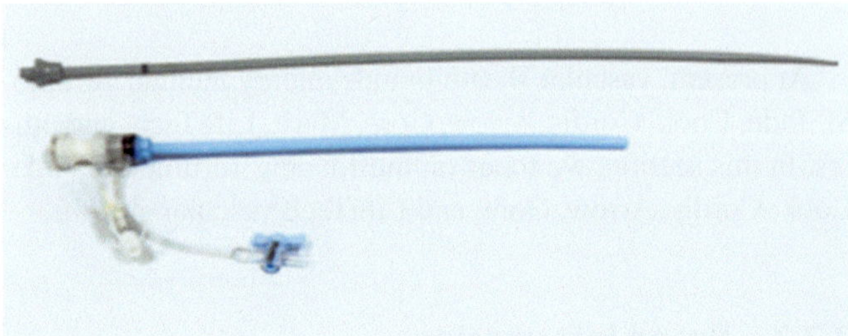

Fig. 2.11 Dryseal long sheath (Gore)

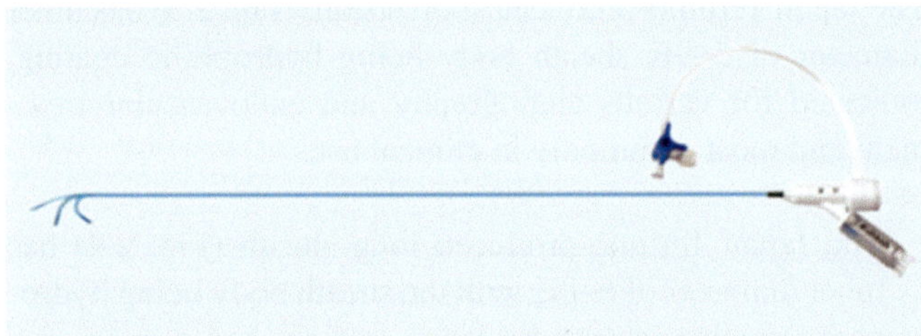

Fig. 2.12 Fustar adjustable curved sheath (LifeTech)

2.2.3.6 Gore Vascular Sheath

The US Gore-produced Dryseal long sheath (Fig. 2.11) is used with Gore aortic stent system at a diameter of 12–26F and a length of 28 cm.

2.2.3.7 LifeTech Adjustable Curved Sheath

A product of Shenzhen LifeTech, Fustar adjustable curved sheath (Fig. 2.12), can make the distal end of the sheath change between 0° and 160° by adjusting its proximal end so as to suit for different forms of blood vessels. The sheath has an inner diameter of 5–14F and a length of 55 cm, 70 cm, 80 cm, and 90 cm, with bendable length of 30 mm and 50 mm and bendable angle of 0–160°. Fustar adjustable curved sheath is used for percutaneous angiography or treatment, which accesses through the vascular system to build a passage by which the devices or drugs are taken into or out of the lesion position, for example, introducing congenital heart defect occlude, balloon catheter, angiography catheter, stent, or leading out temporary vena cava filter and others.

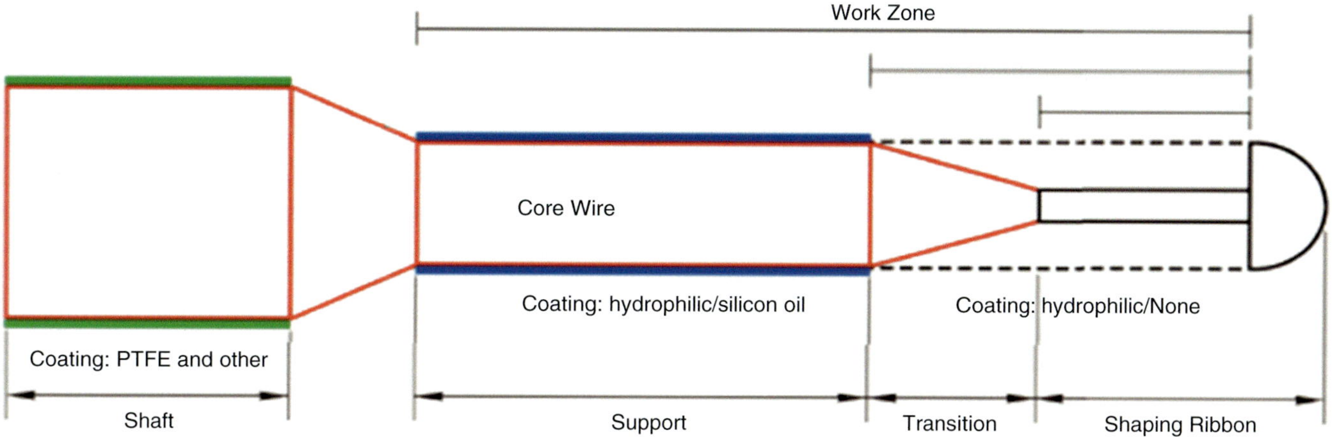

Fig. 2.13 Wire Structure

2.3 Wire

Wire is of vital importance for endovascular therapy. Wire reaching and crossing the lesion can largely affect the success of an operation, and selecting adequate wire can lead to twofold results with half the effort for the operation. However, wire performance differs greatly due to different brand-specific structure designs and material selections. In this section, wire characteristics of different designs for different wire structures and materials are introduced, including a brief description of the influence on their performance.

2.3.1 Product Structure

2.3.1.1 Wire Structure

Wire usually comprises four segments, i.e., shaping, transition, support, and shaft sections (Fig. 2.13).

Shaping Section

1. Tip Design
   - Tip with coil cover (Fig. 2.14): This design features excellent tactile feedback and increased visibility but relatively larger friction which is not conducive to crossing the severely calcified, distorted, and occluded lesions.
   - Tip with polymer cover (Fig. 2.15): This design serves to apply polymer coating (usually hydrophilic coating) on the outside of the coil, enabling smooth wire surface and effectively reducing wire friction. This design is an improvement in coil cover design to certain extent but still has its own shortcomings in design.

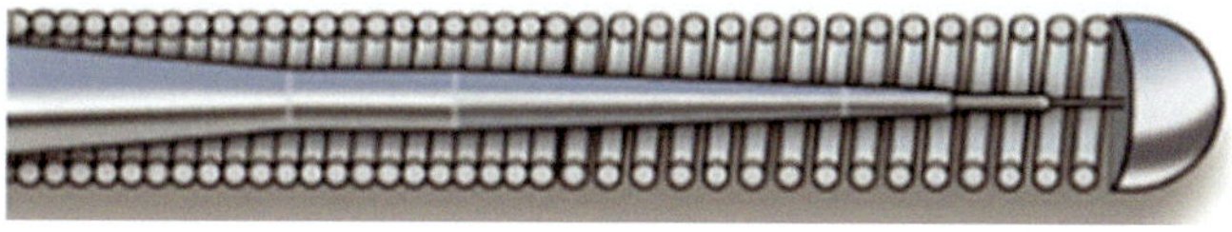

Fig. 2.14 Wire with coil cover tip

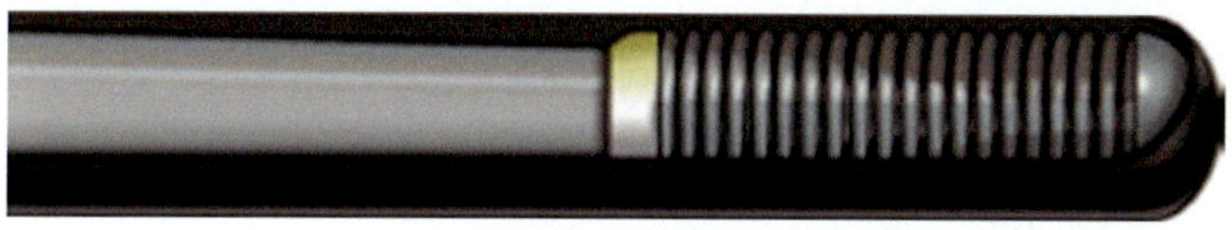

Fig. 2.15 Wire with polymer cover tip

Polymer cover does not provide good tip tactile feedback and increases the risk of intraoperative dissection and perforation.

- Partial polymer cover+ partial coil (Fig. 2.16): Considering the shortcomings inherent with the polymer cover, coil plus polymer cover design has been developed and extensively used. This kind of design comprises partially polymer cover and partially embolization, which, compared with polymer cover that has small friction and easily crosses the lesion, increases some friction so that it improves tactile feedback, reduces the risk of intraoperative dissection and perforation, and ensures safer operation.
- Taper coil design (Fig. 2.17): This special design aims to increase the stiffness of the wire tip so as to cross the occluded lesion, but due to the increased tip stiffness, perforation risk increases as well. This design, mainly for crossing the occluded lesion, is not recommended for use with conventional operation.

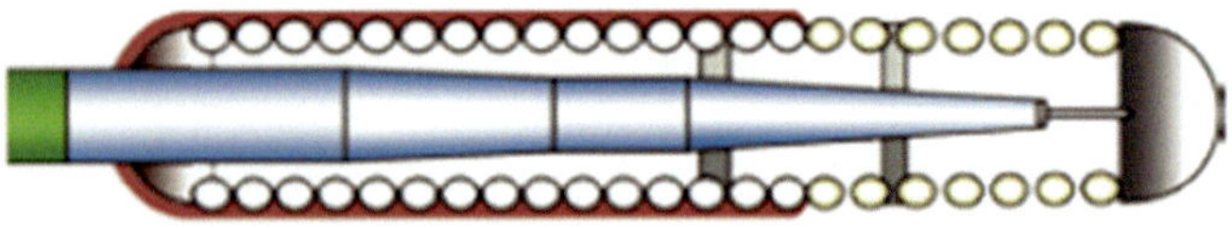

Fig. 2.16 Wire with polymer cover + coil tip

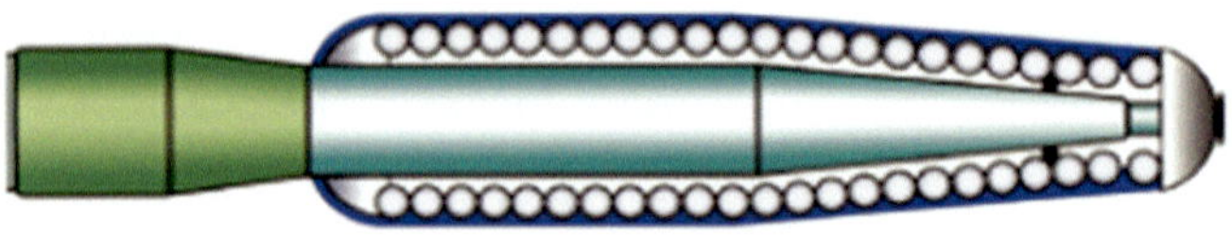

Fig. 2.17 Wire with taper coil tip

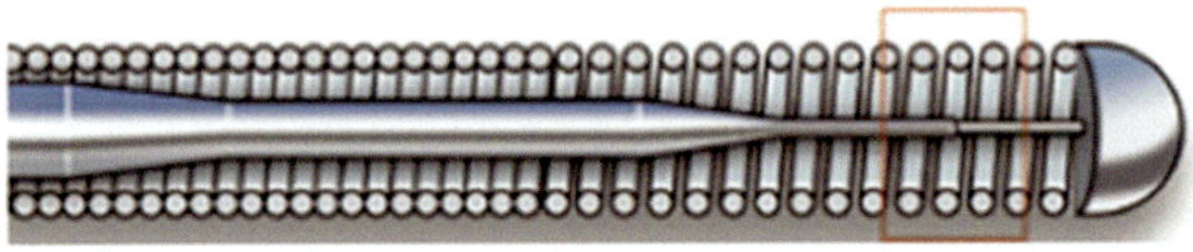

Fig. 2.18 Wire with core to tip design

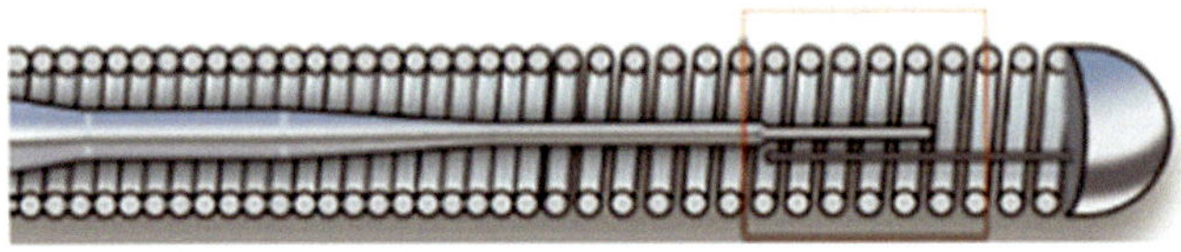

Fig. 2.19 Wire with shaping ribbon design

2. Shaping Section
   - Core to tip design (Fig. 2.18): a design integrating the shaping needle with core wire, which features excellent tactile feedback and steerability with adequate tip stiffness and easy access through highly resistant lesion
   - Shaping ribbon design (Fig. 2.19): a two-piece design of the shaping needle and core wire, which features flexible tip and split shaping needle with core wire, resulting in increased shaping performance after tip shaping

Transition Section

The soft tip facilitates shaping and reduces damage to blood vessels, while the supportive section is the stiff core wire. Therefore, both differ so greatly from each other in stiffness that the guide-wire is liable to bending where its stiffness changes abruptly. For that reason, transition section is used to reduce the difference in stiffness between the two sections so as to ensure smooth transition of stiffness throughout the entire wire and reduce wire bending and damage due to stiffness change.

Transition design mainly reflects in improved taper. The initial taper was rather short, but with the ever-improving technology, the taper becomes longer, further mitigating stiffness change. Gradually, it has been found through physical experiments that the streamlined taper has better transition performance than the linear one, for streamlined tapers and multilayer planar ones are being continuously invented and improved.

Support Section

The material selected and the cross section of the supportive section of a wire decides the supportive force of the wire. For material selection, the initial material selected for wire was stainless steel, but at present some use nickel-titanium alloy or other alloy materials. With the support of improved wire, the delivery of endovascular devices is strengthened, consequently improving the vascular straightening. Usually, the higher the material strength is, the stronger the supportive force will be; the larger the cross section of the support is, the stronger the supportive force will be.

The Shaft

The shaft extends from the support section to the proximal end of a wire, functioning mainly as delivering and supporting the devices. Hydrophobic or hydrophilic coating is usually applied to the shaft section, which is unnecessarily the same with the coating on other sections, aimed mainly to balance the lubrication and tactile feedback of the overall wire.

2.3.1.2 Functions and Performance Parameters of Wire

A wire in endovascular treatment operates as approaching, reaching, and accessing through the lesions and delivering endovascular devices. In consideration of the four roles played by a wire, the performance parameters of a wire are usually evaluated with reference to the following aspects:

- Steerability: the ability of the tip (distal end) of a wire to rotate while the operator rotates its proximal end

- Compliance: the ability of a wire to access through the lesions in compliance with the natural vascular conditions
- Pushability: the ability of a wire to navigate through the lesions under the action of the ex vitro shaft pushed by the operator
- Support: the ability of a wire to retain in place in vascular lesions and to deliver endovascular devices as a guide rail

2.3.1.3 Application of Wire in Different Vascular Lesions

Table 2.1 shows wire applications in different contexts of vascular lesions.

2.3.2 Specifications and Models

Wire outer diameter is customarily expressed in inch, generally including 0.014 in (0.36 mm), 0.018 in (0.46 mm), 0.021 in (0.53 mm), 0.025 in (0.64 mm), 0.028 in (0.71 mm), 0.032 in (0.81 mm), 0.035 in (0.89 mm), and 0.038 in (0.97 mm), among which 0.035 in (0.89 mm) is most commonly used. Wire length is 150 cm and 180 cm; and in vascular sheath, occlusion, and other endovascular devices, wire is of 50 cm, 80 cm, 100 cm, and 125 cm; and other specifications are also used for coordination. Exchanging wire lengths include 260 cm, 300 cm, 400 cm, and others. In selecting wire, the following rules are observed generally.

Table 2.1 Different performance requirements for wire in different vascular lesions (for reference only)

Type of lesion	Definition	Performance requirements for wire
Common vascular lesion	Simple	Ordinary support, soft tip, excellent steerability and flexibility
Tortuous vascular lesion	Target vessel deformed seriously in corrugated shape	Excellent steerability, soft tip, optimum flexibility, ordinary support
Vascular lesion required for super-strong support	Delivery of volumetric devices and large angulation at proximal end	Strong support, soft tip, excellent steerability, ordinary flexibility
Vascular lesion with extremely serious stenosis	Chronic total occlusion (CTO)	Excellent steerability, excellent pushability, ordinary flexibility, strong support

2.3.2.1 Length

Usually, 150 cm or 180 cm wire is used for adult angiography, but it also depends on the length of the catheter used. In implanting catheter, insert the wire tip into the body (at least 10 cm) through the puncture needle. The portion left outside the body shall be longer than the catheter to be inserted so that when the catheter is placed into the blood vessels, the operator can hold the exposed part of the wire for endovascular treatment and prevent the wire from entering into the blood vessels together with the catheter and being unable to be pulled out. If, after placement into certain blood vessels, it is expected to exchange the catheter before placement into the inferior ones, longer exchanging wire is usually used.

2.3.2.2 The Outer Diameter

Wire diameter shall match with the inner diameter of the puncture needle and the catheter. Wire with the diameter larger than the puncture needle core and catheter inner diameter cannot be inserted into the puncture needle and the catheter. And also, excessively thinner wire cannot be closely wrapped around by the catheter and, moreover, has inadequate support so that the catheter often fails to move forward along the wire and enter into the blood vessels easily, but staying against the subcutaneous loose tissue or even pulling out the wire from the blood vessels and entering into the subcutaneous tissue together. Due to separated force action, the pull of the wire to the catheter leads to the rupture of the catheter opening. Therefore, the matching of the wire outer diameter with the catheter inner diameter is of paramount importance, which may even have direct impact on the success of an operation.

2.3.2.3 External Shape

J-tip wire is often used when the puncture needle is inserted into the wire to introduce the catheter and then introduce the catheter to the first vascular branch. Straight-tip wire is only used for the carotid artery or some excessively narrow blood vessels. Straight-tip wire is also used in case of looped wire catheter, and selection shall be made by operators based on the actual situation.

Currently, wire brands mainly include Terumo, Boston Scientific, Cook, Abbott, Merit, Asahi, Cordis, Medtronic, etc. In this section, we will mainly introduce commonly used Terumo, Boston Scientific, Cook, Abbott, and Asahi wires (Table 2.2).

Table 2.2 Commonly used wires (for reference only)

Common name of wire	Brand	OD (in)	Length (cm)	Tip type	Features and use
Common hydrophilic wire	Terumo	0.035	150, 180, 260	Type J	Total hydrophilic coating, supersmooth, soft, suitable for introduction and superselection of all blood vessels, most commonly used in clinical context
Hardened hydrophilic wire		0.035	150, 260	Type J	Total hydrophilic coating, slightly hard, supersmooth, suitable for recanalization and superselection of narrowed or occluded blood vessels
Zipwire hydrophilic wire	Boston Scientific	0.035	150, 180, 260	Straight, Type J	Hydrophilic coating, supersmooth, soft, suitable for introducing various arteries and veins
Amplatz super-stiff wire		0.035	150, 180, 260	Straight, Type J	High supportability, relatively hard, suitable for main arteries with rather straight blood vessels in placement of stents
V-18 control wire	Boston Scientific	0.018	150, 200,300	Shapable, straight	Tip with hydrophilic coating, excellent steerability and supportability, proximal end with PTFE coating, suitable for recanalization and treatment of peripheral arteries
PT2 wire		0.014	185, 300	Shapable, Type J	Tip with hydrophilic coating, proximal end with PTFE coating, suitable for recanalization and treatment of peripheral fine arteries
Amplatz super-stiff wire	Cook	0.035	180, 260	Straight	Ordinary hardness, suitable for placement of peripheral stent graft for tortuous blood vessels
Rosen super-stiff wire		0.035	180, 260	Type G	Bent tip to avoid perforating blood vessels, ordinary hardness, suitable for superselection of renal arteries or placement of peripheral stent for tortuous blood vessels
Lunderquist super-stiff wire		0.035	260	Straight	Stainless steel, high hardness, suitable for placement of stents for main arteries with tortuous blood vessels
Pilot50 wire	Abbott	0.014	300	Straight	Tip with embolization design, soft, easy for shaping, distal end with hydrophilic coating, suitable for superselection of simple vascular lesions
Pilotl50 wire		0.014	300	Straight	Tip with the polymer cover, strong support, hydrophilic coating, suitable for recanalization of vascular stenosis and occluded lesions
Pilot200 wire		0.014	300	Straight	Tip with the polymer cover, strong support, hydrophilic coating, suitable for recanalization of seriously occluded vascular diseases
Command wire		0.014	190, 300	Shapable, straight	Shapable tip, the distal end with hydrophilic coating, ordinary support, suitable for superselection of narrowed or slightly occluded lower extremity arteries
Command ES wire		0.014	190, 300	Shapable, straight	Shapable tip, the distal end with hydrophilic coating, strong support, suitable for recanalization of complex lower extremity occlusion
Progress series wire		0.014	190, 300	Straight	Sharp tip with the taper coil and polymer cover, hydrophilic coating, suitable for recanalization of seriously occluded lesions of the lower extremities
Treasure floppy	Asahi	0.018	190, 300	Shapable, straight	Tip load 4 g, the catheter body with PTFE coating, excellent torqueability, suitable for recanalization and treatment of peripheral blood vessels
Treasure 12		0.018	180, 300	Shapable, straight	Tip load 12 g, the catheter body with PTFE coating, excellent torqueability, suitable for recanalization of chronic total occlusion diseases
Astato 30		0.018	180, 300	Straight	Tip load 30 g, taper tip, high crossability, suitable for accessing the fibrous cap and lesions with calcified deposits
Regalia XS 1.0		0.014	180, 300	Shapable, straight	Tip load 1 g, tip with the multi-polymer cover, suitable for recanalization and treatment of peripheral fine blood vessels
Astato XS 20		0.014	190, 300	Straight	Tip load 20 g, the taper tip, high crossability, suitable for accessing the fibrous cap and calcified deposit lesions
Extension wire		0.014	150	/	0.36 mm (0.014 in) extended wire, suitable for extending the wire that has been placed in human body but needs to be prolonged for operation

2.3.3 Brand Information

2.3.3.1 Terumo Exchanging Wire

The Japan Terumo-produced wire consists of the inner core, tip ring, and tubular container. The inner core is made of Ni-Ti alloy with two layers of coatings: the inner coating of the tungsten-contained polymer and the outer coating of the copolymer of semi-ester methoxyethene and maleic anhydride. This wire is most commonly used in clinical context and can be classified as common loach and hardened hydrophilic wire according to its stiffness.

2.3.3.2 Boston Scientific Wire

The US Boston Scientific-produced wire has multifarious types, like Zipwire hydrophilic wire, Amplatz super-stiff wire, V-18 control wire, PT2 wire, and others. Zipwire hydrophilic wire has Ni-Ti alloy core covered with radiopaque polyurethane cannula applied with hydrophilic coating. Amplatz super-stiff wire has a hard core covered with PTFE coating, featuring strong support but not used as initial wire. V-18 wire is controllable wire, consisting of stainless steel core and plastic noninvasive tip, with hydrophilic coating applied at 8–12 cm at the distal end of the wire and a 2-cm-long soft shaping section at the tip. PT2 wire has a nitinol alloy core, with 30 cm polymer cannula applied with hydrophilic coating at its distal end, a 2 cm soft shaping section at its tip, and PTFE coating at its proximal end. V-18 control wire and PT2 wire are usually used for recanalization and treatment of the lesions of the lower extremities.

2.3.3.3 Cook Wire

The US Cook-produced wire has multifarious varieties, among which Amplatz, Rosen, and Lunderquist super-stiff wires are most commonly used in clinical context. Rosen super-stiff wire has a G-type tip, preventing from perforating the blood vessels and suitable for the superselective treatment for renal arteries and other tortuous arteries.

2.3.3.4 Abbott Wire

The US Abbott-produced wire has diversified types and specifications, including commonly used Pilot series and Command wire in series. Pilot wire has three types: Pilot50, Pilot150 and Pilot200, the hardness of the wire tip is indicated by the suffixed number, where Pilot50 wire has relatively soft tip, Pilot150 moderate and Pilot200 rather hard. Command wire includes two types: Command and Command ES, where Command ES has stronger support than the Command ones. In operation, wire is selected according to the difference in vascular lesions. This kind of wire is usually used for treatment of lower extremity arterial stenosis and recanalization of occluded lesions.

2.3.3.5 Asahi Wire

The Japan Asahi-produced wire has multifarious varieties, among which, Treasure Floppy, Treasure 12, Astato 30, Regalia XS 1.0 and Astato XS 20 wire are mainly used in clinical context, different mainly in their tip hardness. The tip load of Treasure Floppy is 4 g, 12 g for Treasure 12, 30 g for Astato 30, 1 g for Regalia XS 1.0, and 20 g for Astato XS 20. Asahi lower extremity wire uses "core-to-tip" single core design, available for providing 1:1 torque for operators, wherein Regalia XS 1.0 is designed with the multi-polymer protective cover at the tip of the wire so as to provide excellent smoothnes and trackability, while Astato 30 and Astato XS 20 have specially designed taper tip free from hydrophilic coating, which, matched with its super-stiff tip load, features high crossability that facilitates the access through the proximal fibrous cap and lesions with calcified deposits. This kind of wire is indicated for revascularization of (chronic total occlusion, CTO) vessels.

2.4 Catheter

Catheter is a long thin-wall hollow plastic tube, which, after entering into the blood vessels with the wire, can be used as selective and superselective catheter or for endovascular angiography by injecting contrast medium via the catheter, for perfusion treatment by injecting drugs, or for embolotherapy by injecting the embolic agent. Catheter performance is mainly manifested in three aspects: friction coefficient, torque, and elastic memory.

- Friction coefficient: The smaller the friction coefficient is, the more conveniently the catheter moves in and out.
- Torque: Torque represents the ability of a catheter to transmit rotational force. A catheter with excellent torque can transmit the force to the catheter's distal end immediately in the same rotation direction and angle as the proximal end of the catheter rotates, while a catheter with poor torque rotates its distal end suddenly and drastically while its proximal end rotates and loses control.
- Elastic memory: Elastic memory is the ability of a catheter to retain its shape after shaping and to restore its original shape after withdrawal of external force. In selective and superselective catheterization, the catheter of certain shape is required, or catheter has to be shaped so as to access through tortuous and narrow blood vessels. However, a catheter with poor elastic memory may lose its original shape, making selective catheterization unavailable.

2.4.1 Product Structure

The materials used for catheters decide the performance, which is analyzed in detail in the following according to the materials and structures of the catheters.

2.4.1.1 Catheter's Materials

At present, the materials for catheters are classified into the following four categories.

PE

Polyethylene (PE) is commonly used material for the catheter, moderate in hardness, easy for pre-shaping, good at elastic memory, and moderate in friction coefficient. Therefore, the catheter made of this material is smooth, but intolerant of disinfection of high temperature.

PU

Polyurethane (PU) features excellent elastic memory. Compared with PE, it is soft and has small friction coefficient, disadvantaged in high thrombotic probability. Using catheters made of this material requires for systemic heparinization, and it is also intolerant of disinfection of high temperature.

PVC

Polyvinyl chloride (PVC) is relatively soft with high friction coefficient, disadvantaged in poor elastic coefficient. Therefore, it is difficult for pre-shaping and also has high thrombotic probability.

PTFE

Polytetrafluoroethylene (PTFE) catheter features smooth surface and low friction coefficient, disadvantaged in high hardness, poor elastic memory, and difficulty in pre-shaping.

In addition, metal materials such as lead, bismuth, and barium are often added in the production of the catheter so that the catheter is resistant to X-ray and facilitates operators to operate under X-ray.

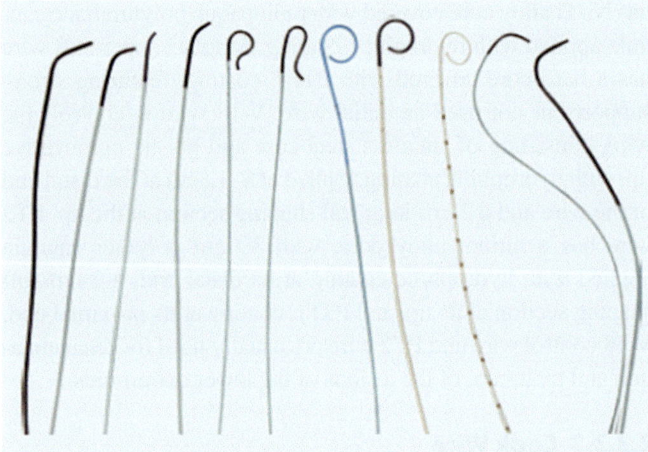

Fig. 2.20 Various catheter tips

2.4.1.2 Catheter Structure

Initially the catheter is made of homogeneous material. In order to enhance the torque effect, extremely fine stainless steel woven fabric is added into the catheter, which is called reticulate catheter.

With the international popularization of fine needle and small-bore catheter technology, especially the use of digital subtraction angiography (DSA), the majority of physicians choose 5F catheters to operate. 5F catheter is usually not a reticulate catheter, which is thin and soft, and is very different in operation from the 7F mesh catheter, and its performance and methods must be understood in operation. One of the more specific classes of catheters is the dilatable catheter. Initially, Dotter et al. designed the dilatable catheter by intertwining several catheters of different sizes to expand the narrowed vessels, usually called as coaxial dilatable catheter. After that, Gruntzig innovatively used a two-cavity balloon catheter, having more significant advantages and quickly replacing the coaxial dilatable catheter. Balloon catheter, as is often called internationally, has two cavities, one of which is the same as the common catheter that introduces the catheter via the wire or performs perfusion treatment by injecting the contrast agent, the other being connected with a balloon around the distal end of the catheter, through which the diluted contrast agent is injected to expand the balloon thus expanding the narrowed vessels. Balloon length and outer diameter differ as the case may be. Some balloons can be bent into an arc shape. Balloon is generally placed at 1–2 cm from the catheter tip. To ensure visibility of the balloon position under X-ray, metal rings are arranged at both ends of the balloon.

In appearance, the distal end or tip of a catheter refers to the end that first enters into human blood vessels along the wire, while the proximal or tail end always remains in vitro. If there are more than two arcs at the tip of a catheter, the arc closest to the tip is called the first arc and then counted in sequence towards the tail end. The peak of the arc is called the knee; the catheter on both sides of which is called side-arm and distal arm, respectively. To selectively or superselectively insert the catheter into target vascular lesions, the catheter must be bent into certain shape according to the diameter, direction, and length of the target vascular lesions. Some catheters are significantly different in appearance, but there is no difference in actual use, such as the left and right coronary artery catheter; some catheters seem exactly identical in appearance, but they cannot be exchanged in use, such as the superior and inferior mesenteric artery catheter, which requires the operator not only to understand their shapes, but also their principles in order to precisely use these catheters, decide shaping by themselves, or "borrow" certain catheter for their own use. Figure 2.20 lists some commonly used catheter tips.

In addition, there are different shapes of catheter; some catheters have a different number of side holes, aimed at preventing catheter loop from whipping the blood vessels or the catheter from exiting from the diseased vessels in injecting the contrast agent under high pressure. The proximal end of various catheters is basically the same, having a flared opening to facilitate fitting with the catheter connectors. Some connectors are made of plastics and completely integrated with the catheter.

2.4.2 Specifications and Models

The catheter is measured in F, the same as the vascular sheath. This section mainly introduces the routinely used catheters (Table 2.3). Special catheters, such as the support catheter, the thrombolytic perfusion catheter, the embolectomy catheter, the balloon dilatation catheter, and others, are described in detail in Section 5 Special Catheters in this

Table 2.3 Commonly used catheters (for reference only)

Common name of catheter	Brand	OD (F)	Length (cm)	Function
Common pigtail catheter	Cook, AngioDynamics, Optimed, Cordis	5, 6	90, 100, 110	Used for various vascular angiographies
Scaled pigtail catheter	Cook, AngioDynamics, Optimed	5	100, 110	Used for various vascular angiography and measurement
Omni Flush catheter	AngioDynamics	4, 5	90, 100	Used for superselection of contralateral limbs for crossing-over operation of lower extremities
Straight-tip catheter	AngioDynamics	4, 5	90	Used for various superselective blood vessels
RIM catheter	Cook	5	80	Used for superselection of contralateral limbs for crossing-over operation of lower extremities
RH hepatic artery catheter	Cook, Cordis	4, 5	80	Used for superselective hepatic arteries
RS splenic artery catheter	Cook, Cordis	4, 5	80	Used for superselective splenic arteries
Cobra catheter (Cl, C2, C3)	Cook, AngioDynamics	4, 5	90	Used for various superselective blood vessels
Sos Omni catheter	AngioDynamics	4, 5	80	Used for superselective renal arteries
Super-slide catheter	Terumo	4, 5	100	Used for superselective tortuous blood vessels
Aqua hydrophilic catheter	Cordis	4, 5	100	Used for superselective narrow lower extremity arteries
Left coronary angiography catheter (AL I, AL II, AL III)	Cordis	6, 7	100	Used for superselective left coronary arteries
Right coronary angiography catheter (AR I, AR II, AR III)	Cordis	6, 7	100	Used for superselective right coronary artery
Vertebral artery catheter	AngioDynamics, Cordis, Cook	4, 5	100	Used for various superselective blood vessels
MPA multifunction catheter	Cordis	4, 5, 6	100, 125	Used for superselective supra-arch branch and lower extremity arteries
HeadHunter catheter (HI)	AngioDynamics	4, 5	100	Used for superselective visceral artery
Simmons catheter (SIM1, SIM2, SIM3)	AngioDynamics, Cordis	4, 5	100	Used for superselective supra-arch branch arteries
Bentson catheter (JB1, JB2, JB3)	AngioDynamics, Cordis	4, 5	100	Used for superselective supra-arch branch arteries
VTK catheter	Cook	4, 5	125	Used for superselective supra-arch branch arteries
Mariner Berenstein catheter	AngioDynamics	4, 5	130, 150	Used for superselective lower extremity arteries (upper limb approach)

chapter and Chap. 3 Balloon Dilatation Catheter. In conventional endovascular treatment, the catheter can be classified as the perfusion angiography catheter and introducer catheter according to the use of catheters. Perfusion angiography catheter refers to the catheter with many side holes at the tip and can be used for angiography, such as the pigtail catheter. The introducer catheter can be further classified as the catheter for abdominal, coronary, and cervical angiography based on the position of treatment, characterized in that catheter's pre-shaping, and length differs from different positions of the blood vessels to ensure quicker and more accurate superselection of various blood vessels by operators, thus reducing damage to vessels. Certainly in special circumstance, the tip can be modified to access through the blood vessels.

Currently, catheter brands mainly include AngioDynamics, Cook, Terumo, Cordis, Optimed, Merit, etc. In this section, we mainly introduce commonly used AngioDynamics, Cook, Terumo, and Cordis catheters.

2.4.3 Brand Information

2.4.3.1 AngioDynamics Catheter

The 4F and 5F catheters at a length of 80–150 cm, the US AngioDynamics-produced, have multifarious varieties, such as the vertebral artery catheter (commonly known as elbowed catheter), Bentson catheter, Sos Omni catheter, and Omni Flush catheter, characterized by moderate hardness and a hydrophilic-coating black section at the tip, facilitating superselected blood vessels.

2.4.3.2 Cook Catheter

The US Cook-produced catheter includes the hepatic artery catheter, the splenic artery catheter, the pigtail catheter, and other catheters of different tips. Its emblematic pigtail catheter is a gold scale, resulting in clearer film, easy for vascular measurement. The catheter has a model of 4–6F at a length of 80–125 cm.

2.4.3.3 Terumo Catheter

The Japan Terumo-produced catheter includes the elbowed catheter, the straight-head catheter, and other catheters of various tips, characterized by total hydrophilic coating, soft and smooth catheter. The catheter has a model of 4–5F at a length of 100 cm.

2.4.3.4 Cordis Catheter

The US Cordis-produced catheter includes Aqua catheter, the left coronary angiography catheter, the right coronary angiography catheter, the introducer catheter, and others, among which Aqua catheter is of total hydrophilic coating, which, compared with Terumo super-smooth catheter, has stronger support and can be superselective for the occluded lesions of lower extremities. Aqua catheter's models include 4F and 5F at a length of 100 cm. The models for left and right coronary artery angiography catheters include 5F, 6F, and 7F. The introducer catheter is of three-layer design, the outer layer being nylon, the middle layer being stainless steel woven fabric, and the inner layer being PFE coating, with various types of tips available for selection, having a model of 6–9F at a length of 55 cm, 90 cm, 95 cm, and 125 cm (special type).

2.5 Special Catheter

2.5.1 Support Catheter

2.5.1.1 Productive Structure

The support catheter consists of the catheter and the catheter seat, an OTW single-lumen catheter (Fig. 2.21), surfaced with hydrophilic coating, having radiopaque marks at its tip for catheter positioning at an interval of 1 cm between the marks that can also be used for measurement.

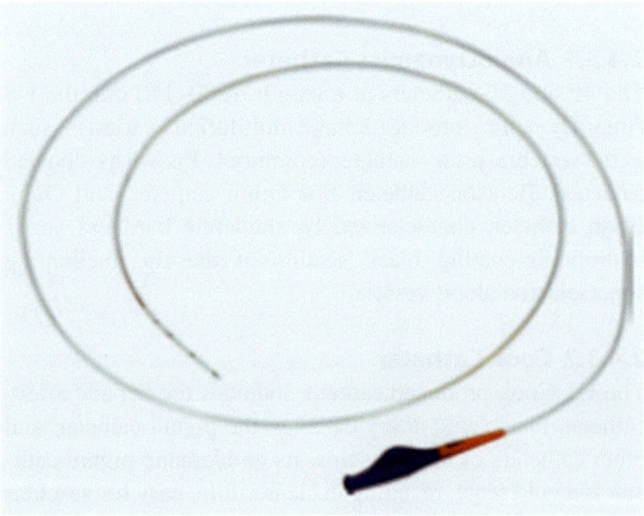

Fig. 2.21 TrailBlazer support catheter (Medtronic)

2.5.1.2 Features and Models

The support catheter features supportability, crossability, and visibility.

- Supportability: Provide strong support for wire, improve lesion repatency rate, and provide the catheter with excellent flexibility for the catheter body made of special polymer materials and easier in shaping along with the wire.
- Crossability: Hydrophilic coating design enhances the ability of the catheter to navigate through tortuous vessels and dense lesions.
- Visibility: Radiopaque mark facilitates measuring vascular diameter and length. Depth marks can clearly indicate the feeding depth of catheter sheath.

Currently, major support catheter brands include Cook, Medtronic, Boston Scientific, Bard, etc. This section focuses on introduction to CXI (Cook) and TrailBlazer (Medtronic) support catheters.

2.5.1.3 Brand Information

CXI Support Catheter

- The US Cook-produced CXI support catheter is seamlessly connected with the wire, with a smooth inner chamber for easing wire exchange. The straight-head catheter provides strong push force, while the elbowed catheter is available for superselective fine blood vessels, improving the crossability of the catheter. CXI support catheter is mainly used for revascularizing the occlusive vascular lesions of lower extremities.
- CXI support catheter has 2.6F and 4F OD, with the tip being straight and elbowed, suitable for matching with 0.46 mm (0.018in) and 0.89 mm (0.035in) wires, the shaft length of 2.6F support catheter is 90 cm and 150 cm, and the shaft length of 4F support catheter includes 90 cm, 130 cm, and 150 cm.

TrailBlazer Support Catheter

- The US Medtronic-produced TrailBlazer support catheter is an OTW single-lumen catheter with noninvasive taper tip, having three radiopaque marks on the catheter axis at the distal end to assist with the catheter positioning. Hydrophilic coating is applied at 40 cm from the distal end of the catheter.
- TrailBlazer support catheter is suitable for matching with 0.36 mm (0.014in), 0.46 mm (0.018in), and 0.89 mm (0.035in) wire, having a straight tip, with a shaft length of 135 cm and 150 cm, maximum matching sheath of 5F.

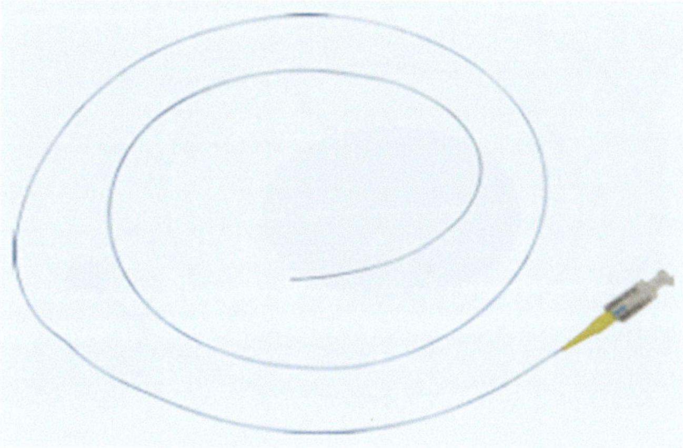

Fig. 2.22 Renegade STC 18 microcatheter (Boston Scientific)

2.5.2 The Microcatheter

2.5.2.1 Product Structure

The microcatheter is a single-lumen catheter with end holes (Fig. 2.22), equipped inside with a shaping needle, having standard seat at the proximal end to be connected with other accessories. The catheter consists of a semihard proximal shaft and a highly flexible distal shaft. There are two radiopaque marks at the distal end of the catheter, and the catheter is surfaced with hydrophilic coating.

2.5.2.2 Features and Models

The microcatheter mainly functions as a delivery catheter for embolization, liquid embolic agent, and other embolic products. Currently, microcatheter brands include Boston Scientific, Medtronic, Cook, Asahi, Terumo, etc. This section focuses on introducing Renegade STC 18 (Boston Scientific) microcatheter and Echelon (Medtronic) microcatheter.

2.5.2.3 Brand Information

Renegade STC 18 Microcatheter

- Renegade STC 18 microcatheter of US Boston Scientific consists of the microcatheter, the shaping needle, and the rotary hemostatic valve (RHV), with an radiopaque mark at its distal end and available for tip shaping via steam heating. The microcatheter is integrated with a standard luer joint at its proximal end. The outer diameter of the microcatheter gradually tapers along the long axle from the 3F proximal semihard area to 2.4F distal flexible area. The maximum inner diameter of the microcatheter is 0.53 mm (0.021 in), and the external surface at the distal section of the microcatheter is applied with Hydro Pass hydrophilic coating.
- Renegade STC 18 microcatheter is specially designed for endovascular embolotherapy of peripheral blood vessels and used in conjunction with Boston Scientific's Interlock embolization. Coaxial tracking of the microcatheter via one controllable wire is available so as to enter distal tortuous blood vessels. After entering the sub-selection zone, the microcatheter can be used to push the embolization and other embolus controllably and selectively into the blood vessels. Renegade STC 18 microcatheter can access through 0.46 mm (0.018in) wire.

Echelon Microcatheter

- Echelon microcatheter is a single-lumen microcatheter with a hole at its tip made by US Medtronic, woven with Ni-Ti alloy fabric, featuring long-lasting and steady support and lumen shape retention, inside which a shaping needle is equipped. The standard seat is available at its proximal end to connect with other accessories, and the catheter is a combination of a semihard proximal shaft and a flexible distal shaft. The catheter is surfaced with hydrophilic coating, thus enhancing catheter's lubrication to ensure improved access to the lesion positions.
- Echelon microcatheter is a support catheter with endovascular embolotherapy for arterial aneurysm and used in conjunction with Onyx liquid embolic agent, consisting of two models: Echelon 14 and Echelon 10.
  1. Echelon 14: distal outer diameter of 1.7F, and proximal 2F, distal inner diameter of 0.43 mm (0.017in). The length of the catheter is 150 cm, matching with 0.36 mm (0.014in) wire. It has straight 45°- and 90°-angled tips.
  2. Echelon 10: distal outer diameter of 1.9F and proximal 2.4F, distal inner diameter of 0.43 mm (0.017in), at a length of 150 cm, matching with 0.36 mm (0.014in) wire. It has straight, 45°- and 90°-angled tips.

2.5.3 Embolectomy Catheter

2.5.3.1 Product Structure

Arterial embolectomy catheter consists of the catheter, the balloon, and the handle, a small rubber balloon equipped at its distal end and connected with the catheter for injection of normal saline from the end of the catheter to fully fill the balloon thus facilitating the removal of the thrombus. Arterial embolectomy catheter can be classified as single-lumen embolectomy catheter (Fig. 2.23) and double-lumen one (Fig. 2.24) on the basis of their structures, differing in that the double-lumen catheter has one more wire lumen than the single-lumen one, where the wire can be first placed into the distal end of occlusive vessels and removal of thrombus can then be performed by introducing the double-lumen embolectomy catheter via the wire under angiography. Currently, commonly used embolectomy catheters are US Edwards-produced Fogarty arterial embolectomy catheters.

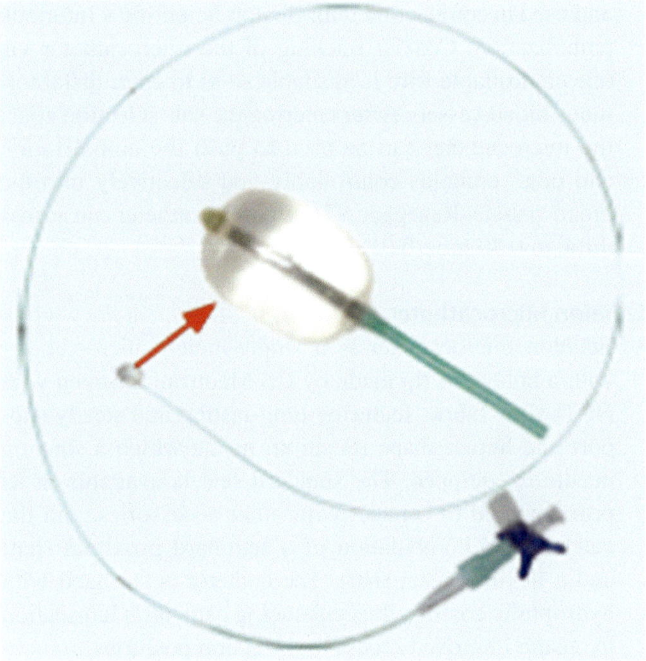

Fig. 2.23 Fogarty single-lumen embolectomy catheter (Edwards)

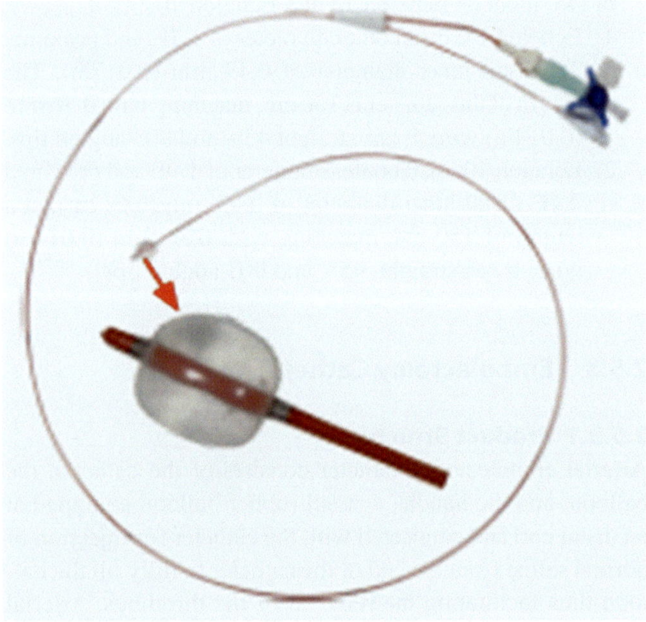

Fig. 2.24 Fogarty double-lumen embolectomy catheter (Edwards)

2.5.3.2 Features and Models

Fogarty arterial embolectomy catheter is indicated for removing newly formed soft embolus and thrombus. The diameter of a single-lumen embolectomy catheter is 2–7F and that of double-lumen 3–7F, matching with 0.46 mm (0.018in), 0.64 mm (0.025in), and 0.89 mm (0.035in) wire. The maximum catheter length is 100 cm.

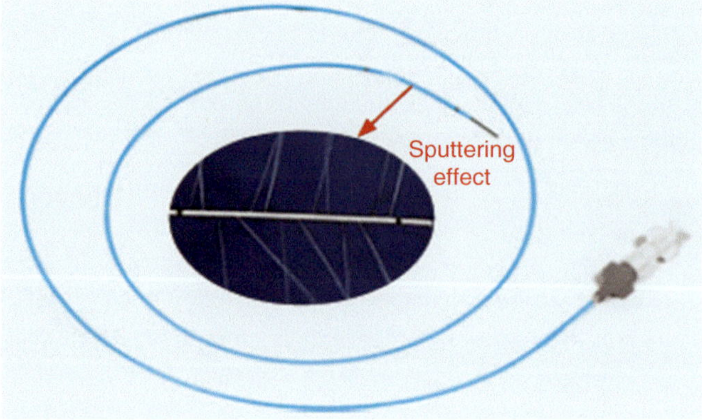

Fig. 2.25 UniFuse thrombolytic catheter (AngioDynamics)

2.5.4 Thrombolytic Catheter

Thrombolytic catheter, also called thrombolytic perfusion catheter, is used to inject liquid (including thrombolytic drugs and contrast agents) into the peripheral vessels. Currently, thrombolytic catheter brands include Cook, AngioDynamics, Merit, etc. This section focuses mainly on US AngioDynamics's UniFuse perfusion system and US Merit's Fountain perfusion system.

2.5.4.1 UniFuse Perfusion System

Product Structure

UniFuse perfusion system produced by US AngioDynamics (Fig. 2.25) uses laser cutting techniques, where four cuts are designed every 0.5 cm and one cut every 90° along the circumferential direction. The perfusion system consists of the outer cannula and the inner core, namely, thrombolytic catheter plus occlusive wire, which can ensure that, when the outer cannula is integrated with the inner core, all thrombolytic drugs can sputter out from the lateral seams. Both ends of the thrombolytic segment are equipped with two radiopaque marks, used for adjusting the position of the thrombolytic segment.

Features and Models

UniFuse perfusion system is indicated for thrombolytic therapy for acute embolism of peripheral arteries and acute thrombosis of peripheral veins. In treatment, intraoperative impulse injection technique and postoperative micropump continuous perfusion technique are usually adopted, which can be used in conjunction with each other, but overdose should be avoided as much as possible.

UniFuse perfusion system is characterized in that:

- Its inner core is occluded wire, fracture resistant, and available for inducing stress reactive perfusion.
- The cutting seam design, compared with side-hole design, is safer. Cutting seam is of one-way opening, where the

side hole is closed when no thrombolytic operation is performed and the thrombolytic drugs enter the vascular lesions through the cutting seams only after drugs are injected under pressure.

- The maximum perfusion segment reaches 50 cm, suitable for the long-segment thrombosis in any part of the blood vessels.

UniFuse perfusion system catheter is 135 cm long, accessible by 0.89 mm (0.035in) wire, the catheter's outer diameter is 4–5F, the perfusion segment is 5–50 cm long, and side seams amount to 400 at most.

2.5.4.2 Fountain Perfusion System

Product Structure

Fountain perfusion system produced by US Merit is a thrombolytic catheter (Fig. 2.26), consisting of Fountain perfusion thrombolytic catheter with the side hole, the occlude wire with snap-fastener cap, Y valve, and Squirt impulse drug-spraying unit. Eight holes every 1 cm are arranged on the Fountain perfusion catheter evenly around the peripheral of the catheter by laser drilling technique, the principle of which is to break the thrombus by the mechanical force from impulse spraying and perform thrombolysis with the help of drugs.

Features and Models

This perfusion system is indicated for thrombolysis therapy for peripheral artery occlusion, deep venous thrombus (DVT), hemodialysis access blocking, and other diseases. There are two ways of perfusion for Fountain perfusion system: one is impulse spraying, while the other is slow infiltration injection. Its catheter is of patented gradient-hole design, with hole diameter enlarging from the proximal end to the distal end gradually along the catheter. Fountain perfusion catheter is 45 cm, 90 cm, and 135 cm long, tip inner diameter being 0.94 mm (0.037 in), with the catheter outer diameter being 4F and 5F, and perfusion segment being 5–50 cm long (among which, the perfusion segment is 5–20 cm long for 45-cm-long perfusion catheter.

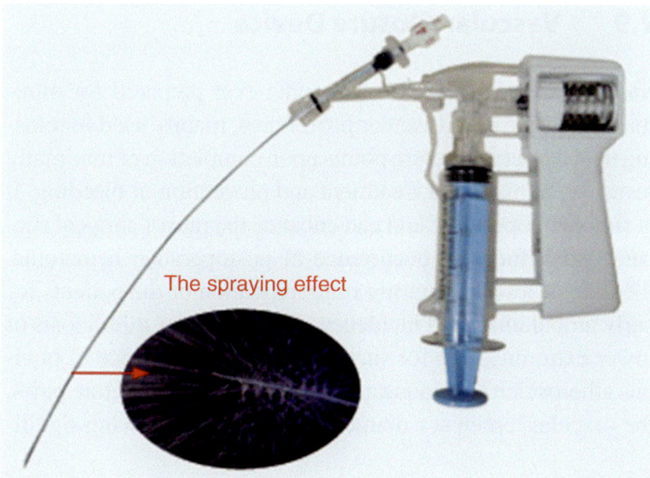

Fig. 2.26 Fountain perfusion system (Merit)

2.6 Y Valve

Y valve is a routine device for minimally invasive endovascular therapy and can be connected with the catheter, vascular sheath, and other endovascular devices, functioning as an alternatively available cavity and usually used in conjunction with T joint. Currently, there are diversified brands of Y valves, and this section mainly introduces Abbott's Y valve accessory kit (Fig. 2.27), composed of three accessories: the rotary hemastatic valve (Y valve), the wire introducer, and the wire controller.

2.6.1 The Rotary Hemostatic Valve

The rotary hemostatic valve (Y valve) is a Tuohy-Borst adapter, keeping tight the area subject to endovascular treatment by the rotary knob so as to avoid liquid leak.

2.6.2 The Wire Introducer

The wire introducer is a device assisting with 0.23–0.46 mm (0.009–0.018in) wire to access through the blood vessels and used in conjunction with the wire.

2.6.3 The Wire Controller

The wire controller can be used in conjunction with 0.23–0.46 mm (0.009–0.018in) guide wire, keep in place the proximal end of the guide wire via its rotary knob and control the guide wire for endovascular operation, facilitating the movement of relatively thinner guide wire in the blood vessels.

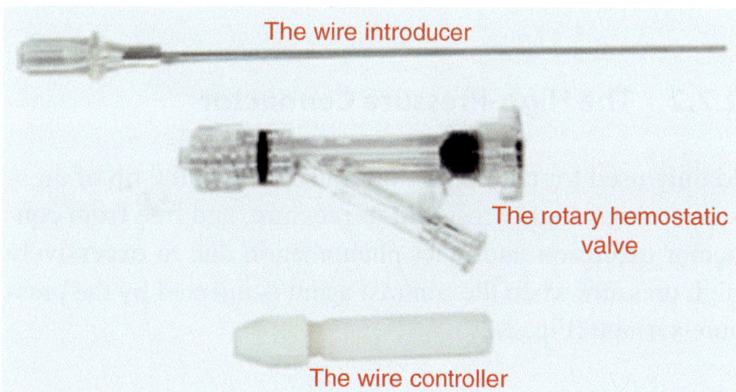

Fig. 2.27 Y valve accessory kit (Abbott)

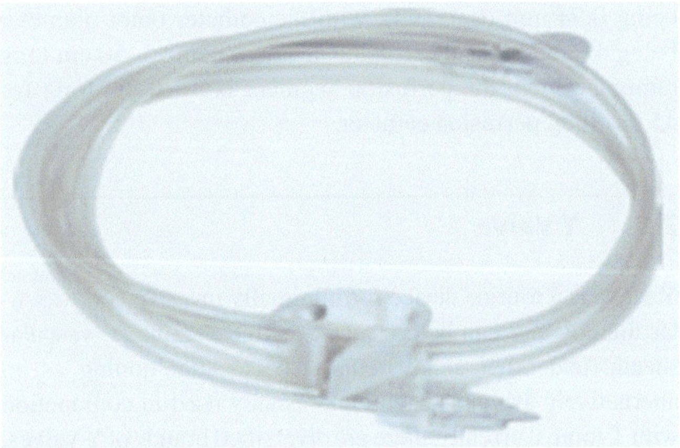

Fig. 2.28 The general connector

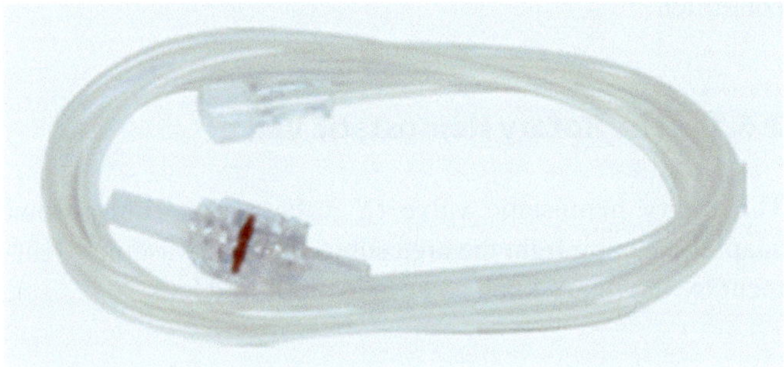

Fig. 2.29 High-pressure connector

2.7 Connector

Commonly used connectors are generally divided into general and high-pressure connectors, the air inside which shall be emptied in use.

2.7.1 General Connector

Usually used as an extension tube to extend the infusion device, having relatively low resistance to pressure (Fig. 2.28).

2.7.2 The High-Pressure Connector

Mainly used for connecting the catheter with the tip of pressure syringe, highly resistant to pressure, and free from connector explosion and other phenomenon due to excessively high pressure when the contrast agent is injected by the pressure syringe (Fig. 2.29).

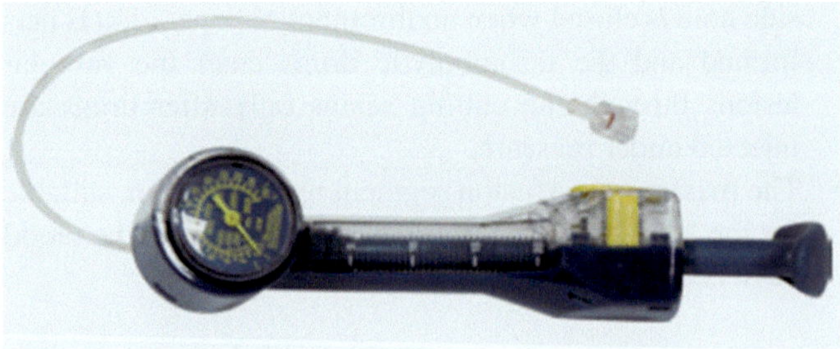

Fig. 2.30 Encore 26 inflation device (Boston Scientific)

2.8 Inflation Device

Inflation device is a threaded embolism locking device, functioning as a device for accurate control and pressure monitoring in connecting with the balloon dilatation catheter. Currently, inflation device brands include Boston Scientific, Cordis, Merit, etc. This section mainly introduces Boston Scientific-produced Encore 26 inflation device (Fig. 2.30). This device is activated by the finger bold (the yellow part). When the finger bolt is pressed down, the threaded embolism will unlock and move back and forward as indicated. When the finger bolt is released, the device is in locking position. The inflation device is integrated with a pressure gauge (0–26 atm dial), through which, atmospheric pressure (atm) and its intensity (kPa) can be produced and monitored.

Encore 26 inflation device is used for balloon dilatation and withdrawal of balloon dilatation catheter and stent, at maximum pressure of 26 atm. In endovascular treatment, 1:1 diluted contrast agent can be used to inflate the balloon so that the pressure inside the balloon can be observed via X-ray. Compared with hand-driven syringe, the inflation device can control the pressure value in balloon dilatation more accurately and will not affect the therapeutic effect due to excessively higher or lower pressure.

2.9 Vascular Closure Device

Vascular closure device has become ever prepared for minimally invasive endovascular procedures, mainly used for closing up the artery puncture points upon completion of minimally invasive endovascular treatment and prevention of bleeding. It is simple in operation and can enhance the rate of surgical success and reduce the occurrence of postoperative hematoma, the time of lower extremity immobilization of the patients for early ambulation, and incidence of deep venous thrombosis of lower extremity. But for such conditions as presence of obvious atherosclerotic plaque at the femoral artery puncture point, the vascular lumen at a diameter < 5 mm, and showing signifi-

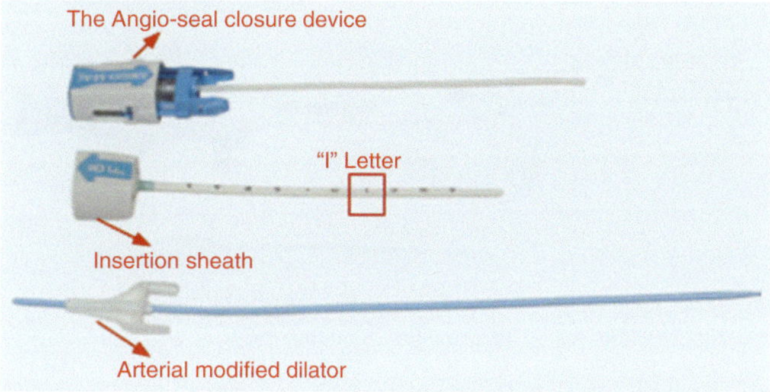

Fig. 2.31 The Angio-Seal vascular closure device (St. Jude)

cantly serious calcification of the narrow femoral artery, tortuous artery, or puncture point located at the distal part of the femoral artery branch (like superficial femoral artery, SFA), using vascular devices shall be prudent.

At present, vascular closure device brands include St. Jude, Abbott, Cordis, Cardiva, PuyiTech, etc. This section will mainly introduce Angio-Seal vascular closure device (St. Jude), Perclose Proglide suture-mediated closure system (Abbott), Starclose SE vascular closure system (Abbott), ExoSeal vascular closure device (Cordis), and Hemostat (PuyiTech).

2.9.1 Angio-Seal Vascular Closure Device

2.9.1.1 Product Structure

The US St. Jude-produced Angio-Seal vascular closure device consists of the Angio-Seal closure device, insertion sheath (6F or 8F), and arterial modified dilator (positioner) (Fig. 2.31). Inside the device are an absorbable collagen gauze and a specially designed absorbable polymer block (anchor), the two being connected by an absorbable positioning suture with a self-tightening running knot. The anchor, collagen, and suture of the closure device can be completely absorbed within 90 days.

2.9.1.2 Features and Models

The Angio-Seal device is indicated for minimally invasive endovascular closure treatment with femoral artery puncture, in two types: 6F and 8F.

2.9.1.3 Operation Procedures

1. Select matching Angio-Seal closure device according to the vascular sheath to be used in operation.
2. First insert the positioner into the sheath cannula, then access the cannula into the blood vessels along the wire, and access further 1–2 cm into the vessels when blood is seen to come out from the hole till the "I" letter appears. When blood stops, pull out the positioner.
3. Insert the closure device into the sheath cannula till the cap of the closure device fits together with the axle of the sheath cannula and clicks (then the anchor stretches out from the sheath cannula).
4. Withdraw the cap of the closure device and click again till there is resistance. At this moment, the resistance is felt to come from the obstruction of the anchor with the tip of the sheath cannula and part of the ribbon on the cuff is exposed.
5. Press the two sides of the puncture point with left hand; continue to withdraw the device cap by the right hand till final locking (at this moment, the left and right hands are under counterbalance), that is, the entire black suture is exposed completely (at this time, the device cap and the cannula axle cannot move separately).
6. Withdraw the entire closure device, retain anchor tension for 10 s, cut the suture when no blood leakage is found at the puncture point, and apply pressure for bandage.

2.9.2 Perclose Proglide Suture-Mediated Closure System

2.9.2.1 Product Structure

The US Abbott-produced Perclose Proglide suture-mediated closure system consists of the vascular suture device and the suture trimmer (Fig. 2.32). The vascular closure device consists of two stainless steel needles and 3-0 PP suture.

2.9.2.2 Features and Models

Perclose Proglide suture-mediated closure system is indicated for vessel suture using 5–21F vascular sheath at common femoral artery puncture point. When the sheath cannula diameter exceeds 12F, two or more closure systems may be used as the case may be. Pre-embedded suture technique may be used in operation according to actual surgical procedures. Its model is 6F.

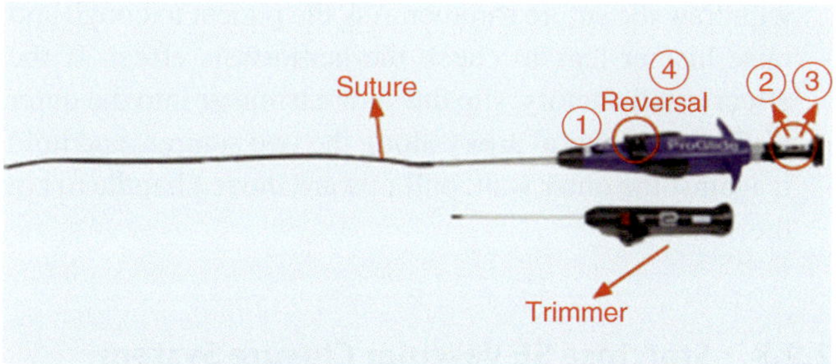

Fig. 2.32 Perclose Proglide suture-mediated closure device (Abbott). (**1**) Pull upward foot control lever, (**2**) push injector; (**3**) pull out injector; (**4**) push downward foot control lever

2.9.2.3 Operation Procedures

1. Angiography: Angiography is performed for the blood vessels to be closed so as to identify availability for suture operation.
2. Positioning: Withdraw the original vascular sheath; place the closure device along the exchange wire (available for pre-embedded or direct suturing technique). Push the closure device forward so that the white wire opening is close to the skin. Withdraw the wire, continue to push the closure device till the blood sprays out in linear throbbing, and then pull up the suture control lever, and at this time, the suture foot opens inside the femoral artery.
3. Injection: Withdraw the closure device till it encounters resistance. At this time, the foot is situated on the inner wall of the femoral artery, and blood stops spraying. Maintain the closure device at a 45° angle with skin surface and keep an up-pulling tension, then push the injector, and keep it for 2 s.
4. Withdrawal: Pull out the injector and we can see two long and thin needles. On the long needles, there is a blue suture attached with a white connector wire, pull tightly the blue suture, pull up the suture, wind it to the opening depression with a scissors marker on the suture body, pull upward the suture, and cut it. Press down the suture foot controller; withdraw the closure device till the white wire opening appears on the surface of the skin. Intertwine two sutures together, find the longer blue suture and wind it around the index finger of the left hand and pull it tightly in the coaxial direction of the suture body. At this time, withdraw the closure device by right hand and the pre-embedded suture knot will enter the outer wall of the femoral artery.
5. Locking: Pull tightly the blue suture wound around the index finger of the left hand in the coaxial direction. Hold against the top of the suture trimmer by the thumb of the left hand; keep the suture at 75° angle with the skin. Adjust it to 45° angle, keep it for about 60 s by left hand alone, pull tightly the short suture by right hand, and withdraw the suture trimmer. Ask the patient to cough and raise his/her legs to check the hemostasis effect. If the effect is satisfactory, slip the suture trimmer into the outer wall of the femoral artery along the two sutures, and hold it against the outer wall; pull upward the red handle to cut the suture.

2.9.3 Starclose SE Vascular Closure System

2.9.3.1 Product Structure

Starclose SE vascular closure system (Fig. 2.33) produced by US Abbott consists of a clip applier with an implantable clip, an exchange sheath, a dilator, and wire. The clip is made of super-elastic nitinol, and the vessel outer wall and tunica media is clipped by the locking pin on the clip to realize hemostasis through closure.

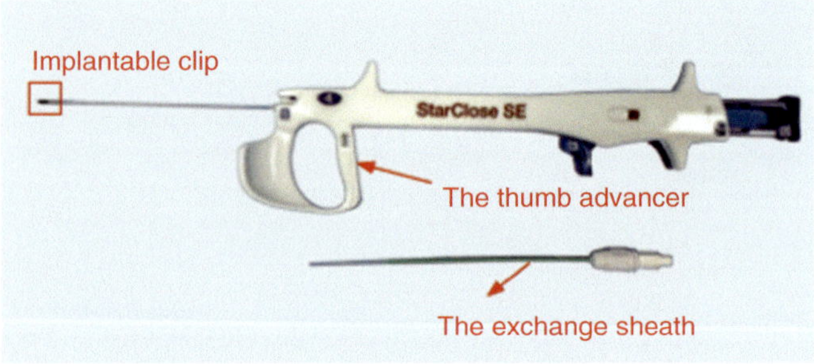

Fig. 2.33 Starclose SE vascular closure system (Abbott)

2.9.3.2 Features and Models

Starclose SE vascular closure system is indicated for the closure of femoral artery puncture sites using a 5-7F vascular sheath, especially for vascular closure procedures requiring for repeated femoral artery puncture. Its model is 6F.

2.9.3.3 Operation Procedures

Starclose SE vascular closure system performs operation procedures through four audible clicks in device deployment.

1. The first click (click1): Connect the exchange sheath with the main port of the clip applier and have the side with "Starclose SE" logo facing upward. In connection, the first audible click is heard and conform its engagement.
2. The second click (click2): Hold the stabilizer with left hand, and stabilize the body of the clip applier at an angle of 30°~40° with the skin surface. With the right thumb on the vessel locator button, with the right index and middle fingers on the thumb advancer, depress the locator button with right thumb; a second click will be heard to conform that the locator button is depressed.
3. The third click (click3): Keep the left hand on the finger loop and stabilize the body of the clip applier at an angle of 30–40° with skin surface; retract the body 2–3 cm, with the right thumb on the thumb advancer, and other four fingers on the upper part of the clip applier; push downward the thumb advancer with the right thumb; pull apart the exchange sheath 2–3 cm; push the plunger with right hand; and gently retract the closure device. When resistance is felt, stop retracting, push downward the thumb advancer with the thumb, pull apart the remaining part of the exchange sheath, and advance the thumb advancer to the ending arrow. At this time, the third click is heard to check if the arrow aligns with the ending arrow.
4. The fourth click (click4): Hold the metal shaft with gauze with the left hand, raise the clip applier up to an angle of

60–75°, and gently push the device about 1 mm downward. After pulsation is felt, depress the clip safety release with right thumb, stabilize the clip applier with left hand for 2 s, move away the clip applier with right hand, and press the percutaneous puncture site with sterile gauze for 1–2 min to confirm that the clip applier restores to its tiled memory state.

2.9.4 ExoSeal Vascular Closure Device

2.9.4.1 Product Structure

The US Cordis-produced ExoSeal vascular closure device consists of a plug applier and an absorbable plug (Fig. 2.34). The plug applier consists of a handle assembly and a delivery shaft, while the absorbable plug is fully enclosed in the distal portion of the delivery shaft. The plug applier made of bioabsorbable materials can be degraded into carbon dioxide and water, most of which are absorbed within 30 days after implantation and completely all within 60–90 days postimplantation.

2.9.4.2 Features and Models

The ExoSeal vascular closure device is indicated for femoral artery puncture site closure. The plug applier positions and deploys the absorbable plug to the extravascular surface of the puncture site through the use of 5F, 6F, or 7F vascular sheath introducer with a work length of up to 12 cm, and hemostasis is achieved when the absorbable plug is deposited on top of the arteriotomy site.

2.9.4.3 Operation Procedures

1. Insert the ExoSeal device into corresponding French-size vascular sheath at an angle of 30°–45° till the marker band reaches the distal hemostasis valve of the sheath.
2. Stabilize the ExoSeal handle assembly with the right hand; retract the sheath with the left hand till the indicator wire cowling fully engages with the handle assembly, during which the pulsatile blood stream can be observed to flow out from the bleed-back indicator.
3. While holding the handle assembly gently with the right hand, make sure not to touch the plug deployment button. Stabilize the left hand on the patient body and slowly retract the sheath. Observe the bleed-back indicator till the pulsatile blood flow significantly slows down or stops.
4. Observe the indicator window, while even more slowly retract the sheath (about 1 cm) with the left hand till the indicator window turns from black-white to black-black.
5. Anchor the left hand on the body surface of the patient, while holding the vascular sheath with the left thumb and index finger, and keep it immovable and stabilize the black-black indication. Deploy the plug and depress it once and for all with the right thumb and stay for 3 s, then slowly retract the ExoSeal and the vascular sheath, and manually press it for 2–4 min.

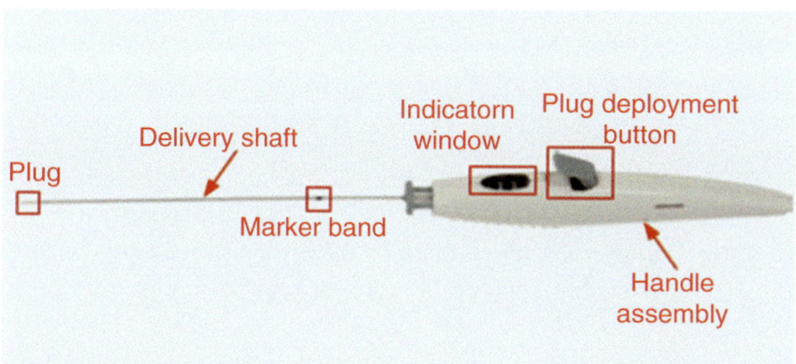

Fig. 2.34 ExoSeal vascular closure system

2.9.5 Hemostat

2.9.5.1 Product Structure

China's PuyiTech-produced hemostat consists of a push-pull lock, a silvery handle, a dilatable catheter, and a hemostasis umbrella (Fig. 2.35). The maximum outer diameter of the device is equal to 18G needle, a deployable memory-alloy hemostasis umbrella being equipped at its distal end enveloped with a biofilm that can perform quick and temporary hemostasis.

2.9.5.2 Features and Models

Hemostat is indicated for vascular hemostasis of artery puncture sites using 6–8F vascular sheath. The diameter of the umbrella is 6 mm when deployed, and the length from the umbrella to the distal end of the dilatable catheter is 15 cm.

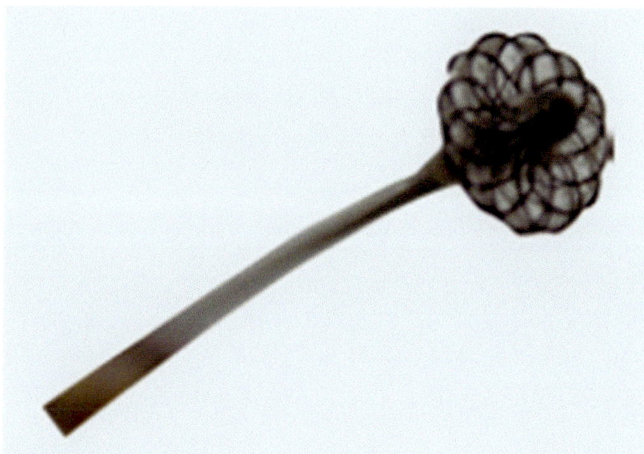

Fig. 2.35 Hemostat (PuyiTech)

2.9.5.3 Operation Procedures

1. Before insertion into the hemostat via the vascular sheath introducer, deploy and retract the umbrella under sterile operation, check if the umbrella is damaged, and observe if the umbrella is of a concentric circle shape.
2. Advance the hemostat into the blood vessels through the hemostasis valve at the end of the vascular sheath till the blue dilatable catheter is fully submerged.
3. Hold the silvery handle and pull the push-pull lock backward to deploy the umbrella till obvious obstruction is felt by the hand, and then the device is locked. Slowly retract the hemostat and when minor resistance is felt, indicating that the umbrella is on the top of sheath introducer.
4. Hold the hemostasis valve of the vascular sheath by the right thumb and index finger; gently withdraw the vascular sheath in the reverse direction of puncture. Don't force to pull any portion of the hemostat while withdrawing the sheath introducer.
5. When the blue dilatable catheter appears, gently pull the blue dilatable catheter with the left thumb and index finger; continue to pull out the vascular sheath completely via the wire of the hemostasis umbrella. Hold the blue dilatable catheter; gently pull the hemostat upward 1–1.5 cm till the vascular bleeding stops completely. Then fix it on the extravascular surface of the femoral artery puncture site with the retaining clip so as to maintain lasting tension.
6. Observe if the puncture site bleeds. If continuous artery bleeding lasts for over 1 min, readjust the tension.
7. Press the device with the proximal end of the finger to remove the retaining clip, maintain proximal compression, retract hemostasis umbrella, withdraw the hemostat, and maintain proximal pressure.
8. Press it with fingers, remove the retaining clip, and find the artery pulsation at the proximal end (upward side) of the artery puncture port. Press it with fingers, don't press on the umbrella directly and maintain proximal pressure while removing the retaining clip.
9. Press the push-pull lock forward and retract the umbrella. When the umbrella is completely retracted, only 1 mm blue marker can be observed. Note: Keep the hemostat free from tension.
10. With the umbrella retracted, withdraw the hemostat safely from within the body. While withdrawing the hemostat, gently rotate it.

Balloon Dilatation Catheter

3

Huajuan Mao, Junmin Bao, Zhiyong Chen, and Jian Dong

Abstract

Balloon catheters are main devices for endovascular treatment, and, based on the features of their delivery systems, they can be classified into two types, i.e., the over-the-wire (OTW) type and the rapid exchange system (RX) type. This chapter provides a tabular summary of the names, brands, compliances, and specifications of balloon catheters, as well as their adapter wires, adapter sheaths, bursting pressures, shafts, and other adapter devices. After that, it elaborates on their structures and features based on balloons of different brands.

Keywords

Balloon catheter · Adapter device · Structure and features Model types

3.1 Introduction

The balloon dilatation catheter, short for balloon, is used for expanding the diseased portion and delivering endovascular devices for stents or as the support catheter to recanalize the diseased segments of the blood vessels. The balloon can be divided into four parts: the tip, balloon body, connecting segment, and delivery shaft.

H. Mao (✉) · J. Bao · J. Dong
Department of Vascular Surgery, Changhai Hospital, Second Military Medical University, Shanghai, China
e-mail: czymm8@163.com

Z. Chen
Department of Vascular Surgery, The First Hospital, Anhui Medical University, Anhui, China

3.1.1 Balloon Performance

Balloon dilatation catheter performance is evaluated usually with reference to the following parameters:

3.1.1.1 The Crossing Profile

The crossing profile refers to the outer diameter when the balloon is not expanded, currently taking the minimum outer diameter that the balloon can cross as the criteria, and it generally refers to the outer diameter of the balloon marker portion.

3.1.1.2 Flexibility

Flexibility refers to the ability that the balloon accesses through the lesions in natural vascular state.

3.1.1.3 Trackability

Trackability refers to the ability of the balloon to reach the lesions under the guidance of the wire.

3.1.1.4 Pushability

Pushability refers to the ability of the balloon tip to navigate through the lesions when the operator manipulates the balloon delivery unit in vitro.

3.1.2 Balloon Compliance

Balloon compliance refers to the ability that the balloon diameter changes along with the pressure change when the balloon is fully inflated, an index indicating the tensile capacity of the balloon. Balloon can be classified as non-compliant, semi-compliant, and compliant balloons according to the ratio of the final diameter with the rated diameter when the balloon reaches rated standard pressure and is continually compressed to the bursting pressure.

Z. Jing et al. (eds.), *Endovascular Surgery and Devices*, https://doi.org/10.1007/978-981-10-8270-2_3

3.1.2.1 The Non-compliant Balloon

The balloon with 100–110% ratio between final diameter and rated one is usually high-pressure balloon, featuring strong and even expansion force, not liable of dog-bone phenomenon (dog-bone phenomenon means that when the balloon is inflated to rated bursting pressure within a stent, both the proximal and distal diameters of the balloon are all larger than those of the stent, showing like a dog-bone under X-ray), and available for expanding hard plaques.

3.1.2.2 The Semi-compliant Balloon

Most balloons with 110–130% ratio between final and rated diameters are semi-compliant balloons, having a crossing profile smaller than that of the non-compliant ones and excellent crossability.

3.1.2.3 The Compliant Balloon

Compliant balloons are the ones with ratio between final and rated diameters exceeding 130% or even reaching several times their own volume. These balloons are mainly used for aortic dilatation and temporary closure or expansion of indwelling vascular prosthesis.

3.1.3 Types and Features of Balloons

Balloons are mainly classified into two categories: over the wire (OTW) and rapid exchange system (RX), according to the delivery system.

3.1.3.1 OTW

OTW (over the wire). The balloon dilatation catheter is mainly used for long-segment occlusive diseases and situations where the wire needs to be exchanged. This kind of balloon features excellent pushability, commonly used for the endovascular treatment for subclavian artery, iliac artery, femoral artery, popliteal artery, and infra-popliteal artery.

3.1.3.2 RX

RX (rapid exchange system). The balloon dilatation catheter often has a smaller outer diameter, facilitating the operator control, available for rapid exchange of the balloons, but disadvantaged in relatively poorer trackability and pushability than the OTW, thus making it inconvenient for wire exchange. This kind of balloon is often used for endovascular treatment of renal artery, carotid artery, and coronary artery, as well as for the retrograde puncture of lower extremity arteries.

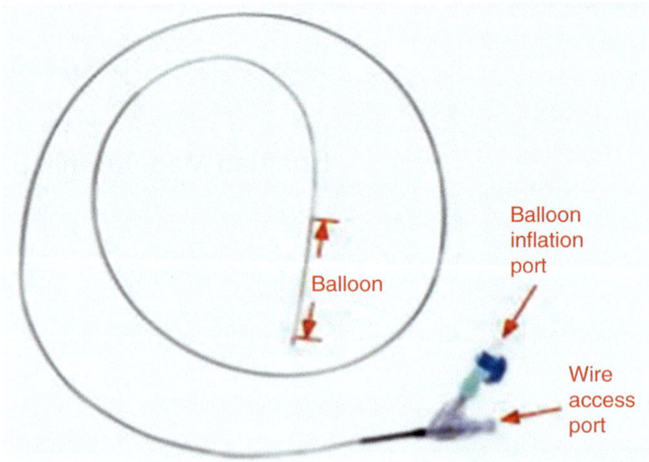

Fig. 3.1 OTW balloon dilatation catheter

3.2 OTW Balloon Dilatation Catheter

3.2.1 Product Structure

OTW balloon dilatation catheter consists of a double-lumen shaft lever with the balloon body connected at its distal end (Fig. 3.1). The double-lumen shaft lever is branched at its proximal end, one of the lumen functions as the port for the wire to enter the central lumen while the other lumen as a pathway to control the inflation and shortening of the balloon with the mixture of the contrast agent and the normal saline. A smooth, flexible, and noninvasive tip is located at the proximal end of the catheter, facilitating the advancement of the catheter through narrow portions. To ensure accurate positioning of the balloon under X-ray, two radiopaque marker bands are equipped on both ends of the work zones of the balloon.

3.2.2 Specifications and Models

At present, the brands of OTW balloon dilatation catheters include Boston Scientific, Medtronic, Bard, Cordis, Medtronic, Abbott, Biotronik, Optimed, Cook, Gore, etc. This section mainly introduces balloon dilatation catheters from such brands as Mustang (Boston Scientific), Admiral Xtreme (Medtronic), Reekross 35 (Bard), Savvy Long (Cordis), Evercross (Medtronic), Fox Sv (Abbott), Passeo-35 (Biotronik), Coda (Cook), and Tri-Lobe (Gore) (Table 3.1).

Table 3.1 Brand-specific OTW balloon specifications (for reference only)

Name	Brand	Compliance	Balloon diameter (mm)	Balloon length (mm)	Matching wire (in)	Matching sheath (F)	Burst pressure (atm)	Shaft (cm)
Mustang	Boston Scientific	Non-compliant	3–12	20–200	0.035	5–7	14–24	40, 75, 135
Sterling OTW	Boston Scientific	Semi-compliant	2–10	20–150	0.018	4	10–14	80, 90, 135, 150
Coyote	Boston Scientific	Semi-compliant	1.5–4	40–220	0.014	4	12–14	90, 150
XXL	Boston Scientific	Non-compliant	12–18	20–60	0.035	7	5–8	75, 120
Admiral Xtreme	Medtronic	Semi-compliant	3–12	20–300	0.035	5–7	17.76	80, 130
Pacific	Medtronic	Semi-compliant	2–7	20–300	0.018	4–5	24.67	90, 130, 180
Deep	Medtronic	Semi-compliant	1.5–4	20–210	0.014	5	15.79	120, 150
Reekross 14	Bard	Semi-compliant	25	40–220	0.014	4	13–16	140
Reekross18	Bard	Semi-compliant	2–5	40–220	0.018	4	13–16	130
Reekross 35	Bard	Semi-compliant	2–6	40–220	0.035	5–6	13–16	75, 110
Bantam	Bard	Semi-compliant	2–9	20–220	0.018	4–6	12–16	75, 90, 130
Bantam α	Bard	Semi-compliant	1.25–5	15–220	0.014	4	13–16	100, 130, 150
Powerflex P3	Cordis	Semi-compliant	4–12	10–100	0.035	5–7	15	40, 80, 110, 135
Powerflex Pro	Cordis	Semi-compliant	3–12	20–220	0.035	5–7	18	80, 135
Maxi LD	Cordis	Semi-compliant	14–25	40–80	0.035	8–12	5–6	40, 80
Savvy	Cordis	Semi-compliant	2–6	20–100	0.018	4–5	10	80, 120, 150
Savvy Long	Cordis	Semi-compliant	2–6	120–220	0.018	4–5	12–15	80, 120, 150
Sleek	Cordis	Semi-compliant	1.5–5	15–280	0.014	4	10–16	150
Evercross	Medtronic	Semi-compliant	3–12	20–200	0.035	5–7	10–20	80, 135
Powercross	Medtronic	Semi-compliant	2–6	20–200	0.018	4–6	14	90, 150
Nanocross	Medtronic	Semi-compliant	1.5–4	20–210	0.014	4	14	90, 150
Fox Sv	Abbott	Semi-compliant	2–5	15–120	0.018	4	16–22	90, 135, 150
Fox cross	Abbott	Semi-compliant	3–14	20–120	0.035	5–7	8–18	50, 80, 135
Armada 14	Abbott	Semi-compliant	1.5–4	20–200	0.014	4	14	90, 150
Armada 35	Abbott	Semi-compliant	4–14	20–250	0.035	5–7	7–25	80, 135
Passeo-35	Biotronik	Semi-compliant	3–10	20–200	0.035	5–6	16	80, 90, 130
Passeo-18	Biotronik	Semi-compliant	2–7	20–220	0.018	4–5	15	90, 130, 150
Passeo-14	Biotronik	Semi-compliant	1.5–4	20 ~ 220	0.014	4	14	90, 120, 150
Mars	Optimed	Non-compliant	3–10	40–100	0.035	5–6	17.76	75, 120
Coda	Cook	Compliant	32	40	0.035	10	/	100
Sanye	Gore	Compliant	16–45	40	0.035	18	/	104

3.2.3 Brand Information

3.2.3.1 Mustang Balloon Dilatation Catheter

Product Structure

Mustang balloon dilatation catheter, the US Boston Scientific-produced high-pressure non-compliant balloon, consists of a balloon, bumper tip, an inner tip, a reducer tube, a stain relief, Y connector, and the catheter shaft. The balloon has hydrophilic coating applied on both ends of the work zones and platinum-iridium radiopaque marker bands.

Features and Models

The Mustang balloon dilatation catheter is indicated for percutaneous transluminal angioplasty (PTA) in the peripheral vasculature. The balloon matches well with 0.89 mm (0.035 in) wire and 5–7F vascular sheath, available with 3–12 mm in diameter, 20–200 mm in length, 14–24 atm of bursting pressure, and 40 cm, 75 cm, and 130 cm in shaft length.

3.2.3.2 Admiral Xtreme Balloon Dilatation Catheter

Product Structure

Admiral Xtreme balloon dilatation catheter, the US Medtronic-produced semi-compliant balloon, consists of a coaxial dual-lumen catheter and a balloon, wherein the coaxial dual-lumen catheter is made of the polyamide elastomer, and the balloon of polyamide material, surfaced with hydrophilic coating. On both ends of the work zones of the balloon are two radiopaque metal marker bands.

Features and Models

The balloon dilatation catheter is indicated for percutaneous transluminal angioplasty (PTA) in the peripheral vasculature. The balloon matches well with 0.89 mm (0.035in) wire, and 5–7F vascular sheath, available with 3–12 mm in diameter, 20–300 mm in length, 17.76 atm of bursting pressure, and 80 cm and 130 cm in shaft length.

3.2.3.3 Reekross 35 Balloon Dilatation Catheter

Product Structure

Reekross 35 balloon dilatation catheter, the US Bard-produced semi-compliant balloon, consists of a rigid shaft (extending from the proximal handle to the distal tip) with a separate rigid inflation lumen. The balloon is made of a blend of nylon and polyamide elastomer and the rigid shaft of 304 V stainless steel. The catheter shaft is surfaced with Silx hydrophilic coating, and by virtue of Quadflex Technology, the balloon can perform multiple inflations, while the catheter is advanced through long, occluded lesions. Platiniridium marker bands are equipped on both ends of the work zone of the balloon, ensuring accurate positioning under X-ray.

Features and Models

The balloon dilatation catheter is indicated specially for the treatment of highly difficult seriously calcified artery lesions of lower extremity, suitable for both transluminal and endovascular angioplasty. The balloon matches well with 0.89 mm (0.035 in) wire and 5–6F vascular sheath. The balloon diameter is 2–6 mm, length 40–220 mm, burst pressure 13–16 atm, and 75 cm and 110 cm in shaft length.

3.2.3.4 Savvy Long Balloon Dilatation Catheter

Product Structure

The Savvy Long balloon dilatation catheter, the US Cordis-produced semi-compliant balloon, consists of a seat, strain relief, a catheter, and a balloon (2 mm balloon is twofold and 3–6 mm threefold). The catheter is surfaced with Silx hydrophilic coating. The catheter is made of nylon blend, balloon of nylon blend and Pebax. On both ends of the work zones of the balloon are hydrophilic coating and radiopaque platiniridium marker bands.

Features and Models

The balloon dilatation catheter is indicated for endovascular dilatation treatment for the superficial femoral artery of lower extremity, deep femoral artery, popliteal artery, and infrapopliteal artery. The balloon matches well with 0.46 mm (0.018in) wire and 4–5F vascular sheath. The balloon diameter is 2–6 mm, length 120–220 mm, burst pressure 12–15 atm, and 80 cm, 120 cm and 150 cm in shaft length.

3.2.3.5 Evercross Balloon Dilatation Catheter

Product Structure

The Evercross balloon dilatation catheter, the US Medtronic-produced semi-compliant balloon, consists of a dual-lumen catheter with a distally mounted semi-compliant inflatable balloon. The material for the balloon is polyamide and that for the catheter is polyamide and Pebax. A layer of hydrophilic coating of light-sensitive sodium sulfonate and polyvinylpyrrolidone is applied at the distal portion of the catheter. On both ends of the work zones of the balloon are a radiopaque marker band used for balloon positioning.

Features and Models

The balloon dilatation catheter is indicated for endovascular dilatation treatment of lower extremity artery and renal artery and other vascular stenoses. The balloon matches well with 0.89 mm (0.035in) wire and 5–7F vascular sheath. The diameter of the balloon is 3–12 mm, the length 20–200 mm, the burst pressure 10–20 atm, and 80 cm and 135 cm in shaft length.

3.2.3.6 Fox Sv Balloon Dilatation Catheter

Product Structure

The Fox Sv balloon dilatation catheter, the US Abbott-produced semi-compliant balloon, consists of a dual-lumen catheter and a balloon, made of polyamide, and surfaced with hydrophilic coating on the catheter, a balloon tip and wire lumen, except on the balloon. On both ends of the work zones of the balloon are platiniridium marker bands used for positioning the relative position of the balloon and vascular stenosis.

Features and Models

The balloon dilatation catheter is indicated for endovascular dilatation treatment for atherosclerosis obliteration of lower extremity and restenosis following the stent placement. The balloon is suitable with 0.46 mm (0.018in) wire and 4F vascular sheath and available with 2–5 mm diameter, 15–120 mm length, 16–22 atm burst pressure, and 90 cm, 135 cm and 150 cm in shaft length.

3.2.3.7 Passeo-35 Balloon Dilatation Catheter

Product Structure

The Passeo-35 balloon dilatation catheter, the German Biotronik-produced semi-compliant balloon, consists of a balloon, a catheter, and an operation handle. The material for the balloon is polylaurylamide, and that for the catheter is Pebax and that for the Y joint portion of the operation handle is Polycarbonate. The catheter is surfaced with hydrophilic silicon coating and the balloon with hydrophilic patching coating. On both ends of the work zones of the balloon is a radiopaque marker band used for balloon positioning.

Features and Models

The balloon dilatation catheter is indicated for endovascular dilatation treatment of lower extremity artery, renal artery, and other vascular stenoses. The balloon fits well with 0.89 mm (0.035in) wire and 5–6F vascular sheath. The balloon is available with 3–10 mm diameter, 20–200 mm length, 16 atm burst pressure, and 80 cm, 90 cm, and 130 cm in shaft length.

3.2.3.8 Coda Balloon Dilatation Catheter

Product Structure

The Coda balloon dilatation catheter, the US Cook-produced compliant balloon, consists of a balloon, a catheter, and a catheter seat (Fig. 3.2). The material for the balloon is polyurethane, and that for the catheter is polyurethane, barium sulfate, and yellow dye, that for the catheter seat is polyurethane, and that for the balloon lumen joint is polycarbonate. On both ends of the work zones of the balloon is a radiopaque platiniridium marker band used for balloon positioning under X-ray.

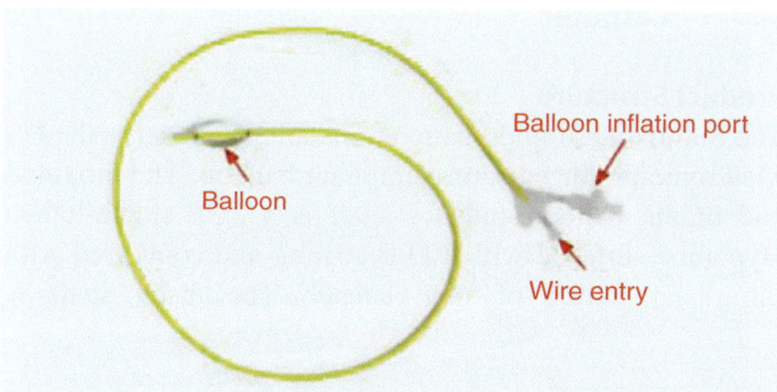

Fig. 3.2 Coda balloon dilatation catheter (Cook)

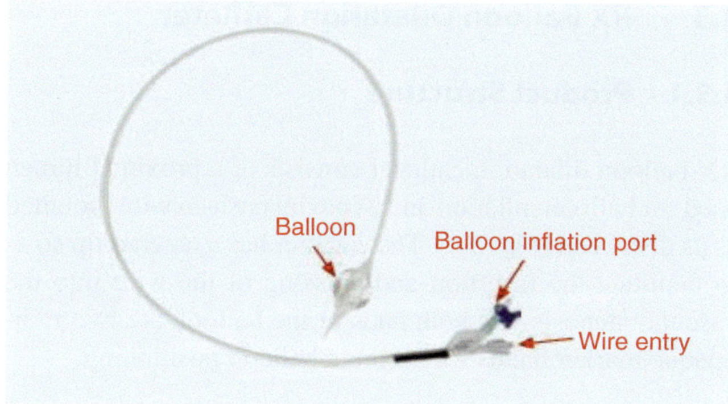

Fig. 3.3 Tri-lobe balloon catheter (Gore)

Features and Models

The balloon is indicated mainly for aortic (thoracic and abdominal aorta) dilatation and temporary closure or endovascular dilatation treatment of vascular prosthesis. The balloon is used in conjunction with 0.89 mm (0.035in) wire and 10F vascular sheath (11–12F recommended according to clinical experience). The balloon is 32 mm in diameter, 40 mm in length, and 100 cm in delivery shaft length.

3.2.3.9 Tri-Lobe Balloon Dilatation Catheter

Product Structure

The Tri-Lobe balloon dilatation catheter, the US Gore-produced compliant balloon (Fig. 3.3), consists of three polyurethane balloons distally mounted on a dual-lumen catheter and radiopaque marker bands along the edge of the balloon. The three inflation lumens are connected with a balloon, and the proximal inflation port is connected with all inflation lumens by a Luer joint. The tri-lobe design of the balloon dilatation catheter ensures that the aortic blood flow will not be completely obstructed when the balloon is fully inflated.

Features and Models

The balloon dilatation catheter is indicated for assisting the self-expanding stent graft with endovascular dilatation treatment for large-diameter blood vessels (thoracic and abdominal aorta). The balloon is used in conjunction with 0.89 mm (0.035in) wire and 18F vascular sheath. The balloon can be divided into large and small ones: the inflated diameter of the small balloon is 16–34 mm and that for large balloon 26–45 mm, with 104 cm in delivery shaft length.

3.3 RX Balloon Dilatation Catheter

3.3.1 Product Structure

RX balloon dilatation catheter consists of a proximal lumen used for balloon inflation and a coaxial push-in wire mounted at its distal end (Fig. 3.4). The catheter has a tapered tip so as to facilitate the insertion and crossing of the wire into the vascular stenosis. On both ends of the balloon are two radiopaque marker bands for accurate balloon positioning.

3.3.2 Specifications and Models

At present, the brands for RX balloon dilatation catheters mainly include Boston Scientific, Bard, Medtronic, Cordis, etc.; the features and models of which are shown in Table 3.2. This section mainly introduces Sterling Monorail (Boston Scientific), LitePAC (Bard), and Submarine Rapido (Medtronic) balloon dilatation catheters.

3.3.3 Brand Information

3.3.3.1 Sterling Monorail Balloon Dilatation Catheter

Product Structure

The Sterling Monorail balloon dilatation catheter, the US Boston Scientific-produced semi-compliant balloon, has a thin tip fixed on the distal RX catheter. The inner layer material of the wire lumen is made of high density polyethylene (hdpe) and dye. The balloon catheter has a tapered tip, facilitating the access through vascular stenosis. On both ends of the balloon are two marker bands available for observation and balloon catheter positioning under X-ray.

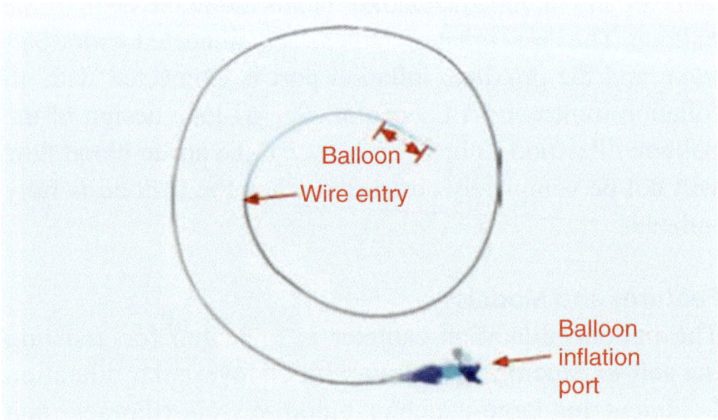

Fig. 3.4 RX balloon dilatation catheter

Features and Models

The balloon dilatation catheter is indicated for percutaneous transluminal angioplasty of such peripheral vessels as carotid, vertebral, and renal arteries. The balloon matches with 0.46 mm (0.018in) wire and 4–5F vascular sheath. The balloon is available with 5–8 mm diameter, 10–60 mm length, 14 atm burst pressure, and 80 cm and 135 cm in delivery shaft length.

3.3.3.2 LitePAC Balloon Dilatation Catheter

Product Structure

The LitePAC balloon dilatation catheter, the US Bard-produced semi-compliant balloon, has its proximal end made of 304 stainless steel and distal coaxial catheter made of nylon mixture. There are two radiopaque platiniridium markers on the balloon, facilitating balloon positioning under X-ray. A transparent axle is mounted at the proximal end of the catheter, facilitating the observation of air bubbles and removal of air bubbles during balloon preparation.

Features and Models

The balloon dilatation catheter is indicated for endovascular dilatation treatment for such peripheral vessels as carotid, vertebral, and renal arteries. The balloon matches with 0.36 mm (0.014 in) wire and 4–5F vascular sheath. The balloon is 2–7 mm in diameter and 15–220 mm in length, available with 12–16 atm burst pressure and 150 cm and 155 cm in delivery shaft length.

3.3.3.3 Submarine Rapido Balloon Dilatation Catheter

Product Structure

The Submarine Rapido balloon dilatation catheter is the US Medtronic-produced semi-compliant balloon. The proximal end of the balloon catheter shaft is a 2.3F single-lumen Hypotube surfaced with PTFE coating and connected with the distal lumen of the catheter. The distal shaft is

Table 3.2 Brand-specific RX balloon specifications (for reference only)

Name	Brand	Compliance	Balloon diameter (mm)	Balloon length (mm)	Matching wire (in)	Matching sheath (F)	Burst pressure (atm)	Delivery shaft (cm)
Sterling Monorail	Boston scientific	Semi-compliant	5–8	10–60	0.018	4–5	14	80, 135
LitePAC	Bard	Semi-compliant	2–7	15–220	0.014	4–5	12–16	150, 155
Submarine Rapido	Medtronic	Semi-compliant	2–7	20–80	0.018	4–5	16.7	135
Aviator plus	Cordis	Semi-compliant	4–7	15–40	0.014	4	12–14	142

3.5F. Catheter shaft and the balloon are all applied with hydrophilic coating. When the catheter gets moist, the hydrophilic coating functions as lubrication to the catheter.

Features and Models

The balloon dilatation catheter is specially used for endovascular dilatation treatment for carotid and renal artery lesions. The balloon matches with 0.46 mm (0.018in) wire and 4–5F vascular sheath. The balloon is 2–7 mm in diameter and 20–80 mm in length, available with 16.7 atm burst pressure and 135 cm in delivery shaft length.

3.4 Special Balloon Dilatation Catheter

3.4.1 Peripheral Cutting Balloon Dilatation Catheter

3.4.1.1 Product Structure

The Peripheral Cutting Balloon dilatation catheter (Fig. 3.5), the US Boston Scientific-produced non-compliant balloon, consists of 3–4 atherotome blades (microsurgical blade) mounted lengthwise on the balloon surface. The balloon is made of nylon. When the peripheral cutting balloon inflates, atherotome blades can cut the angiosclerosis plaque, thus forming the starting point for crack propagation.

The main body of the OTW type cutting balloon dilatation catheter is of dual-lumen design, the outer lumen being the balloon inflation lumen, and the inner lumen delivering the cutting balloon to the lesion portion to be expanded via the wire. At the end of the atherotome blades are radiopaque marker bands, providing a reference point after the placement of the balloon inside the blood vessels.

RX-type cutting balloon dilatation catheter contains two lumens. The proximal catheter handle is made of hypotube containing balloon inflation lumen. The distal handle is made of flexible material. The balloon tip and wire lumen are coated green, facilitating the observation and fast balloon exchange. Wire exit is located 24 cm from the catheter tip.

3.4.1.2 Features and Models

The balloon dilatation catheter is indicated for endovascular treatment of seriously calcified plaque, hard plaque, in-stent restenosis, and other vascular stenoses. At 6 atm pressure, the balloon will inflate to a specified diameter and length at a rated burst pressure of 10–12 atm. The balloon dilatation catheter can be divided into two types: OTW and RX.

- Cutting balloon with 5–8 mm diameter is OTW type balloon, suitable for matching with 0.46 mm (0.018in) wire; the balloon (including blade) is 20 mm in length, with four blades and 50 cm, 90 cm, and 135 cm in delivery shaft length.
- Cutting balloon with 2–4 mm diameter is RX type balloon, suitable for matching with 0.36 mm (0.014in) wire; the balloon (including balde) is 15 mm in length, with 3–4 blades and 140 cm in delivery shaft length.

3.4.2 VascuTrak Dual-Wire Balloon Dilatation Catheter

3.4.2.1 Product Structure

The VascuTrak Dual-Wire balloon dilatation catheter is the US Bard-produced RX-type semi-compliant balloon (Fig. 3.6). A steel wire is attached outside the balloon portion of the catheter. When the balloon inflates, the steel wire and the balloon attach with the vascular wall, playing a role of cutting the inner membrane inside the vascular lumen.

3.4.2.2 Features and Models

The balloon dilatation catheter is characterized by a small outer diameter, high lesion crossability, and ability of cutting the plaque, suitable for endovascular dilatation treatment for calcified vessels or in-stent restenosis. The burst pressure of the balloon is 12 atm, with 80 cm and 140 cm in delivery shaft length, and it can be divided into two types: VascuTrak 14 and

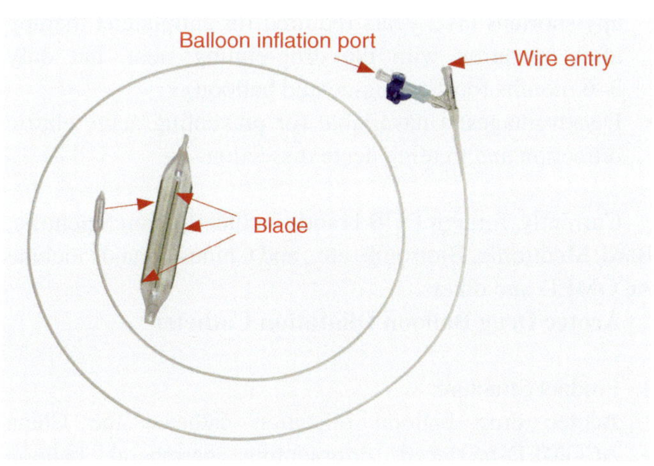

Fig. 3.5 Peripheral Cutting balloon dilatation catheter (Boston Scientific)

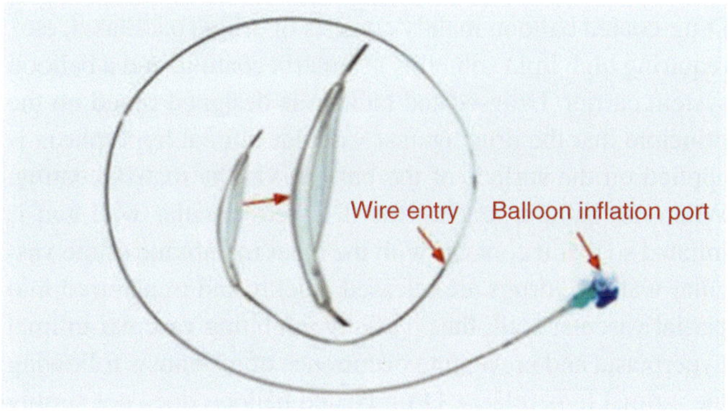

Fig. 3.6 VascuTrak dual-wire balloon dilatation catheter (Bard)

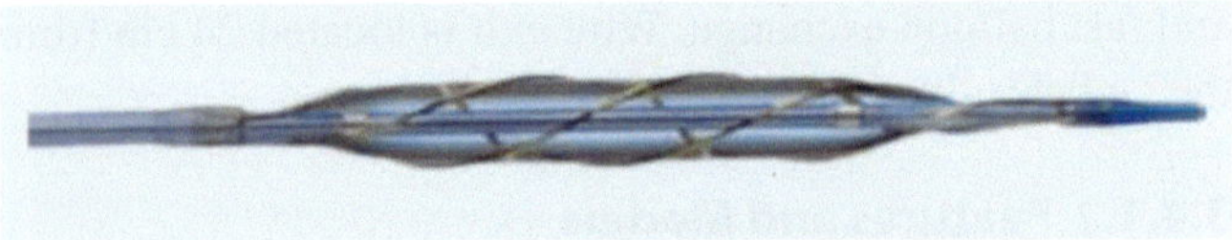

Fig. 3.7 AngioSculpt scoring balloon (Spectranetics)

VascuTrak 18 balloons. VascuTrak 14 is suitable for matching with 0.36 mm (0.014in) wire and 5–7F vascular sheath, with 2–3.5 mm in diameter and 20–300 mm in length. VascuTrak 18 balloon matches with 0.46 mm (0.018in) wire and 5F vascular sheath, available with 4–7 mm diameter and 20–30 mm length.

3.4.3 AngioSculpt Scoring Balloon

3.4.3.1 Product Structure

The AngioSculpt scoring balloon, the US Spectranetics-produced OTW semi-compliant balloon, consists of a balloon catheter with a triple-helical hollow tube laser engraved from Ni-Ti alloy (Fig. 3.7). When the balloon opens, an expansion force of 15–25 times larger than the balloon itself produces via the three helical Ni-Ti steel wires mounted outside the balloon, where the diameter of the steel wire is 0.18 mm. The expansion force, like a scoring, changes the tension of lesion tissue so that it can expand under very low balloon pressure.

3.4.3.2 Features and Models

The balloon is indicated for endovascular treatment for such lesions as calcified peripheral arteries and in-stent restenosis. The triple helical design of the AngioScuplt scoring balloon takes into account the balloon crossability, scoring function, and consistency in lumen diameter after expansion. The balloon is suitable for matching with 0.36 mm (0.014 in) and 0.46 mm (0.018 in) wires and 5–6F vascular sheath. The balloon is 2–8 mm in diameter and 20–200 mm in length, available with 12–20 atm burst pressure and 50 cm, 90 cm, 137 cm, and 155 cm in delivery length.

3.4.4 Drug-Coated Balloon

Drug-coated balloon mainly consists of drugs (paclitaxel, etc., requiring high lipid solubility), a matrix coating, and a balloon system carrier. Drug-coated balloon is designed based on the principle that the drug against vascular intimal hyperplasia is applied on the surface of the balloon via the matrix coating. When the balloon reaches the diseased vascular wall and is inflated so that it contacts with the inner membrane of the vascular wall, the drugs are released quickly and transferred into partial vascular wall, thus partially inhibiting vascular intimal hyperplasia and preventing occurrence of restenosis following the intimal hyperplasia. Drug-coated balloon does not simply mean to apply drugs on the balloon drug, but rather, it differs in various aspects, such as types of catheter drugs, the coating technique, and the release technique, from conventional balloon technology. For the drug-coated balloon, it is necessary to prevent as much as possible the drug from being flushed away by the blood flow during expansion, and the drug can be quickly released to vascular wall tissues shortly after the expansion (usually less than 60 s), rather than slowly eluted, where the role of the matrix coating technique is mainly reflected and where the difference with the drug-eluting stent lies. Therefore, many experts propose to change the name of the drug-coated balloon from its original drug-eluting balloon (DEB) to the present drug-coated balloon (DCB).

The drug-coated balloon acts primarily as a drug-loading system to resist intimal hyperplasia and prevent restenosis. In order to better retain the drug from eluting from the balloon before dilatation, it is necessary to carry out conventional balloon pre-expansion before the deployment of the drug-coated balloon. Drug-coated balloon has no continuous resistance against elastic retraction, which is mainly achieved by the stent. Therefore, the concept of using drug-coated ball and metal bare stents and drug-eluting stent is not contradictory, but rather a good complementary treatment program. At the same time, if serious dissection occurs after DCB dilatation, stent is stilled necessary for covering the dissection without exceeding the both ends of the drug-coated balloon. Currently, drug-coated balloons have extensive indications, including in-stent restenosis, bifurcation lesions, small blood vessels lesions, or positions unsuitable for or unable of placement of stents. Meanwhile, even if the drug-eluting stent is used, there will still be occurrence of restenosis, where the drug-coated balloon can well distinguish itself.

The drug-coated balloon is mainly characterized by:

- Advantages: Drugs are evenly distributed on the specific vascular wall areas (while for the drug-eluting stent, drugs are distributed on the stent beam structure). No metal remnants remain, retaining the original anatomical morphology of the blood vessels; the time of antiplatelet therapy shortens (1–2 years required for antiplatelet therapy after operation with the drug-eluting stent, but only 3–6 months for the drug-coated balloon).
- Disadvantages: Unavailable for preventing acute elastic retraction and treating acute dissection.

Currently, foreign DCB brands include Boston Scientific, Bard, Medtronic, Biotronik, etc., and Chinese brands include ACOMED and others.

Acotec Drug Balloon Dilatation Catheter

1. Product Structure
   Acotec drug balloon dilatation catheter, the China ACOMED-produced drug-eluting peripheral balloon

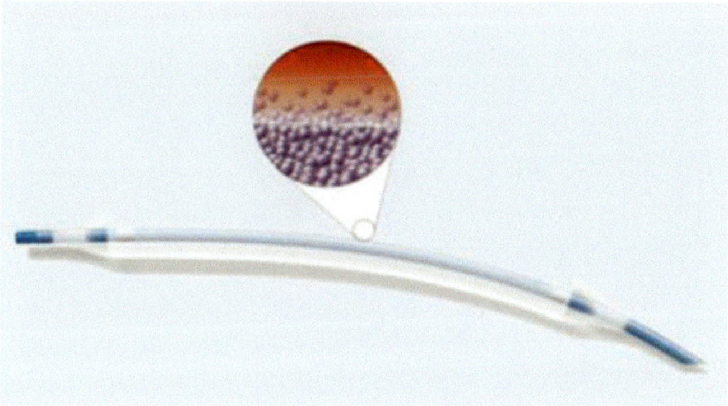

Fig. 3.8 Acotec drug balloon dilatation catheter (ACOMED)

(Fig. 3.8), consists of a balloon, a catheter tip, a dual-lumen shaft, Y connector, and radiopaque marker bands. The balloon is made of polyamide 12, surfaced with drug coating by way of solvent bonding. The coating contains paclitaxel at a dose of 3.3 μg per square millimeter, and the drug-loading matrix is magnesium stearate. This OTW-type balloon dilatation catheter can be classified as orchid type and dahlia type according to its matching wire.

2. Features and Models

This drug balloon dilatation catheter is indicated for percutaneous transluminal angioplasty of femoral artery and arteries. Orchid-type drug balloon adapts to 0.89 mm (0.035in) wire and 5–6F vascular sheath, available with 3–12 mm in balloon diameter and 20–300 mm in length. Dahlia-type drug balloon adapts to 0.46 mm (0.018in) wire and 5–6F vascular sheath, available with 3–12 mm in balloon diameter and 20–300 mm in length. The burst pressure of the balloon is 6–17 bar, with 80 cm and 120 cm in delivery shaft length.

Embolic Protection Device

4

Huajuan Mao, Junmin Bao, and Yu Xiao

Abstract

Anti-embolism protection devices are the most common instruments used in endovascular treatment for carotid artery diseases, and they can be classified into two types, i.e., the distal type and the proximal blocking type. This chapter introduces distal anti-embolism protection devices of different brands and provides a conclusion and summary about their structures, features, and model types.

Keywords

Anti-embolism protection device · Structure and features
Model types

4.1 Introduction

Embolic protection device, also called protective umbrella, is indicated for percutaneous transluminal angioplasty to capture the embolus and avoidance of distal arteriole occlusion, mostly used for endovascular therapy for the carotid artery lesions.

Common embolic protection device is classified into two categories: distal embolic protection device and proximal occlusive embolic protection device. The brands of distal embolic protection devices include Boston Scientific, Cordis, Abbott, Medtronic, Gore, Medtronic, etc., and those of proximal occlusive one include Medtronic, Silk Road, etc.

This section mainly introduces Angioguard(Cordis), Filterwire EZ(Boston Scientific), Spider FX(Medtronic), Embolished NAV6(Abbott) and Mo.Ma(Medtronic) embolic protection devices.

4.2 Angioguard Embolic Protection Device

4.2.1 Product Structure

The Angioguard embolic protection device of US Cordis consists of Angioguard embolus capture guide wire, a delivery sheath, a retrieval sheath, a controller, a filter basket introducer, and a peel-away wire introducer. At the distal end of the guide wire is a filter basket (Fig. 4.1) with a porous membrane supported by a pure metal skeleton. The guide wire is made of 304 V stainless steel and the filter of nickel alloy. The delivery system is made of nylon, and there are two radiopaque markers on the proximal shaft ends of the delivery and the retrieval sheaths.

4.2.2 Features and Models

Angioguard embolic protection device is indicated for endovascular treatment of peripheral arteries such as carotid artery, vertebral artery, and lower extremity arteries. The protection device is available with two models: 5–6 mm, the former is used for distal artery diameter at 3.5–4.5 mm; the latter at 4.5–5.5 mm. The device is compatible with 8F guide catheter and 6F long vascular sheath.

H. Mao (✉) · J. Bao · Y. Xiao
Department of Vascular Surgery, Changhai Hospital, Second Military Medical University, Shanghai, China
e-mail: czymm8@163.com

Z. Jing et al. (eds.), *Endovascular Surgery and Devices*, https://doi.org/10.1007/978-981-10-8270-2_4

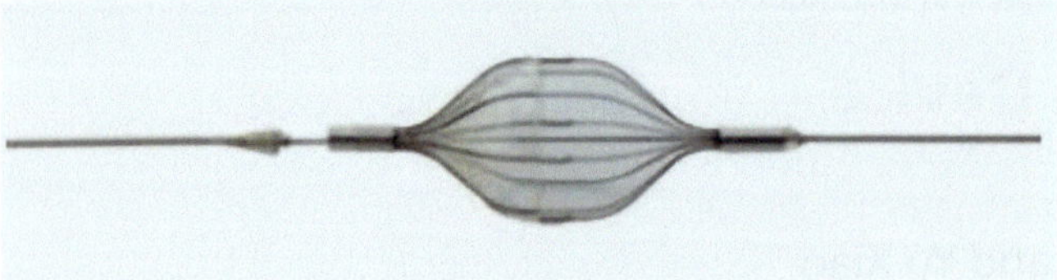

Fig. 4.1 Angioguard embolic protection device (Cordis)

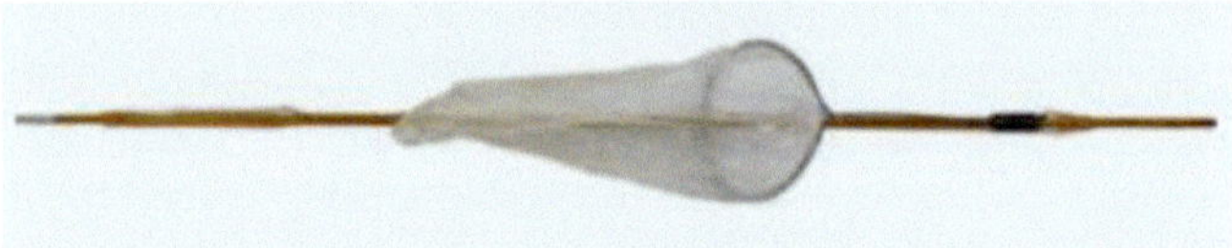

Fig. 4.2 Filterwire EZ embolic protection device (Boston Scientific)

4.3 Filterwire EZ Embolic Protection Device

4.3.1 Product Structure

The US Boston Scientific-produced Filterwire EZ embolic protection device consists of a thrombosis filter bag (Fig. 4.2), a protective wire, a sheath, a retrieval sheath, and a controller. The tip of the device is wrapped with a noninvasive 3 cm platinum spiral coil, soft and shapable. The mesh is made of polyurethane arranged at a gap of 110 μm. When deployed, the filter bag of the protective wire can contain and remove the embolic materials that may be liberated during the endovascular treatment. PTFE-coated stainless steel protective wire is used as a standard 0.36 mm (0.014in) wire, protecting the soft tip of the wire, and the filter ring is radiopaque.

4.3.2 Features and Models

The Filterwire EZ embolic protection device is indicated for angioplasty in the peripheral vascular system, carotid artery, coronary artery, and saphenous vein graft, as well as for containing and removing the thrombus or debris in stent operations. The protection device is suitable for placement in arteries with a diameter of 3.5–5.5 mm; the self-contained protective wire diameter is 0.36 mm (0.014in), with lengths of 190 cm (RX type) and 300 cm (OTW type). The device is compatible with 8Fguide catheter and 6F long vascular sheath.

4.4 SpiderFX Embolic Protection Device

4.4.1 Product Structure

The US Medtronic-produced SpiderFX embolic protection device consists of capture wire, a mesh filter with a distal soft tip (Fig. 4.3), and SpiderFX catheter. The nitinol filter is surfaced with Applause heparin molecular coating covalently attached with nitinol. The filter is mounted on a 0.36 mm (0.014in) PTFE-coated stainless steel wire with a length of 190–320 cm, where in operation the 320 cm wire can be broken off to 190 cm along the scoring mark for the purpose of quick exchange. The distal portion of the wire for quick exchange is golden, and the proximal portion used as standard OTW is black.

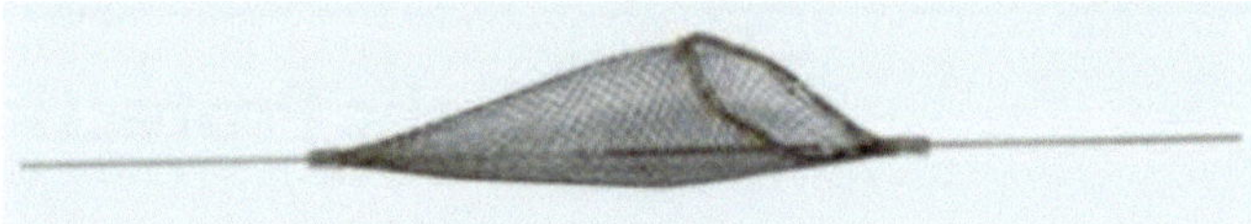

Fig. 4.3 SpiderFX embolic protection device (Medtronic)

4.4.2 Features and Models

SpiderFX embolic protection device is used first by accessing the vascular lesions through superselection via a 0.36 mm (0.014 in) wire and then delivered to distal end of the vascular lesions along the wire. After the wire is withdrawn, push the mesh filter of the protective umbrella to the preset position and release it. This device is suitable for capturing and removing the debris dislodged inside the distal artery during interventional procedures, especially suitable for such superselectively difficult lesions as seriously tortuous and severe stenosis. The mesh filter has a diameter of 3–7 mm, suitable for placement in the arteries with a diameter of 2–7 mm. The capture wire diameter is 0.014in, available with a length of 190–320 cm, compatible with 8F guide catheter and 6F long vascular sheath.

4.5 Emboshield NAV6 Embolic Protection Device

4.5.1 Product Structure

The US Abbott-produced Emboshield NAV6 embolic protection device consists of a mesh filter (Fig. 4.4), BareWire Filter Delivery Wire, an RX delivery catheter, and an RX retrieval catheter. The mesh filter consists of a nylon membrane wrapped on a nickel skeleton with two proximal ports and several distal perfusion ports. In order to improve the visibility, the proximal and distal ends of the filter are all equipped with marker bands, and the filter skeleton is radiopaque. BareWire Filter Delivery Wire is a 0.36 mm (0.014in) PTFE-coated stainless steel wire with a 3 cm radiopaque platinum-nickel alloy at its distal end, available with a length of 190–315 cm and hardness of different degrees.

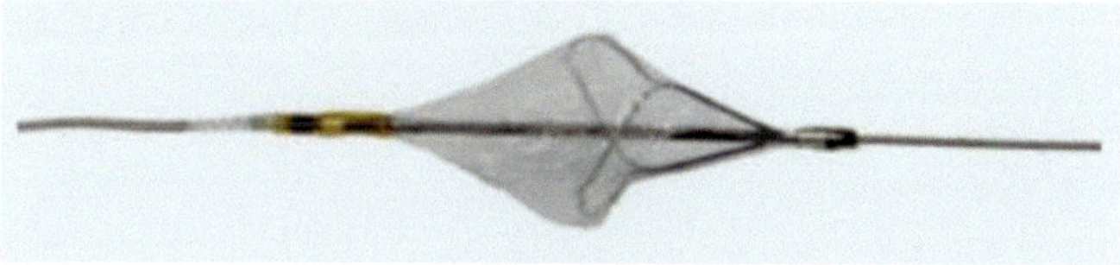

Fig. 4.4 Emboshield NAV6 embolic protection device (Abbott)

4.5.2 Features and Models

Embossed NAV6 embolic protection device has separated wire and umbrella, allowing relative mobility of the wire with the umbrella filter. During operation, certain degree of the wire mobility can assure that the protective umbrella filter remains steady and immobilized, suitable for containing and removing embolic materials during carotid angioplasty and stent implantation process. The protection device has two specifications for option: 5–7.2 mm, 5 mm protection device suitable for 2.5–4.8 mm diameter of distal blood vessels and 7.2 mm for 4.0–7.0 mm. The diameter of BareWire Filter Delivery Wire is 0.36 mm (0.014in), and the length is 190–315 cm. The device is compatible with 8F guide catheter and 6F long vascular sheath.

4.6 Mo.Ma Embolic Protection Device

4.6.1 Product Structure

The US Medtronic-produced Mo.Ma embolic protection device consists of a triple-lumen tube (including a work channel and two expansion or shortening lumens), two compliant balloons, and a handle at the end (Fig. 4.5). The two compliant balloons can be expanded separately: the proximal balloon (maximally expandable to 13 mm) is located in the common carotid artery and the distal balloon (maximally expandable to 6 mm) is located in the external carotid artery. The balloon is located at the distal portion of the triple lumen, where the distal balloon is near its tip, and the proximal balloon is located just behind the exit of the work channel, approximately 6 cm from the distal balloon (relative distance between the balloon markers). There is also a hollow shaft in the package, accessible through 0.89 mm (0.035in) wire to increase the thrust of the device when it is inserted.

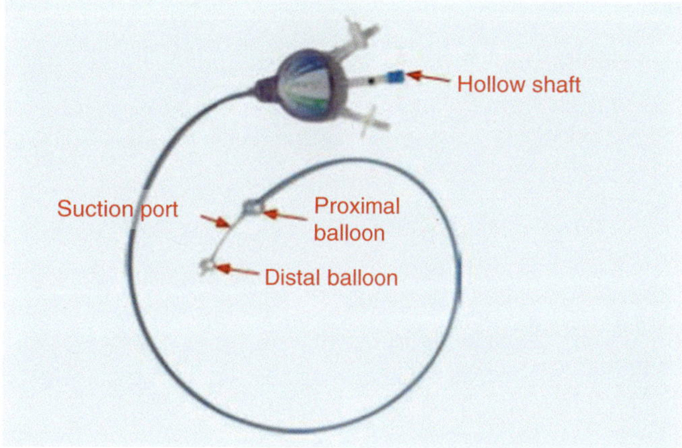

Fig. 4.5 Mo.Ma embolic protection device (Medtronic)

4.6.2 Features and Models

Mo.Ma embolic protection device is a proximal occlusive embolic protection device, which does not need to pass through the diseased blood vessels and can prevent plaque defluvium while the device navigates through the vascular lesions, suitable for protection therapies of blood vessels where stenosis involves the internal carotid artery and/or carotid bifurcation, but carotid artery angioplasty and/or stent implantation procedure can be performed, especially for nearly occlusive. However, because of the need to block the cranial blood flow, it may be intolerable for the patients with poor contralateral blood flow compensation. The thrombus protection device is used for the external carotid arteries with a diameter of 3–6 mm and the common carotid arteries with a diameter of 5–13 mm; the total length from the hemostatic valve to the catheter tip is 111 cm, and the device adapts to 0.89 mm (0.035in) wire and 8F and 9F vascular sheath.

5 Peripheral Stent

Huajuan Mao, Junmin Bao, and Guangqin Liu

Abstract

Peripheral stents are main devices used in endovascular treatment for peripheral vascular diseases. Based on their release modes, they can be classified into self-expanding peripheral stents and balloon-expanding peripheral stents. This chapter mainly provides a tabular conclusion and summary about the names, brands, materials, structures, manufacturing processes, diameters, lengths, adapter wires, adapter sheaths, delivery system lengths, and other details of peripheral stents and elaborates on their structures, features, and model types based on peripheral stents of different brands.

Keywords

Peripheral stent · Structure and features · Model types

5.1 Introduction

Stent is mainly used to solve such problems as elastic vascular retraction following endovascular balloon dilatation, residual stenosis, and dissection. The performance of the stent is mainly related to the material, structure, expansion mode, production process, etc. Due to the diversity of peripheral blood vessels, the stent should be selected on the basis of the anatomical location, stent material, function, and the experience of surgeons.

H. Mao (✉) · J. Bao · G. Liu
Department of Vascular Surgery, Changhai Hospital, Second Military Medical University, Shanghai, China
e-mail: czymm8@163.com

5.1.1 Classifications of Stents

5.1.1.1 By Stent's Release Mode

Self-Expanding Stent

Stent expansion and support are achieved through self-expansion of the stent. The advantages of this type of stent are to strike a balance between the self-expanding tension and the elastic constraint of the vascular wall so as to attach itself to the vascular wall, featuring excellent flexibility, resistance to deformation under compression, and lasting expansion force, mostly used for the carotid artery, iliac artery, femoral artery, and other blood vessels.

Balloon-Expandable Stent

Stent expansion and support are achieved through balloon dilatation. This kind of stent is characterized by accurate positioning in release, no obvious shortening after release, and strong radial support. The disadvantages are that the stent itself lacks elasticity and is liable of collapse after compression, unsuitable for carotid, femoral, and popliteal arteries and other sites vulnerable to compression or movement. Balloon-expandable stent is often used for subclavian arteries, coronary arteries, renal arteries, iliac arteries, and other blood vessels.

5.1.1.2 By Availability of Stent Graft

Stent Graft

This kind of stent is covered with PTFE or PET and other materials, mainly used for aneurysm repair, aortic dissection, arteriovenous fistula, AVF, post-traumatic arteriorrhexis, and some occlusive peripheral artery diseases. Most stents of this kind are self-expanding, and balloon-expandable ones are available in foreign countries.

Bare Stent

This kind of stent can be both self-expanding and balloon-expandable. Related to the stent graft, bare stent is advantaged

Z. Jing et al. (eds.), *Endovascular Surgery and Devices*, https://doi.org/10.1007/978-981-10-8270-2_5

in thinner delivery system, impossibility to cover the branch vessels where the branch vessels are much developed, and is mostly used in clinical context for treatment of vascular stenosis and occlusion.

5.1.1.3 By Production Process of the Stent

Braided Stent

At present, the typical braided stents in clinical practice include Wallstent stent (Boston Scientific), and Supera stent (Abbott). The initial materials used for the stents are stainless steel wire. At present, the stents are braided from cobalt-chrome wire, advantaged in good development effect and availability for retraction even when the stent is 50% released during operation, but disadvantaged in poor wall adhesion and more than 30% stent shortening that leads to poor stent release accuracy and affects the therapeutic effect.

Laser-Engraved Stent

Currently most common in clinical practice, this kind of stent is laser-engraved from cobalt-chromium or nickel-titanium alloy tubes, advantaged in low shortening rate, accurate release positioning, excellent support strength, and sound wall adhesion.

5.1.1.4 By the Structure of the Engraved Cells

Closed-Cell Stent

This kind of stent has small mesh size and low degree of freedom, providing better support and plaque coverage, but with relatively low flexibility.

Open-Cell Stent

This kind of stent has large mesh size and big degree of freedom, with better flexibility than the closed one and not liable of straightening the blood vessels, but poorer plaque coverage than the closed one.

Open- and Closed-Cell Hybrid Stent

This kind of stent combines the characteristics of the above-mentioned two stents, with better flexibility and accurate positioning and preventing stent shortening and forward jump.

5.1.1.5 By Availability with Drugs on the Stent

Non-drug-Eluting Stent

At present, the peripheral bare stents in clinical practice are basically non-drug-eluting ones.

Drug-Eluting Stent

This kind of stent is mainly used for coronary arteries, usually balloon-expandable stents. In clinical practice, this stent is also used for blood vessels below the popliteal artery. Internationally used self-expanding drug-eluting stents exclusively for lower extremity (femoral and popliteal arteries) include Zilver PTX (Cook) and Eluvia (Boston Scientific). The drugs are loaded mainly through the polymer carrier or microporous design. The polymer carrier functions as the target release and controlled release of the drugs. The stent can prevent the proliferation of vascular endothelial cells, thus ensuring unobstructed blood vessels under the action of the drugs. The drugs used with this kind of stent are mostly paclitaxel, rapamycin, and in their derivatives at present.

5.1.2 Stent Materials

5.1.2.1 316L Stainless Steel

The stent made of this material features strong radial support, sound biocompatibility, and excellent development effect, but with the presence of nickel ions. Therefore, care shall be taken in use with those allergic to nickel. This kind of stent is often used as the balloon-expandable stent.

5.1.2.2 Cobalt-Chromium Alloy

The stent made of this material features strong radial support, sound biocompatibility, excellent development effect, and lower content of nickel than 316L stainless steel. It is also thinner than the stainless steel under the same mechanical properties and commonly used as balloon-expandable stent and braided self-expanding stent.

5.1.2.3 Nickel-Titanium Alloy

The stent made of this material is marked by shape memory and sound flexibility, but ordinary development effect and radial support. Therefore, other metal markers should be added in general. The stent is surfaced with titanium oxide layer, preventing the release of nickel ions, with superior fatigue resistance to 316L stainless steel and cobalt-chromium alloy and usually used as self-expanding stent.

5.1.2.4 Degradable Polymer Materials

Materials, mainly poly-L-lactic acid (PLLA), are featured by inferior mechanical properties and development effect to metal materials but are degradable in human bodies, resulting in zero remnants of foreign articles in human bodies and mainly used as the balloon-expandable stent.

5.1.2.5 Absorbable Metal Materials

Materials, mainly iron and magnesium, have better mechanical properties but ordinary development effect and are also absorbable, resulting in zero remnants in human bodies. This kind of stent is currently under development.

5.2 Self-Expanding Peripheral Stent

5.2.1 Product Structure

Self-expanding peripheral stent is mainly made of nitinol, and its stent delivery system is OTW. The lesion sites of peripheral vessels are very complicated, and the stent should be chosen according to actual requirements.

5.2.2 Features and Models

Self-expanding peripheral stent is multifarious, mainly indicated for endovascular treatment of peripheral vascular diseases. This kind of stent is advantageous of long stent, excellent flexibility, and accurate positioning. Currently, the brands of the self-expanding peripheral stent system include Medtronic, Bard, Optimed, Cordis, Biotronik, Boston Scientific, Abbott, etc., the features and models of which are shown in Table 5.1. This section mainly introduces Complete SE (Medtronic), E-Luminexx (Bard), Lifestent (Bard), Smart Control (Cordis), Smart Flex (Cordis), Pulsar-18 (Biotronik), Everflex (Medtronic), Innova (Boston Scientific), Wallstent (Boston Scientific), Absolute Pro (Abbott), and Supera Peripheral Stent Systems (Abbott).

5.2.3 Brand Information

5.2.3.1 Complete SE Peripheral Stent

Product Structure

Complete SE peripheral stent (Fig. 5.1) is the US Medtronic-produced laser-engraved open-cell self-expanding nitinol stent, cutting off from a non-welded nitinol memory tube by laser-engraving technique, expanding the stent to its maximum diameter under heating and then performing electropolishing to the stent so as to provide smooth surface

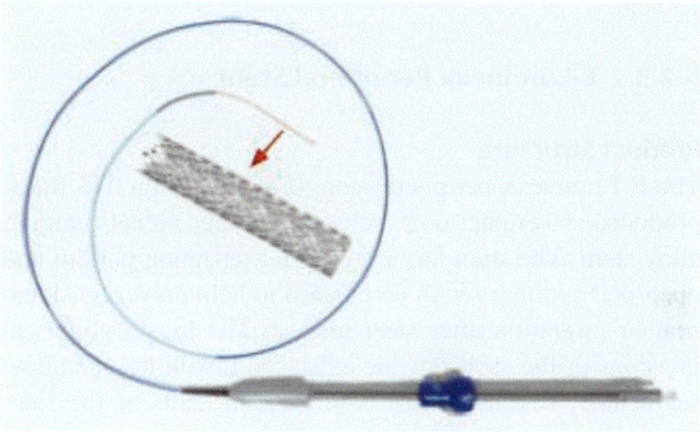

Fig. 5.1 Complete SE peripheral stent (Medtronic)

Table 5.1 Brand-specific self-expanding peripheral stent specifications (for reference only)

Name	Brand	Material	Structure	Production process	Diameter (mm)	Length (mm)	Matching wire (in)	Matching sheath(F)	Shaft (cm)
Complete SE	Medtronic	Nitinol	Open cell	Laser engraved	4–10	20–150	0.035	6	80, 130
Lifestent	Bard	Nitinol	Open cell	Laser engraved	5–8	20–170	0.035	6	80, 130
E-Luminexx	Bard	Nitinol	Open cell	Laser engraved	4–14	20–120	0.035	6	135
Superflex-635	Optimed	Nitinol	Open cell in the middle and closed cell on both ends	Laser engraved	6–12	40–200	0.035	6	75, 120
Visual-XL	Optimed	Nitinol	Closed cell	Laser engraved	12–34	30–100	0.035	10	75, 100
Smart flex	Cordis	Nitinol	Closed cell	Laser engraved	5–8	30–200	0.035	6	80, 120
Smart control	Cordis	Nitinol	Open cell	Laser engraved	6–14	20–100	0.035	6–7	80, 120
Smart long	Cordis	Nitinol	Open cell	Laser engraved	6–8	120–150	0.035	6–7	80, 120
Pulsar-18	Biotronik	Nitinol	Open cell	Laser engraved	4–7	20–200	0.018	4	90, 135
Astron	Biotronik	Nitinol	Open cell	Laser engraved	7–10	30–80	0.035	6	70, 120
Everflex	Medtronic	Nitinol	Open cell	Laser engraved	4–10	20–200	0.035	6	80, 120
Innova	Boston Scientific	Nitinol	Open cell in the middle and closed cell on both ends	Laser engraved	5–8	20–200	0.035	6	75, 130
Wallstent	Boston Scientific	Nitinol	Closed cell	Braided	10–24	20–94	0.035	9–11	75, 100
Absolute pro	Abbott	Nitinol	Open cell	Laser engraved	5–10	20–100	0.035	6	80, 135
Absolute pro LL	Abbott	Nitinol	Open cell	Laser engraved	5–8	120–150	0.035	6	80, 135
Supera	Abbott	Nitinol	Closed cell	Braided	4.5–6.5	20–150	0.018	6	80, 120

with no overlapping fulcrums. On both ends of the stent are four X-ray-resistant tantalum markers, facilitating accurate stent positioning.

Features and Models

The stent is indicated for the endovascular treatment of peripheral atherosclerotic vascular disease. The delivery system of the stent has a dual release mechanism for the purpose of simple and precise release. The stent is compatible with 0.89 mm (0.035 in) wire, 6F vascular sheath, available with diameter ranging from 4 to 10 mm, length from 20 to 150 mm, and the stent's delivery system length of 80 cm and 130 cm.

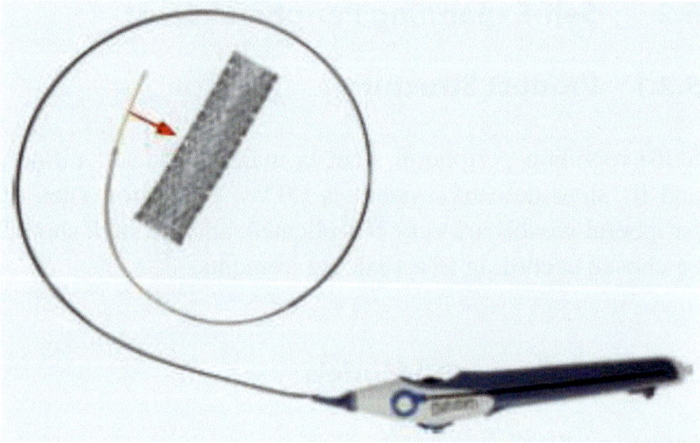

Fig. 5.3 Lifestent peripheral stent (Bard)

5.2.3.2 E-Luminexx Peripheral Stent

Product Structure

The E-Luminexx peripheral stent (Fig. 5.2) is the US Bard-produced laser-engraved self-expandable nickel-titanium alloy stent. The stent has a segmental repeating pattern and open-cell geometry with flared ends to help prevent dislocation or migration after stent release. The local cylindrical incisions of the stent provide enhanced flexibility and allow segment-by-segment expansion. On both ends of the stent are four radiopaque tantalum markers, facilitating accurate stent placement.

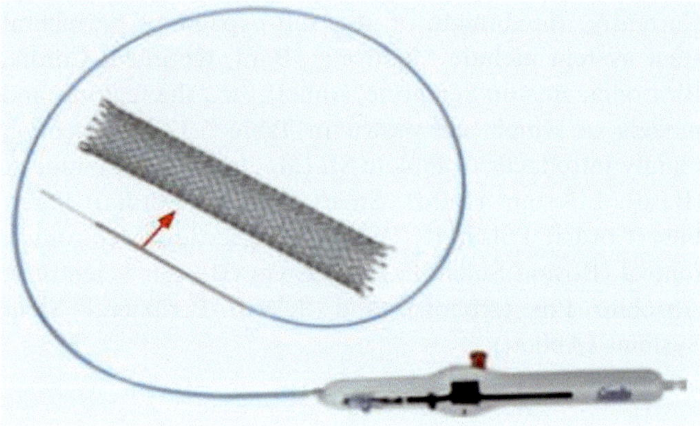

Fig. 5.4 Smart Control peripheral stent (Cordis)

Features and Models

This stent is indicated for endovascular treatment for revascularization of peripheral vascular stenosis and occlusion. The stent system is compatible with 0.89 mm (0.035in) wire and 6F vascular sheath, available with diameter ranging 4–14 mm, length from 20 cm to 120 cm, and the delivery system length of 135 cm.

5.2.3.3 Lifestent Peripheral Stent

Product Structure

The Lifestent peripheral stent (Fig. 5.3) is the US Bard-produced laser-engraved self-expandable nickel-titanium alloy stent, as an upgrade for the E-Luminexx stent. The stent with a helical structure design features excellent flexibility. Upon deployment, the stent imparts an outward radial force on the luminal surface of the vessel to achieve the preset diameter. On both ends of the stent are six radiopaque tantalum markers, facilitating accurate stent placement.

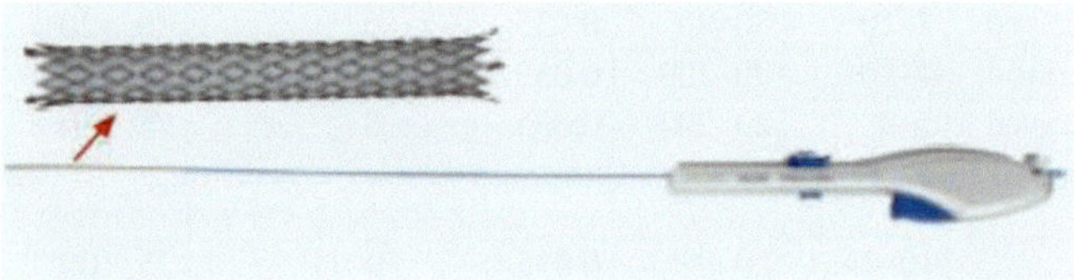

Fig. 5.2 E-Luminexx peripheral stent (Bard)

Features and Models

The stent is indicated for endovascular treatment of new peripheral artery diseases or restenosis and other vascular lesions. The stent is compatible with 0.89 mm (0.035in) wire and 6F vascular sheath, available with diameter ranging from 5 mm to 8 mm, length from 20 cm to 170 cm, and the delivery system length of 80 cm and 130 cm.

5.2.3.4 Smart Control Peripheral Stent

Product Structure

The Smart Control peripheral stent (Fig. 5.4) is the US Cordis-produced laser-engraved open-cell self-expanding nickel-titanium alloy stent. The stent is a flexible fine-mesh tubular prosthesis. Upon its deployment, the stent will form a supportive force on the luminal surface of the blood vessels to achieve vascular patency. On both ends of the stent are six radiopaque tantalum markers, facilitating stent placement.

Features and Models

The stent is indicated for endovascular treatment of peripheral atherosclerosis. The stent is compatible with 0.89 mm (0.035in) wire and 6–7F vascular sheath, available with diameters ranging from 6 mm to 14 mm, length from 20 cm to 100 cm, and the delivery system length of 80 cm and 120 cm.

5.2.3.5 Smart Flex Peripheral Stent

Product Structure

The Smart Flex peripheral stent (Fig. 5.5) is the US Cordis-produced laser-engraved self-expanding nitinol stent, which is an upgrade for the Smart Control stent. The stent is an almost fully connected stent made from super elastic nitinol tubing and is constructed through the integration of helically wound struts with helical flexible coils. Both the strut elements and the helical coils provide radial stiffness and an expansion-oriented mechanism. The stent is very bendable and almost has no fish scaling. Upon deployment, the stent achieves its predetermined diameter and exerts a constant, gentle outward force to achieve endovascular patency. On both ends of the stent is a radiopaque marker for easy stent placement.

Features and Models

The stent is indicated for endovascular treatment of atherosclerotic lesions of the superficial femoral arteries and proximal popliteal arteries. The stent is compatible with 0.89 mm (0.035in) wire and 6F vascular sheath, available with diameters ranging from 5 mm to 8 mm, lengths from 30 m to 200 m, and the delivery system length of 80 cm and 120 cm.

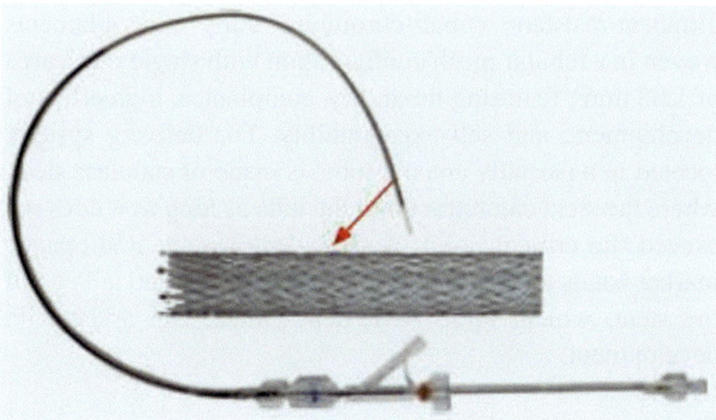

Fig. 5.5 Smart Flex peripheral stent (Cordis)

5.2.3.6 Pulsar-18 Peripheral Stent System

Product Structure

Pulsar-18 peripheral stent (Fig. 5.6) is the German Biotronik-produced laser-engraved open-cell self-expanding nitinol stent. The stent is made of nitinol tubing through laser cutting and on both ends of the stent are six radiopaque extenders covered with amorphous silicon carbide, facilitating accurate stent placement.

Features and Models

The stent is indicated for endovascular treatment of atherosclerotic stenosis or occlusion of lower extremities and other vascular diseases, especially for the patients suffering from lower extremity diseases treated with retrograde popliteal puncture. The stent is compatible with 0.46 mm (0.018in) wire and 4F vascular sheath, available with diameter ranging from 4 mm to 7 mm, length from 20 mm to 200 mm, and the delivery system length of 90 cm and 135 cm.

5.2.3.7 Everflex Peripheral Stent

Product Structure

The Everflex peripheral stent (Fig. 5.7) is the US Medtronic-produced laser-engraved self-expandable nitinol stent. The stent is made of a nickel-titanium tube cut into an open grid structure via laser, with radiopaque tantalum markers at both ends of the stent to achieve accurate stent placement.

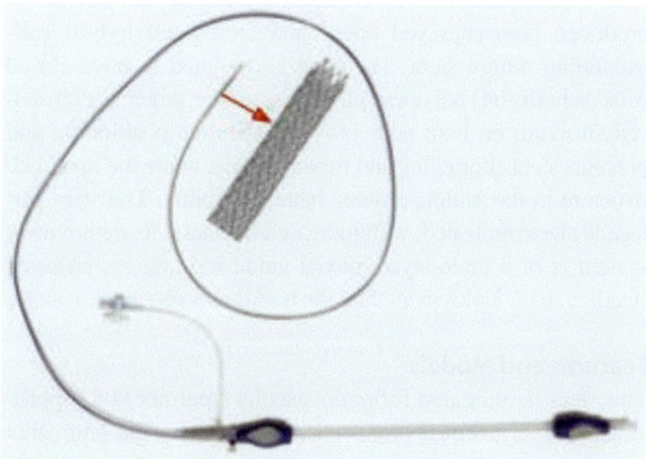

Fig. 5.6 Pulsar-18 peripheral stent (Biotronik)

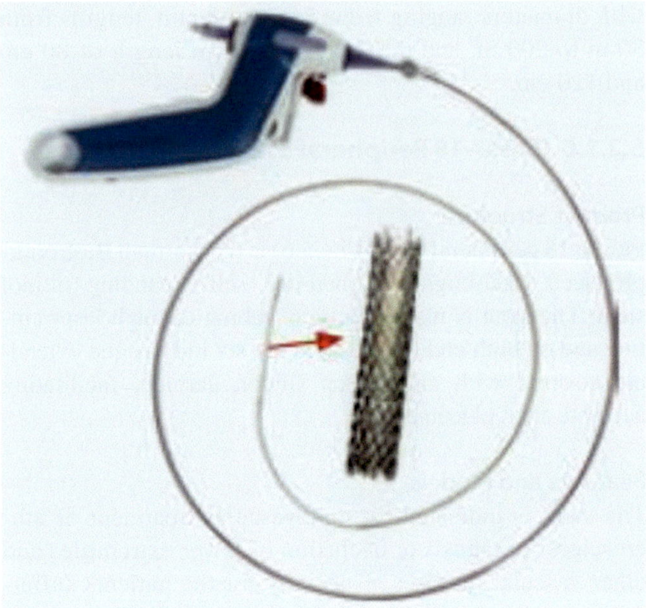

Fig. 5.7 Everflex peripheral stent (Medtronic)

Features and Models

The stent is indicated for endovascular treatment of peripheral vascular stenosis, occlusion, and other lesions, featuring excellent flexibility and accessibility to tortuous vessels. The stent is compatible with 0.89 mm (0.035in) wires and 6F vascular sheath, available with diameters ranging from 4 mm to 10 mm, length from 20 mm to 200 mm, and the delivery system of 80 cm and 120 cm.

5.2.3.8 Innova Peripheral Stent

Product Structure

Innova peripheral stent (Fig. 5.8) is the US Boston Scientific-produced laser-engraved open- and closed-cell hybrid self-expanding nitinol stent. The stent is designed to have closed cells on both ends but open cells in the middle, where the closed-cell structure on both ends provides accurate positioning and prevents stent shortening and forward jump, while the open-cell structure in the middle ensures better flexibility. The stent surface is electropolished, with increased firmness. Its deployment system is of a three-layer coaxial guide rod system, ensuring steadier stent deployment than the traditional version.

Features and Models

The stent is indicated for endovascular treatment of superficial femoral arteries, proximal popliteal arteries, and other blood vessels. The stent is compatible with 0.89 mm (0.035 in) wire and 6F vascular sheath, having diameters ranging from 5 mm to 8 mm, length from 20 mm to 200 mm, and the delivery system length of 75 cm and 130 cm.

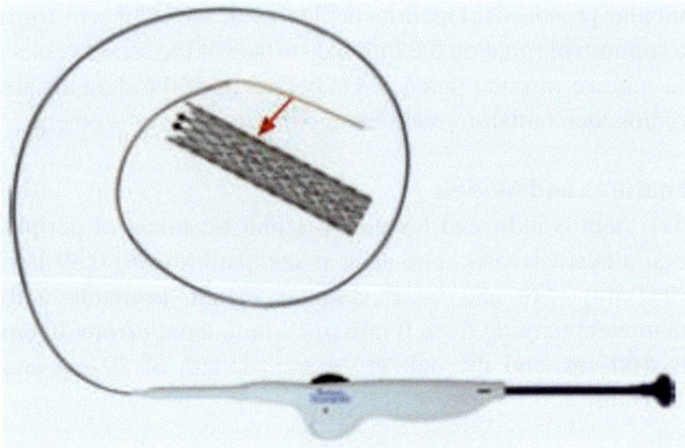

Fig. 5.8 Innova peripheral stent (Boston Scientific)

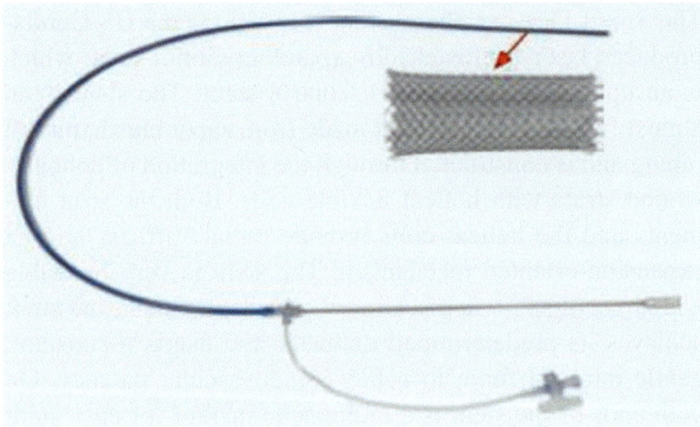

Fig. 5.9 Wallstent peripheral stent (Boston Scientific)

5.2.3.9 Wallstent Peripheral Stent

Product Structure

The Wallstent peripheral stent (Fig. 5.9) is the US Boston Scientific-produced braided closed-cell self-expanding cobalt-chromium alloy stent. The stent is made of radiopaque ultraheat-resistant cobalt-chromium alloy monofilaments woven in a tubular mesh configuration with single mesh area of 1.08 mm^2, featuring flexibility, compliance, high effect of development, and self-expandability. The delivery system, located in a partially coaxial tube, is made of stainless steel, where the stent can retract into the tube as long as it does not exceed the critical point of stent deployment. Radiopaque marker bands are equipped near the guide end and tail end of the stent, which, upon stent deployment, can assist with development.

Features and Models

This stent is indicated for endovascular treatment of peripheral venous diseases, characterized in that the stent can be retrieved at 50% deployment and can be repositioned and

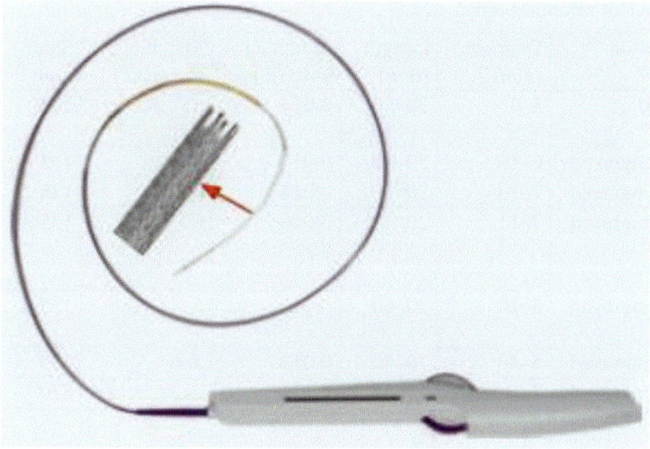

Fig. 5.10 Absolute Pro peripheral stent (Abbott)

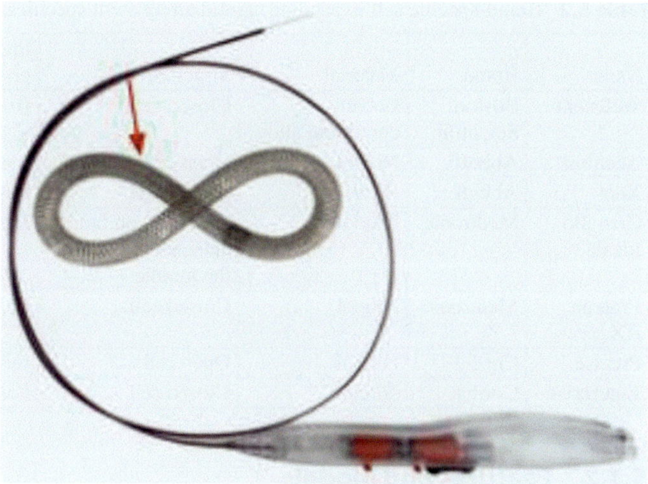

Fig. 5.11 Supera Peripheral Stent (Abbott)

redeployed to achieve accurate stent placement. The stent is compatible with 0.89 mm (0.035in) wire and 9–11F vascular sheath, available with diameter ranging from 10 mm to 24 mm, length from 20 mm to 94 mm, and the delivery system length of 75 cm and 100 cm.

5.2.3.10 Absolute Pro Peripheral Stent

Product Structure
Absolute Pro peripheral stent (Fig. 5.10) is the US Abbott-produced laser-engraved open-cell self-expanding nitinol stent. The stent is made of flexible nitinol, equipped with six nitinol markers, respectively, on both ends of the stent to achieve accurate stent positioning. The stent adopts a 3-axle delivery system, consisting of a retractable sheath, a tip, an I beam with wire lumen (for supporting the stent during stent deployment), a detachable outer jacket, and handle assembly with safety lock. Accurate stent placement is ensured by moving the thumbwheel.

Features and Models
The stent is indicated for endovascular treatment of peripheral artery diseases. The stent is compatible with 0.89 mm (0.035in) wire and 6F vascular sheath, with diameter ranging from 5 mm to 10 mm, length from 20 mm to 100 mm, and the delivery system length of 80 cm and 135 cm.

5.2.3.11 Supera Peripheral Stent

Product Structure
Supera peripheral stent (Fig. 5.11) is the US Abbott-produced braided closed-cell self-expanding nitinol stent. The stent is a braided stent interwoven with six closed nitinol wire. Because it can better adapt itself to the anatomic form and flow direction of the blood vessels, it is also called vascular mimetic implant (VMI). Compared with traditional laser-engraved nitinol stent, this stent features excellent radial support and flexibility, smaller chronic expansion force, and excellent fracture resistance. The delivery system of the stent is of coaxial monolithic exchange, and its delivery shaft has hydrophilic coating.

Features and Models
The stent is indicated for endovascular treatment of symptomatic primary or restenotic lesions or occlusions of superficial femoral arteries and/or proximal popliteal arteries with vascular diameters ranging from 4.0 mm to 6.5 mm. As revealed by clinical studies, this stent has a good therapeutic effect for occlusive femoral and popliteal lesions, especially for long-segment and severely calcified lesions. The stent is compatible with 0.014in and 0.018in wires and 6F vascular sheath, available with stent diameter ranging from 4.5 mm to 6.5 mm, length from 20 mm to 150 mm, and the delivery system length of 80 cm and 120 cm.

5.3 Self-Expanding Carotid Artery Stent

5.3.1 Product Structure

The self-expanding carotid artery stent is mostly made of nitinol and cobalt-chromium alloy, with a RX-type delivery system, and usually used in conjunction with the protective umbrella. The stent can be classified as straight type and tapered type by their forms, open-cell, closed-cell, and open-closed-cell hybrid by their structures, and laser-engraved and braided by their production process.

Table 5.2 Brand-specific self-expanding carotid artery stent specifications (for reference only)

Name	Brand	Material	Structure	Production process	Diameter (mm)	Length (mm)	Matching wire (in)	Matching sheath (F)	Shaft (cm)
Wallstent	Boston Scientific	Cobalt-chromium alloy	Closed cell	Braided	5–9	30–50	0.014	6	135
Acculink	Abbott	Nitinol	Open cell	Laser engraved	6–10	20–40	0.014	6	132
Xact	Abbott	Nitinol	Closed cell	Laser engraved	7–10	20–40	0.014	6	136
Cristallo Ideale	Medtronic	Nitinol	Open cell on both ends, closed cell in the middle	Laser engraved	7–11	20–40	0.014	6	135
Protege RX	Medtronic	Nitinol	Closed cell	Laser engraved	6–10	20–60	0.014	6	135
Precise	Cordis	Nitinol	Open cell	Laser engraved	5–10	20–40	0.014	5–6	135
Enterprise	Cordis	Nitinol	Closed cell	Laser engraved	4.5	14–37	0.021	2, 3	220

5.3.2 Features and Models

At present, the brands of the Self-expanding carotid artery stent include Boston Scientific, Abbott, Medtronic, Cordis, etc., the features and models of which are shown in Table 5.2. This section mainly introduces Wallstent (Boston Scientific), Acculink (Abbott), and Cristallo Ideale (Medtronic) carotid artery stent system and Enterprise (Cordis) revascularization device.

5.3.3 Brand Information

5.3.3.1 Wallstent Carotid Artery Stent

Product Structure

Wallstent carotid artery stent (Fig. 5.12) is the US Boston Scientific-produced braided closed-cell self-expanding stent, made of alloy monofilament wire braided in a tubular mesh configuration. The wire is manufactured from a biomedical grade cobalt-chromium-iron-nickel-molybdenum alloy containing an enhanced radiopaque tantalum core. The stent with closed-cell braided design can better cover the lesions, protect the plaques, and facilitate the retrieval of the thrombus protection device with an excellent effect of development. The stent delivery system is composed of two coaxially arranged shafts, the proximal end of the inner shaft is made of stainless steel and its distal end and the outer sheath made of thermoplast. There are two radiopaque markers on the inner shaft and one on the retractable outer sheath, which are used to assist with stent placement.

Features and Models

The stent is indicated for endovascular treatment of vascular stenosis diseases of common carotid artery, internal carotid artery, and carotid bifurcation. The stent is compatible with 0.36 mm (0.014in) wire and 6F long vascular sheath or 8F guide catheter, available with diameter ranging from 5 mm to 9 mm, length from 30 mm to 50 mm, and the delivery system length of 135 cm.

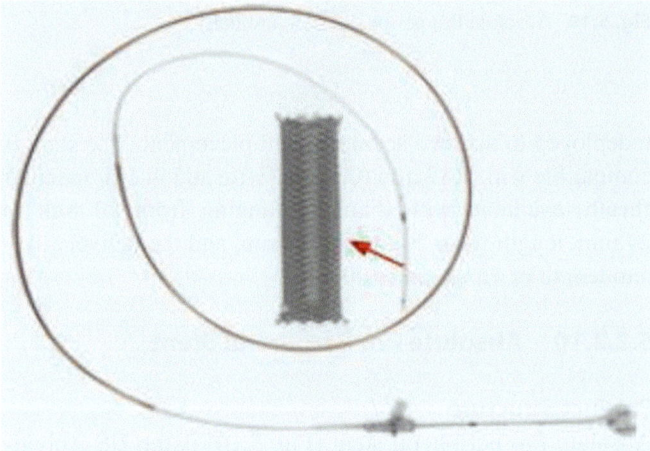

Fig. 5.12 Wallstent carotid artery stent (Boston Scientific)

5.3.3.2 Acculink Carotid Artery Stent

Product Structure

Acculink carotid artery stent (Fig. 5.13) is the US Abbott-produced laser-engraved open-cell self-expanding nitinol stent. The specially designed stent ensures high flexibility both before deployment and after vascular implantation of the stent while imparting radial support force to achieve vascular patency. The stent system consists of a delivery sheath, a stent, a radiopaque tip, an internal wire lumen, handle assembly with safety lock, and a pullback handle for stent deployment. With the handle in the unlocked position, retract the pullback handle to deploy the stent. Two radiopaque markers are mounted on the stent catheter to facilitate stent placement.

Features and Models

The stent is indicated for endovascular treatment of carotid arteries stenosis diseases, compatible with 0.36 mm (0.014in) wire and 6F long vascular sheath or 8F guide catheter. The stent is available in straight and tapered configuration: the

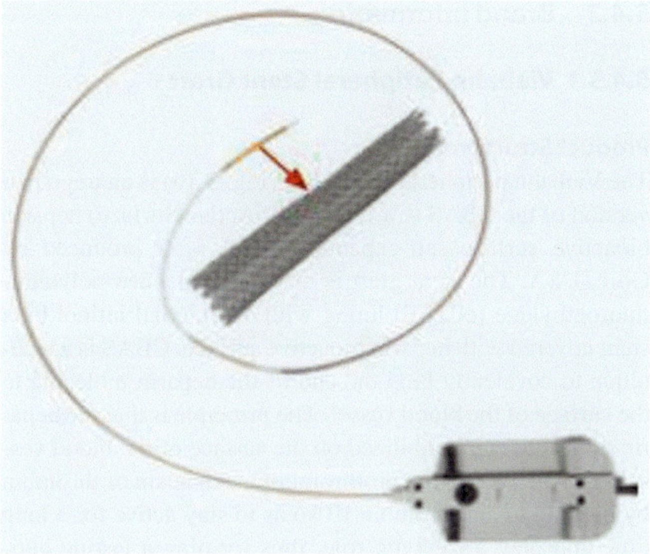

Fig. 5.13 Acculink carotid artery stent (Abbott)

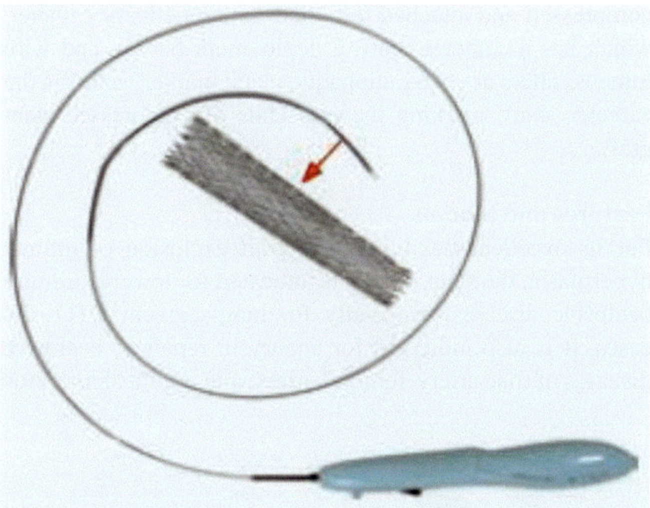

Fig. 5.14 Cristallo Ideale carotid artery stent (Medtronic)

straight stent has a diameter ranging from 6 mm to 10 mm and a length from 20 mm to 40 mm. The proximal diameter of the tapered stent ranges from 8 mm to 10 mm and distal diameter from 6 mm to 7 mm, at a length of 30–40 mm, and the delivery system length of 132 cm.

5.3.3.3 Cristallo Ideale Carotid Artery Stent

Product Structure

Cristallo Ideale carotid artery stent (Fig. 5.14) is a laser-engraved self-expanding nitinol stent combined with open-cell and closed-cell design by Medtronic, USA. The stent is designed to be a central closed cell and an open cell at the proximal and distal ends. The stent is laser cut from non-welded nitinol tubing, which is heated to dilate the stent to a larger diameter, thus determining its ultimate diameter. The end of the stent is electropolished to provide a smooth surface without obvious protrusion.

On both ends of the stent is a radiopaque tantalum marker to enhance its visibility under X-ray. The stent delivery system consists of an internal shaft and an outer jacket. The internal shaft consists of a distal coil, platiniridium markers, a lock, and proximally tapered wire. The stent can be delivered to place via retracting the outer sheath.

Features and Models

The stent is indicated for endovascular treatment of carotid atherosclerosis and other vascular diseases. The stent is compatible with a 0.36 mm (0.014in) wire and 6F long vascular sheath or 8F guide catheter. The stent is available in straight and tapered configuration: the straight stent has a diameter ranging from 7 mm to 11 mm and a length from 20 mm to 40 mm. The distal and proximal diameters of the tapered stent range from 6 mm to 7 mm and 9 mm to 10 mm, respectively, and length from 30 mm to 40 mm. The delivery system length is of 135 cm.

5.3.3.4 Enterprise Revascularization Device

Product Structure

Enterprise revascularization device (Fig. 5.15) is the US Cordis-produced laser-engraved closed-cell self-expanding nickel-titanium alloy stent. The stent is preloaded on a delivery system consisting of an introducer and a delivery wire for

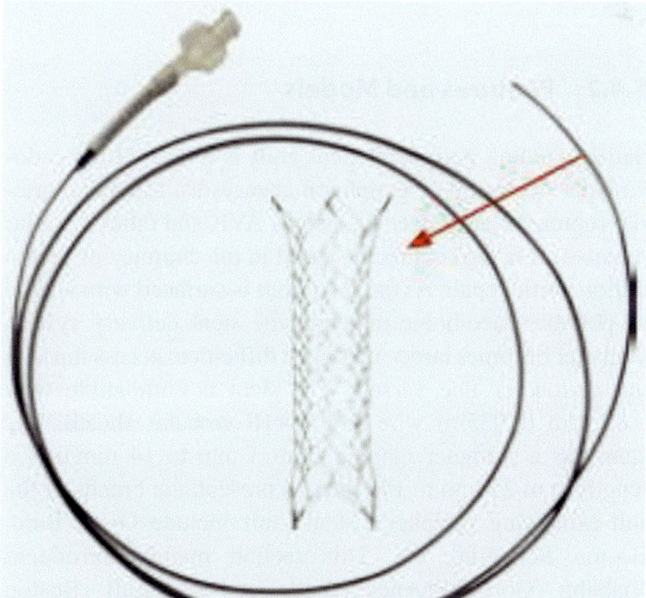

Fig. 5.15 Enterprise revascularization and delivery system (Cordis)

use with PROWLER® SELECT® Plus microcatheter. The inner circle diameter of the mesh of the stent in 2.5 mm blood vessels averages 3.2F, minimally 2.6F. Four radiopaque markers are mounted on each of the stent end, respectively, covered with a polymer layer. The introducer is made of distally tapered polymer.

Features and Models

The stent is indicated for the treatment of diseases such as wide-necked intracranial saccular or fusiform aneurysms with parent artery diameter ≥ 2.5 mm and ≤ 4 mm, often used in conjunction with aneurysm embolization devices (e.g., embolization, Onyx, etc.). The stent can be retracted once during its deployment. The stent is compatible with 0.53 mm (0.021in) wire and its adapted PROWLER® SELECT® Plus microcatheter with proximal diameter of 2.8F and the distal diameter of 2.3F; the stent has a diameter of 4.5 mm and a length of 14–37 mm, with the delivery system length of 220 cm.

5.4 Self-Expanding Peripheral Stent Graft

5.4.1 Product Structure

Self-expanding peripheral stent graft means to cover special polymeric membrane materials on the self-expanding bare metal stents. The bare metal stents are mostly made of nitinol or cobalt-chromium alloy surfaced with mostly expanded polytetrafluoroethylene (ePTFE) or polyethylene terephthalate (PET). The stent delivery system is of OTW type.

5.4.2 Features and Models

Self-expanding peripheral stent graft is indicated for endovascular exclusion of peripheral aneurysms, traumatic arterial rupture or arteriovenous fistula, AVF, and other vascular diseases. It is also commonly used in the chimney or fenestration aortic repair. As the stent graft is surfaced with a layer of polymer membrane material, the stent delivery system diameter becomes larger, making it difficult to access through the narrow or fine vessels. The stent is compatible with 0.89 mm (0.035in) wire and 7–11F vascular sheath. The stent has a diameter ranging from 5 mm to 14 mm and a length from 25 mm to 150 mm. At present, the brands of the self-expanding peripheral stent graft include Gore, Bard, Boston Scientific, etc. This section mainly introduces Viabahn (Gore), Fluency (Bard), and Wallgraft (Boston Scientific) peripheral stent grafts.

5.4.3 Brand Information

5.4.3.1 Viabahn Peripheral Stent Graft

Product Structure

The Viabahn peripheral stent graft (Fig. 5.16) is an upgraded version of the CBAS (Carmeda® BioActive Surface) heparin bioactive surface self-expanding stent graft produced by Gore, USA. The stent graft is made of expanded polytetrafluoroethylene (ePTFE) lining with an external nitinol bare stent covered with heparin bioactive surface. CBAS is a technique to covalently bind the end of the heparin molecule to the surface of the blood vessel. The principle is that the heparin molecule is immobilized on the surface of the blood vessels by inactivating the prothrombin mechanism of thrombin by binding to antithrombin III so as to stay active for a long time and play a catalytic role, thus forming a lasting antithrombotic ability. The stent surface provides sustained bioactivity of at least 12 weeks to the blood vessel through the heparin molecular terminal covalent bond; the stent graft is compressed and attached to a dual-lumen delivery catheter, which has a catheter shaft, a deployment button, and wire lumens. There are two radiopaque metal marker bands on the catheter shaft, marking the two ends of compressed stent graft.

Features and Models

For its excellent flexibility and graft exclusion of intimal hyperplasia, the stent system is indicated for lower extremity occlusive diseases, especially for long-segment CTO diseases. It is also indicated for aneurysm repair of occlusive diseases of iliac artery, femoral artery, and popliteal artery, as

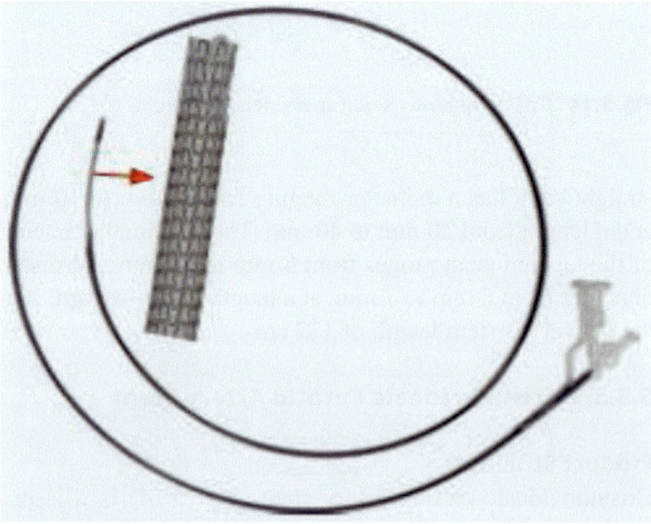

Fig. 5.16 Viabahn peripheral stent graft (Gore)

well as peripheral artery aneurysms, arteriovenous fistula, AVF, arteriorrhexis, and other peripheral artery diseases. The stent is compatible with 0.89 mm (0.035in) wire and 7–12F vascular sheath. The stent has a diameter ranging from 5 mm to 13 mm, length from 25 mm to 150 mm, and the delivery system length of 75 cm and 120 cm.

5.4.3.2 Fluency Peripheral Stent Graft

Product Structure

Fluency peripheral stent graft (Fig. 5.17) is the US Bard-produced self-expanding nitinol stent graft. The inner and outer layers of the stent are covered with a film of expanded polytetrafluoroethylene (ePTFE) with 2 mm metal bare stent area (excluding the length of tantalum mark) and four radiopaque tantalum markers to assist with the placement of the stent graft.

Features and Models

The stent is indicated for aneurysm repair of subclavian, iliac, and femoral arteries and restenotic or reocclusive vascular lesions. The stent is compatible with 0.89 mm (0.035in) wire and 8–10F vascular sheath, at a diameter ranging from 5 mm to 13.5 mm, a length from 20 mm to 120 mm, and the delivery system length of 80 cm and 117 cm.

5.4.3.3 Wallgraft Peripheral Stent Graft

Product Structure

Wallgraft peripheral stent graft (Fig. 5.18) is the US Boston Scientific-produced braided self-expanding stent graft made of cobalt-chromium alloy. The stent is made of radiopaque ultraheat-resistant alloy monofilaments woven in a tubular mesh configuration, with its outer layer being covered with polyethylene terephthalate (PET) film. On both ends of the stent is a radiopaque marker band, facilitating accurate placement during delivery.

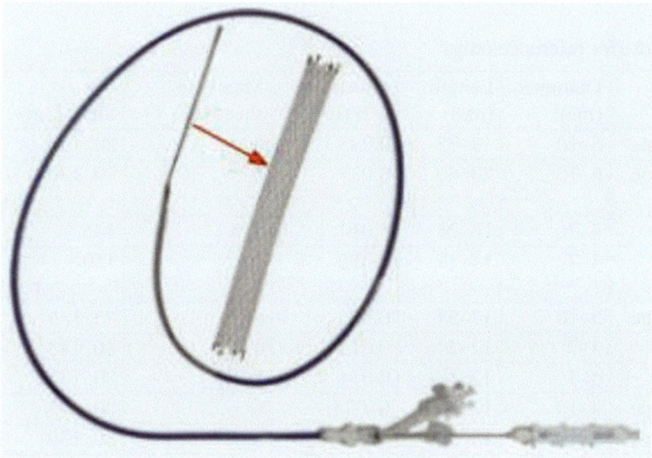

Fig. 5.17 Fluency peripheral stent graft (Bard)

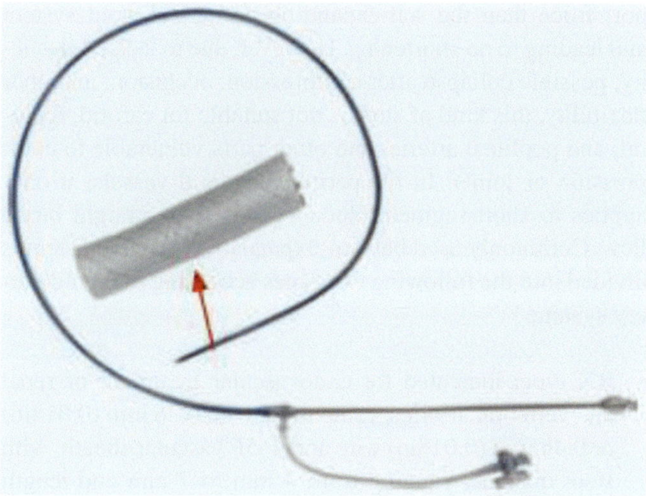

Fig. 5.18 Wallgraft peripheral stent graft (Boston Scientific)

Features and Models

The stent is indicated for the aneurysm repair of atberosclerotic aneurysm and traumatic vascular rupture of peripheral blood vessels. The stent is indicated for 0.89 mm (0.035in) wire and 9–12F vascular sheath, with a diameter ranging from 6 mm to 14 mm, a length from 20 mm to 70 mm, and the delivery system length of 75 cm.

5.5 Balloon-Expandable Peripheral Stent

5.5.1 Product Structure

Balloon-expandable peripheral stent is to preload the bare metal stent on matching balloon and deliver the balloon and the stent to the vascular lesions along the blood vessels till the balloon dilates to the preset diameter, and the stent is attached to the vascular wall without producing sustained expansion tension to the vascular wall. The stent is mainly made of cobalt-chromium alloy or stainless steel.

5.5.2 Features and Models

Balloon-expandable peripheral stent is accurate in positioning when deployed and is indicated for vascular ostial lesions of vertebral artery and renal artery, with stronger radial support force than the self-expanding peripheral stent system and leading to no shortening. However, due to lack of elasticity, possible collapse after compression, occlusion, and poor flexibility, this kind of stent is not suitable for carotid, femoral, and popliteal arteries and other parts vulnerable to compression or joints. In the peripheral blood vessels, it only applies to short-segment blood vessels with straight blood flow. Commonly used balloon-expandable peripheral stent is divided into the following two types according to their delivery system.

- RX type: indicated for endovascular treatment of renal and vertebral arteries, compatible with 0.36 mm (0.014in) or 0.46 mm (0.018in) wire and 4–5F vascular sheath, with stent diameter ranging from 4 mm to 7 mm and length from 10 mm to 24 mm. At present, the brands of RX-type balloon-expandable peripheral stent system in clinical practice include Medtronic, Boston Scientific, Cordis, Abbott, Biotronik, etc., whose features and models are shown in Table 5.3. This section mainly introduces Hippocampus (Medtronic), Express SD (Boston Scientific), and Palmaz Blue (Cordis) balloon-expandable peripheral stents.
- OTW type: Indicated for endovascular treatment of subclavian and iliac arteries, compatible with 0.89 mm (0.035in) wire and 6–7F vascular sheath, with stent diameter ranging from 4 mm to 10 mm and length from 12 mm to 60 mm. Currently, the brands of OTW balloon-expandable peripheral stent system in clinical use include Medtronic, Boston Scientific, Abbott, etc., whose features and models are shown in Table 5.3. This section mainly introduces Express LD (Boston Scientific) and Omnilink Elite (Abbott) balloon-expandable peripheral stents.

5.5.3 Brand Information

5.5.3.1 Hippocampus Balloon-Expandable Stent

Product Structure

Hippocampus balloon-expandable stent (Fig. 5.19) is the US Medtronic-produced stainless steel RX-type stent, consisting of a tail end, a shaft, a RX segment, and a balloon strut segment. The stent is preloaded onto the RX delivery system along with the matching balloon. Two radiopaque marker bands are mounted on the shaft levers on both ends of balloon, facilitating stent placement under X-ray.

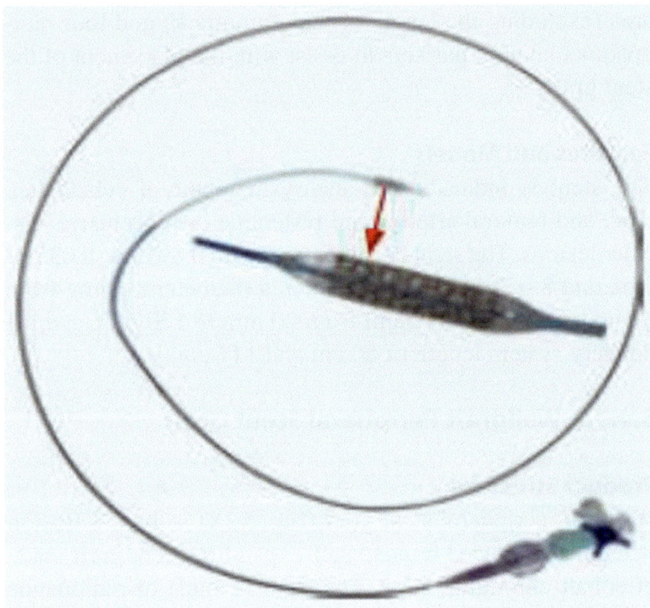

Fig. 5.19 Hippocampus balloon-expandable stent (Medtronic)

Table 5.3 Brand-specific balloon-expandable peripheral stent specifications (for reference only)

Name	Brand	Material	Delivery system	Diameter (mm)	Length (mm)	Matching wire(in)	Matching sheath (F)	Shaft (cm)
Scuba	Medtronic	Nickel-chromium alloy	OTW type	5–10	18–75	0.035	6	80, 130
Assurant	Medtronic	Nickel-chromium-molybdenum alloy	OTW type	6–10	20–60	0.035	6	80, 130
Hippocampus	Medtronic	Stainless steel	RX type	4–7	10–24	0.014	4–5	145
Express SD	Boston Scientific	Nickel-chromium-molybdenum alloy	RX type	4–7	14–19	0.018	5	150
Express LD	Boston Scientific	Stainless steel	OTW type	5–10	17–57	0.035	6–7	75, 135
Palmaz Blue	Cordis	Nickel-chromium alloy	RX type	4–7	12–24	0.014	4–5	80, 142
Herculink	Abbott	Nickel-chromium alloy	RX type	4–7	12–18	0.014	5	80, 135
Omnilink Elite	Abbott	Nickel-chromium alloy	OTW type	4–10	12–59	0–035	6	80, 135
Dynamic	Biotronik	Stainless steel	OTW type	5–10	15–56	0–035	6	80, 130
Dynamic renal	Biotronik	Nickel-chromium alloy	RX type	4.5–7	12–19	0.014	4–5	80, 140
PRO-kinetic energy explorer	Biotronik	Nickel-chromium alloy	RX type	2–5	9–40	0.014	4	140

Features and Models

The stent is indicated for endovascular treatment of renal and vertebral artery stenosis and other vascular diseases. The stent is compatible with 0.36 mm (0.014in) wire and 4–5F vascular sheath, with a diameter ranging from 4 mm to 7 mm, a length from 10 mm to 24 mm, and the delivery system length of 145 mm.

5.5.3.2 Express SD Balloon-Expandable Stent

Product Structure

Express SD balloon-expandable stent (Fig. 5.20), the US Boston Scientific-produced stainless steel RX-type stent, is premounted on a RX-type stent delivery system (SDS) equipped with a semi-compliant balloon, which, through patented tandem architecture design, provides additional luminal support on the proximal ends of the stent, featuring excellent radial action, low retraction, certain flexibility while providing proximal support, and increased support for proximal lumens of the stent. The stent has two radiopaque marker bands embedded in the shaft on both ends of the balloon to assist with accurate stent placement.

Features and Models

The stent is indicated for endovascular treatment of renal artery, vertebral artery, and other small-diameter peripheral vascular lesions. The stent is compatible with 0.46 mm (0.018in) wire and 5F vascular sheath, available with diameter ranging from 4 mm to 7 mm, length from 14 mm to 19 mm, and the delivery system length of 150 cm.

5.5.3.3 Palmaz Blue Balloon-Expandable Stent

Product Structure

Palmaz Blue balloon-expandable stent (Fig. 5.21) is the US Cordis-produced RX-type stent made of cobalt-chromium alloy. The stent is a hollow tubular configuration laser engraved from a monolithic L605 cobalt-chromium alloy, premounted on the Aviator Plus balloon dilation catheter, wherein the catheter's tip is in conical shape so as to pass through the stenotic lesion sites, and the proximal axis is used as balloon dilation hole. There are two radiopaque marker bands on the inner shafts of both ends of the balloon to ensure accurate stent placement.

Features and Models

The stent is indicated for endovascular treatment of other smaller-diameter peripheral arterial lesions such as the renal artery, vertebral artery, and the like. The stent is compatible with 0.36 mm (0.014in) wire and 4–5F vascular sheath, available with diameter ranging from 4 mm to 7 mm, length from 12 mm to 24 mm, and the delivery system length of 80 cm and 142 cm.

5.5.3.4 Express LD Balloon-Expandable Stent

Product Structure

Express LD balloon-expandable stent (Fig. 5.22), the US Boston Scientific-produced OTW-type stainless steel stent, is preloaded on a stent delivery system (SDS) with a non-compliant balloon, which, through patented tandem architecture design, provides additional luminal support on the proximal ends of the stent, featuring excellent radial strength,

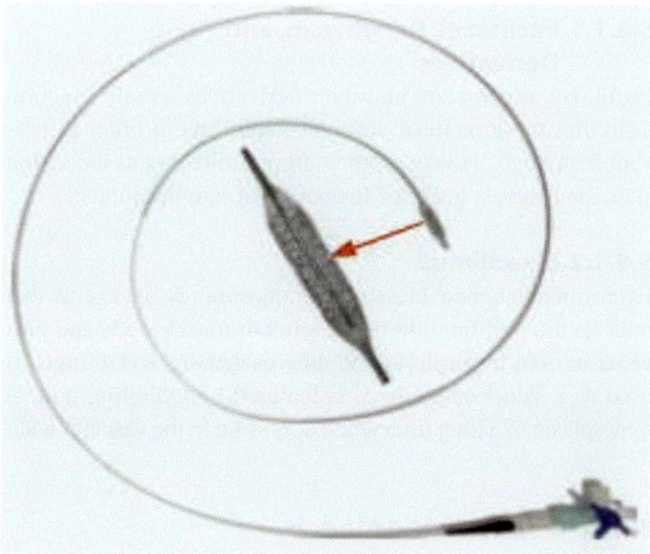

Fig. 5.20 Express SD balloon-expandable stent (Boston Scientific)

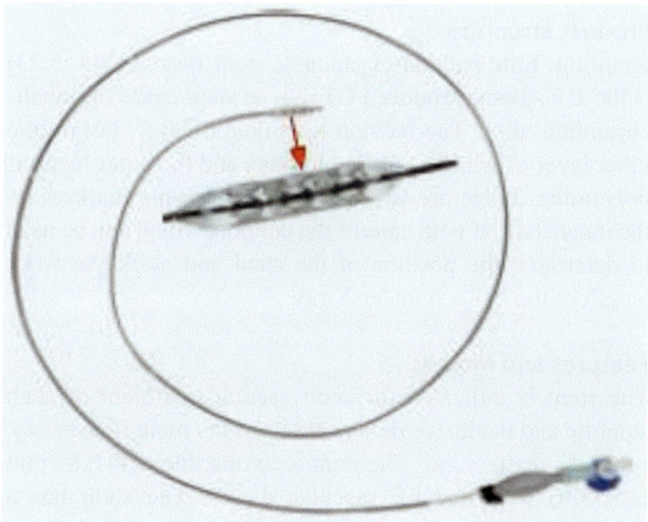

Fig. 5.21 Palmaz Blue balloon-expandable stent (Cordis)

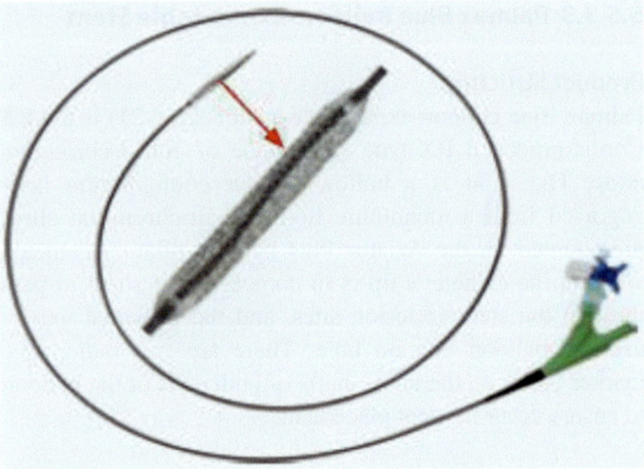

Fig. 5.22 Express LD balloon-expandable stent (Boston Scientific)

low retraction, certain flexibility while providing proximal support, and increased support for proximal lumens of the stent. The stent has two bands of radiopaque markers embedded in the shaft on both ends of the balloon to assist with accurate stent placement.

Features and Models
The stent is indicated for endovascular treatment of diseased blood vessels at a diameter ranging from 7 mm to 10 mm such as the subclavian artery, iliac artery, etc. The stent is compatible with 0.89 mm (0.035in) wire and 6–7F vascular sheath, available with a diameter ranging from 5 mm to 10 mm, a length from 17 mm to 57 mm, and the delivery system length of 75 cm and 135 cm.

5.5.3.5 Omnilink Elite Balloon-Expandable Stent

Product Structure
Omnilink Elite balloon-expandable stent system (Fig. 5.23) is the US Abbott-produced OTW-type stent made of cobalt-chromium alloy. The balloon is of double-layer design, the inner layer of which is made of Pebax and the outer layer of polyamide. There are two bands of radiopaque markers on the inner shaft of both ends of the balloon, which can be used to determine the position of the stent and mark the work length of the balloon under X-ray.

Features and Models
The stent is indicated for endovascular treatment of such stenotic and occlusive blood vessels as the main iliac artery, subclavian artery, etc. The stent is compatible with 0.89 mm (0.035in) wire and 6F vascular sheath. The stent has a diameter ranging from 4 mm to 10 mm, a length from 12 mm to 59 mm, and the delivery system length of 80 cm and 135 cm.

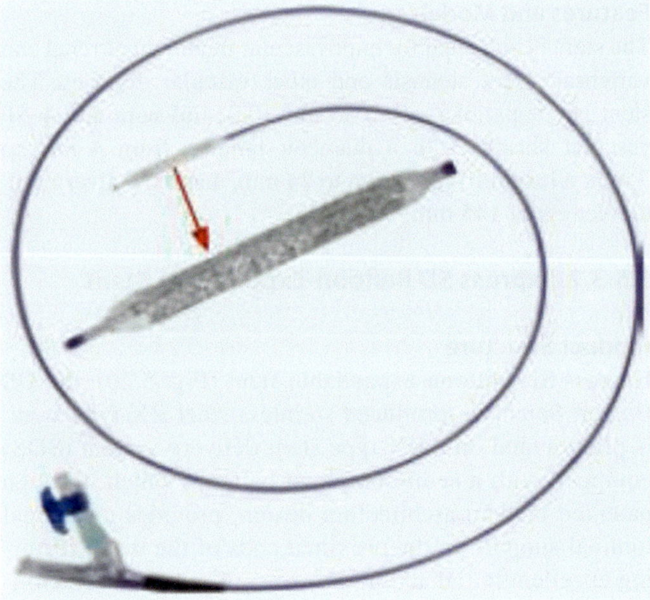

Fig. 5.23 Omnilink Elite balloon-expandable stent (Abbott)

5.6 Balloon-Expandable Drug-Eluting Stent

5.6.1 Product Structure

Balloon-expandable drug-eluting stent is to load drugs via a polymer carrier or microporous design, where the polymer carrier functions as targeted drug release and controlled release. The stent can, with the action of the drugs, prevent the proliferation of vascular endothelial cells to achieve vascular patency. At present, the drugs loaded on such stents are mostly paclitaxel, everolimus, rapamycin, and their derivatives.

5.6.1.1 Paclitaxel, Rapamycin, and Their Derivatives

Paclitaxel, rapamycin, and their derivatives mainly function to inhibit the growth of vascular neointima in order to prevent restenosis. However, they are not directed at the lesion sites themselves, liable of formation of late thrombosis.

5.6.1.2 Everolimus

Everolimus is a new class of immunosuppressive agents that inhibits the proliferation of the smooth muscle cells and prevents intimal hyperplasia and atherosclerosis. Everolimus, if used as a stent-coated drug, is featured by inhibiting intimal hyperplasia of a long time when accessing to the vascular wall.

5.6.2 Features and Models

Balloon-expandable drug-eluting stent is mainly indicated for endovascular treatment of coronary artery, infra-popliteal artery and other diseased vessels. This kind of stents is compatible with 0.36 mm (0.014in) wire and 5F vascular sheath at a diameter ranging from 2.25 mm to 4 mm and a length from 8 mm to 38 mm. At present, foreign brands of balloon-expandable DES include Abbott, Medtronic, Boston Scientific, etc. Chinese brands include MicroPort (Shanghai), Jiwei (Shandong), Lepu (Beijing), and Kinhely (Shenzhen). This section mainly introduces Xience Prime (Abbott) and Firebird2 (MicroPort) balloon-expandable DES.

5.6.3 Brand Information

5.6.3.1 Xience Prime Balloon-Expandable Drug-Eluting Stent

Product Structure

Xience Prime balloon-expandable drug-eluting stent (Fig. 5.24) is the US Abbott-produced RX-type stent made of cobalt-chromium alloy. The stent is made of L605 cobalt-chromium alloy undercoated with n-butyl polymethacrylate, and its drug-coating consists of everolimus and vinylidene fluoride-hexafluoropropylene copolymer with everolimus dose of 100 μg/cm^2 and drug loading dosage of 40–232 μg. The balloon is made of Pebax 7233 at a hardness of 72D. Hydrophilic coating is applied within 30 cm from the proximal tip of the catheter, except for the balloon portion.

Features and Models

The stent is mainly indicated for endovascular treatment of diseased coronary artery and infra-popliteal short-segment blood vessels, compatible with 0.36 mm (0.014 in) wire and 5F vascular sheath, available with stent diameters ranging from 2.25 mm to 4 mm, length from 8 mm to 38 mm, and the delivery system length of 150 cm.

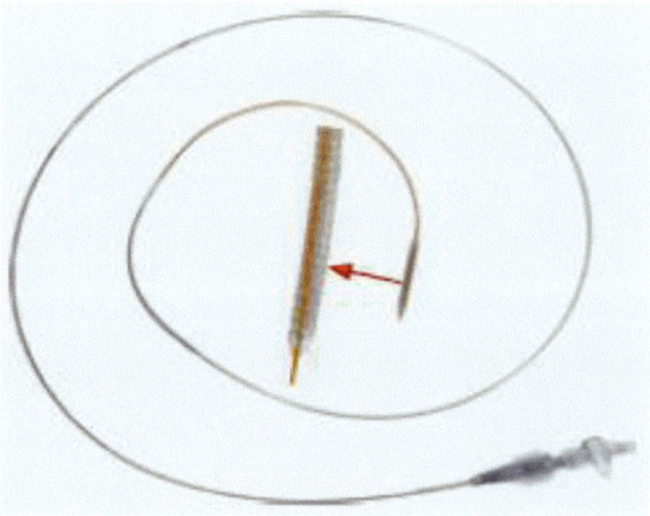

Fig. 5.24 Xience Prime balloon-expandable drug-eluting stent (Abbott)

5.6.3.2 Firebird2 Balloon-Expandable Drug-Eluting Stent

Product Structure

Firebird2 balloon-expandable drug-eluting stent (Fig. 5.25) is the China Microport-produced RX-type stent made of cobalt-based alloy. The stent is made of L605 cobalt-chromium alloy, and its coating consists of a drug storage layer and an external controlled release layer, wherein the storage layer consists of a copolymer of rapamycin and styrene isobutene copolymer with a rapamycin content of 120–305 μg; the controlled release layer is made of styrene-isobutylene copolymer. The balloon is made of 72D block polyether amide resin (Pebax7233), and the catheter portion is applied with a hydrophilic coating.

Features and Models

The stent is indicated for endovascular treatment of coronary and peripheral artery atherosclerosis and other vascular diseases. The stent is compatible with 0.36 mm (0.014 in) wire and 5F vascular sheath. The stent has a diameter ranging from 2.5 mm to 4 mm, a length from 13 mm to 33 mm, and the delivery system length of 140 cm.

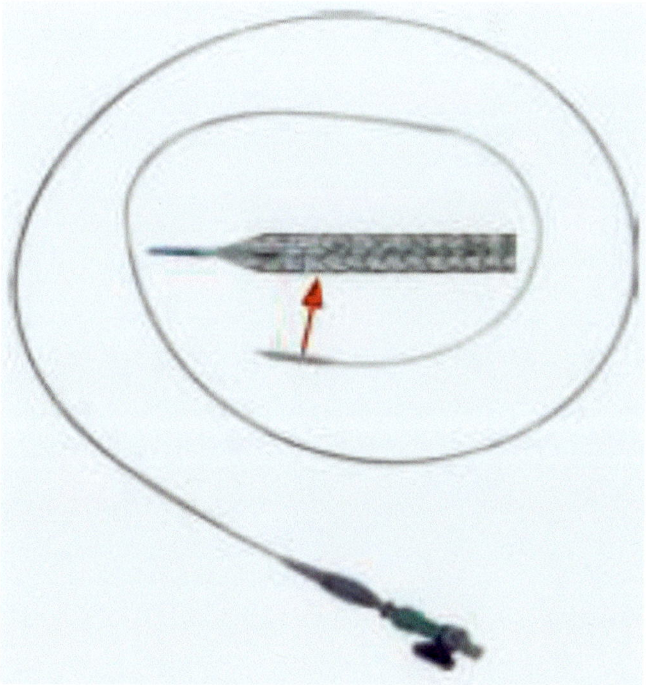

Fig. 5.25 Firebird2 balloon-expandable DES (MicroPort)

6 Aortic Endograft

Huajuan Mao, Qingsheng Lu, Lei Zhang, and Zaiping Jing

Abstract
Aortic endovascular grafts are main endovascular devices used for treating aortic diseases. They include thoracic aortic stent graft system, abdominal aortic stent graft system, CP (Cheatham-Platinum) stent, etc. This chapter mainly provides a tabular conclusion and summary about the names, brands, metal stent materials, coating materials, head-end bare stents, barbs, reinforcing ribs, rear release positioning, delivery sheaths, and other details of aortic stent graft systems and elaborates on their structures, features, and model types based on stent graft systems of different brands.

Keywords
Aortic endovascular graft · Structure and features · Model types

6.1 Introduction

Aortic endograft refers to implants delivered into the diseased aortic segments via superficial arteries, such as stent grafts for aortic aneurysms, stent for aortic stenosis or occlusion, occluder of atrial septal defect (ASD), and metal embolization for aortic aneurysm embolization, etc. As the name suggests, aortic endograft refers to a series of endovascular devices used in the aortic portion. This chapter introduces mainly three aspects: TAA stent graft, AAA stent graft, and CP (Cheatham-Platinum) stent. At present, the Castor branch TAA stent graft, which is mainly developed and used in clinical context by the Department of Vascular Surgery, Changhai Hospital, affiliated to the Naval Medical University, is going to be launched into the market, thus opening up a new path for the treatment of aortic arch "forbidden zone."

H. Mao (✉) · Q. Lu · L. Zhang · Z. Jing
Department of Vascular Surgery, Changhai Hospital, Second Military Medical University, Shanghai, China
e-mail: czymm8@163.com

6.2 TAA Stent Graft

6.2.1 Product Structure

The TAA stent graft belongs to the aortic endograft, which is composed of a stent graft and a delivery system. The stent graft is a self-expanding stent graft where the bare metal stent is covered with polymer-specific film material. According to the stent pattern, it can be morphologically divided into two kinds: straight type and tapered type.

6.2.2 Features and Models

TAA stent graft is used for major artery vascular diseases, such as minimally invasive endovascular exclusion of thoracic aortic aneurysms, aortic dissection, etc. There are currently a variety of brands on the market, each having its own advantages. Brand-specific performance of the TAA stent graft is shown in Table 6.1. At present, foreign brands of the TAA stent graft include Bolton Medical, Cook, Medtronic, etc. Chinese brands include MicroPort (Shanghai), LifeTech (Shenzhen), Aortec (Beijing), Grikin (Beijing), etc. This section mainly introduces Hercules (MicroPort), Ankura (LifeTech), Zenith TX2 (Cook), Valiant (Medtronic), C-TAG (Gore), and Relay (Bolton Medical) TAA stent grafts.

Z. Jing et al. (eds.), *Endovascular Surgery and Devices*, https://doi.org/10.1007/978-981-10-8270-2_6

Table 6.1 Brand-specific TAA stent graft performance (for reference only)

Name	Brand	Material of metal stent	Coating material	Tip bare stent	Barb	Stiffener	Post-release positioning	Delivery sheath (F)
Hercules	MicroPort	Nitinol and 316L stainless steel	PET	Y	N	Y	N	18–20
Ankura	LifeTech	Nitinol	ePTFE	Y	N	Y	Y	21–24
Zenith TX2	Cook	Stainless steel	PET	N	Y	N	Y	20–22
Valiant	Medtronic	Nitinol	PET	Y	N	N	Y	20–24
C-TAG	Gore	Nitinol	ePTFE	Y	N	N	N	20–24
Relay	Bolton Medical	Nitinol	PET	Y	N	Y	Y	22–26
Castor	Microport	Nitinol	PET	N	N	N	Y	24

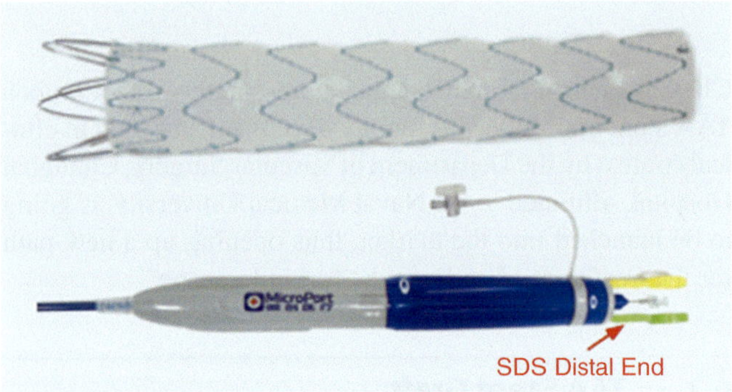

Fig. 6.1 Hercules TAA stent graft (MicroPort)

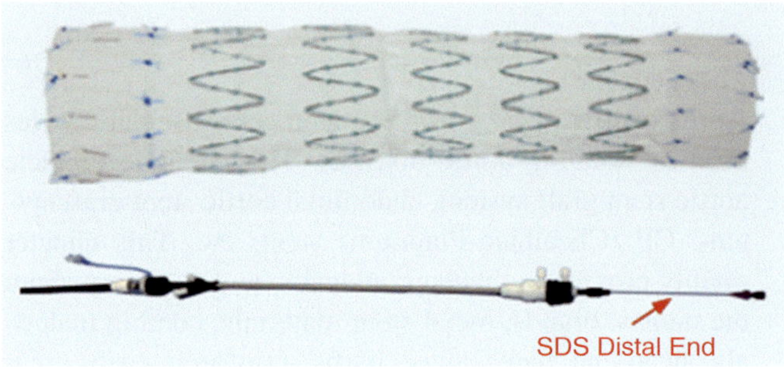

Fig. 6.2 Zenith TX2 TAA stent graft (Cook)

6.2.3 Brand Information

6.2.3.1 Hercules TAA Stent Graft

Product Structure

Hercules TAA stent graft is the China Microport-produced self-expanding stent graft made of nitinol and 316L stainless steel (Fig. 6.1). The stent graft is a sutured combination of a proximal bare stent segment, a proximal high-profile stent segment, a high-profile main stent segment, and a coated tube. The metal stent is made of nitinol and 316L stainless steel, and the coating material is polyethylene terephthalate (PET). The stent has five developing points: two markers on each end of the stent and one on the stiffener side. The stent applies low-profile delivery system, the delivery system adopts bare segment post-release mechanism, and its inner tube uses the same nitinol material as the stent. As compared with the inner tube made of polymeric materials, nitinol inner tube can provide better rigidity while ensuring excellent bending performance. The combined use of the inner tube with the superhard wire ensures that the entire system remains immobilized upon stent deployment and avoids forward jump and back movement of the stent system, thus making the subsequent release more accurate.

Features and Models

The stent graft system is indicated for aneurysm repair of thoracic aortic diseases. The stent system consists of a tapered body and a straight extension (cuff), compatible with 0.89 mm (0.035in) superhard wire and 14–20F vascular sheath. The proximal end diameter of the tapered body is 14–44 mm, and its distal end diameter is 12–42 mm, available with 2–10 mm in taper and 160 mm in length. The diameter of the straight extension of the covered stent is 12–44 mm, and its length is 45–80 mm.

6.2.3.2 Zenith TX2 TAA Stent Graft

Product Structure

Zenith TX2 TAA stent graft (Fig. 6.2), the US Cook-produced stainless steel self-expanding stent graft, is sewn onto the stent with braided polyester (PET) and monofilament polypropylene sutures. The TAA stent graft is morphologically divided into straight type and tapered type. Barbs at the proximal end of the stent are arranged at 2 mm increment and can be directly fixed onto the vascular wall. On both ends of the stent are four radiopaque markers, respectively, which are placed in the circumferential direction within 1 mm of both ends of the covered stent. Stent delivery system uses a single-trigger metal wire release unit and adopts a procedure of sequential deployment to provide continuous control over the release of the TAA stent graft throughout its deployment and ensure accurate stent positioning before stent deployment.

Features and Models

The stent graft is mainly indicated for thoracic aortic aneurysm (TAA) repair. The stent is compatible with 0.89 mm (0.035in) superhard wire and 20–22F vascular sheath. The diameter of the straight-type TAA stent is 28–42 mm, and the length is 120–216 mm. The diameter of the proximal end of the tapered TAA stent is 32–42 mm, the diameter of the distal end is 28–38 mm, the taper at both ends is 4 mm, and the length is 152–208 mm.

6.2.3.3 Valiant TAA Stent Graft

Product Structure

Valiant TAA stent graft (Fig. 6.3), the US Medtronic-produced nitinol self-expanding stent graft, is composed of a spring scaffold made from nitinol wire (55% nickel and 45% titanium and trace elements) sewn to a fabric graft with non-resorbable sutures. The metal scaffold is composed of a series of serpentine springs stacked in a tubular configuration. The proximal end of the covered stent consists of a proximal bare stent with miniature bearing spring. During and after the deployment of the TAA stent graft, the miniature bearing spring can prevent the stent graft from being retracted. Its distal end is a stent not exceeding the edge of the stent graft. The TAA stent graft is divided morphologically into straight and tapered types. The stent uses Captivia delivery system, which consists of a disposable catheter with an integrated handle and a tip capture device. The TAA stent graft can be deployed by two steps: (1) TAA stent graft is deployed, but the tip bare stent is still under constraint; (2) the bare stent is released. This special delivery system ensures controllable implantation of the stent graft into the thoracic artery.

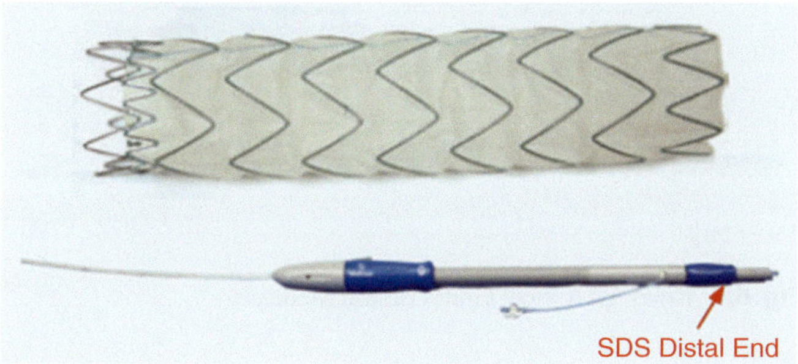

Fig. 6.3 Valiant TAA stent graft (Medtronic)

Features and Models

This stent graft is indicated for endovascular treatment of thoracic aortic diseases. The system is compatible with 0.89 mm (0.035in) superhard wire and 20–25F vascular sheath. The diameter of the straight-type TAA stent is 22–46 mm and the length is 107–212 mm; the diameter of the proximal end of TAA stent is 26–46 mm, and the distal end diameter is 22–42 mm, with 4 mm taper at both ends and a length of 107–155 mm (tapered stent has not been marketed in China).

6.2.3.4 C-TAG TAA Stent Graft

Product Specifications

C-TAG TAA stent graft (Fig. 6.4), the US Gore-produced self-expanding stent graft, is made of nitinol memory alloy with dual-layer coating design, where the contact face with the blood flow is made of ePTFE reinforced with fluorinated ethylene propylene (FEP) membrane. The stent graft is free from suture. The TAA stent graft body can be morphologically divided as straight type and tapered type. A bare stent with nine peak structures is placed at the proximal end of the covered stent, on both ends of which are equipped with anti-leak sleeves for sealing and fixation. Two gold radiopaque marker rings are placed on both ends of the stent, where the marker ring at the proximal end is located at the bottom of the peak-structured bare stent. The stent is deployed via pulling the wire in a sequence starting from the center of the stent and extending toward both ends of the stent.

Features and Models

The stent graft system is mainly indicated for endovascular treatment of patients with thoracic aortic aneurysm. The stent is compatible with 0.89 mm (0.035in) superhard wire and 18–24F vascular sheath. The diameter of the straight-type TAA stent is 21–45 mm, and the length 100–200 mm. The diameter of the proximal end of the tapered-type TAA stent is 26–31 mm, the distal end diameter 21–26 mm, and the taper on both ends 5 mm and the length 100 mm.

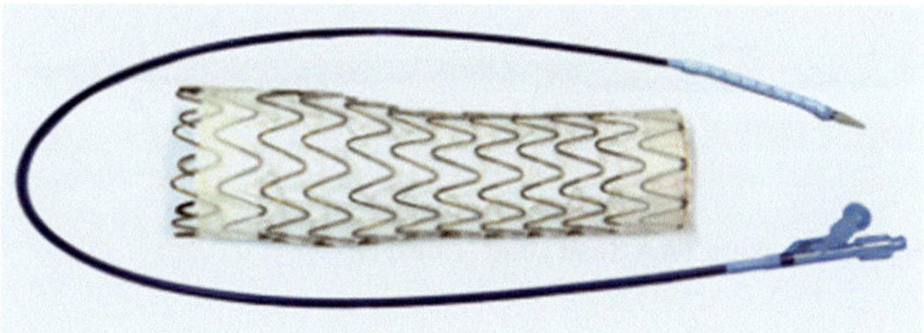

Fig. 6.4 C-TAG TAA Stent Graft (Gore)

6.2.3.5 Ankura TAA Stent Graft

Product Structure

Ankura TAA stent graft (Fig. 6.5), a self-expanding stent graft manufactured by LifeTech, China, is made of nitinol coated with ePTFE membrane which is integrated with the stent through heat treatment. The covered stent with its axial keel design enhances the stability of the overall stent skeleton and prevents the stent graft from shortening under long-time pulsation. The axial support can prevent the proximal and distal ends of the stent graft from being displaced under the impact of blood flow. The proximal end of the covered stent with its mini-wave design can provide radial support and excellent wall adhesion and thus avoid of Type I endoleak. The nitinol wire of the bare stent is thinner than that of the main body segment and can alleviate damage to the blood vessels on the aortic arch. The TAA stent graft can be morphologically divided into straight type and tapered type. Totally three radiopaque markers are placed on the stent: an "8"-like marker on the proximal keel of the stent, an "O" marker at the lesser curvature side, and a "V" marker at the distal end. The stent uses tip-capture post-release delivery system, which consists of a front handle, a safety trigger, a rear handle, a proximal release, and a safety catch. The delivery system is surfaced with hydrophilic coating.

Features and Models

The stent graft is mainly indicated for thoracic aortic aneurysm repair. The stent is compatible with 0.89 mm (0.035in) superhard wire and 21–24F vascular sheath. The diameter of the straight-type TAA stent is 28–44 mm and the length 40–200 mm. The diameter of the proximal end of the tapered-type TAA stent ranges from 28 mm to 44 mm, the diameter of the distal end from 20 mm to 40 mm, the taper on both ends from 4 mm to 8 mm, and the length from 120 mm to 200 mm.

6.2.3.6 Relay TAA Stent Graft

Product Structure

Relay TAA stent graft (Fig. 6.6), the France Bolton Medical-produced self-expanding stent graft, is made of nitinol sewn with polyester vascular graft (PET), on which an oblique nitinol wire provides vertical support for the stent. This TAA stent graft can be morphologically divided into straight-type and tapered-type stent. Totally four "D" platiniridium markers are placed on both ends and the center of the covered stent. The stent uses the transport delivery system, which consists of a series of coaxially arranged outer sheath, a catheter, and a tubular handle control system. The outer sheath can be bent to ensure that the stent system can track the thoracic aorta, especially the bending portion of the arch area.

Features and Models

The stent graft is mainly indicated for endovascular treatment of patients with true or false thoracic aortic aneurysm, aortic dissection, penetrating ulcer, intramural edema, and other aortic lesions. The stent is compatible with 0.89 mm (0.035in) superhard wire and 22–26F vascular sheath. The diameter of the straight-type TAA stent is 22–46 mm and the length 100–200 mm. The diameter of the proximal end of the tapered-type stent is 28–46 mm, the distal end diameter 24–42 mm, the taper on both ends 4 mm, and the length 150–200 mm.

6.2.3.7 Castor TAA Stent Graft

Product Structure

Castor TAA stent graft (Fig. 6.7), a self-expanding stent graft manufactured by MicroPort, China, is made from a plurality of self-expanding nitinol stent segments sewn to a polyester

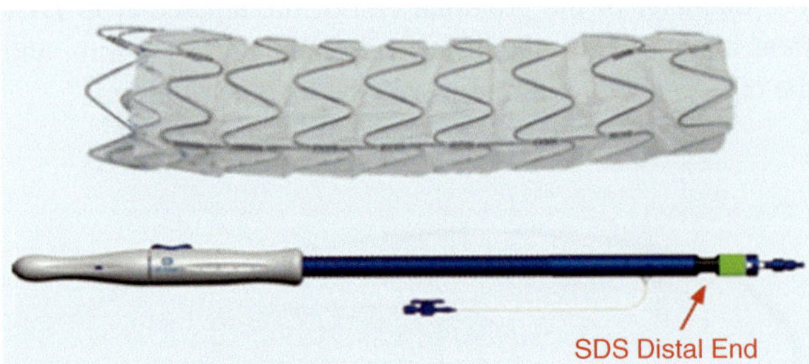

Fig. 6.5 Ankura TAA Stent Graft (LifeTech)

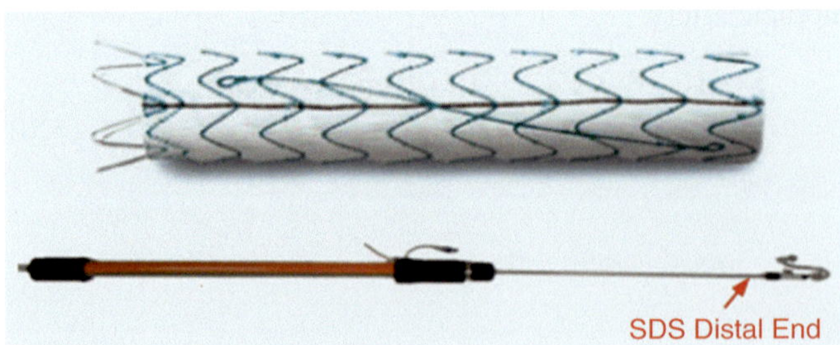

Fig. 6.6 Relay TAA Stent Graft (Bolton Medical)

membrane (PET) with non-resorbable sutures. Castor stent graft consists of a main body stent graft sewn with a collateral limb, all being sewn with platiniridium developing markers. The Castor delivery system consists of an outer tube, flexible sleeve, and inner tube. The inner tube is accessible to 0.035in wire, the flexible sleeve enables the stent system to navigate through the aortic arch, and the outer tube is anti-bending designed. The delivery system has two pieces of control wire to control the deployment of the main body stent and the bifurcated stent, respectively.

Features and Models

The stent graft is mainly indicated for endovascular treatment of patients with complicated aortic dissection aneurysm involving the branch arteries. The stent system is compatible with 0.89 mm (0.035in) superhard wire and 24F vascular sheath. The diameter of the proximal end of the covered stent ranges from 26 mm to 44 mm, the distal end diameter from 20 mm to 44 mm, the distal end diameter of the collateral limb from 6 mm to 14 mm, the length of the main body stent from 60 mm to 210 mm, the length of the collateral limb from 25 mm to 45 mm, and the backward length of the collateral limb from 0 mm to 30 mm.

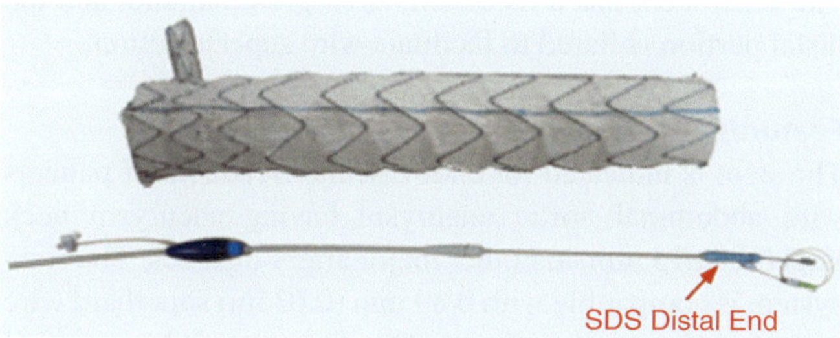

Fig. 6.7 Castor TAA Stent Graft (Shanghai MicroPort)

6.3 AAA Stent Graft

6.3.1 Product Structure

AAA (abdominal aortic aneurysm) stent graft is a kind of aortic endograft, divided into split type (short for "split-type AAA stent") and integrated type (short for "integrated AAA stent"). The split-type AAA stent consists of split-type AAA main body stent ("abdominal aortic main body stent") and iliac limb components ("abdominal aortoiliac stent"). The abdominal aortic main body stent is of a single-leg form that can be accurately placed into the abdominal aorta and one side of the iliac arteries, and the abdominal aortoiliac stent is placed contralaterally into the short leg of the abdominal aortic main body stent, thus forming an integrated stent.

6.3.2 Features and Models

AAA stent graft system is indicated for minimally invasive endovascular treatment of patients with abdominal aortic aneurysm, iliac artery aneurysm, abdominal aortic dissection aneurysm, and other diseases. At present, there are various brands of AAA stent grafts on the market, each with its own advantages. The brand-specific performance of the AAA stent grafts is shown in Table 6.2. Currently, the international brands of AAA stent grafts include Bolton Medical, Cook, Medtronic, Gore, Cordis, etc., and Chinese brands include MicroPort, LifeTech, Aortec, etc. This section mainly introduces Aegis (MicroPort), Hercules (MicroPort), Ankura (LifeTech), Zenith Flex (Cook), Endurant (Medtronic), and Excluder (Gore) AAA stent grafts.

Table 6.2 Brand-specific performance of AAA stent grafts (for reference only)

Name	Brand	Stent material	Coating material	Stent structure	Tip bare stent	Barb	Post-release positioning	Delivery sheath diameter(F)
Aegis	MicroPort	Nitinol	ePTFE	Integrated	Y	N	N	22
Hercules	MicroPort	Nitinol and 316L stainless steel	PET	Split type	Y	N	N	16–24
Ankura	LifeTech	Nitinol	ePTFE	Split type	Y	N	Y	18–23
Zenith Flex	Cook	Stainless steel	PET	Split type	Y	Y	Y	14–20
Endurant	Medtronic	Nitinol	PET	Split type	Y	Y	Y	14–20
Excluder	Gore	Nitinol	ePTFE	Split type	N	Y	Y	12–18
Treovance	Bolton Medical	Nitinol	PET	Split type	Y	Y	Y	15–19
InCraft	Cordis	Nitinol	PET	Split type	Y	Y	Y	12–16

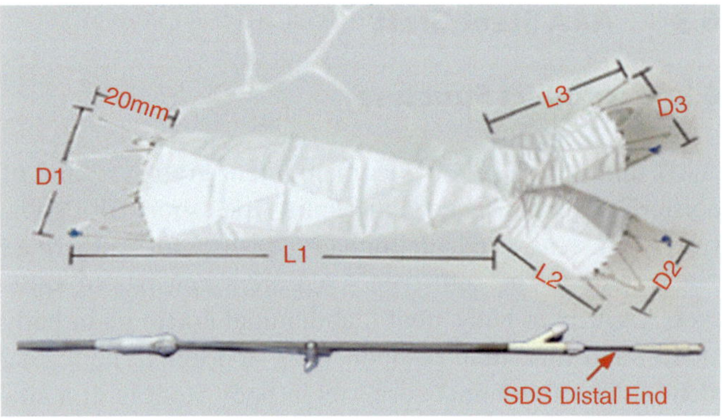

Fig. 6.8 Aegis AAA stent graft (MicroPort)

6.3.3 Brand Information

6.3.3.1 Aegis AAA Stent Graft

Product Structure

Aegis AAA stent graft (Fig. 6.8), the China MicroPort-produced nitinol self-expanding stent graft, adopts integrated design to fix the aortic main body stent with the aortoiliac limb components. The stent is made of woven radiopaque nitinol wire coated with expanded polytetrafluoroethylene (ePTFE), and a 20 mm bare stent is designed at the proximal end of the stent graft.

Features and Models

The stent graft is indicated for endovascular treatment of patients with abdominal aortic or aortoiliac artery aneurysms. The stent system is compatible with 0.89 mm (0.035in) superhard wire and 22F vascular sheath. The length from the proximal bare stent of the integrated stent to the bifurcation (L1) is 60–150 mm, and its proximal end diameter (D1) is 20–36 mm. The length of the short legs (L2, L3) at the distal end of the integrated stent is 40–100 mm, and its distal end diameter (D2, D3) is 12–20 mm. The effective length of the stent delivery system is 60 cm.

The stent's models are very complicated in actual use, and an example is given here for detailed illustration. AB [28][12][14] – [90][40][50] – [20][10][05], where A represents the stent graft, B the bifurcated type, 28 the diameter of the main body stent, 12 the diameter of the ipsilateral bifurcated stent, 14 the diameter of the contralateral bifurcated stent, 90 the coated segment length of the main body stent graft, 40 the coated segment length of the ipsilateral bifurcated stent, 50 the coated segment length of the contralateral bifurcated stent, 20 the bare segment length of the main body stent, 10 the bare segment length of the ipsilateral bifurcated stent, and 05 the bare segment length of the contralateral bifurcated stent.

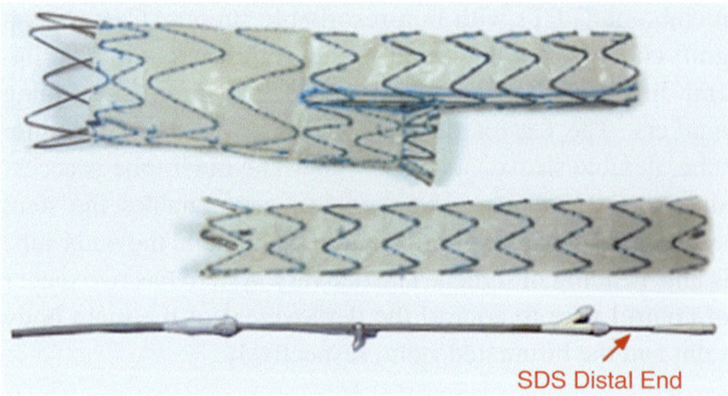

Fig. 6.9 Hercules AAA Stent Graft (MicroPort)

6.3.3.2 Hercules AAA Stent Graft

Product Structure

Hercules AAA stent graft (Fig. 6.9), a self-expanding stent graft made of nitinol and 316L stainless steel by MicroPort, China, consists of a tubular-coated pipe and a nitinol skeleton. Using split-type configuration, the stent graft consists of the aortic main body stent (HBB) and the aortoiliac limb component (HBL). The stent is made of nitinol and 316L stainless steel coated with polyester fiber material (PET). The HBB stent has a bare stent at its proximal end, and the distal portion is flared to facilitate wire superselection.

Features and Models

The stent is indicated for endovascular treatment of patients with abdominal aortic aneurysm having aneurysm neck larger than 15 mm and other major artery diseases. The stent system is compatible with 0.89 mm (0.035in) superhard wire and 16–24F vascular sheath. The diameter of the proximal end of the aortic main body stent is 20–34 mm, its distal end diameter is 12–18 mm, and bare stent length is 15–20 mm. The length from the coated portion at the proximal end to the distal end of the ipsilateral iliac limb is 130–170 mm. The aortoiliac limb component has a diameter ranging from 12 mm to 18 mm and a length from 50 mm to 120 mm.

6.3.3.3 Zenith Flex AAA Stent Graft

Product Structure

Zenith Flex AAA stent graft, the US Cook-produced stainless steel self-expanding stent graft (Fig. 6.10), consists of an aortic main body stent and two aortic iliac limb components. The stent graft is constructed of full-thickness woven polyester fabric sewn to a stainless steel stent with braided polyester and monofilament polypropylene suture. In addition, the covered stent is also equipped with an independent extension (cuff). The bare stent at the proximal end of the main body graft contains barbs placed at 3 mm increment for direct

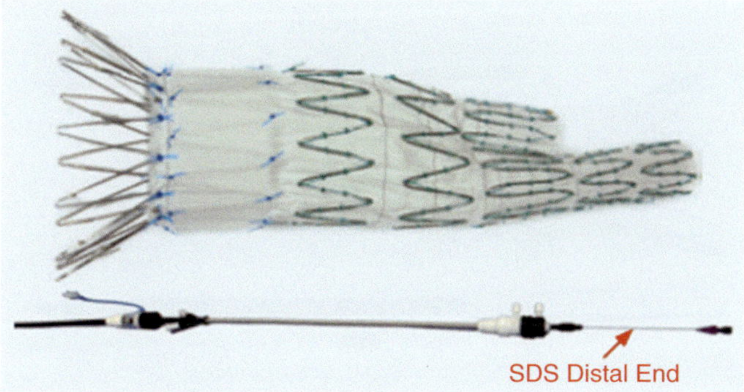

Fig. 6.10 Zenith Flex AAA Stent Graft (Cook)

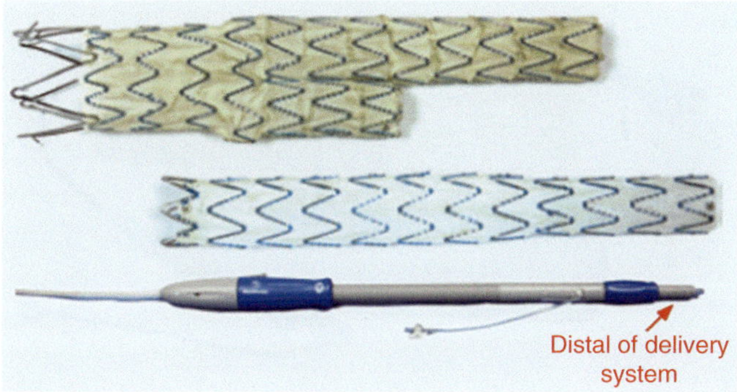

Fig. 6.11 Endurant AAA Stent Graft (Medtronic)

adhesion to and fixation with the vascular wall. Totally five radiopaque markers are arranged on the graft, one of which is placed on the lateral aspect of the distal end of the "short leg" of the aortic main body stent and the other four in a circumferential orientation within 2 mm of the proximal end of the graft material of the main body stent. The stent delivery system (SDS) adopts a procedure of sequential deployment to provide continuous control over the release of the stent graft throughout its deployment and ensure accurate stent positioning before stent deployment.

Features and Models

The stent graft is indicated for endovascular treatment of patients with abdominal aortic or aortoiliac aneurysms. The stent is compatible with 0.89 mm (0.035in) superhard wire and 14–20F vascular sheath. The aortic main body stent has its proximal end diameter ranging from 22 mm to 32 mm, and its distal iliac limb diameter of 12 mm, available with stent length of 82–140 mm; the aortic iliac limb component has its proximal end diameter of 12 mm and distal end diameter of 8–24 mm, available with a length of 37–122 mm. The stent extension has a diameter of 22–32 mm and a length of 39 mm.

6.3.3.4 Endurant AAA Stent Graft

Product Structure

Endurant AAA stent graft (Fig. 6.11) is the US Medtronic-produced nitinol self-expanding stent graft, which is divided into aortic main body stent, aortic iliac stent, extender, and aortic uni-iliac stent (AUI). A one-piece polyethylene terephthalate (PET) fabric is sewn onto the nitinol stent framework by using polyester and polyethylene sutures. On the proximal end of the aortic main body stent is a bare stent, which has barbs that can be anchored on the vascular wall to prevent stent displacement upon implantation into the blood vessels. Six radiopaque markers are sewn onto the stent to help development, one of which is located at the bifurcation of the aortic main body stent, one at the distal end of the ipsilateral aortic iliac stent, and the other four on the proximal graft of the aortic main body stent evenly distributed in a circle. The aortic iliac stent has no bare stent at its proximal end and is in an open mesh configuration, reducing the possible endoleak. A radiopaque marker is placed on each end of the stent. The extender has bare stent with barbs at its proximal end, and four radiopaque markers are placed at the proximal graft of the stent and one at its distal end. AUI stent proximal end is the same as the aortic main body stent, but with a distal end being gradually tapered, and four radiopaque markers are placed at the proximal graft of the stent and two at its distal end.

Features and Models

The stent is indicated for infrarenal abdominal aortic aneurysm repair or aortic iliac artery aneurysm repair, compatible with 0.89 mm (0.035in) superhard wire and 14–20F vascular sheath. The proximal end diameter of the aortic main body stent is 23–36 mm, and its distal iliac stent diameter is 13–20 mm, at a length of 124–166 mm. The proximal end diameter of the aortic iliac stent is 16 mm and its distal diameter is 10–28 mm, at a length of 82–199 mm. The extender has a diameter ranging from 23 mm to 36 mm and a length from 49 mm to 70 mm. AUI stent has 23–36 mm proximal end diameter and 14 mm distal end diameter, at a length of 102 mm.

6.3.3.5 Excluder AAA Endoprosthesis

Product Structure

Excluder AAA endoprosthesis (Fig. 6.12) is the US Gore-produced nitinol self-expanding stent graft, which is divided into aortic main body stent, aortic iliac stent, and extender. The graft materials of the stent are expanded polytetrafluoroethylene and fluorinated ethylene propylene (ePTFE and FEP) and are supported by nitinol wire along its external surface. An ePTFE/FEP sealing cuff and barbs are located near

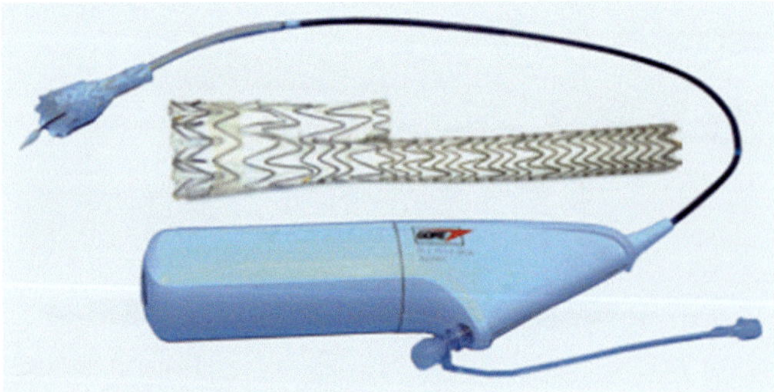

Fig. 6.12 Excluder AAA Endoprosthesis (Gore)

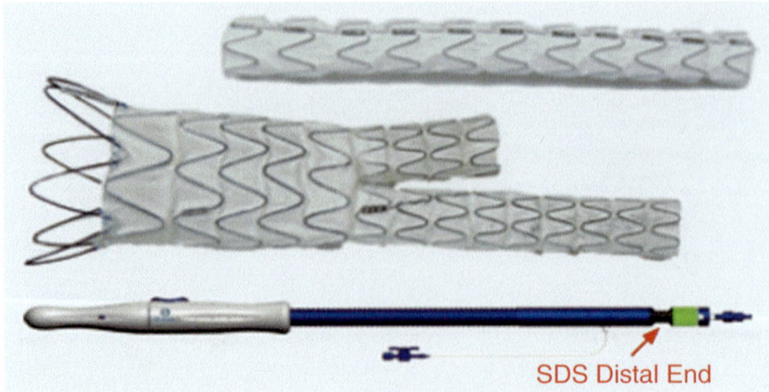

Fig. 6.13 Ankura AAA Stent Graft (Shenzhen LifeTech)

the proximal end of the endoprosthesis, along with three radiopaque markers: a radiopaque marker on the distal end of the ipsilateral iliac limb of the aortic main body stent, and on both ends of the bifurcation are two markers, one long and one short; a radiopaque marker ring on the distal end of the contralateral iliac limb of the aortic main body stent; a radiopaque marker on both ends of the aortic iliac stent, respectively; three radiopaque markers on the proximal end of the extender and one on its distal end. The stent adopts C3 delivery system, consisting of black nut, red safety lock, transparent button, gray compressor turntable, and white external deployment button, and the delivery system releases the stent by pulling the wire through micro-adjusting of the aortic main body stent.

Features and Models

The stent graft is indicated for repair of infrarenal abdominal aortic aneurysm, compatible with 0.89 mm (0.035in) superhard wire and 12–18F vascular sheath. The proximal end diameter of the aortic main body stent is 23–35 mm, and its distal iliac stent diameter is 12–14.5 mm, at a length of 120–180 mm. The proximal end diameter of the aortic iliac stent is 16 mm, its distal end diameter 12–27 mm, and at a length of 95–140 mm. The extender diameter is 23–36 mm at a length of 33–45 mm.

6.3.3.6 Ankura AAA Stent Graft

Product Structure

Ankura AAA stent graft (Fig. 6.13) is the China LifeTech-produced nitinol self-expanding stent graft, which can be divided into aortic main body stent, aortic iliac stent, and aortic uni-iliac (AUI) stent. The stent is made of nitinol with a double-layer compressed ePTFE membrane which is integrated with the stent through thermal treatment, having flared bare stent design at its proximal end and featuring radial strength and better wall adhesion and anchoring capacity. The aortic main body stent is sutured with five radiopaque markers to help development. Two "8"-like markers are placed on the proximal membrane and one "V"-like marker on the distal end of the iliac stent on the same side of main body stent, a "√" marker on the distal end of the opposite iliac stent, and a "V" marker on the bifurcation of the main body stent. There is no bare stent at the proximal end of aortic iliac stent, but with a stiffener to prevent the stent from being shortened in tortuous blood vessels, and two radiopaque V-like markers on the stent. AUI stent has the same proximal end design as the aortic main body stent, with its distal end being gradually tapered.

Features and Models

The stent graft is indicated for abdominal aortic aneurysm (AAA) repair, compatible with 0.89 mm (0.035in) superhard wire and 18–23F vascular sheath. The proximal end diameter of the aortic main body stent is 24–34 mm, and its distal iliac stent diameter is 12 mm, with membrane length of 120 mm. The proximal end diameter of aortic iliac stent is 14 mm and its distal diameter 12–16 mm, at a length of 60–100 mm. AUI proximal end diameter is 24–28 mm and distal end diameter 12–14 mm, at a length of 140–160 mm.

6.3.3.7 Incraft AAA Stent Graft

Product Structure

Incraft AAA stent graft (Fig. 6.14) is the US Cordis-produced nitinol self-expanding stent graft, which consists of the aortic main body stent and aortic bifurcated iliac prosthesis. The stent is constructed of a seamless, low-porosity, woven polyester graft supported by a series of self-expanding, laser-cut, and electropolished nickel-titanium (nitinol) short stent rings which are sutured to the inner surface of the graft material. Eight or ten barbs are mounted on the proximal bare stent (the actual number of barbs depends on the tip diameter). Several radiopaque markers are sutured onto the stent to achieve stent placement accuracy.

Features and Models

The stent is indicated for the treatment of infrarenal abdominal aortic aneurysm and other aorta diseases. The stent is compatible with 0.89 mm (0.035in) superhard wire. The

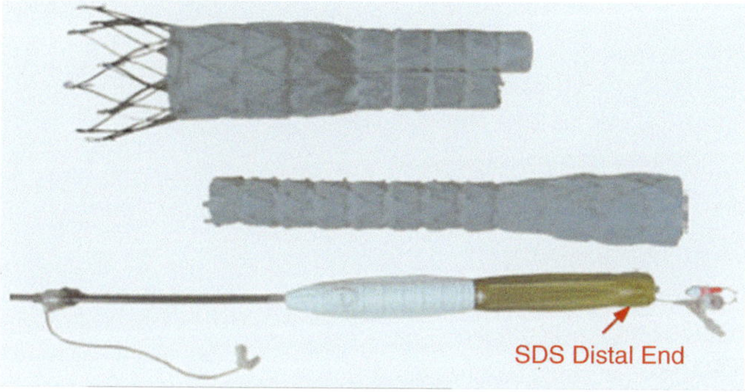

Fig. 6.14 Incraft AAA Stent Graft (Cordis)

proximal diameter of the aortic main body stent is 22–34 mm, and the distal iliac diameter is 11 mm, at a length of 94 mm and compatible with 14–16F vascular sheath. The proximal diameter of the aortic bifurcated iliac prosthesis is 13 mm and the distal diameter 10–24 mm, at a length of 82–138 mm and compatible with 12–13F vascular sheath.

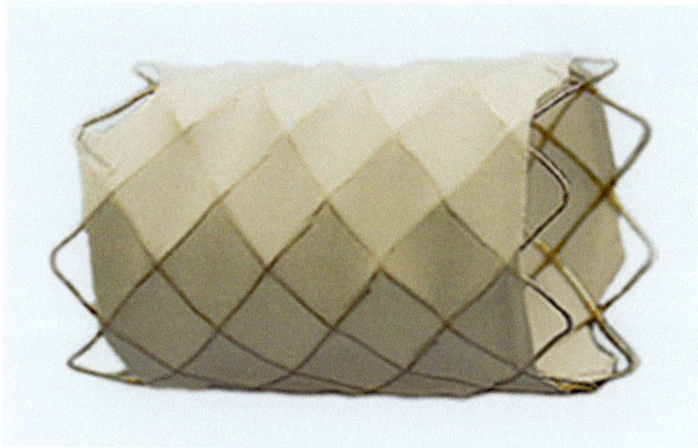

Fig. 6.15 CP Stent (NuMED)

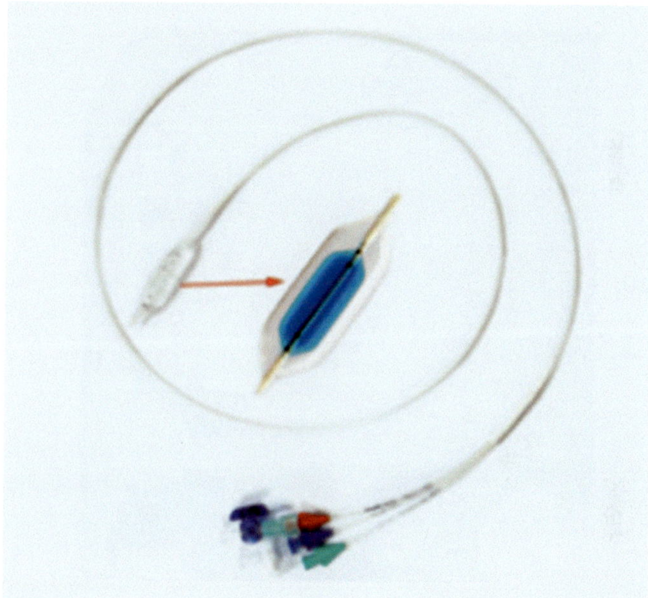

Fig. 6.16 BIB (NuMED)

6.4 CP Stent

6.4.1 Product Structure

CP Stent is a balloon-expandable stent made of platiniridium by NuMED, USA, available with two varieties: bare metal stent (Fig. 6.15) and stent graft. The bare metal stent is made of platiniridium wire arranged in rows of zigzag pattern (90% platinum and 10% iridium through thermal treatment) with its joints laser welded with 24 K gold. The stent graft is a bare metal stent covered with an extendable porous PTFE tube. CP stent is delivered to the target blood vessel via NuMED's BIB (balloon in balloon) (Fig. 6.16). The balloon is a dual-balloon design, where the diameter of the inner balloon is ½ of the outer balloon diameter and 1 cm shorter. The dual-balloon design ensures uniform inflation of the stent. The inner balloon provides initial expansion of the stent and also acts as a tool to hold the stent in place, while the outer balloon is inflated. The delivery system of the balloon uses a triaxial design, two lumens of which are used to inflate the balloon while the other functions as the wire lumen and flushing lumen. Two radiopaque platinum marker bands are placed on both ends of the work area of the inner balloon.

6.4.2 Features and Models

CP stent graft is indicated for endovascular treatment of congenital coarctation of the aorta, and aortic coarctation caused by aorto-arteritis and whose stenosis diameter is 20% larger than the adjacent blood vessels. CP bare stent is indicated for endovascular treatment of pulmonary artery, vena cava stenosis, and other vascular diseases. The stent system is compatible with 0.89 mm (0.035 in) wire and 10–14F vascular sheath, available with diameters ranging from 12 mm to 24 mm and length from 16 mm to 45 mm. The diameter of the inner balloon is 6–12 mm and that of the outer one is 12–24 mm, at length ranging from 25 mm to 55 mm. The rated burst pressure of the inner balloon is 4–5 atm and that of the outer one is 3–7 atm and the delivery system length is 112 cm.

Cardiac Aortic Valved Stent

7

Huajuan Mao, Qingsheng Lu, Jian Zhou, and Zaiping Jing

Abstract

Cardiac aortic valved stents are endovascular treatment devices for senior patients with severe calcific aortic valve stenosis. They can be classified into balloon-expanding aortic valved stents and self-expanding aortic valved stents. This chapter elaborates on their structures, features, and model types based on valved stents of different brands.

Keywords

Cardiac aortic valved stent · Structure and features · Model types

7.1 Introduction

There are two kinds of cardiac aortic valved stent systems: the balloon-expandable aortic valved stent and the self-expanding aortic valved stent. The balloon-expandable aortic valved stent is a device compressed onto a release system with a balloon, then delivered to the aortic stenosis sites via a delivery system, and injected with diluted contrast agent into the balloon via an inflation device so that the aortic valved stent is dilated to be attached to the aortic valves, thus improving the aortic blood flow. This kind of stent is advantaged in accurate positioning and less possibility of displacement. The self-expanding aortic valved stent is a device compressed onto a specific delivery device, by which the valved stent is delivered to the aortic stenosis sites and released in place, and then self-expanded to adhere to the vascular wall, thus improving the aortic blood flow. This kind of stent is advantaged in that it prevents damage to the biovalves due to balloon dilatation, and the self-expanding mechanism at superior segment of the valved stent can be more steadily fixed onto the ascending aorta, featuring strong self-expanding capacity.

Cardiac aortic valved stent is composed of a metal stent and biovalves. The metal stent can be made of stainless steel, nitinol, and cobalt-chromium alloy, and the biovalve can be bovine or porcine pericardium valves and porcine aortic valves, which differ in that the porcine aortic valves originate from porcine pericardium tissue and the porcine pericardium tissues can be cut arbitrarily after treatment, being more beneficial for bioengineering design. By virtue of unique bioengineering design, bovine or porcine pericardium valves have more superior effective orifice areas (EOA) to that of the porcine aortic valve of the same type, reduce damage to the valves caused by the turbulent flow running through the valves, and increase the service life of the valves.

At present, the foreign brands of the cardiac aortic valved stent include Edwards, Medtronic, Boston Scientific, Sadra, Direct Flow, Hansen, etc., but only Edwards and Medtronic aortic valved stents are FDA certified. Based on this, the two companies have launched their upgrade models and also passed through FDA certification in 2015. For example, outside the Sapien three-valved stent (Edwards) is an "apron" made of polyethylene glycol terephthalate (PET), which can reduce perivalvular leakage (PVL). For another example, CoreValve stent (Medtronic) allows the valve to be retracted after 2/3 having been released and has extended "apron" structure to extend the adhesion zone and reduce perivalvular leakage. Moreover, the emerging new technologies allow the use of larger valves so as to be attached more closely to the inner wall of the heart and ensure more accurate stent placement. Also, the delivery catheter further boils down to such an extent that it can access through 5 mm diameter artery, reducing vascular damage and alleviating the risk of intraoperative angiorrhexis and cerebral apoplexy.

Chinese brands include Venus Medtech, JieCheng, MicroPort, etc. At present, multicenter clinical trial has been

H. Mao · Q. Lu · J. Zhou · Z. Jing (✉)
Department of Vascular Surgery, Changhai Hospital, Second Military Medical University, Shanghai, China
e-mail: zhoujian1-2@163.com; jingzp@xueguan.net

Z. Jing et al. (eds.), *Endovascular Surgery and Devices*, https://doi.org/10.1007/978-981-10-8270-2_7

completed by Venus Medtech and JieCheng, which have been launched into the market application. This chapter mainly introduces Sapien XT balloon-expandable valved stent (Edwards), CoreValve self-expanding valved stent (Medtronic), Venus A self-expanding valved stent (Venus Medtech), J-Valve self-expanding valved stent (Jiecheng).

7.2 Sapien XT Balloon-Expandable Valved Stent

7.2.1 Product Structure

Sapien XT balloon-expandable valved stent (Fig. 7.1), the US Edwards-produced second-generation valved stent, consists of a Sapien XT valved stent, a NovaFlex delivery system, a NovaFlex catheter introducer kit, an Edwards balloon catheter, an inflation device, and a crimping device. Sapien XT valved stent uses the bovine pericardial tissue that has long been clinically evidenced for its durability, which features excellent tissue durability and is sewn onto a cobalt-chromium stent with high radial strength that can provide hemodynamic performance and consistent leaflet bonding. The Sapien XT valved stent is delivered accurately to the aortic valve lesion sites through the femoral artery by balloon dilation technique with the NovaFlex delivery system. This delivery system can guide, control, smoothly bridge, and reliably perform minimally invasive endovascular replacement of the aortic heart valves.

7.2.2 Features and Models

This valved stent system is indicated for minimally invasive endovascular replacement for the aged patients with severely calcified aortic valve stenosis. Sapien XT balloon-expandable valved stent is compatible with 0.89 mm (0.035 in) super hardwire and 18–24F vascular sheath, available with 20, 23, 26, and 29 mm specifications.

7.3 Core Valve Self-Expanding Valved Stent

7.3.1 Product Structure

Core valve self-expanding valved stent system (Fig. 7.2) is the US Medtronic-produced second-generation valved stent, manufactured by suturing three-valve leaflets made from a porcine pericardium onto a self-expanding nitinol frame which is directly laser-cut from a 50 mm nitinol tube. The inferior segment of the device has higher radial tension that it expands itself to squeeze the calcified aortic valve onto the wall at the aortic root and prevent deformation of the device itself. The middle segment is narrow supportive leaflet, avoiding influence on the incision of the coronary artery. The superior segment is rather wide so that the device can be anchored inside the ascending artery and ensures the stability of the long axle. The stent is made of nitinol, and the valve becomes flexible and liable of deformation in iced water. The valve can be compressed into the delivery system, and it can expand itself under normal body temperature,

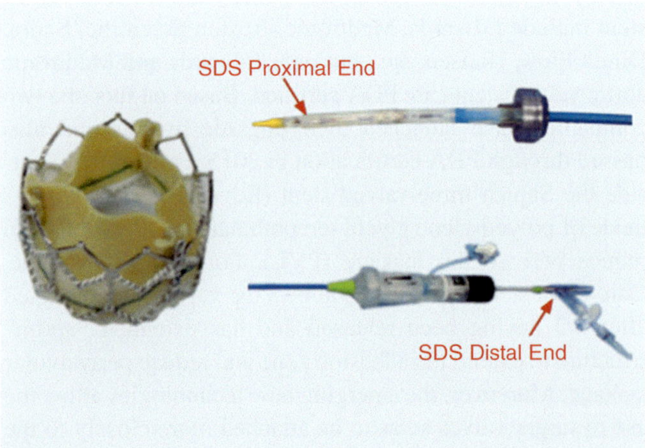

Fig. 7.1 Sapien XT balloon-expandable valved stent (Edwards)

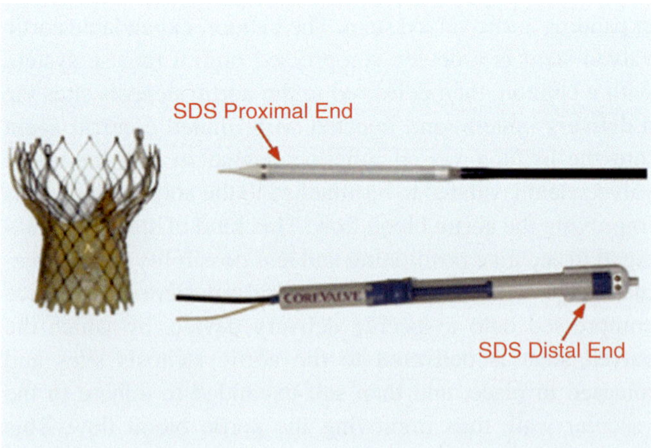

Fig. 7.2 Core valve self-expanding valved stent (Medtronic)

which has higher radial tension to make the device anchored at specified sites. The long axle of the stent can be self-adjusted to certain extent, being beneficial for postoperative device stability and ensuring stable hemodynamic stability of the patients. When the distal end of the device is released by 2/3, and if the device positioning is unsatisfactory (hyponasty position), the device can be readjusted. If the device fails to expand in place, especially in severely calcified aortic valves, the valve can be further dilated through the balloon, preventing damage to the sewn valves in the stent.

7.3.2 Features and Models

This valved stent system is indicated for minimally invasive endovascular replacement for the aged patients with severely calcified aortic valve stenosis. Core valve self-expanding valved stent system is compatible with 0.89 mm (0.035in) super hardwire and 18–20F vascular sheath, available with 23 mm, 26 mm, 29mm, and 31 mm specifications.

7.4 Venus A Self-Expanding Valved Stent

7.4.1 Product Structure

Venus A self-expanding valved stent system (Fig. 7.3), the China's Venus Medtech-produced first-generation valved stent, consists of an aortic valved stent (PAV), a vascular delivery catheter system (DCS), and a compression loading system (CLS). The PAV is a biovalve sewn into the self-expanding stent and can be retracted when being released to 2/3, but it cannot be retracted when being fully released. The valve tissue is made of a single-layer porcine pericardium sewn onto a nitinol frame consisting of three parts. The self-expanding nitinol stent system features excellent biocompatibility. The frame is a simple diamond structure, where the trabeculae of the stent have different lengths and widths to suit for heterogeneous cylindrical expansion. The central part is molded to accommodate the artificial valve tissue and prevent influence on the incision of the coronary artery. The entire frame can be fully visualized under X-ray. PAV valve is a tri-leaflet structure made of a single-layer porcine pericardium, where the tri-leaflets are attached onto a fan-shaped skirt (also made of single-layer pericardium) and sutured with PTFE suture in the vascular flow direction of the valve. Subsequently, this part of the device is sewn onto the PAV support frame (with 5.0 PTFE suture). The flow-in skirt design is the same as the stent form.

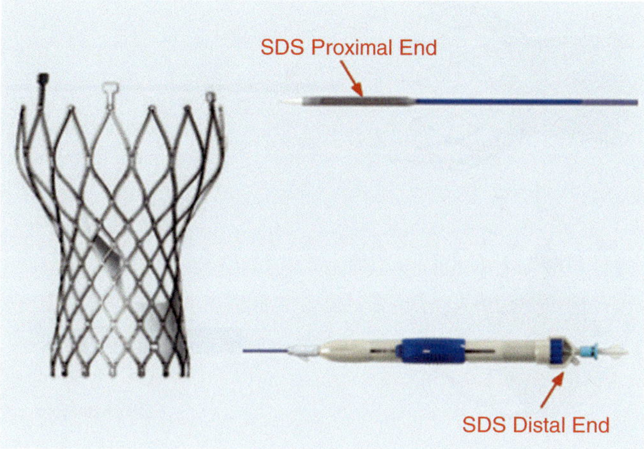

Fig. 7.3 Venus A self-expanding valved stent (Venus Medtech)

7.4.2 Features and Models

This valved stent system is indicated for minimally invasive endovascular replacement for the aged patients with severely calcified aortic valve stenosis. Venus A self-expanding valved stent is compatible with 0.89 mm (0.035in) super hardwire and 18–20F vascular sheath, available with 20 mm, 23 mm, 26 mm, 29 mm, and 32 mm specifications.

7.5 J-Valve Self-Expanding Valved Stent

7.5.1 Product Structure

J-Valve self-expanding valved stent system (Fig. 7.4),the China's Jiecheng-produced first-generation valved stent,consist of a valved stent and a trans-apical implant of artificial bioprosthetic heart valve, among which the valved stent consists of a medical fabric tube, a porcine aortic heart valve leaflet, positioning piece, support and medical suture line. The transapical implant of artificial bioprosthetic heart valve consists of a valve loading system, an operating system and other accessories. The valve loading system contains a nose cone and a cannula, of which the nose cone is made of acetal resin and the cannula PEBAX. The operating system contains three control buttons, one release button and one handle.

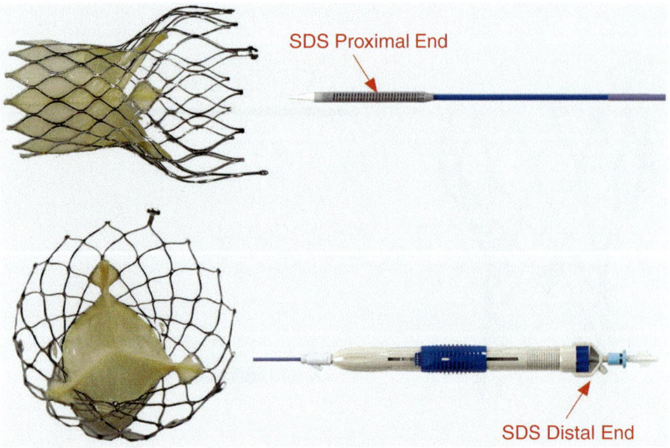

Fig. 7.4 J-Valve Self-Expanding Valved Stent (Jiecheng)

7.5.2 Features and Models

The valved stent system is suitable for the replacement therapy for the elderly patients complicated with severely calcified stenotic aortic valves, aortic insufficiency or the combination thereof. The valve bioprothesis is compatible with 0.89 mm (0.035 in.) super-stiff wire, 27–33F vascular sheath and available with models of 21 mm, 23 mm, 25 mm, 27 mm and 29 mm.

8 Vena Cava Filter

Huajuan Mao, Junmin Bao, and Wenping Hu

Abstract

Vena cava filters are filter units designed to prevent the dropped embolus of the inferior vena cava system from pulmonary artery embolism. They are classified into temporary filters and permanent filters. Based on different brands, this chapter elaborates on the structures, features, and model types of filters.

Keywords

Vena cava filter · Structure and features · Model types

8.1 Introduction

Vena cava filter is a filter device designed to prevent pulmonary embolism caused by dislocation of the inferior vena cava system. Vena cava filter mainly includes temporary filters and permanent filters. In recent years, the retrievable filter has become more and more widely used in clinical practice, which can be used as a permanent filter for long-term placement or as a temporary filter. However, the retrievable filter has certain time requirement for body implantation, which, if recovered within the specified time limit, has a high retrieval rate, hence reducing risks originated from long-term in vivo retention as well as the occurrence of related complications. At the same time, vena cava filter's prevention of pulmonary embolism is not limited to the prevention of emboli from the inferior vena cava system source but extends to its possible use in the superior vena cava.

At present, vena cava filter brands include B. Braun, Cordis, Cook, Boston Scientific, Bard, LifeTech, etc. This section mainly introduces TempofilterII (B. Braun), VenaTech Convertible (B. Braun), Denali (Bard), Optease (Cordis), and Aegisy (LifeTech) vena cava filters.

8.2 Tempofilter II Vena Cava Filter

8.2.1 Product Structure

Tempofilter II vena cava filter system (Fig. 8.1), the German B. Braun-produced temporary filter, consists of a wire, a catheter, an introducer, and a filter device. The wire is made of PTFE-coated AISI304V stainless steel. The introducer is composed of an introducer sheath, a ring, a dilator, and a Luer lock. The filter material is ductile cold-formed cobalt-nickel-chromium-molybdenum alloy. The material of the indwelling catheter is fluorinated ethylene propylene (FEP) containing barium sulfate, and the fixation device is made of silicon resin. The introducer system of Tempofilter II consists of a 10F dilator and a 12F catheter sheath, made of chromium-cobalt-nickel alloy.

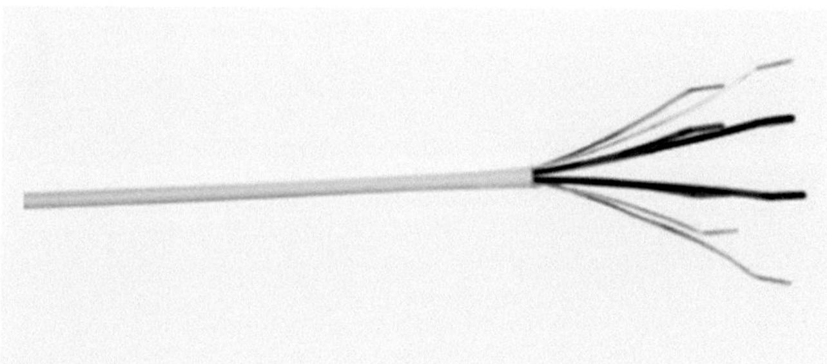

Fig. 8.1 Tempofilter II vena cava filter (B. Braun)

H. Mao (✉) · J. Bao · W. Hu
Department of Vascular Surgery, Changhai Hospital, Second Military Medical University, Shanghai, China
e-mail: czymm8@163.com

Z. Jing et al. (eds.), *Endovascular Surgery and Devices*, https://doi.org/10.1007/978-981-10-8270-2_8

8.2.2 Features and Models

The filter system is indicated for preventing temporary pulmonary embolism and other endovascular treatment. The filter is implanted through the right internal jugular vein at an indwelling time of 12 weeks maximum. The maximum diameter of the filter is 28 mm. Capture is not required and it is withdrawn just by directly pulling out the filter rod. The delivery sheath is 70 cm in length, equipped with a 150-cm long type J PTFE-coated wire.

8.3 VenaTech Convertible Vena Cava Filter

8.3.1 Product Structure

VenaTech Convertible vena cava filter system (Fig. 8.2), the German B. Braun-produced convertible vena cava filter, consists of a convertible filter, an introducer sheath system, and a shaft. The taper-designed filter is made of cobalt-chromium alloy, with a small hook at the upper portion of the filter and a mechanical lock device at its lower portion, where the small hook is caught by the snare and the introducer sheath faces downward to hold against the tip of the filter and maintain certain tension to function as a temporary filter.

Pull outward the snare and open the safety lock. When the safety lock opens, maintain tension and pull upward the small hook. The filter device can also be used as a permanent filter to be placed in the vena cava (similar to a stent). On the filter are four upward and downward barbs, respectively, which are used to prevent filter displacement and are parallel to the vena cava vascular wall which will not cause damage to the vena cava wall. This convertible filter is pre-loaded into the cartridge through femoral or jugular vein approach.

8.3.2 Features and Models

This filter system is indicated for endovascular treatment for the prevention of pulmonary embolism and vena cava stenosis and can be used as a permanent or temporary filter through mechanical lock conversion. The filter is suitable for vena cava vessels in maximum 32 mm diameter with a 12.9F ID introducer sheath. Additional 0.89 mm (0.035 in) type J wire, snare, and 9F catheter need to be equipped for removal of the small hook at the top of the filter.

8.4 Denali Vena Cava Filter

8.4.1 Product Structure

Denali vena cava filter system (Fig. 8.3) is the US Bard-produced recyclable filter and can be used as a permanent or temporary filter. The filter consists of 12 shape-memory laser-cut nickel-titanium appendages. These 12 appendages form two levels of filtration with the filter arm providing the upper level of filtration together with its wedged shoulder design available for autonomous center positioning and avoiding filter inclination and the lower leg providing the lower level of filtration in tri-paired length design, anchored on the vena cava wall, being beneficial for separation upon retrieval. The anchors of the filter are puncture-protected, preventing the filter leg line from coming out.

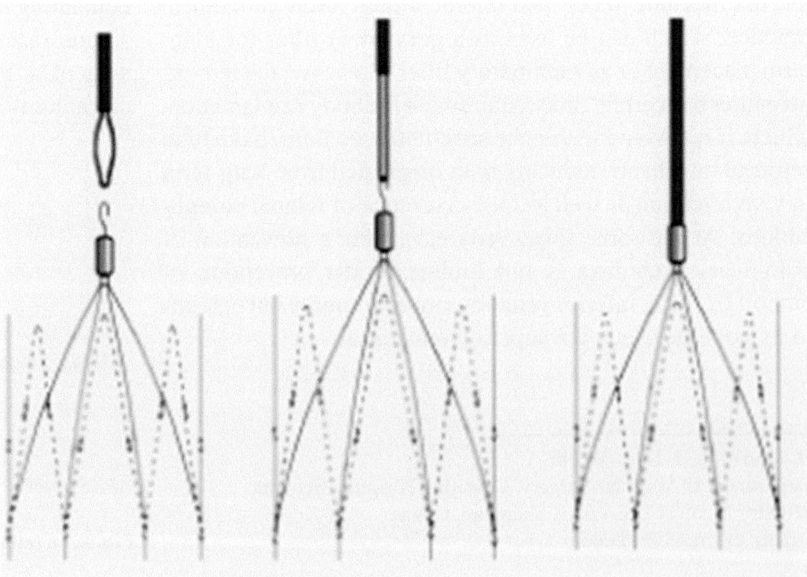

Fig. 8.2 VenaTech Convertible vena cava filter (B. Braun)

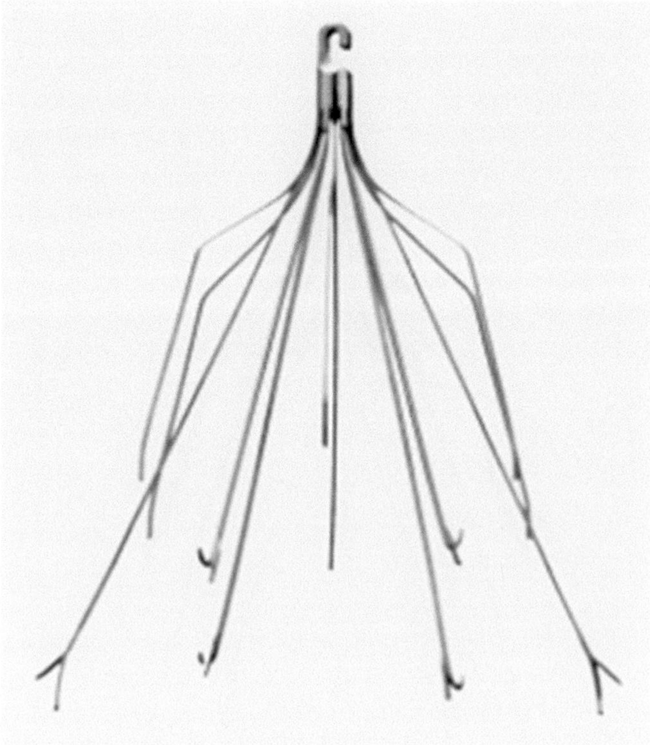

Fig. 8.3 Denali vena cava filter (Bard)

8.4.2 Features and Models

Denali vena cava filter is indicated for preventive treatment of pulmonary artery embolism and other diseases with inferior vena cava diameter of less than or equal to 28 mm and can be delivered through femoral, jugular, and subclavian vein approach, each of which has a separate delivery system. This filter is a vena cava filter with ultra-long time window at maximum 454 days upon in vivo implantation, averaging 136 days. US FDA-approved maximum retrieval time window is 632 days.

8.5 Optease Vena Cava Filter

8.5.1 Product Structure

Optease vena cava filter system (Fig. 8.4), the US Cordis-produced temporary filter, is made of laser-cut nitinol tube, with six diamond struts on both ends, for capturing blood clots and fixing it to the vascular wall. At the distal end of the filter is a retrieval hook, facilitating filter recovery and snaring. The filter, upon deployment, will exert outward expanding force on the luminal surface of the inferior vena cava, and the self-centering design ensures accurate positioning and stable structure that avoids filter tilting.

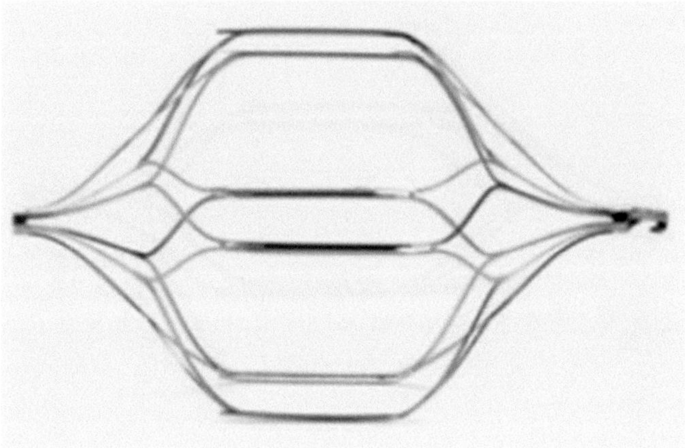

Fig. 8.4 Optease vena cava filter (Cordis)

8.5.2 Features and Models

This filter system is indicated for preventive treatment of pulmonary artery embolism, inserted via jugular, femoral, and antecubital veins with maximum in vivo indwelling time of 14 days, while FDA-approved retrieval time is 23 days. This filter suits with vena cava vessels with 30 mm diameter or below, compatible with 0.89 mm (0.035in) wire and available with 55–90-cm long delivery sheath.

8.6 Aegisy Vena Cava Filter

8.6.1 Product Structure

Aegisy vena cava filter system (Fig. 8.5), the China LifeTech-produced retrievable filter, consists of a 6F delivery sheath, a sheath core, a 6F introducer sheath, a delivery cable, and a filter. The filter is made of nitinol tube and the delivery system of Pebax. The tip and the end have embedded threads, respectively, which can be connected with the delivery cable, controllable in rotation and release, thus avoiding filter's forward jump during deployment.

This filter is of horizontally symmetric basket design with single-layer filtration and vertically asymmetric structure, which poses limited influence on hemodynamics after emboli capturing. The filter is fixed on the vascular wall by anchors, and the symmetric vertical support is attached closely to the vascular wall, not liable of tilting.

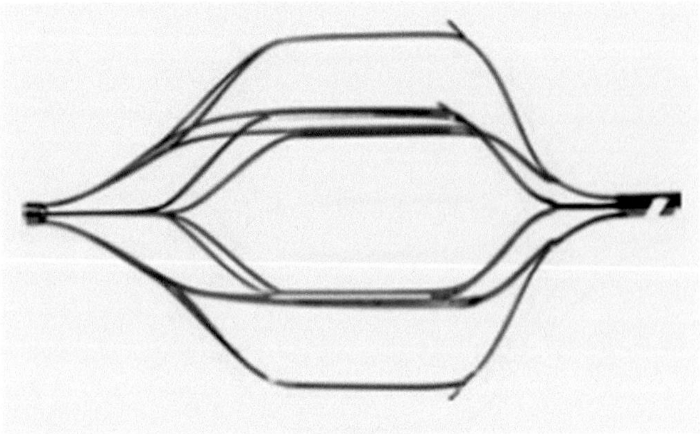

Fig. 8.5 Aegisy vena cava filter (LifeTech)

8.6.2 Features and Models

This filter adopts asymmetric lantern design with single-layer design, featuring controlled release and accurate placement in clinical practice. The filter is indicated for preventive treatment of pulmonary artery embolism by insertion via femoral or jugular artery. The retrievable time of the filter is generally 12–14 days, exceeding which, retrieval may be inadequate. Otherwise, it may lead to difficult retrieval and damage to the inferior vena cava. The filter is compatible with 0.89 mm (0.035in) wire and available with 18 mm × 40 mm, 25 mm × 50 mm (the former two models need to be ordered in advance), and 32 mm × 60 mm (conventional order), among which the maximum diameter of the filter is 32 mm and delivery sheath length is 55 cm.

8.7 Celect Vena Cava Filter

8.7.1 Product Structure

Celect vena cava filter system (Fig. 8.6), the US Cook-produced selectively retrievable filter, consists of a filter, an introducer, a coaxial introducer sheath, and a dilator with hydrophilic coating. The coaxial sheath dilator has eight side ports and two radiopaque markers arranged at 30 mm increment (end-end). The filter is made of cobalt-chromium alloy, and the filter looks like a cone upon deployment with its four major struts and eight accessory wire. There are two kinds of introducers: the femoral or the jugular vein approach. The NavAlign delivery system of a new generation has a single-key release handle, with side ports and markers on its tip to facilitate imaging and measurement of vena cava lumens.

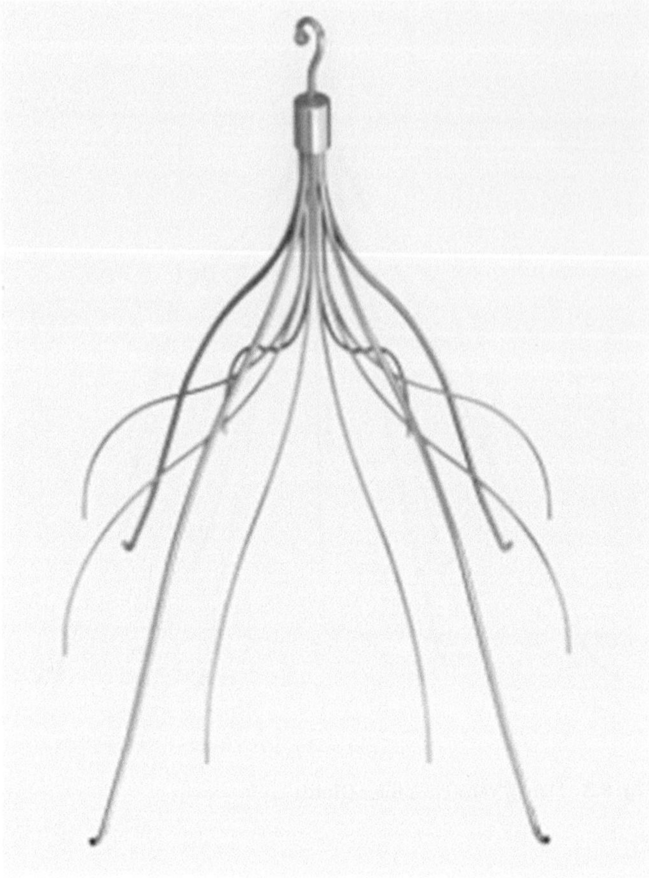

Fig. 8.6 Celect vena cava filter (Cook)

8.7.2 Features and Models

This filter system is indicated for holding up venous thrombus and preventing pulmonary embolism, suitable for vena cava vessels with an implantation diameter of 15–30 mm. The NavAlign delivery system is available with 7F introducer sheath at a length of 65 cm.

8.8 Option Vena Cava Filter

8.8.1 Product Structure

Option vena cava filter system (Fig. 8.7), the US Argon-produced retrievable filter, consists of a catheter sheath, an angiographic vessel dilator, a pusher with deployment marker, an Option filter, and a sheath cap. The Option filter is laser-cut from nitinol alloy tubing, consisting of shape-memory nitinol struts emanating from a central location, with a retrieval hook located at the caudal portion of the filter. Letters and arrows are printed on the filter storage tube for identifying the filter approach direction, where the femoral artery approach is marked green and the jugular artery approach blue.

8.8.2 Features and Models

This filter system is indicated for preventive treatment of pulmonary embolism, characterized by the hollow body design of the filter to facilitate wire access, by which the filter is delivered in place along the wire and released without removing the wire so as to enhance the stability of the filter and reduce the occurrence of shifting. Option vena cava filter suits for vena cava with implantation diameter up to 30 mm, available for maximum 175 days of in vivo indwelling time, compatible with 0.89 mm (0.035 in) wire at 6.5F delivery sheath O.D. and 70 cm in length.

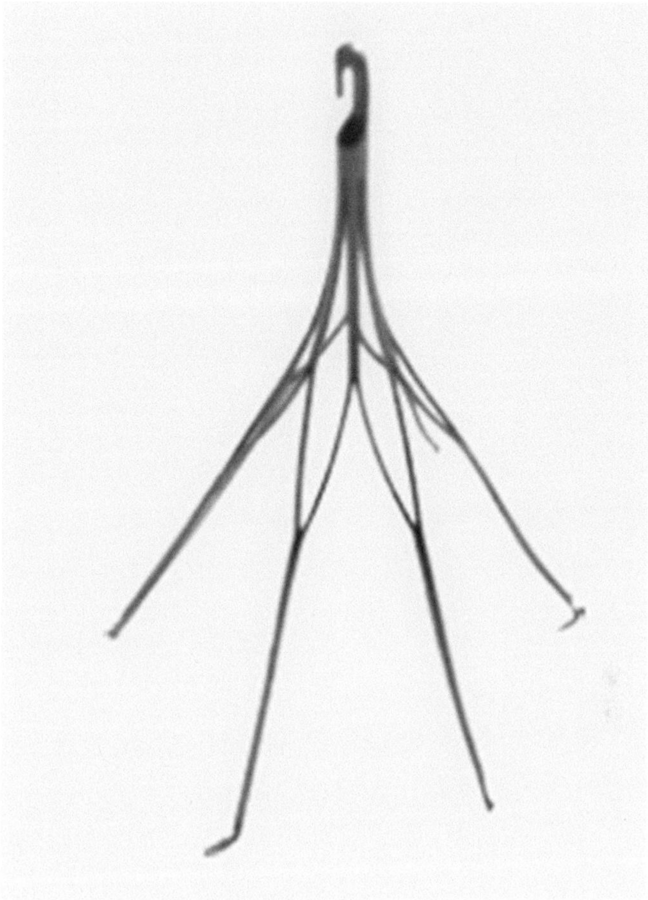

Fig. 8.7 Option vena cava filter (Argon)

Vascular Prosthesis

9

Huajuan Mao, Fuxiang Wang, and Junmin Bao

Abstract

Vascular prostheses are vascular grafts used for severe vascular stenosis, occlusion, and interpositional transplantation. They are mainly made of nylon, Dacron, ePTFE, PU, and other polymer-composite materials. This chapter elaborates on their structures, features, and model types based on vascular prostheses of different brands.

Keywords

Vascular prosthesis · Structure and features · Materials and model types

9.1 Introduction

Vascular prosthesis is a vascular graft for the treatment of severe vascular stenosis, occlusion, and indirect transplantation, mainly composed of nylon, Dacron, expanded polytetrafluoroethylene (ePTFE), and polyurethane (PU). At present, vascular prosthesis is mainly indicated for systemic vascular bypass surgery. The vascular grafts mainly originate from autogenous vein and vascular prosthesis. Autogenous vein will not produce rejection upon in vivo implantation and has natural anticoagulation function and biocompatibility. However, not everyone is qualified for autogenous vein transplantation, and vascular prosthesis is still needed for adjuvant therapy.

H. Mao (✉) · F. Wang · J. Bao
Department of Vascular Surgery, Changhai Hospital, Second Military Medical University, Shanghai, China
e-mail: czymm8@163.com

9.1.1 Materials of Vascular Prosthesis

9.1.1.1 Dacron

Vascular prosthesis made of this material is liable of reaction with peripheral tissues, resulting in extensive platelet aggregation, liable of formation of thrombus, with low biocompatibility. This is the material used in early time. Anticoagulation measures should be taken before the use of this kind of vascular prosthesis, and it is usually used for high-profile vascular transplantation.

9.1.1.2 ePTFE

Vascular prosthesis made of this material shows excellent biocompatibility, withstands artery pressure, and has superior antithrombosis performance to the vascular prosthesis made of other materials. Its peculiar micropore structure enables the human tissue cells and blood vessels to grow into the micropores and form tissue bonding like the autogenous tissues. However, it is disadvantaged in low compliance and lower graft patency as compared with the autogenous vein graft. This kind of material is often used to produce vascular prosthesis with 6–10 mm aperture and mostly used in clinical practice.

9.1.1.3 PU

Vascular prosthesis made of this material shows similar compliance to natural blood vessels, featuring excellent rebound resilience, wear resistance, and aging resistance and is available for faster endothelialization. However, as an in vivo graft, it will still cause inflammatory response to human bodies and result in such reactions as blood clotting and endotheliosis when contacting with blood. Therefore, the performance should be further improved while using this kind of material. PU is the optimum material for making vascular prosthesis with aperture of less than 6 mm.

Z. Jing et al. (eds.), *Endovascular Surgery and Devices*, https://doi.org/10.1007/978-981-10-8270-2_9

9.1.2 Characteristics of Vascular Prosthesis

- Histocompatibility and hemocompatibility
- Similar dynamic performance with blood vessels
- Effective close-up with blood vessels
- Ability to maintain vascular patency and not liable of formation of thrombus
- Stable performance
- Tolerance to artery pressure
- Excellent fracture resistance, free from deformation under compression
- Without rejection reaction
- Anti-inflammation
- Easy suturing, without endoleak

At present, vascular prosthesis brands include Gore, Bard, Terumo, etc. This chapter mainly introduces Gore-Tex (Gore) and Impra (Bard) vascular prosthesis.

9.2 Gore-Tex Vascular Prosthesis

9.2.1 Product Structure

The US Gore-produced Gore-Tex vascular prosthesis (Fig. 9.1) is made of ePTFE with FEP rings, and the graft materials contains silica gel and blue dyes.

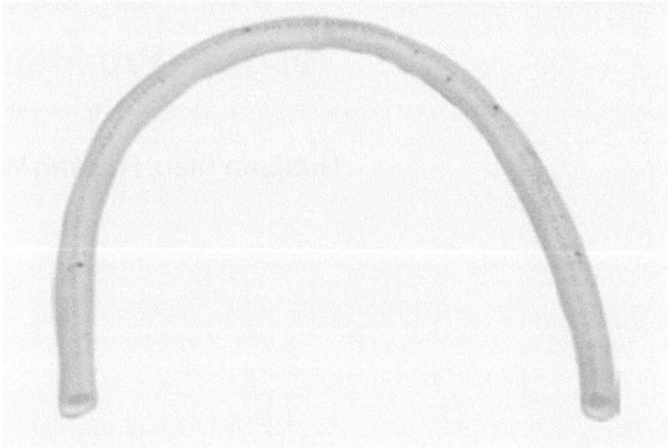

Fig. 9.1 Gore-Tex vascular prosthesis

9.2.2 Features and Models

Gore-Tex vascular prosthesis is characterized by:

1. Outer reinforcement film: Enhance vascular burst resistance and suture pull resistance, enable tissue cells to grow in and gradually vascularize with its microporous structure, reduce formation and adhesion of thrombus, and focalize any infection once upon occurrence.
2. Longitudinal stretch: Refers to the ability of the vascular prosthesis to rebound longitudinally upon adequate stretching, so as to reduce anastomotic bleeding, provide length tolerance for vascular prosthesis cutting, improve anastomotic consistency, and reduce bending and twisting of vascular prosthesis.
3. Bending resistance and twisting resistance: Retractable FEP outer support ring can increase the bending and twisting resistance of vascular prosthesis. The outer supportive ring can be retracted during operation according to actual intraoperative requirements, causing no damage to the outer reinforcement film. The thin-wall vascular prosthesis is more similar to human vascular wall thickness, ensuring more convenient surgical suturing. The blue marker line serves intraoperative positioning and provides reference for avoiding vascular twisting.

Gore-Tex vascular prosthesis can be used for angiorrhaphy or for treatment of vascular occlusion or aneurysm, trauma, dianalysis, etc. At present, the clinically used vascular prosthesis has rings or no rings, and the vascular prosthesis with rings is further classified as the inner ring and the outer ring. The commonly used vascular prosthesis at present is of 6–8 mm inner diameter and 300–500 mm in length.

9.3 Impra Vascular Prosthesis

9.3.1 Product Structure

The US Bard-produced Impra vascular prosthesis (Fig. 9.2) is made of ePTFE, with its inner wall added with carbon element and overall external helical design (support ring).

9.3.2 Features and Models

This vascular prosthesis is indicated for bypass or reconstruction surgery for peripheral artery vessels. At present, the commonly used vascular prosthesis is available with 6–8 mm in diameter and 300–500 mm in length.

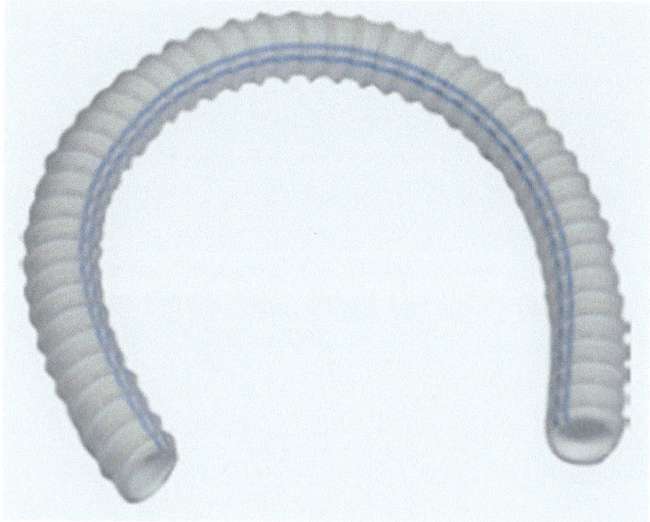

Fig. 9.2 Impra vascular prosthesis (Bard)

Other Endovascular Devices

10

Huajuan Mao, Fuxiang Wang, Junmin Bao, and Ye Lu

Abstract

Other endovascular devices refer to endovascular treatment devices that are related to therapeutic equipment or that cannot be properly classified, like the thrombus aspiration system, mechanical thrombectomy system, peripheral atherectomy system, true lumen reentry catheter, spring ring, liquid embolism system, snare, cerebrospinal fluid drainage kit, Turbo Elite laser fiber-catheter system, memory ASDO atrial septal defect occlusion device, etc. This chapter introduces the abovementioned devices from the perspectives of their structures, features, model types, brands, and so forth and offers a series of conclusion and summary about the operating steps of therapeutic equipment.

Keywords

Other endovascular devices · Structure and features · Model types · Usage in operation

10.1 Aspiration Thrombectomy System

10.1.1 Product Structure

AngioJet aspiration thrombectomy system of US Boston Scientific consists of the Ultra console and thrombectomy device. The aspiration thrombectomy system and its consumable items make use of the Bernoulli principle of fluid mechanics, that is, high-speed fluid or gas can produce low pressure, thus generating a vacuum effect. This device can be used to remove thrombus ≥3 mm in diameter.

H. Mao (✉) · F. Wang · J. Bao · Y. Lu
Department of Vascular Surgery, Changhai Hospital, Second Military Medical University, Shanghai, China
e-mail: czymm8@163.com

The Ultra console is used to control the thrombectomy device (Fig. 10.1), drive the running of the pump, and regulate fluid flow in and out. After having been energized, the LCD console panel will show the total saline content and

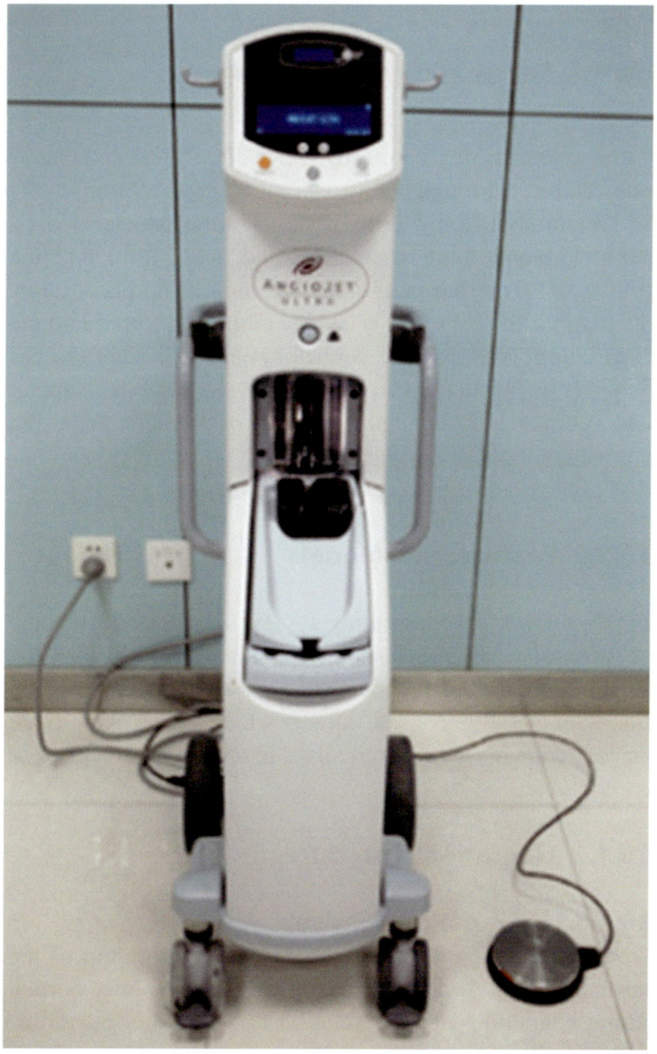

Fig. 10.1 Ultra console

Z. Jing et al. (eds.), *Endovascular Surgery and Devices*, https://doi.org/10.1007/978-981-10-8270-2_10

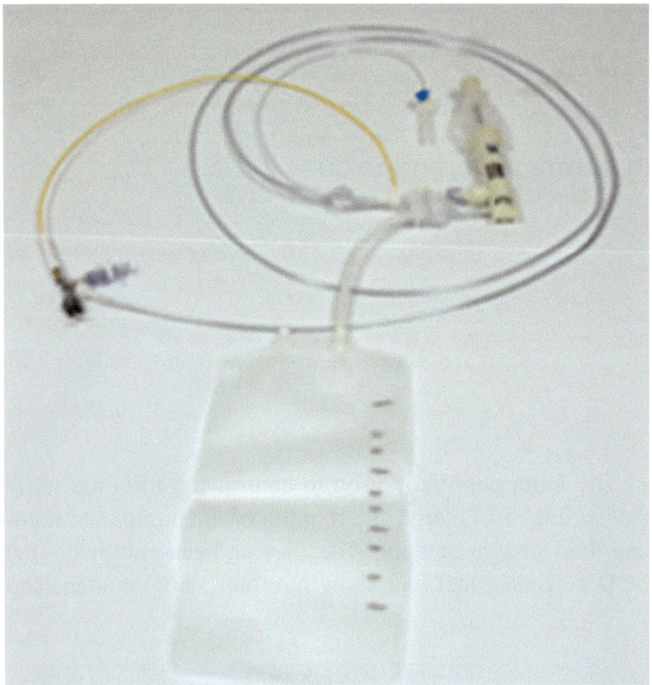

Fig. 10.2 Thrombectomy device (Boston Scientific)

Ultra system failure reports, by which adjustment and operation can be performed before aspiration thrombectomy.

The thrombectomy device consists of the catheter body, a pump, a waste fluid bag, saline, and waste fluid pipeline (Fig. 10.2). The four parts constitute an integral part. Below the pump is the bar code. When the pump is inserted into the Ultra control system, the control system will scan the bar code via its infrared ray to identify the model of the catheter and automatically configure relevant parameters, requiring no manual input of any parameter.

10.1.2 Features and Models

This aspiration thrombectomy system is indicated for acute or subacute venous and artery thromboembolic vascular diseases. There are seven models of catheters used in conjunction with the Ultra console, among which 4F, 5F, and 6F are currently the most commonly used in clinical practice.

10.1.3 Operation Procedures

10.1.3.1 Prepare the Console

Open and check the Ultra console, insert the pump of the thrombectomy device, prepare a bag of 500 mL normal saline containing heparin solution (500 mL normal saline +50 mg heparin sodium injection), and insert the syringe needle of the thrombectomy device fluid bag into the prepared diluted heparin saline bag.

10.1.3.2 Load the Catheter

Fully immerse the catheter tip of the thrombectomy device into the heparinized saline, and step down the foot pedal to load the catheter till the console screen displays "0," and then loosen the foot pedal. At this time, the display system is ready. During the aspiration procedure, total time and total perfusion volume will be displayed on the screen.

10.1.3.3 Aspiration Mode

Aspiration can be performed upon completion of Step 2.

10.1.3.4 Thrombolysis Mode

6F thrombectomy device can also be used for drug-spraying thrombolysis. Hang a bag of normal saline mixed with urokinase drugs (100 mL normal saline + 250,000 units of urokinase, or adjust preparation proportion according to actual intraoperative situations) on the other side, and insert the needle of the fluid bag of the thrombectomy device. Double-click the "Catheter" button on the console, then press the "∨" button, and choose to enter thrombolysis mode ("∨" indicates yes and "∧" no), and double-click the "Catheter" button on the console again to confirm the selection. At this time, the screen displays "PP." Step on the foot pedal to spray the diluted urokinase solution into the vascular thrombus site. Upon completion of thrombolysis, insert the needle of the fluid bag of the thrombectomy device into the prepared heparin saline diluent. Double-click the "Catheter" button on the console, and then press "∧" button to select to enter the aspiration mode, click the "Catheter" button, and repeat the aspiration operation.

10.2 Mechanical Thrombectomy System

10.2.1 Product Structure

The Swiss Straub-produced Straub Mechanical Thrombectomy System consists of a Rotarex catheter (Fig. 10.3), an Aspirex catheter (Fig. 10.4), and a Straub medical power system (Fig. 10.5), where the Rotarex catheter is indicated for mechanical thrombectomy of artery thrombus and the Aspirex catheter for that of venous thrombus.

The rotating Rotarex catheter contains a rotating tip driven by a rotary spiral. The rotating tip consists of two stacked metal cylinders with a pair of side holes. The outer cylinder is connected with the rotary spiral and the inner one

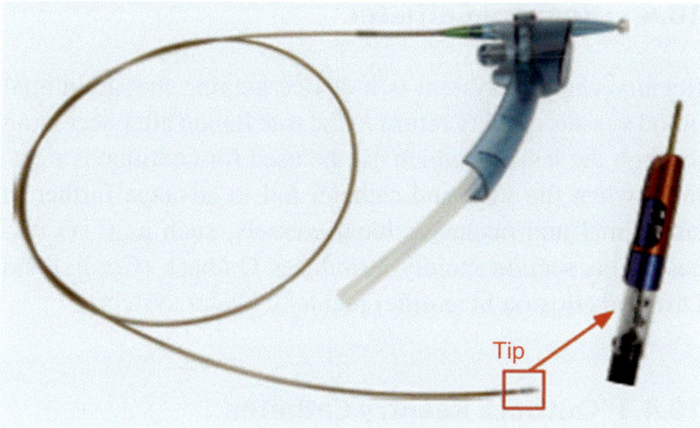

Fig. 10.3 Rotarex aspiration catheter (Straub)

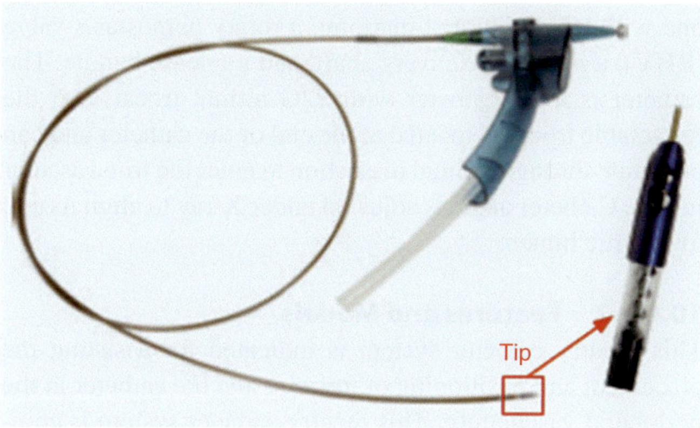

Fig. 10.4 Aspirex aspiration catheter (Straub)

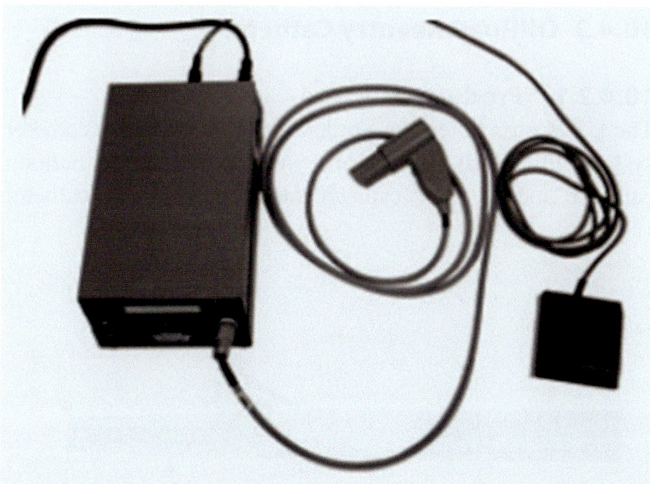

Fig. 10.5 Straub medical power system

with the catheter axle. The rotary outer cylinder has several sections at its front-most end, which constitute the rotary structure and by which the catheter tip grinds the embolus in front. Meanwhile, the rotary outer cylinder produces strong vortex in the blood vessels, and all dislocated emboli subsequently enter the side holes of the cylinder. Inside the rotary tip, the debris of various sizes is broken into microparticles and carried away by the transfer screw into the in vitro collection bag via the inner lumen. During this process, the vascular wall will not be affected, for there is no sharp edge outside the rotary tip and the catheter needs not to and also should not contact the vascular wall during operation.

The Aspirex catheter contains a catheter tip, inside which is a rotary spiral that can access through a window inside the catheter tip for catheter aspiration to break up and remove fresh acute thrombus or emboli. The catheter tip is a smooth circle, and the catheter is designed to ensure that when the wire is placed in the lumen and sufficient blood flow runs across the neighboring zones, any accidental contact with the vascular wall will not cause damage to the wall. Compared with Rotarex catheter, it differs in that the Aspirex catheter tip is not equipped with several rotary sections to avoid the scratching of venous valves when placed in the veins.

The power transmission between the Straub medical power system and the rotary catheter is realized via a magnetic clutch. This noncontact power transmission mechanism between the medical power system and the catheter enables the system to completely cover the unsterilized motor with the sterilized cloth of the catheter kit and connect the sterilized motor with the sterilized rotary catheter.

10.2.2 Features and Models

This mechanical thrombectomy system is indicated for mechanical thrombectomy of any acute, subacute, and chronic occlusive thrombus, emboli, and atherosclerotic materials in blood vessels except for the heart, pulmonary and coronary arteries, and cerebral circulation, at 60000RPM speed and maximum aspiration capacity (i.e., maximum blood loss) of 45–180 mL/min. The wire equipped within the Straub medical power system goes through special fusing process and can be used under high temperature due to the high-speed rotation of the rotary spiral. The Rotarex catheter is compatible with 6F and 8F (10F not available on Chinese market) 0.46 mm (0.018 in) wire, at a length available ranging from 85 to 135 cm. The Aspirex catheter is compatible with 8F and 10F 0.46 mm (0.018 in) wire, at a length available ranging from 85 to 135 cm.

10.3 Peripheral Plaque Excision System

10.3.1 Product Structure

The US Medtronic-produced SilverHawk (first generation)/TurboHawk (second generation) peripheral plaque excision system (Fig. 10.6) consists of a cutter catheter and a cutter driver, wherein the distal end of the cutter catheter is the embedded miniature rotary blade mounted inside the catheter sheath. At the proximal end of the catheter are a connector and a positioning handle. The handle can be connected with the accompanying batteries to drive the embedded rotary blade. When the catheter is connected with the cutter driver, retract the positioning handle and start the motor simultaneously to offset the distal end of the cutter sheath and reach the target lesion sites. This will make the embedded rotary blade stretch out. When the blade rotates, the catheter is pushed forward slowly to access through the lesion sites and then to scratch out the occlusive materials in arteries. The excised tissues are captured and then stored in the proximal catheter tip. If excision work needs to be terminated, push forward the positioning handle to retract the embedded blade into the sheath, and restore the cutter to its "No Offset" position to automatically turn off the system.

10.3.2 Features and Models

SilverHawk plaque excision system is indicated for endovascular treatment of primary and restenotic atherosclerotic lesion in the peripheral arteries (femoral, iliac, and infrapopliteal arteries). TurboHawk, an upgrade of the SilverHawk, has stronger cutting performance and suits more for the excision of severely calcified lesions. The system is compatible with 0.36 mm (0.014 in) wire; the catheter tip is 4.3–9 cm in length; the catheter is 6–8F in diameter and 135 cm in length.

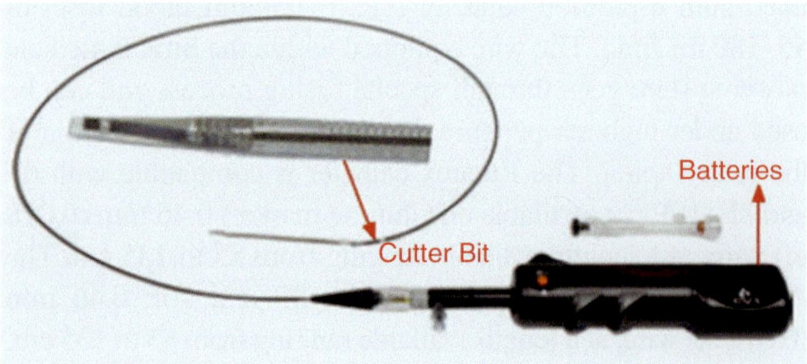

Fig. 10.6 SilverHawk peripheral plaque excision system (Medtronic)

10.4 Reentry Catheter

Reentry catheter system is a device helping the subintimal blood vessels quickly return to the true lumen after accessing through the lesions, which can be used for continuous treatment when the wire and catheter fail to advance further in subintimal and occlusive blood vessels, such as CTO disease. This section mainly introduces Outback (Cordis) and OffRoad (Boston Scientific) reentry catheter systems.

10.4.1 Outback Reentry Catheter

10.4.1.1 Product Structure

The US Cordis-produced Outback reentry catheter system (Fig. 10.7) consists of a 22G trocar, a catheter shaft, a nosecone with LT directional marking, a rotary hemostasis valve (RHV), a proximal delivery shaft, and a release handle. The catheter is a 5F catheter with 22G nitinol trocar, and the retractable trocar is located at the end of the catheter and can penetrate through intimal dissection to enter the true vascular lumen. Catheter angle is adjusted under X-ray to align its end to the true lumen.

10.4.1.2 Features and Models

This reentry catheter system is indicated for assisting the placement and positioning of the wire and the catheter in the peripheral vasculature. This reentry catheter system is compatible with 0.36 mm (0.014in) wire and 6F vascular sheath, with effective catheter length of 120 cm.

10.4.2 OffRoad Reentry Catheter

10.4.2.1 Product Structure

The US Boston Scientific-produced OffRoad reentry catheter system (Fig. 10.8) consists of a wedged positioning balloon catheter and a micro-catheter lancet. The micro-catheter

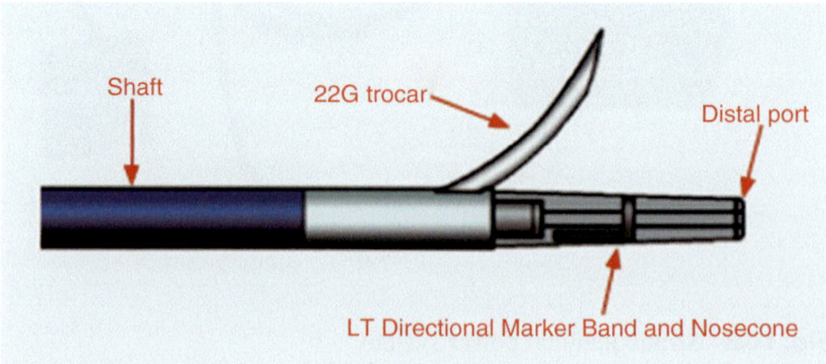

Fig. 10.7 Outback reentry catheter (Cordis)

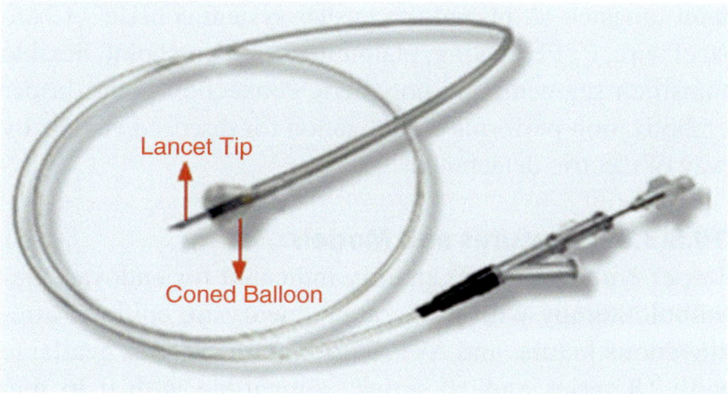

Fig. 10.8 OffRoad reentry catheter system (Boston Scientific)

lancet is a single-lumen hypotube catheter with a lancet, which is advanced coaxially to the preset position inside the lumen of the positioning balloon catheter and passes through the distal tip of the dilated balloon. The OTW-type wedged positioning balloon catheter has 5F delivery shaft and balloon mounted at its distal end. Because the intima and the media have different stress, the round shape and flexible neck of the wedged balloon ensure the balloon to enter the true lumen from the vascular intima by natural rotation or tilting. There is a radiopaque marker band inside the balloon body.

10.4.2.2 Features and Models

This reentry catheter system is indicated for vascular reentry operation for peripheral lesion sites with inner diameter ≥ 4 mm. The OffRoad balloon catheter is available with 5.4 mm in diameter and 70–100 cm in length. The micro-catheter lancet is 0.79 mm (0.031in) in outer diameter and 79–109 cm in length, compatible with 0.36 mm (0.014 in) wire.

10.5 Embolization

Embolization is mainly indicated for endovascular embolotherapy for aneurysms, arteriovenous malformations, arteriovenous fistula, AVF, as well as endoleak following endovascular aortic repair and other vascular diseases. Currently on the market, embolization is mainly divided into free embolization, electric detachable ring, mechanical detachable ring, water detachable ring, etc. Free embolization has no connection with the pusher unit, and additional wire is needed to push the embolization, while electric, mechanical, and water detachable rings are connected with the pusher unit, available for repeated adjustment of the placement position and form of the embolization. The embolization can be detached via various methods after position adjustment. Therefore, these three kinds of embolizations are controllable rings. At present, embolization brands mainly include Cook, Boston Scientific, Medtronic, MicroVention (already purchased by Terumo), Achieva, etc. This section mainly introduces Cook, Interlock (Boston Scientific), and Jasper (Achieva) embolizations.

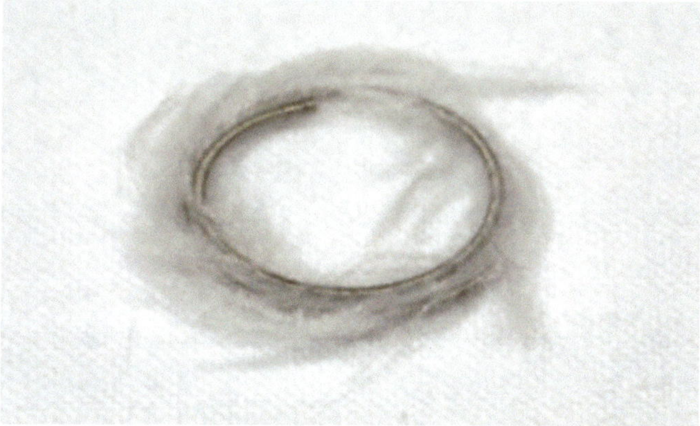

Fig. 10.9 Embolization (Cook)

10.5.1 Cook Embolization

10.5.1.1 Product Structure

The US Cook-produced embolization (Fig. 10.9) is a free coil, consisting of stainless steel wire and synthetic fiber. The supportive force of stainless steel coil is superior to that of platinum one. Moreover, the fibrous hair outside the coil can accelerate thrombogenesis of the embolism site and enhance the effect of embolization. Under fluoroscopy, 0.89 mm (0.035in) hardened wire can be used to be inserted from the end of the loading tube and advance the embolization into the catheter till it reaches the position to be embolized.

10.5.1.2 Features and Models

Cook's embolization is indicated for embolotherapy for complicated medium and small blood vessels. The coil is compatible with 0.89 mm (0.035 in) wire and 5F catheter. The embolization has 2–15 mm diameter upon deployment, at a length ranging from 20 mm to 140 mm.

10.5.2 Interlock Embolization

10.5.2.1 Product Structure

The US Boston Scientific-produced Interlock embolization (Fig. 10.10) is a controllable coil, consisting of platinum tungsten alloy wire and synthetic fiber. The coil is mechanically connected with a coil delivery wire via the interlock

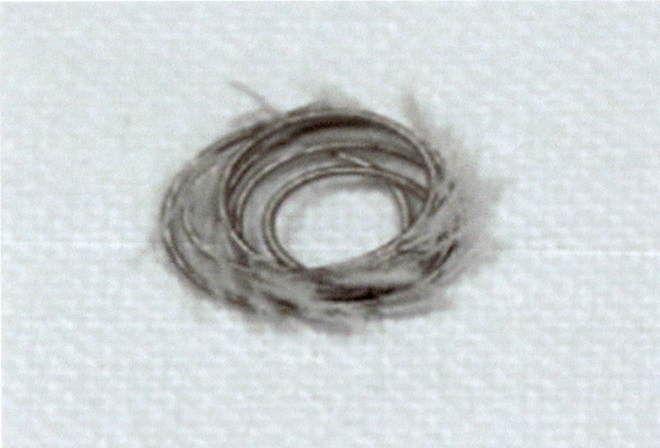

Fig. 10.10 Interlock embolization (Boston Scientific)

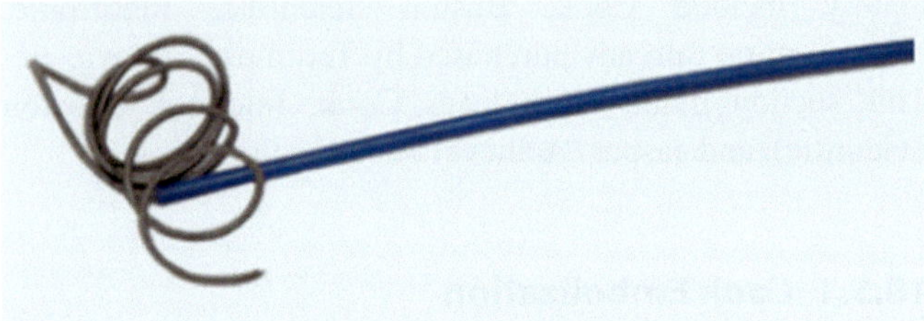

Fig. 10.11 Jasper embolization (Achieva Shanghai)

arm and is sealed within a sheath introducer. The coil is made of platinum tungsten alloy, and the synthetic fiber contained in the coil can achieve better coagulation effect. Under fluoroscopy, the coil system is advanced by a micro-catheter with inner diameter ≥ 0.53 mm (0.021 in). The interlock delivery wire enables the coil position to be adjusted before finally advancing to the embolized vessels. The coil can be repeatedly retracted for repositioning before detachment.

10.5.2.2 Features and Models

Interlock embolization is indicated for endovascular embolotherapy for visceral artery aneurysm, arteriovenous fistula, AVF, aortic endoleak, and other diseases. The embolization coil is available with 35 series and 18 series. The 35 series products are compatible with 0.89 mm (0.035 in) wire, at a diameter of 3–20 mm upon deployment and a length of 40–400 mm. The products of 18 series are compatible with 0.46 mm (0.018 in) wire, at a diameter of 3–14 mm upon deployment and a length of 60–300 mm.

10.5.3 Jasper Embolization

10.5.3.1 Product Structure

The China's Achieva-produced Jasper embolization (Fig. 10.11) is a controllable coil, consisting of an embolization and a pusher system. The embolization is made of platinum tungsten alloy, and the pusher system consists of bare steel wire, PTFE coating, platinum developing point, flexible transition segment, and polymeric connection point. Jasper embolization performs embolization for diseased vessels by way of electric detachment.

10.5.3.2 Features and Models

Jasper embolization is mainly indicated for endovascular embolotherapy with intracranial aneurysm, epidural arteriovenous fistula, and AVF. This embolization is available with 18 series and 10 series, compatible with 0.36 mm (0.014 in) and 0.46 mm (0.018 in) wires, with compatible micro-catheter diameter larger than 1.7F. The coils of 18 series are 6–20 mm in diameter upon deployment, available with a length ranging from 20 mm to 300 mm, and the 10 series coils are 3–10 mm in diameter upon deployment, available with a length ranging from 4 mm to 300 mm.

10.6 Liquid Embolic System

10.6.1 Onyx Liquid Embolic System

10.6.1.1 Product Structure

The US Medtronic-produced Onyx liquid embolic system (Fig. 10.12) is composed of a 1.5 mL vial of Onyx liquid embolic agent, a 1.5 mL vial of DMSO (dimethyl sulfoxide), and two 1 mL Onyx syringes and one 1 mL DMSO syringe. DMSO is a special solvent, and a DMSO-compatible delivery micro-catheter is used to access the embolization site (catheters of other materials may be corroded with the DMSO solvent). The DMSO solvent will dissipate in blood and tissue fluid. Onyx® is a nonadhesive liquid embolic agent composed of EVOH (ethylene vinyl alcohol) copolymer dissolved in DMSO (dimethyl sulfoxide) solvents and sus-

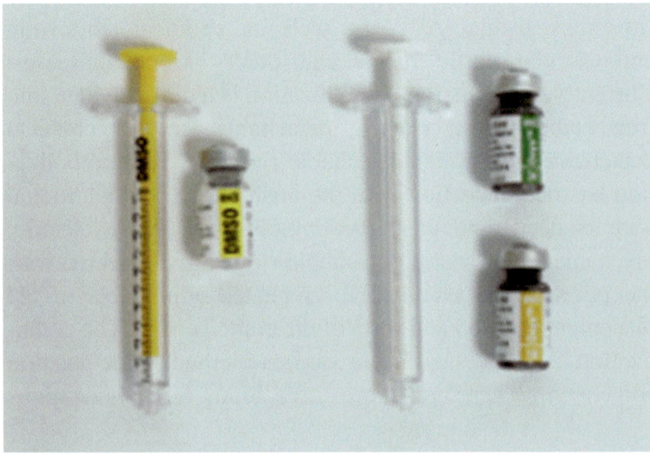

Fig. 10.12 Onyx liquid embolic system (Medtronic)

pended micronized tantalum powder to provide contrast for visualization under fluoroscopy. The EVOH copolymer and suspended tantalum precipitate in situ into a spongy and coherent embolus. The polymeric embolus solidifies and immediately forms a kin from the outside to the inside while traveling more distally in the lesion. The Onyx liquid embolic agent should be heated and shaken before being slowly and controllably injected to the embolic sites from the micro-catheter.

10.6.1.2 Features and Models

Onyx liquid embolic system is indicated for endovascular embolotherapy for arteriovenous malformation and highly vascular tumors. Onyx liquid embolic agents are available in three formulations: Onyx-18 (6% EVOH), Onyx-20 (6.5% EVOH), and Onyx-34 (8% EVOH).

10.6.2 Human Fibrin Sealant

10.6.2.1 Product Structure

The China's RAAS-produced human fibrin sealant (Fig. 10.13) is composed of lyophilized human fibrinogen, lyophilized human thrombin, sterilized injection water, and calcium chloride water, wherein the sterilized injection water and calcium chloride water are used for diluents in preparation. The excipients of the human fibrinogen are sodium chloride, sodium citrate, and sucrose, while the excipients of human thrombin are glycine and trismetyl aminomethane.

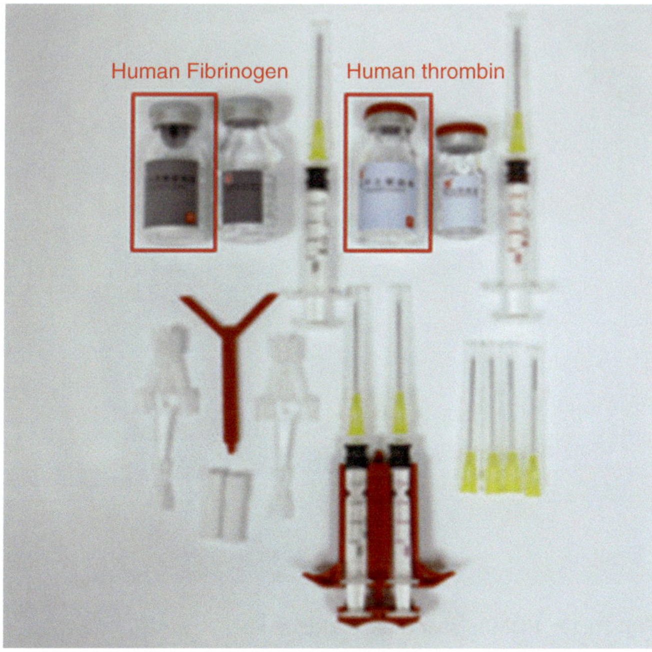

Fig. 10.13 Human fibrin sealant

10.6.2.2 Features and Models

This product is indicated for treatment of errhysis with general surgical abdominal incision, hepatic surgery wound and vascular surgical wound, and also for aneurysm repair. There is only one formulation available for this product.

10.7 Snare

10.7.1 Single-Loop Snare

10.7.1.1 Product Structure

The China's shape-memory alloy-produced single-loop snare (Fig. 10.14) consists of memory nitinol alloy wire, 304 stainless steel pipe, gold-plated tungsten loop, and PTFE catheter. The front end of the snare is circular loop, and the portion connected with the circular loop is the extension of the loop wire angled at about 90°. The snare looks like a stretched line under tensile force. When the external force is removed, it recovers automatically to its preset shape.

10.7.1.2 Features and Models

This snare is indicated for the removal of vascular foreign bodies and recovery of the temporary filter. The snare is available with 15–20 mm deployment diameters, compatible with 6F catheter.

10.7.2 Three-Loop Snare

10.7.2.1 Product Structure

The US Argon-produced Atrieve three-loop snare (Fig. 10.15) consists of a dislodge with three loops, an introducer catheter, an introducer, and a torque device. The dislodge with three loops is made of nitinol alloy, the sheath material of the snare is 304 stainless steel, the introducer catheter and the introducer are made of medical-grade FEP and medical-grade HDPE, and the catheter tip is mounted with radiopaque platiniridium marker ring. The three-loop design of the snare increases the success of foreign body capture in blood vessels.

10.7.2.2 Features and Models

The snare is indicated for the removal of vascular foreign bodies and recovery of the temporary filter. The three-loop snare is available with a diameter ranging from 2 mm to 45 mm, compatible with 3.2F–7F catheters.

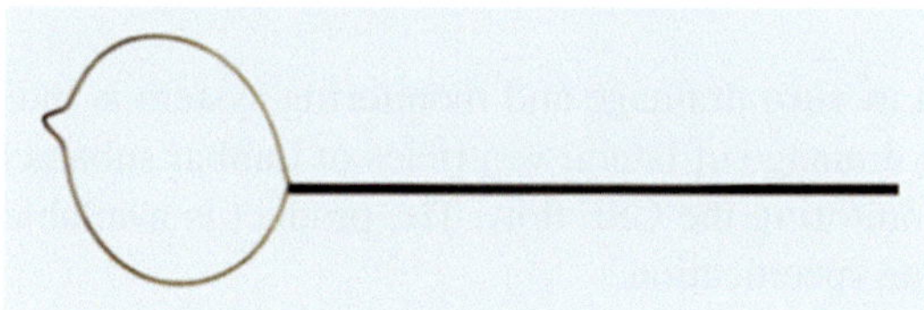

Fig. 10.14 Shape-memory single-loop snare

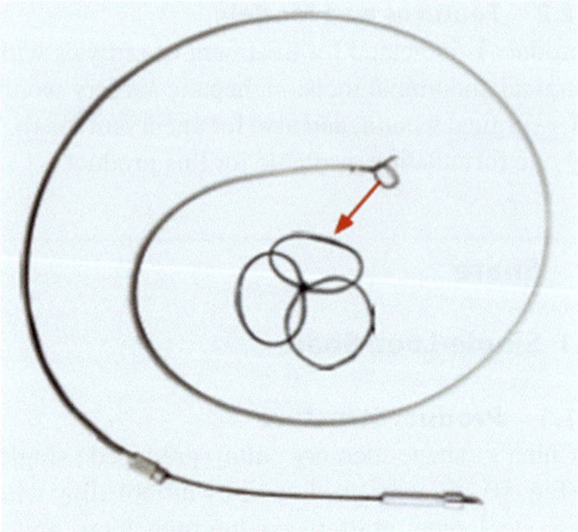

Fig. 10.15 Atrieve three-loop snare (Argon)

10.8 Cerebrospinal Fluid (CSF) Drainage Kit

Exacta In Vitro Drainage and Monitoring System

10.8.1 Product Structure

The US Medtronic-produced Exacta in vitro drainage and monitoring system consists of Exacta in vitro drainage and monitoring system (Fig. 10.16) and the EDM lumbar catheter (Fig. 10.17). Exacta in vitro drainage and monitoring system is mainly indicated for external drainage and monitoring cerebrospinal fluid (CSF) and intracranial pressure while EDM lumbar catheter for CSF drainage and/or proximal component for monitoring from the lumbar subarachnoid.

Exacta in vitro drainage and monitoring system consists of a graduated cylinder with a stopcock and microbial filtration membrane air holes, non-stretchable colored connector with a stopcock, zero reference stopcock attached to the graduated pole clamp, and detachable collection bag close to the volume scale and with microbial filtration air holes.

10.8.2 Features and Models

Exacta in vitro drainage and monitoring system is indicated for the drainage of lateral ventricles or lumbar subarachnoid and monitoring the CSF flow. The product is available only with one specification.

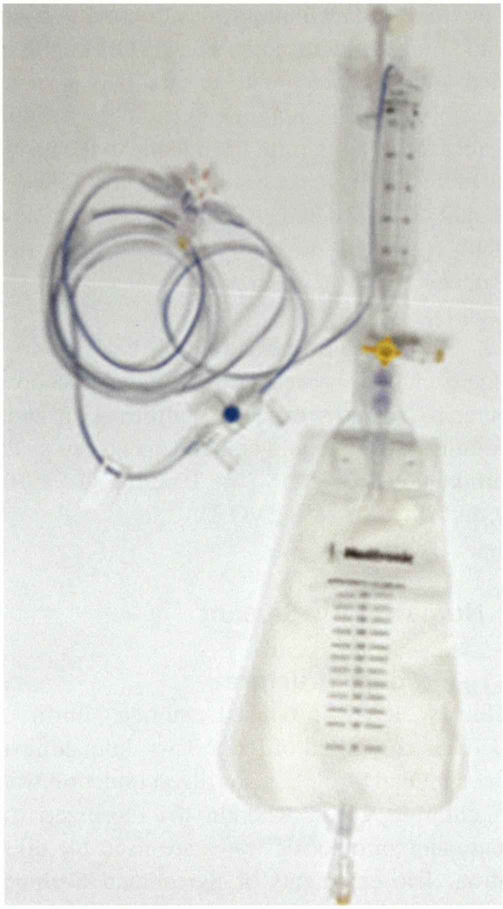

Fig. 10.16 Exacta in vitro drainage and monitoring system (Medtronic)

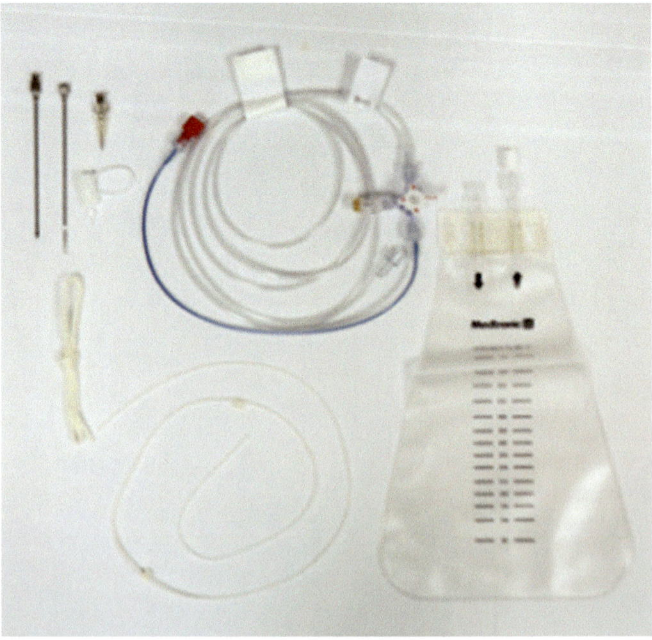

Fig. 10.17 EDM lumbar catheter (Medtronic)

10.9 Turbo Elite Laser Fiber-Optic Catheter System

10.9.1 Product Structure

The US Spectranetics-produced Turbo Elite laser fiber-optic catheter consists of CVX300 excimer laser system (Fig. 10.18) and Turbo Elite laser fiber-optic catheter (Fig. 10.19). Turbo Elite catheter consists of a bundle of optical fibers centered with a wire lumen for transmitting excimer laser light at 308 nm. Each catheter consists of a large bundle of optical fibers. Therefore, Turbo Elite catheter with different diameters will produce different magnitudes of energy. The catheter with 0.9 mm diameter provides about 0.83 W power while that of 2.0 mm about 3.79 W.

The emission wavelength of the laser transmitter of the CVX300 excimer laser system is 308 nm ultraviolet, and this wavelength is similar to that of the laser transmitter used on LASIK surgery. This wavelength is different from the wavelength emitted by CO2 laser transmitter (infrared ray at 10000 nm wavelength) or holmium-YAG laser transmitter (infrared ray at 2100 nm wavelength). When high voltage is applied to the mixture of xenon and hydrogen chloride, ultraviolet at 308 nm wavelength will be emitted. Under this circumstance, the inert xenon gas is ionized to form a molecule containing a chloridion. The molecule (excited dimer or excimer) exists only several nanoseconds before being separated into other elements. This separation will emit molecular bond energy by way of 308 nm ultraviolet photon.

The light at 308 nm wavelength emitted by the Turbo Elite catheter works on the tissue via three kinds of mechanism:

1. Photochemical effect: Billions of molecules of the plaque tissue absorb 308 nm photon energy. This energy absorption will cause molecular vibration and subsequently disconnect the chemical bond that binds the molecules together. This process takes 125 ns.
2. Photothermal effect: The secondary effect of the molecular vibration due to energy absorption by photons is to heat and evaporate the moisture in the adjacent cells, and this process takes 100 μs.

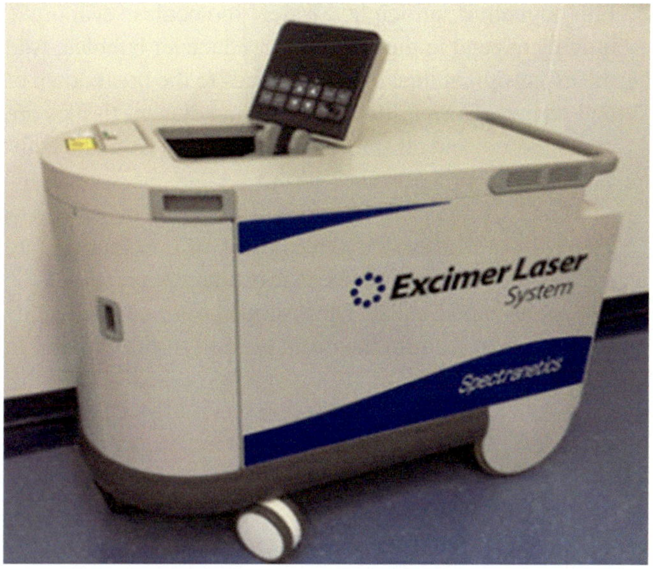

Fig. 10.18 CVX300 excimer laser system (Spectranetics)

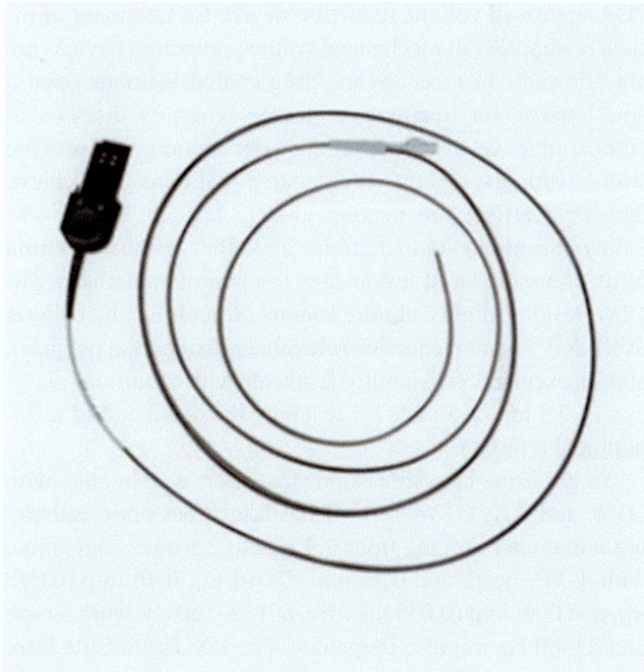

Fig. 10.19 Turbo Elite laser fiber-optic catheter (Spectranetics)

3. Photodynamic principle: Water molecules evaporate, quickly expand in the cells, and produce air bubbles. And the expansion of the air bubbles leads to the breakdown of cell tissues. During this process, the adjacent tissues are decomposed, and all spin-offs are removed from the catheter tip. This process takes 400 μs.

The spin-offs after the three kinds of mechanism are water, gas, and small particles of less than 25 μm (twice the size of white blood cells). During operation, normal saline needs to be injected into the distal portion of the catheter to remove these spin-offs.

10.9.2 Features and Models

This laser fiber-optic catheter is indicated for minimally invasive endovascular recanalization treatment of patients with severe atherosclerotic stenosis and occlusion of lower extremities. Turbo Elite laser fiber-optic catheter is the only FDA-approved volume reduction device for treatment of in-stent restenosis (all mechanical volume reduction devices are not allowed). In recent years, drug-coated balloons open a new horizon for treatment of lower extremity diseases in clinical practice, and the excimer laser therapy will provide strong support for the drug-coated balloons to achieve long-term efficacy in treating in-stent restenosis and ischemia of severe lower extremities and other lesions by virtue of its pretreatment of lesion sites (including moderately calcified lesions, highly fibrotic lesions difficult for the balloon to access), volume reduction role (ablation of partial plaques), and its excellent crossability (catheter with minimum diameter of 0.9 mm available for reaching the distal end of infrapopliteal arteries).

Turbo Elite laser fiber-optic catheter is available with OTW and RX: OTW Turbo Elite laser fiber-optic catheter has a diameter ranging from 0.9 mm to 2.5 mm, compatible with 4–8F sheath and 0.36 mm (0.014 in), 0.46 mm (0.018 in), and 0.89 mm (0.035 in) wire, at 112–150 cm work length and 25–80 Hz impulse frequency. The RX Turbo Elite laser fiber-optic catheter has a diameter ranging from 0.9 mm to 2.0 mm, compatible with 4–7F sheath and 0.36 mm (0.014 in)wire, at 150 cm work length and 25–80 Hz impulse frequency.

10.10 Memory ASDO (Atrial Septal Defect Occluder)

10.10.1 Product Structure

The China's shape-memory alloy-produced memory ASDO (atrial septal defect occluder) (Fig. 10.20) is an occluder in dual-disc shape made of braided shape-memory nitinol wire. Inside the nitinol stent is filled with polyester fiber membrane, and on both ends of the stent is a steel sleeve made of A31723 stainless steel for fixation of the nitinol wires on both ends. On the end of the other steel sleeve is a nut to be matched with the screw on the pusher tip of the delivery device.

10.10.2 Features and Models

This occluder is indicated for the treatment of patients with congenital heart disease with secondary secundum atrial septal defects. The disc diameter of the occluder is 6–34 mm upon deployment, compatible with 7–14F sheath.

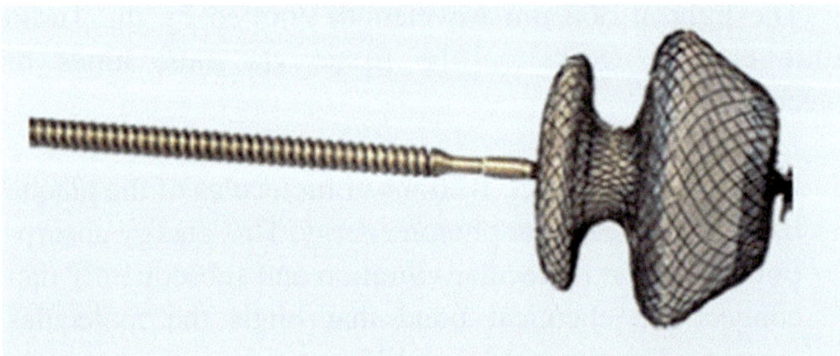

Fig. 10.20 Memory ASD (atrial septal defect) occluder (shape memory)

Part II

Application of Endovascular Surgery and Devices

11 Angiography

Zaiping Jing, Huajuan Mao, Junmin Bao, Yifei Pei, and Xiaolong Wei

Abstract

Angiography is a very important auxiliary examination widely applied to the clinical diagnosis and treatment of many vascular diseases. By virtue of its accuracy, efficiency, a high detection rate, and other advantages, it is usually regarded as the golden standard on the diagnosis of vascular diseases. However, as an invasive examination, it faces puncture point-related complications and other problems which have attracted the attention of vascular surgeons. This chapter mainly gives an introduction to angiography's indications, contraindications and preoperative preparations, arteriopuncture technique, venipuncture technique, etc.

Keywords

Angiography · Puncture · Indication

11.1 Introduction

Angiography is an auxiliary technique of examination that injects radiopaque contrast media into the blood vessel to accurately reflect the location and extent of vascular lesions according to the contrast image displayed under the X-ray, helping the physician to identify the cause, control the progression of the disease, and improve the prognosis of patients, hence improving the survival rate. Angiography is now widely used in clinical diagnosis and treatment of various vascular diseases. But as an invasive operation, angiography also poses risks. Therefore, in clinical practice, the indications and contraindications of angiography should be strictly observed.

Z. Jing (✉) · H. Mao · J. Bao · Y. Pei · X. Wei
Department of Vascular Surgery, Changhai Hospital, Second Military Medical University, Shanghai, China
e-mail: Jingzp@xueguan.net

11.1.1 Indications for Angiography

- Intrinsic vascular lesions, such as primary or secondary hemorrhage, vascular stenosis, thrombosis, aneurysms, arteriovenous fistula, AVF, etc.
- Differential diagnosis of soft tissues or organ lesions with vascular lesions
- Understanding blood supply or relationship with major blood vessels before performing some tumor operations
- Postoperative follow-ups for vascular lesions
- Minimally invasive endovascular treatment for vascular lesions

11.1.2 Contraindications for Angiography

- Patients showing positive or obvious allergic constitution in iodine allergy test
- Patients with severe heart, liver, and renal failure
- Patients with severe disorder of coagulation
- Patients with malignant thyroid hyperfunction and multiple myeloma
- Patients with severe systematic infection or inflammatory puncture site
- Patients of 3-month pregnancy

11.1.3 Preoperative Preparation of Angiography

11.1.3.1 Physicians Who Perform the Angiography Should

- Get familiar with the case history of the patients, and understand in detail various laboratory tests and auxiliary information on examination, with particular attention paid to liver, kidney, and coagulation functions.
- Explain to the patients the purpose of imaging and possible imaging process, dispel their misgivings, and obtain their cooperation.

Z. Jing et al. (eds.), *Endovascular Surgery and Devices*, https://doi.org/10.1007/978-981-10-8270-2_11

- Before the angiography, explain to the patients' family members the purpose of imaging and any possible accidents, including any possible complications during and after the angiography and angiography failure, obtain understanding of their family members, and ask them to sign the informed consent for operation.
- According to the specific clinical requirements, refer to the site, nature, and scope of the lesion and other relevant information, and design optimum angiography program.
- Check if the X-ray machine and auxiliary device function normally and if the equipment is complete and compatible.

11.1.3.2 Preparation of Patients

- Before angiography, perform necessary laboratory tests and other auxiliary examinations for the patients (including conventional chest radiographs, ECG, and ultrasound examination, if necessary).
- Before angiography, perform the test of iodine allergy in the patients.
- Prepare skin of the puncture site, and clean and reduce the possibility of local injection.
- Before angiography, decide whether the patients need to be prohibited from drinking water according to their actual situations (patients with general anesthesia or lumbar anesthesia are prohibited from drinking water 8 h before operation).
- Thirty minutes before angiography, administrate the patients with 10 mg diazepam (valium) via intramuscular injection (if necessary).

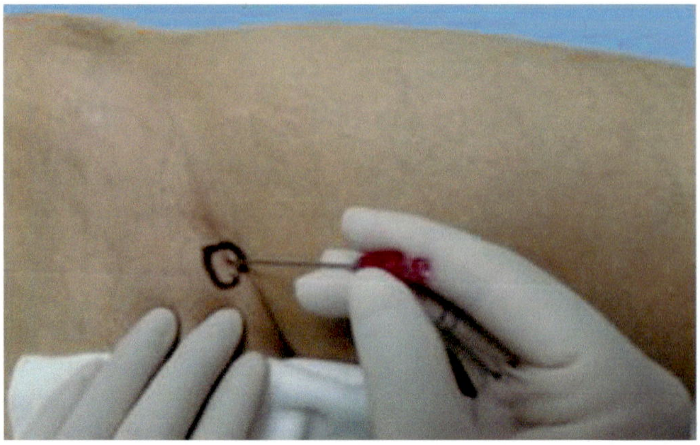

Fig. 11.1 Common femoral artery retrograde puncture (source: Changhai Hospital, for reference only)

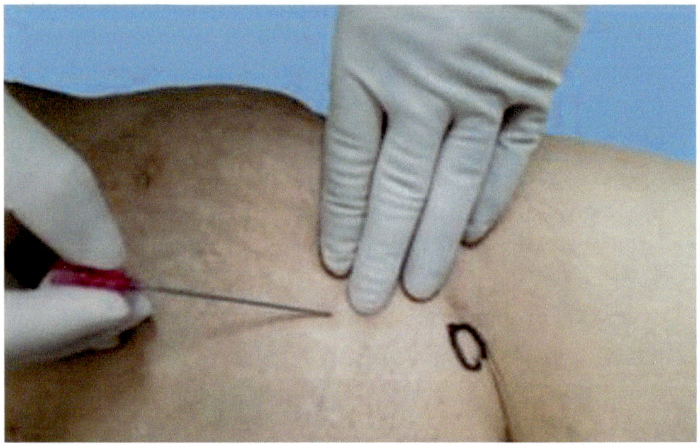

Fig. 11.2 Common femoral artery anterograde puncture (source: Changhai Hospital, for reference only)

11.1.4 Angiographic Puncture Technique

The modified Seldinger puncture technique is currently the most frequently used catheterization technique in clinical practice. Percutaneous transluminal angioplasty (PTA) is performed by a trocar without core, and when the trocar tip penetrates through the anterior wall of the blood vessels and blood sprays out from the end of the trocar, stop advancing the trocar and stop penetrating through the posterior wall of the vessel, and subsequently insert the wire and catheter.

11.2 Arteriopuncture

11.2.1 Puncture Site

Choosing the right puncture site reduces hemorrhage risks, which is important for reducing complications and requires physicians to master the anatomy of the arteries and their surrounding structures. Common percutaneous arterial puncture sites include common femoral artery, brachial artery, popliteal artery, and also puncture carotid artery or auxiliary artery [1]. The following describes the commonly used arterial puncture sites.

11.2.1.1 Common Femoral Artery Puncture

Common femoral artery puncture is the preferred approach for arteriography and minimally invasive endovascular surgery. Common femoral artery puncture site is generally located 1–2 cm below the inguinal ligament, at the punctum maximum of the pulse, mostly by the retrograde puncture to the proximal end of the artery (Fig. 11.1) and, alternatively, by anterograde puncture to its distal end (Fig. 11.2).

11.2.1.2 Brachial Artery Puncture

Brachial artery puncture is the second choice for minimally invasive endovascular treatment, advisable for the left brachial artery (Fig. 11.3), for the right brachial artery puncture requires access through the anonymous artery. In this case, if

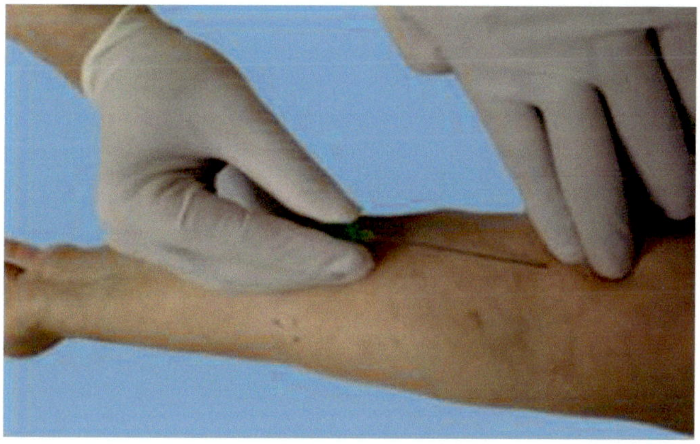

Fig. 11.3 Brachial artery puncture (source: Changhai Hospital, for reference only)

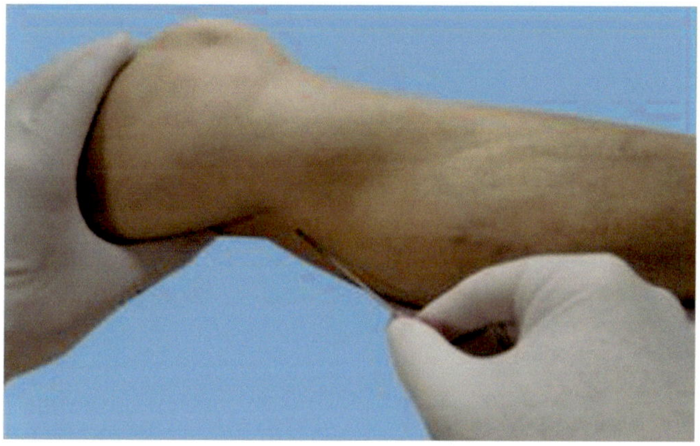

Fig. 11.4 Popliteal artery puncture (source: Changhai Hospital, for reference only)

the lateral thrombus breaks off, it can flow into the intracranial blood vessels along the flow direction, leading to cerebral infarction. For the upper arm puncture, the arm should be extended at 30° angle of abduction, and needle is inserted at the brachial artery pulsating position 0.5–1 cm above the skin-fold in the medial of the elbow joint, because the artery at this place is the most superficial and easy for fixation, facilitating the puncture and hemostasis by compression bandage.

11.2.1.3 Popliteal Artery Puncture

Popliteal artery puncture approach is not commonly used, but for patients with iliofemoral artery lesions and not indicated for common femoral artery puncture or patients unavailable for anterograde technique but for retrograde technique, it is a very useful minimally invasive approach (Fig. 11.4). In performing popliteal artery puncture, the patient can take prone position or supine position. Prone position puncture is relatively simple but needs to repeatedly change the position, more cumbersome and rather intolerable for the elderly

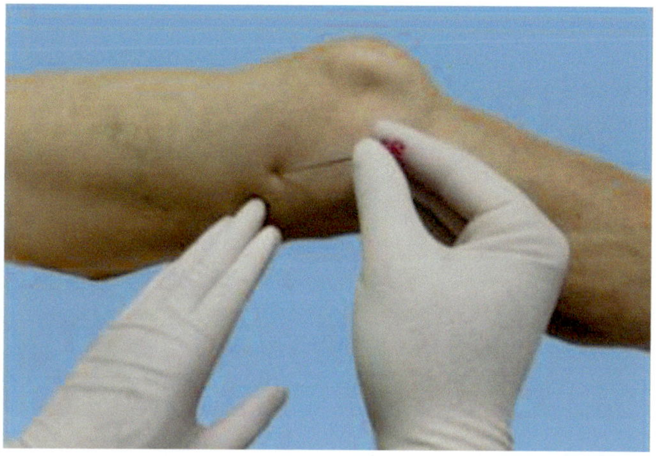

Fig. 11.5 Above-knee popliteal puncture (source: Changhai Hospital, for reference only)

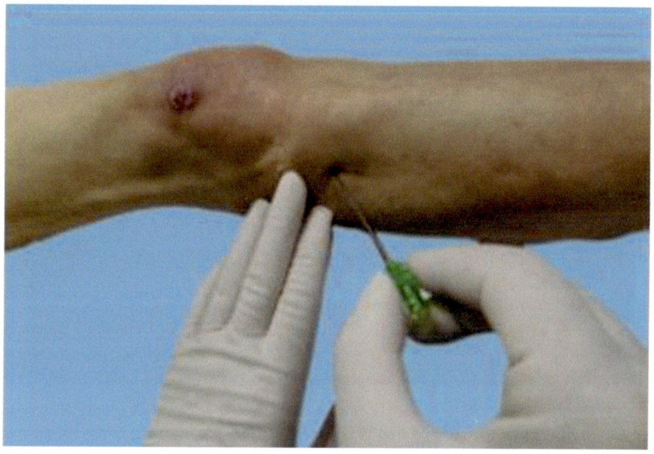

Fig. 11.6 Below-knee popliteal puncture (source: Changhai Hospital, for reference only)

patients. Therefore, supine position is preferred. The patient is asked to slightly bend his/her joints and turn outward. Puncture site is chosen on the knee (Fig. 11.5) or the infra-popliteal (Fig. 11.6). Preparation for popliteal artery puncture site is very important. If poorly prepared, it is liable of hemorrhage and popliteal fossa hematomas. Large hematoma can oppress the nerve and even cause fascia space syndrome.

11.2.1.4 Infra-popliteal Distal Vascular Puncture

For complex lesions, such as patients with occlusive lesion from superficial femoral artery to popliteal artery long segment, if the lesion cannot be accessed via the common femoral artery puncture, popliteal artery distal blood vessels (such as anterior tibial artery (Fig. 11.7), posterior tibial artery (Fig. 11.8), peroneal artery (Fig. 11.9), or dorsalis pedis artery (Fig. 11.10)) can be chosen for retrograde recanalization treatment.

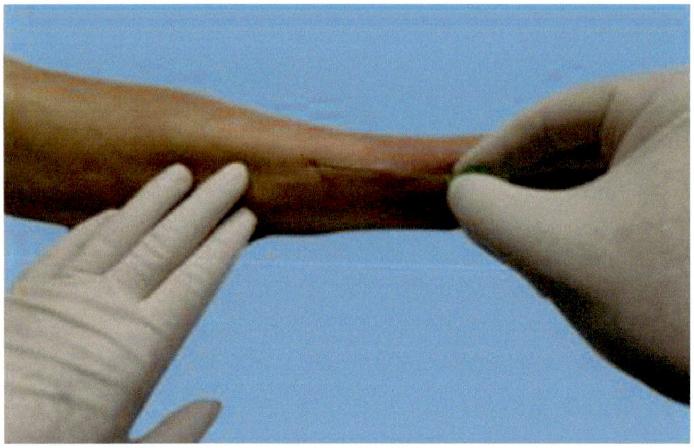

Fig. 11.7 Anterior tibial artery puncture (source: Changhai Hospital, for reference only)

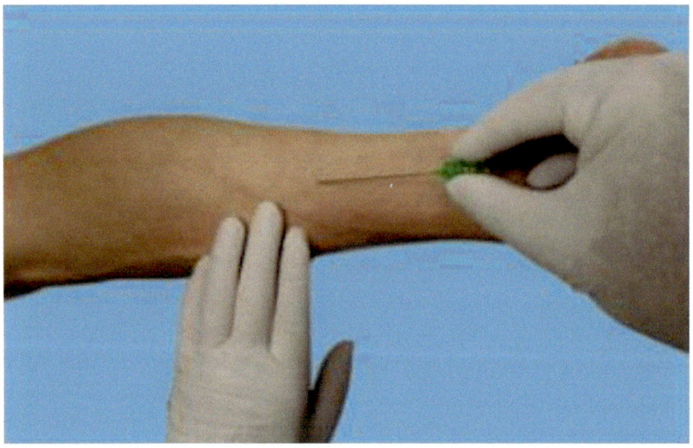

Fig. 11.8 Posterior tibial artery puncture (source: Changhai Hospital, for reference only)

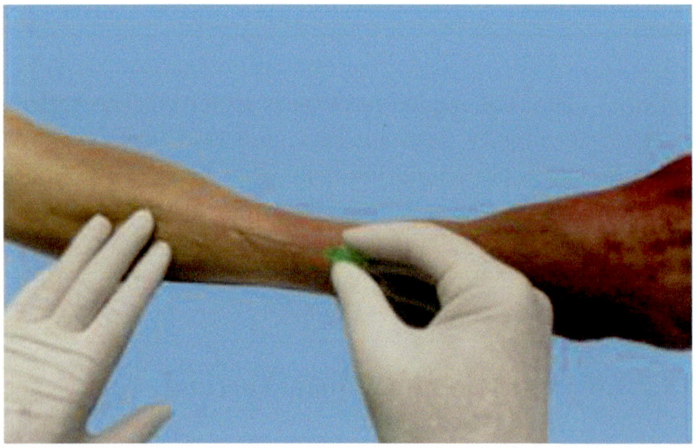

Fig. 11.9 Peroneal artery puncture (source: Changhai Hospital, for reference only)

11.2.1.5 Special Artery Puncture

For patients with in-stent long-segment re-occlusion of the lower extremities, and when it is difficult for them to take common femoral artery puncture, superficial artery direct stent puncture technique (DSPT) can be chosen for revascularization treatment.

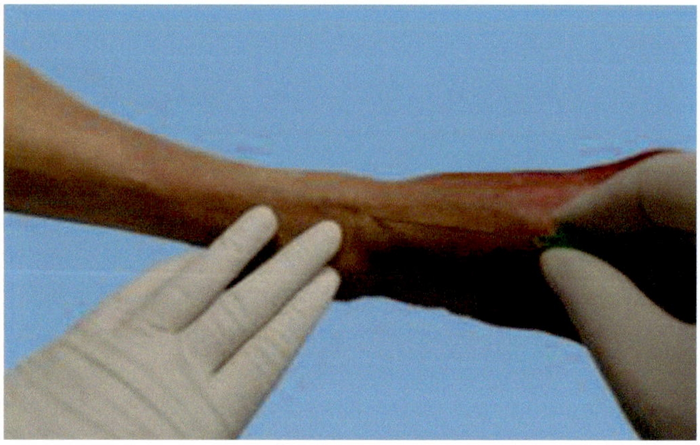

Fig. 11.10 Dorsalis pedis artery puncture (source: Changhai Hospital, for reference only)

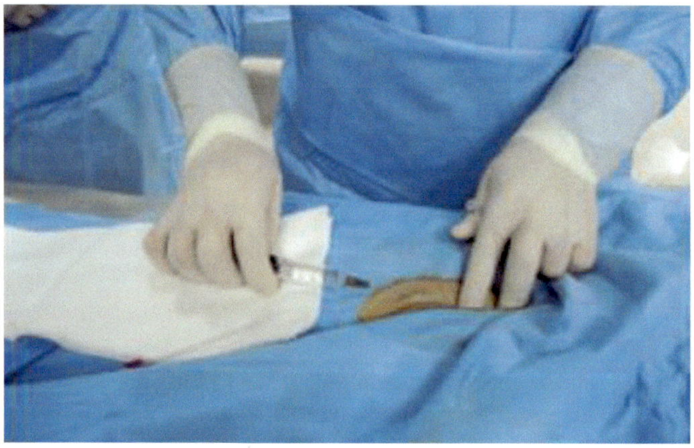

Fig. 11.11 Inject anesthetic (source: Changhai Hospital)

11.2.2 Puncture and Catheterization Methods

Puncture and catheterization methods are presented below with retrograde puncture and catheterization of common femoral artery as an example.

- Perform routine skin disinfection, palpate at the punctum maximum of the pulse about 1.5–2.0 cm below the inguinal ligament (Fig. 11.10) by the left index finger and the middle finger, and take it as the puncture site. Fix the site and administer anesthetic (infants or uncooperative patients can be administered with general anesthesia) (Fig. 11.11). Cut open the skin 2–3 mm with a pointed blade (Fig. 11.12).
- Make the puncture needle tip at 45° angle with the skin (Fig. 11.13), pass through the cut, and insert the needle quickly against the blood flow direction to puncture the common femoral artery. When fresh blood sprays out from the end of the needle, lay flat the puncture needle and keep it at 15–20° angle with the skin, and immediately insert the wire from the end of the needle (Fig. 11.14).
- When the wire is inserted 20–40 cm into the artery, pull out the puncture needle, compress the puncture site of the

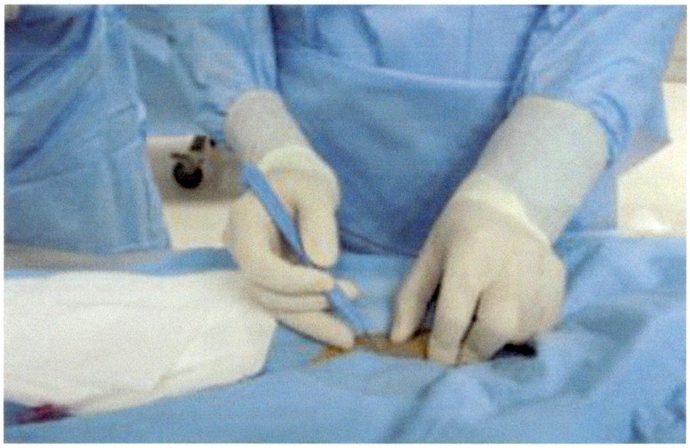

Fig. 11.12 Cut open skin by pointed blade (source: Changhai Hospital)

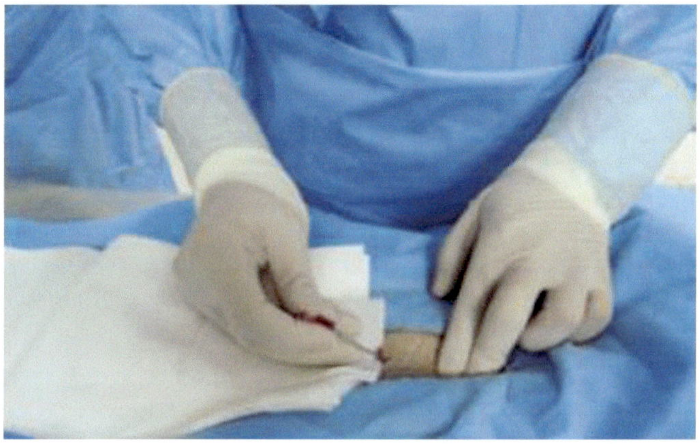

Fig. 11.13 Puncture common femoral artery (source: Changhai Hospital)

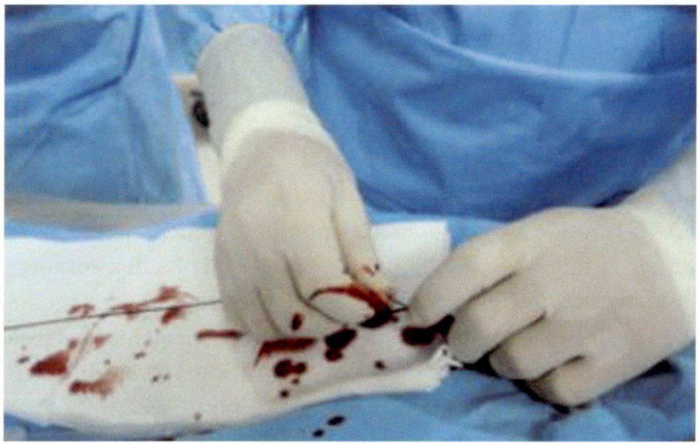

Fig. 11.14 Slightly press down needle end and advance the wire (source: Changhai Hospital)

common femoral artery by the left hand to stop bleeding and fix the wire, insert the vascular sheath with a dilator along the wire (Fig. 11.15), withdraw the dilator and keep the sheath in place, inject heparin diluent from the interface of the T valve of the vascular sheath, and advance the catheter via the sheath along the wire. When the catheter is advanced to certain length, withdraw the wire.

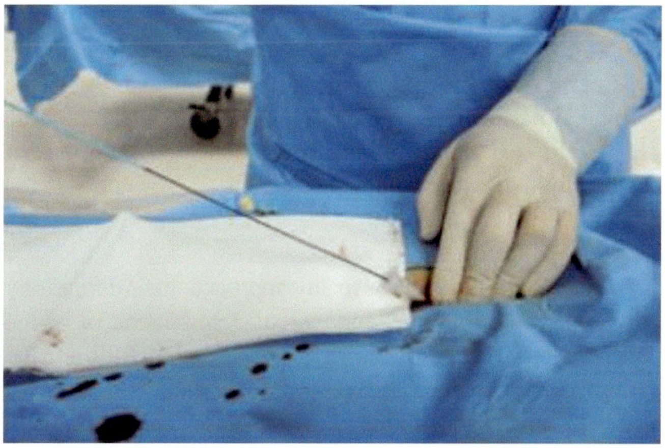

Fig. 11.15 Advance the short sheath with a dilator along the wire (source: Changhai Hospital)

- Under X-ray fluoroscopy, advance the catheter tip to the desired artery or its branch. As required by radiography, determine the contrast dosage and imaging procedures. When the position is decided, connect the tail end of the catheter with the high-pressure syringe and start imaging.
- Upon completion of the examination, and according to the imaging situation, choose an appropriate vascular closure device to block the puncture site, or directly pull out the vascular sheath and compress locally for 15–20 min to stop bleeding. If the hemostatic effect is not good, additionally apply a hemostatic patch, and cover it with a piece of large gauze, and then pack it up with an elastic bandage under pressure. In compressing the puncture site, make sure the compression is moderate. Excessively heavy compression may lead to closed blood vessels under pressure, affecting the blood flow of lower extremities; excessively light compression may lead to the bleeding of the puncture site, local hematoma, formation of false aneurysm, etc.

11.3 Venepuncture Technique

11.3.1 Percutaneous Venepuncture Technique

11.3.1.1 Puncture Site

Commonly used sites for percutaneous venography include femoral vein, popliteal vein, jugular vein, or superficial vein of upper limbs [2]. The following describes the commonly used venepuncture sites.

Femoral Venepuncture

Femoral venepuncture is indicated for angiography of the inferior vena cava and its branches, veins of lower extremity, right atrium, right ventricle, pulmonary artery, and other blood vessels, mostly represented by the femoral artery. Palpate the pulse of the femoral artery, and insert the needle

0.5–1.0 cm inside the puncture site. Upon successful puncture, venous blood slowly flows out from the distal end of the needle, or a core-free puncture needle is connected with the syringe to perform insertion and aspiration at the same time till blood is extracted. Or adjust the puncture direction for in-depth puncture or re-puncture.

Jugular Venepuncture

Jugular venepuncture is also an approach for venography and minimally invasive endovascular treatment of some venous diseases. The puncture is performed as follows: the patient takes a supine position, with the head bending down at 20–30° angle or with the shoulder pillow at hypertension position and turning to the contralateral side (generally puncture is performed mostly on the right side). Find out the trigonum formed among the clavicular head, the sternal head, and the clavicle of the sternocleidomastoid muscle, the top of which is the puncture site. Insert from the puncture site, and keep the needle parallel to the sagittal plane and at 30° angle with the coronal plane. Advance the needle downward, backward, and slightly outward toward the lower rear of the sternoclavicular joint. Advance the needle while aspirating till blood is seen, indicating the entry into the jugular vein. Jugular venepuncture is indicated for the angiography of the superior vena cava, right atrium, right ventricle, pulmonary, inferior vena cava, and their branches.

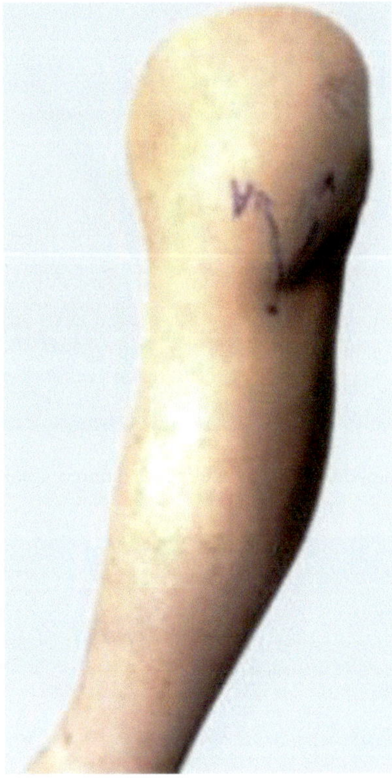

Fig. 11.16 Knee joint medial puncture site (source: Changhai Hospital)

11.3.1.2 Popliteal Venepuncture

Popliteal venepuncture is a common approach for minimally invasive endovascular treatment of lower extremities, especially in the case of deep venous thrombolysis or mechanical thrombus aspiration of the lower limbs or treatment of iliofemoral vein balloon dilatation and stent implantation surgery, popliteal venepuncture is the most effective approach [2]. Popliteal venepuncture can be carried out under ultrasound guidance, or preceded by venous anterograde angiography of lower extremities to visualize the popliteal vein, and then carried out by using Seldinger technique under fluoroscopy or roadmap guidance. Popliteal venepuncture can be performed at both prone position and supine position. The beginners can choose relatively simple prone position to perform puncture under the guidance of the venous anterograde angiogram of lower extremities or conduct blind puncture one finger away from the lateral of the popliteal fossa midline, for popliteal vein has a relatively high profile, easier to succeed in puncture [2].

For patients with supine position, they need not to change their position frequently during catheterization, and its puncture method is similar to the popliteal artery puncture, where the diseased limb is abducted and supinated; needle is inserted 2 cm medial inferior to the popliteal fossa and advanced lateral superior to the popliteal fossa midpoint till dark red venous blood is visibly drawn or popliteal venepuncture proves successful by injecting a little radiocontrast, and, subsequently, the vascular sheath and wire are inserted. In case of prone position in percutaneous popliteal venepuncture, it is safe to conduct horizontal puncture at the popliteal transverse line; in case of supine position, puncture site is chosen on the medial of the knee joint (Fig. 11.16). Popliteal venepuncture is indicated for patients with diseases of lower extremity but difficult for femoral venous catheterization.

11.3.1.3 Venepuncture and Catheterization Methods (with Femoral Venepuncture as an Example)

- In routine skin disinfection, keep the lower limb of the puncture side slightly at abduction and extortion, locate the puncture site at 1.5–3.0 cm of the medial inferior to the center of the inguinal ligament and 0.5–1.0 cm of the medial of the femoral artery pulse, and inject anesthetic (infants or uncooperative patients can be administered with general anesthesia). Prepare an incision of 2–3 mm with a pointed blade.
- Hold the syringe with the right hand, and insert it into the puncture site secured by the left index finger and the middle finger at an angle of 30°–45° with the skin surface along the blood flow direction; advance the needle with aspiration performed simultaneously and slowly.
- Upon entry into the femoral vein, the puncture needle should be withdrawn slowly till dark red venous blood comes out continuously, and then the puncture succeeds. Unfortunately, if bright red blood comes out, it indicates that the needle is wrongly inserted into the artery, and the needle should be withdrawn immediately. Then compress the puncture site for about 20 min till no blood comes out, and repeat puncturing the vein.
- Secure the puncture needle by the left hand, hold the wire in the right hand and insert it from the needle end, secure the wire, and withdraw the puncture needle.
- Insert the vascular sheath with a dilator along the wire, withdraw the dilator, inject heparin diluent via the T-valve interface of the vascular sheath, deliver the catheter along the wire to certain length, and then withdraw the wire. Connect high-pressure syringe at the end of the catheter and then start to take angiogram.
- Upon completion of the examination, withdraw the catheter and vascular sheath, routinely compress the puncture site for 5 min, then cover it with large gauze, and conduct compression dressing for 6 h with elastic bandage.

11.3.2 Anterograde Puncture Technique for Veins of Lower Extremity

Anterograde angiography of lower extremities refers to a rapidly diagnostic and invasive examination method where, by means of dorsal vein puncture, a high-pressure connector is attached to a high-pressure syringe to inject the diluted radiocontrast into the deep vein which visualizes immediately. This method is highly targeted and safe.

The advantage is that the lesion site, scope, and anatomic variation of the lower extremity vein are clearly visualized. It is of great significance for correct diagnosis, selection of appropriate treatment, and the observation of the curative effect and is therefore more and more widely used in the treatment of lower limb venous diseases. But some patients fail in such puncture technique due to leg swelling and ulcers or for other reasons. In view of the above problems, technical and methodological improvements can be made in the following aspects, thereby enhancing the success rate of puncture.

11.3.2.1 Body Position

According to the principle of venous hemodynamics, the venous pressure of lower extremities is about 10 mmHg (1 mmHg ≈ 133.3 Pa) when at supine position, and when at sitting position, the venous pressure of lower extremity can reach 90 mmHg with two legs hanging down. The increased venous pressure increases the dorsal vein filling, thereby increasing the success rate of puncture. The bed-ridden patients can choose supine position, with the diseased limb hanging down to one side, and appropriate position should be chosen according to the actual situation of the patients.

11.3.2.2 Selection of Puncture Needles

The puncture needle has three colors: red, blue, and yellow (Fig. 11.17). Different diameters result in different fluid flow

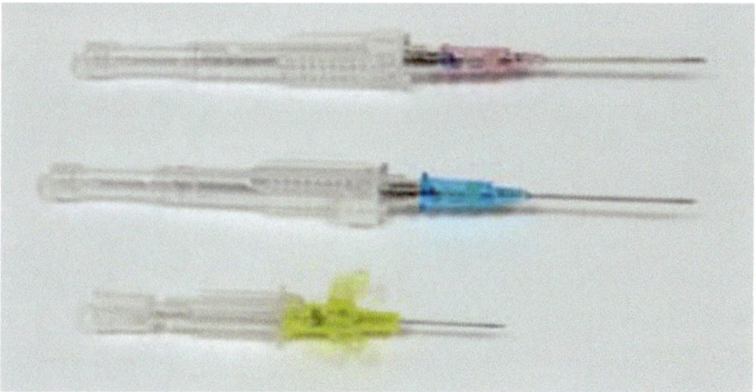

Fig. 11.17 Puncture needle in three colors

Table 11.1 Features of color-specific puncture needles

Color	Diameter(G)	Flow(mL/min)	Scope of application
Red	20	60	Suitable for patients with venous diseases that are definitely indicated for treatment, this puncture needle can directly access through 0.81 mm (0.032in) wire
Blue	22	35	Indicated for patients with obvious swelling for venographic examination
Yellow	24	22	Indicated for patients with insignificant swelling and with thin and fragile vessels for venographic examination

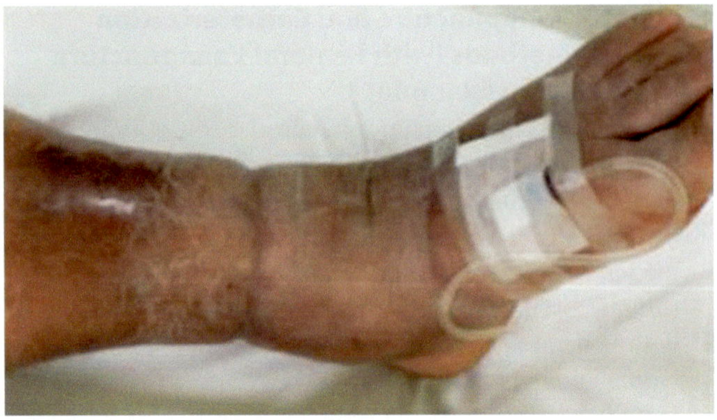

Fig. 11.18 Secure puncture needle (source: Changhai Hospital)

and different scopes of application. Refer to Table 11.1 for the features in details.

11.3.2.3 Selection of Insertion Angle

The veins for such venous diseases are superficial with thin and fragile wall; the insertion angle is generally 10–15°. When the outflow is visible, the needle can no longer be advanced. Otherwise, the venous wall is liable of penetration.

11.3.2.4 Method for Securing Puncture Needle

Securing the puncture needle is the last step for the success of venepuncture. If improperly secured, all that have been previously done will come to naught. According to the clinical experience of the author for more than a decade, the best way is to cover the needle hole with a 3 M patch with its front end being secured, use transparent tape to secure the needle and the high-pressure connector on the dorsum pedis, and then reversely secure the high-pressure connector on the dorsum pedis (Fig. 11.18).

References

1. Jing Z. Endovascular therapy. Beijing: People's Medical Publishing House; 2003.
2. Ye G, Cheng Z, Hu L, et al. Clinical study on 39 cases of diagnosis and treatment of deep venous thrombus of lower extremities with percutaneous popliteal Venepuncture technique. J Clin Int Med. 2006;23(5):328–30.

Cardiac Aortic Valve Stenosis

12

Zaiping Jing, Huajuan Mao, Qingsheng Lu, Chao Song, and Lei Zhang

Abstract

Cardiac aortic valve stenosis refers to related clinical symptoms when the aortic valve cannot fully open in the cardiac systolic phase and the blood of the left ventricular cannot fully shoot out; it can be classified into congenital, rheumatic, and senile arteriosclerosis types. With the improvement of people's living standards and the aging of the population, degenerative aortic valve stenosis has become an important disease influencing the health of senior patients. Its disability rate and fatality rate are even higher among those above 70 years old. Traditional aortic valve replacement is marked by the disadvantages of severe invasion and high blood loss and requires extracorporeal circulation, for which it is intolerable for most senior patients. Catheter-assisted aortic valve replacement is characterized by minimal invasion, fast recovery, and many other advantages and is being more and more frequently used to treat senior patients. The vascular surgery of Changhai Hospital has taken the lead in China to perform transfemoral coronary balloon-expanding aortic valve replacement, having achieved remarkable results. This chapter gives a brief introduction to the clinical manifestations, surgical process, and other details of aortic valve stenosis.

Keywords

Aortic valve stenosis · Minimally invasive · Endovascular surgery

Z. Jing (✉) · H. Mao · Q. Lu · C. Song · L. Zhang
Department of Vascular Surgery, Changhai Hospital, Second Military Medical University, Shanghai, China
e-mail: Jingzp@xueguan.net

12.1 Introduction

Cardiac aortic valve stenosis refers to relevant clinical symptoms as a result of incomplete opening of the heart valve during systole due to aortic valve lesions caused by congenital or acquired factors, mainly because of congenital aortic valve structure abnormalities, commissural lobular fusion stricture due to rheumatic fever, or senile aortic valve calcification. Adult aortic valve opening is ≥ 3.0 cm^2, with systolic trans-valve pressure gradient at 5 mmHg.

Blood flow can be obstructed only when the aortic valve opening is reduced to 1/3 or more of its normal size. When the aortic valve opening decreases to 1.5–3.0 cm^2, it is mild stenosis; to 1.0–1.5 cm^2, moderate stenosis; and less than 1.0 cm^2, severe stenosis [1] (Fig. 12.1).

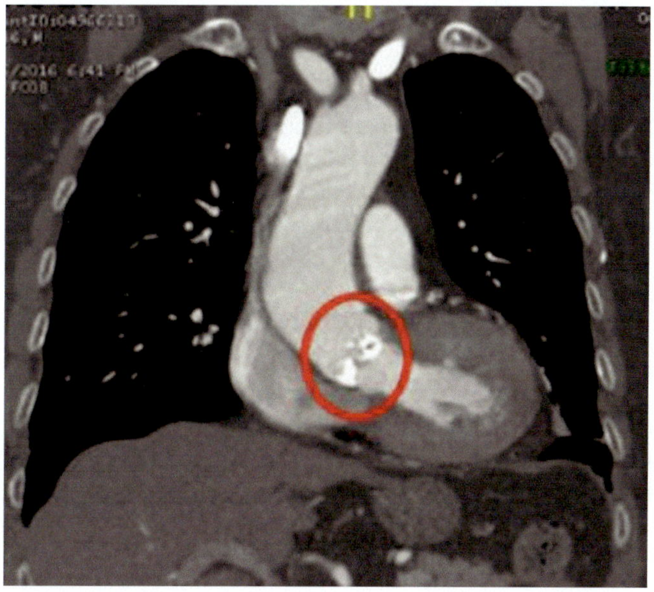

Fig. 12.1 Cardiac Aortic valve stenosis

Z. Jing et al. (eds.), *Endovascular Surgery and Devices*, https://doi.org/10.1007/978-981-10-8270-2_12

12.2 Clinical Manifestations

12.2.1 Angina Pectoris

About 60% of patients with cardiac aortic valve stenosis have angina symptoms, often induced by exercise and relieved after rest. But angina symptoms can also occur at rest, indicating that it is not necessarily related to exertion and physical activities. Its generation mechanism may be due to cardiac hypertrophy, increased myocardial oxygen demand, reduced oxygen supply secondary to excessive coronary pressure, and high ventricular wall tension during left ventricular systole.

12.2.2 Vertigo or Syncope

About 30% of patients with cardiac aortic valve stenosis have vertigo or syncope, lasting from 1 min to half an hour. Some patients are associated with Alzheimer's syndrome or arrhythmia. Relevant symptoms often occur after physical activity and also in the state of rest due to the sudden change in position or induced by sublingual nitroglycerin treatment of angina. Its generation mechanism is not clear and may be related to the following factors: (1) blood vessels expand due to physical activity, while the narrow aortic valve opening restricts the increase in cardiac output, resulting in insufficient intracranial blood supply, and (2) brief and serious arrhythmia, leading to hemodynamic disorders.

12.2.3 Dyspnea

Exertional dyspnea is often a manifestation of cardiac insufficiency, often accompanied by fatigue. With the progress of heart failure, aortic valve stenosis patients may have nocturnal paroxysmal dyspnea, orthopnea, pink bubble sputum cough, and other related symptoms.

12.2.4 Hidrosis and Palpitation

Due to increased myocardial contraction and arrhythmia, aortic valve stenosis patients often feel palpitations and sweating often after the palpitations which are associated with autonomic nervous system dysfunction and increased sympathetic tone.

12.2.5 Sudden Death

Aortic valve stenosis patients with sudden death account for 10–20%. Most patients with sudden death suffer from repeated angina or syncope attack, but sudden death could be the first symptom. The causes may be related to fatal arrhythmia induced by aortic valve stenosis, ventricular fibrillation, etc.

12.3 Intraoperative Coordination

Vascular Surgery Department of Changhai Hospital affiliated to the Second Military Medical University takes the lead in aortic valve replacement via transfemoral balloon dilation, which, for high-risk patients intolerable of thoracotomy, not only provides an opportunity for treatment but also reduces the risk of intraoperative anesthesia and the amount of bleeding, promotes postoperative recovery, and shortens the time of hospitalization [2–4].

12.3.1 Anesthesia and Surgical Position

General anesthesia at supine position

12.3.2 Preparation of Items and Instruments

1. Preparation of routine items and instruments: refer to Table 12.1.
2. Instrument preparation: centralized oxygen supply station, aspirator, anesthesia machine, defibrillator, esophageal ultrasound, ECG monitor, temporary pacemaker, micropump, invasive arterial pressure monitor, extracorporeal circulation device system, large DSA (digital subtraction angiography) machine, PACS image transmission system, high-frequency electrotome, shadowless lamp, etc., all of which should function normally and remain ready for use.

12.3.3 Preparation of Devices

Refer to Table 12.2.

12.3.4 Procedures and Intraoperative Coordination Process

Refer to Table 12.3.

Table 12.1 Preparation of routine items

Name	Qty.	Name	Qty.
Disposable operation kits	2	Appendix retractor	2
Disposable 10–20 mL syringes	1 each	Mastoid retractor	2
Disposable gloves	5 pairs	Needle holder	3
Large gauze	10 patches	Noninvasive vascular clamp	2
Trocar, infusion set	1 each	Mosquito clamp	8
T valve	3	Electrotome bit	1
Normal saline 500 mL	2 bags	Electrotome	1
Heparin sodium injection 100 mg	2	Separating pliers	2
Iodixanol injection 100 mL	1 bottle	Triangular handle	1
Thyroid retractor	2	CV-6 vascular suture	1
Medium-curved nose pliers	4 pairs	Skin suture 4–0	1
Subcutaneous suture 2-0	1	Aspiration tube and head	1 each
Silk suture(1#, 4#, 7#)	1 each	Round needle (9 × 24,7 × 17)	1 each
Blade (11#, 23#)	1 each	Electrode plate	1

Table 12.2 Preparation of devices

Name	Qty.	Name	Qty.
Puncture needle	1	6F short sheath	3
High-pressure connector	2	Edwards balloon	1
Novaflex vascular sheath(18–24 F)	1	Sapien XT balloon-expandable valved stent	1
0.035 in common hydrophilic wire 180 cm	1	Novaflex delivery system	1
0.035 in straight-tip wire 180 cm	1	Temporary pacing electrode catheter	1
6F common pigtail catheter	2	Disposable 50 ml syringe (helical tip)	1 pair
6F left coronary angiography catheter	1	Vascular closure device	1
0.035in Amplatz super-stiff wire 260 cm	1	Inflation device	2
Compressor	1		

Table 12.3 Procedures and intraoperative coordination process

Procedures	Intraoperative coordination process
1. Patient enters the operation room and receives general anesthesia	(1) Mental nursing; (2) keep the patient warm; (3) help to lie at supine position, with two lower limbs slightly at abduction and extortion position;(4) connect ECG to observe changes in blood pressure, heart rate and oxygen saturation; (5) establish intravenous infusion and place indwelling central venous catheter; (6) puncture the radial artery and monitor invasive artery pressure; (7) place indwelling urinary catheter
2. Routinely sterilize the bilateral groins from the umbilical down to mid-thigh, exposing the groins	Prepare disinfectant (heated to 98.6 °F with incubator) and assist with draping; deliver iodixanol injection; prepare heparin diluent (1000 ml normal saline +100 mg heparin sodium injection) – full-time instrument nurse should flush in advance Novaflex vascular sheath (18–24F), Edwards balloon, and Novaflex delivery system on sterilized operation table – prepare for the installation of Sapien XT balloon-expandable aortic valve stent system (Fig. 12.2)
3. Conduct femoral venepuncture on one side, insert a 6F short sheath and a 0.035 in common hydrophilic wire 180 cm, insert temporary pacing electrode catheter into the right ventricle along the common hydrophilic wire, withdraw the common hydrophilic wire, and connect the temporary pacemaker for standby use	Deliver the 6F short sheath, 0.035 in common hydrophilic wire 180 cm and temporary pacing electrode catheter; perform systemic heparinization (initial administered dose is 0.67 mg/kg based on body weight; subsequent dose is administered according to the actual intraoperative situations); endovascular devices should be flushed with the prepared heparin diluent; connect a temporary pacemaker and pacing electrode catheter, check if the parameters and functions of the temporary pacemaker are normal
4. Conduct ipsilateral common femoral artery puncture, insert a 6F short sheath and a 0.035in common hydrophilic wire 180 cm, insert a 6F common pigtail catheter into the aortic valve opening for visualization along the common hydrophilic wire	Deliver the 6F short sheath and 6F common pigtail catheter

(continued)

Table 12.3 (continued)

Procedures	Intraoperative coordination process
5. Cut open (or directly puncture) the common femoral artery on the other side, insert a 6F short sheath and a 0.035in straight-tip wire 180 cm, insert a 6F left coronary angiography catheter into the aortic valve opening along the wire, advance the wire into the left ventricle via the aortic valve opening, advance the catheter via the aortic valve opening and exchange for the 0.035 in Amplatz super-stiff wire 260 cm, withdraw the catheter	Deliver the scalpels, large tweezers (flat tweezers or fine tweezers), separating pliers, mosquito pliers, vascular pliers and 0# silk suture, 6F short sheath, 0.035in straight-tip wire 180 cm, 6F left coronary angiography catheter, 0.035in Amplatz super-stiff wire 260 cm
6. Exchange Novaflex vascular sheath (18–24F) along the 0.035 in Amplatz super-stiff wire 260 cm; place Edwards balloon into the aortic valve stricture site along the wire for pre-expansion	Device nurse delivers the flushed Novaflex vascular sheath (18–24F), inflation device, and Edwards balloon; full-time device nurse verifies with the responsible physician the size and opening direction of balloon-expandable valve stent (18–24F)
7. Manually pump the patient's heart rate to 180–200 beats per minute, and reduce systolic pressure to about 60 mmHg till the pulse-pressure difference is less than 10 mmHg, fully inflate the balloon, then deflate the balloon to restore to autonomous cardiac rhythm and blood pressure, withdraw the balloon	As instructed by the physician, start or stop pumping, quickly change pumping frequency, check if the indicator of the temporary pacemaker flashes, and confirm if the systolic pressure lowers down to about 60 mHg
8. Insert the Sapien XT balloon-expandable valve stent system along the 0.035in Amplatz super-stiff wire 260 cm, position the Sapien XT stent accurately to the diseased aortic valve, manually pump the patient's heart rate to 180–200beats per minute again with systolic pressure decreased to about 60mHg and pulse-pressure difference of less than 10 mmHg, instantly inflate the balloon in full, release the valve stent, retract the balloon, restore to autonomous cardiac rhythm and blood pressure, withdraw the delivery system. Check if the valve stent is placed properly with desired morphology under X-ray visualization	Full-time device nurse delivers the readily assembled Sapien XT valve stent (Fig. 12.3) to the physician and re-verify with the responsible physician the opening direction of the stent; upon placement of the stent, stop pumping as instructed by the physician, closely observe the patient's change in blood pressure, heart rate, and oxyhemoglobin saturation
9. Withdraw the Novaflex delivery system, the 0.035in Amplatz super-stiff wire 260 cm, and the Novaflex vascular sheath(18–24F); suture the surgical incision	Deliver the vascular pliers, CV suture for vascular incision suturing; deliver small round and angled needles and 1# silk suture to suture the incision layer by layer
10. Withdraw common femoral artery and femoral vein catheter's wire and vascular sheath on the other side, select appropriate vascular closure device to occlude the common femoral artery puncture site	Deliver the vascular closure device; deliver gauze and elastic bandage and assist with bandaging
11. Anesthesia completed	Withdraw the radial artery puncture needle, press for 5 min, and bandage it with compression; safely escort the patient back to the ward

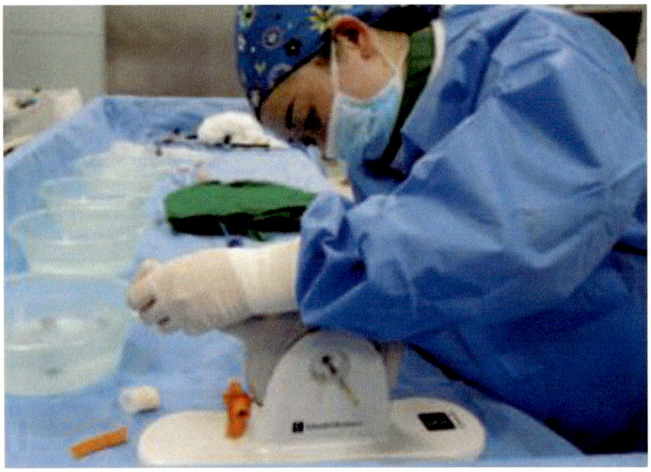

Fig. 12.2 Valves assembled by full-time device specialist

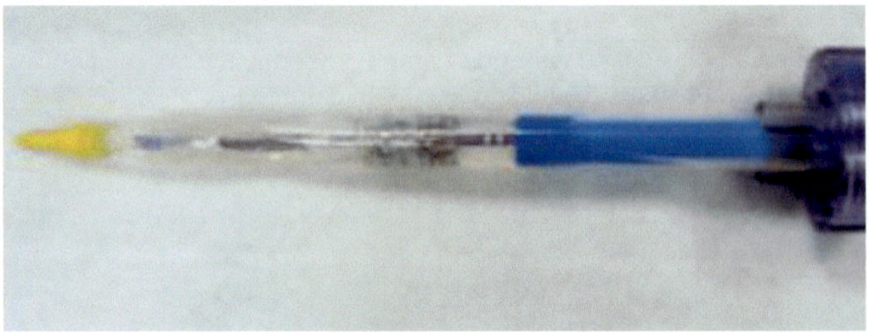

Fig. 12.3 Valves already assembled

12.4 Key for Intraoperative Observation

12.4.1 Observation of Vital Signs

The period of particular concern during operation is the process during which the balloon is quickly inflated and deflated by the right ventricular rapid pacing technique after the Sapien XT balloon-expandable valve stent system is delivered by wire till the balloon is completely deflated and stops rapid pacing. At this time, the patient is in a state of tachycardia and his ECG changes need to be closely monitored. Any occurrence of supraventricular tachycardia, ventricular tachycardia, atrial fibrillation or atrial flutter, and other non-sinus tachycardia should be observed; and whether normal sinus rhythm (NSR) can be restored when the surgeon stops rapid pacing should be checked [4].

12.4.2 Intraoperative Monitoring of Active Coagulation Time (ACT)

Systematic heparinization should be administered to the patient according to his/her body weight after placement of vascular sheath and wire into the patient's body. Heparin dose should be adjusted promptly according to the half-life of heparin and ACT value monitored during operation so as to prevent excessive anticoagulation or thrombosis.

12.4.3 Observation of Puncture Site

Aortic valve stenosis patient is implanted with the indwelling radial artery catheter and common femoral artery sheath during operation. The radial artery catheter is used to monitor arterial blood pressure change, and the common femoral artery sheath is used for endovascular surgery. The sheath should be firmly secured during operation, especially at the puncture site of the common femoral artery. Upon completion of surgical operation, vascular closure device is used to occlude the puncture site, but due to systematic heparinization during the operation, the puncture site still needs to be covered with five medium gauzes and elastic bandage for compression dressing for 12 h. Closely observe the skin temperature, color, and dorsalis pedis artery pulse of the patient's lower extremities.

References

1. Qinsheng L, Hong Y, Wu H, et al. Experience in 5 cases of aortic valve stenosis treatment via balloon expandable aortic valve endovascular replacement technique. J Intervent Radiol. 2013;22(4):274–8.
2. Li H, Mao H, Jing Z, et al. Perioperative nursing approaches for 3 cases of aortic valve stenosis treatment via percutaneous arotic valve replacement technique. Chin J Nurs. 2012;47(2):125–6.
3. Li H, Qinsheng L, Jing Z, et al. 3 Nursing cases of high-risk patients with aortic valve stenosis via percutaneous aortic valve replacement technique. Nurs J Chin People's Liberation Army. 2011;28(12A):43–4.
4. Mao H, Li H, Lu Q, et al. Perioperative nursing approaches for aortic valve stenosis patients with aortic valve replacement via transfemoral artery balloon dilation technique. Nurs J Chin People's Liberation Army. 2015;19:49–51.

Arteriectasia

13

Zaiping Jing, Huajuan Mao, Meiqin Shi, Qingsheng Lu, Rui Feng, Xiaolong Wei, and Chao Song

Abstract

Dilatations of the artery, based on specific pathological forms, can be classified into artery dissection and aneurysm. Based on specific invasion sites, they can be classified into aortic dilatations and peripheral artery dilatations. Promoted by progress in devices and techniques, most dilatations of the artery can now be fixed by minimally invasive methods. The aim of endovascular treatment is to isolate dissection rupture or aneurysm and restore normal blood flow. This chapter mainly introduces clinical manifestations, surgical process, and intraoperative observation points of aortic dissection, abdominal aortic aneurysm, extracranial carotid artery aneurysm, renal artery aneurysm, splenic artery aneurysm, and iliac artery aneurysm.

Keywords

Dilatations of the artery · Dissection · Aneurysm · Minimally invasive endovascular surgery

13.1 Aortic Dissection

13.1.1 Introduction

Aortic dissection refers to a pathologic condition when a tear occurs in the intima of the aortic wall due to various reasons and causes blood to flow from the tear into the media of the aorta, forcing the media apart lengthwise and demonstrating true and false lumens in the aortic lumen (Fig. 13.1). Its major risk factors include hypertension, Marfan syndrome, congenital cardiovascular malformation, idiopathic medial degeneration of the aorta, aortic atherosclerosis, aortic inflammatory diseases, and others. The aorta is the main

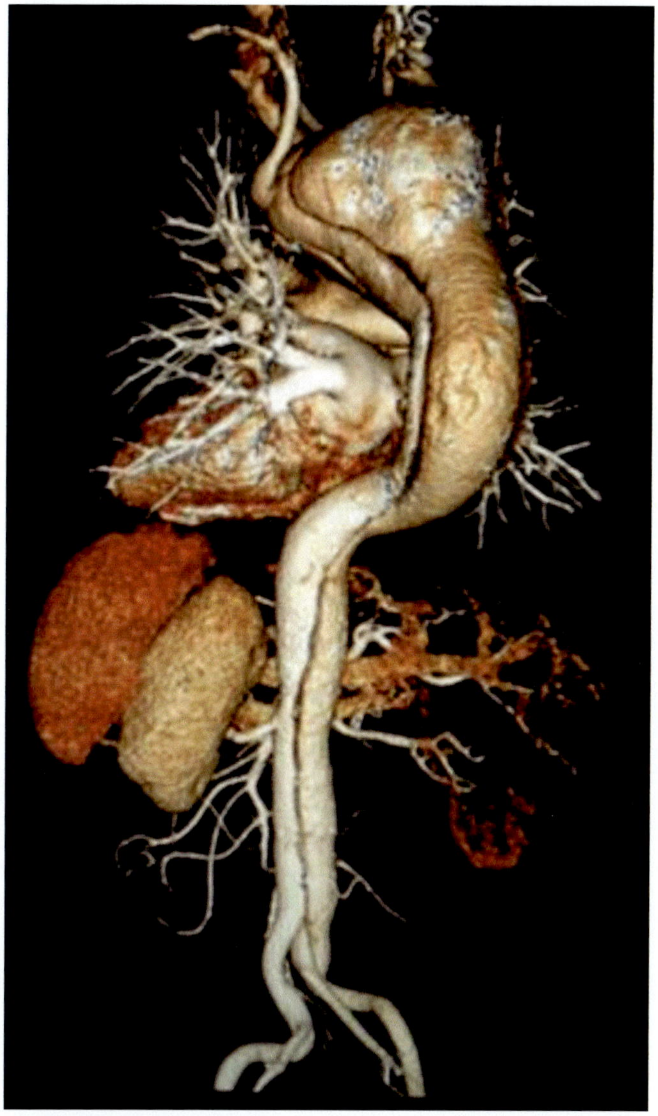

Fig. 13.1 Aortic dissection

Z. Jing (✉) · H. Mao · M. Shi · Q. Lu · R. Feng · X. Wei · C. Song
Department of Vascular Surgery, Changhai Hospital, Second Military Medical University, Shanghai, China
e-mail: Jingzp@xueguan.net

Z. Jing et al. (eds.), *Endovascular Surgery and Devices*, https://doi.org/10.1007/978-981-10-8270-2_13

blood vessel of the body, bearing the pressure directly from the heart beating and having high blood flow, once intimal rupture occurs.

Appropriate and timely treatment is required.

13.1.2 Clinical Manifestations

The clinical symptoms for aortic dissection mainly include:

- Patients with typical acute aortic dissection usually manifest sudden and severe tearing chest and back pains or, more seriously, heart failure, syncope, and even sudden death. Most patients are accompanied with uncontrollable hypertension.
- Aortic branch artery occlusion may cause ischemic symptoms in the brain, limbs, and abdominal organs, such as cerebral infarction, oliguria, abdominal pain, pale legs, weakness, piebald, and even paraplegia.
- Considering the extensive blood supply of the aorta, the manifestations, apart from the aforesaid symptoms and signs, are different according to the cumulative range of the dissection. Other conditions also include absent peripheral arterial pulsation, possible vocal cord paralysis occurring to the left recurrent laryngeal nerve under compression, possible hemoptysis and hematemesis when dissection penetrates through trachea and esophagus, superior vena cava syndrome when dissection compresses the superior vena cava, dyspnea when compressing the tracheas, homer syndrome when compressing the cervicothoracic ganglion, pulmonary embolism when compressing the pulmonary artery or other related symptoms, or enteroplegia and even renal infarction when dissection involves the mesentery and renal artery. Pleural effusion is a common sign for aortic dissection and mostly involves the left.

13.1.3 Intraoperative Coordination

In recent years, with the development of endovascular technique and the upgrading of endografts, many contraindications for aneurysm repair have been gradually broken, so is the case with aneurysm repair forbidden zones [1]. At present, there are two minimally invasive endovascular therapies for aortic dissection: one is TAA stent graft, and the other is multilayer self-expanding bare stent [2]. The former is preferred, while the later still requires more clinical evidences to support its selection of indications and clinical efficacy [2].

13.1.3.1 Intraoperative Coordination for Minimally Invasive Endovascular Aortic Dissection Therapy by TAA Stent Graft

Anesthesia and Surgical Position

Spinal anesthesia or general anesthesia is commonly used, but, with the development in endovascular devices and technology, TEVAR (thoracic endovascular aortic repair) operation with percutaneous puncture under local anesthesia has increasingly become a more minimally invasive and more acceptable treatment. With this technique, there is no need to cut open the common femoral artery, but, instead, two ProGlide vascular closure devices are pre-placed after percutaneous puncture. The pre-placed sutures are tightened upon completion of the endovascular operation, so as to suture the artery wound and stop bleeding. The patient lies in supine position, with both lower limbs staying apart and extending outside (the position to be adjusted in operation based on the patient condition).

Preparation of Routine Items and Instruments

Refer to Table 13.1.

Preparation of Devices

Refer to Table 13.2.

Table 13.1 Preparation of routine items and instruments

Name	Qty.	Name	Qty.
Disposable operation kit (Fig. 13.2)	1	Vascular devices (if necessary)	1 set
Disposable 10 mL syringe	1	Small bypass device	1 set
Disposable 20 mL syringe	1	Aspiration tube	1
Disposable gloves	4 pairs	Aspiration tube head	1
100 mL iodixanol injection	2 vials	Electrotome	1
100 mg heparin sodium injection	1	CV6 or CV7	1 each
500 mL normal saline	2 bags	VCP311(3/0)	1
Central venipuncture kit	1 set	VCP422(4/0)	1
Disposable syringe	2	Sterile blade (23#)	1
Disposable venipuncture needle	1	Red common catheter (as scalp clamp)	1
T valve	1	Extension tube (as sling)	1
Saline gauze	5 pieces	Hui Han Shu Tai	1 vial
Gauze	10 pieces	Round needle, angled needle	1 each
Medium patch	2 pieces	Lyophilized human fibrin sealant (if necessary)	Several
Absorbable hemostatic gauze (if necessary)	2 pieces		

Table 13.2 Preparation of devices

Name	Qty.	Name	Qty.
Puncture needle	1	5F scaled pigtail catheter	1
High-pressure connector	2	TAA stent graft system	Several
0.035 in common hydrophilic wire 180 cm	1	Self-expanding peripheral bare stent (if necessary)	Several
0.035 in Lunderquist super-stiff wire 260 cm	1	Peripheral stent graft (if necessary)	Several
Coda balloon catheter (if necessary)	1	Cuff (if necessary)	1
5F Berenstein catheter (if necessary)	1	Onyx liquid embolic agent (if necessary)	Several
0.035 in common hydrophilic wire 260 cm (if necessary)	Several	Embolization (if necessary)	Several
0.035 in hardened hydrophilic wire 260 cm (if necessary)	Several	Vascular closure device (if necessary)	Several
6–12F short sheath (if necessary)	Several		

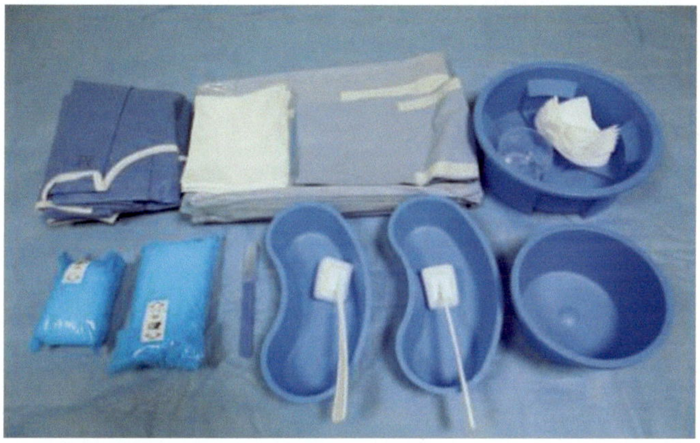

Fig. 13.2 Disposable operation kit

Selection of Minimally Invasive Endovascular Surgery

Different minimally invasive endovascular surgeries can be worked out according to the opening position and shape of the aortic dissection:

(a) Aortic dissection treatment with thoracic aortic endovascular graft exclusion technique: thoracic aortic endovascular graft exclusion technique can be used to treat aortic dissection without involving the supra-arch branch arteries. The thoracic endovascular stent grafts for clinical practice mainly include Hercules (MicroPort), Ankura (LifeTech), Captivia (Medtronic), C-TAG (Gore), Zenith TX2 (Cook), Relay (Bolton Medical), and others. If internal hemorrhage still exists after the placement of thoracic endovascular stent graft, the extension (cuff) can be implanted for further exclusion, or Coda balloon is selected for balloon dilatation, or embolization, lyophilized human fibrin sealant for topical use, or Onyx liquid embolic agent is used for embolotherapy [3–6].

(b) Aortic dissection treatment with chimney-like endovascular exclusion technique: Chimney-like endovascular exclusion technique can be used for aortic dissection involving supra-arch branch arteries. Single- (Fig. 13.3), double-, or triple-chimney technique (Fig. 13.4) can be selected according to the arteries involved with the rupture of the aortic dissection in actual operation. Chimney-like stents can be self-expanding peripheral bare stents or peripheral stent grafts [3–6].

(c) Aortic dissection treatment with endovascular exclusion technique by branched TAA stent graft (Fig. 13.5): Branched TAA stent graft can be used for treating aortic dissection involving three aortic arch branches. Single-, double-, or triple-branch stent graft can be selected according to the branched arteries involved with the rupture of the aortic dissection in operation. At present, Castor (MicroPort) branched TAA stent graft developed and researched mainly by the Vascular Surgery of Changhai Hospital affiliated to Naval Medical University has been transformed and is approved to be put into market [3–6].

(d) Aortic dissection treatment with endovascular exclusion technique by restrictive self-expanding bare stent and TAA stent graft (Fig. 13.6): For aortic dissection whose distal diameter differs greatly from the proximal one, a self-expanding bare stent (such as 16–36 mm Optimed Visual-XL self-expanding bare stent, the size of which is determined according to the distal artery) can be implanted into the distal end of the dissection and then a TAA stent graft into the proximal end, thus avoiding fresh rupture occurring to the distal aortic wall due to direct implanting of the TAA stent graft [3–6].

Procedures and Intraoperative Coordination Process

Endovascular repair of aortic dissection by TAA stent graft technique under general anesthesia is taken as an example, as shown in Table 13.3.

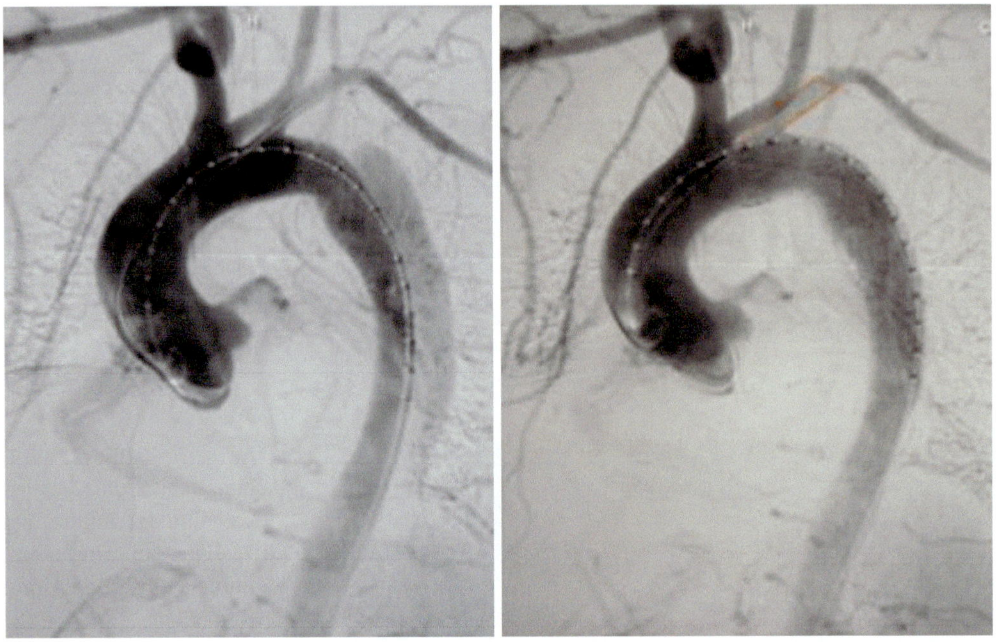

Fig. 13.3 Aortic dissection treatment with single-chimney endovascular exclusion technique

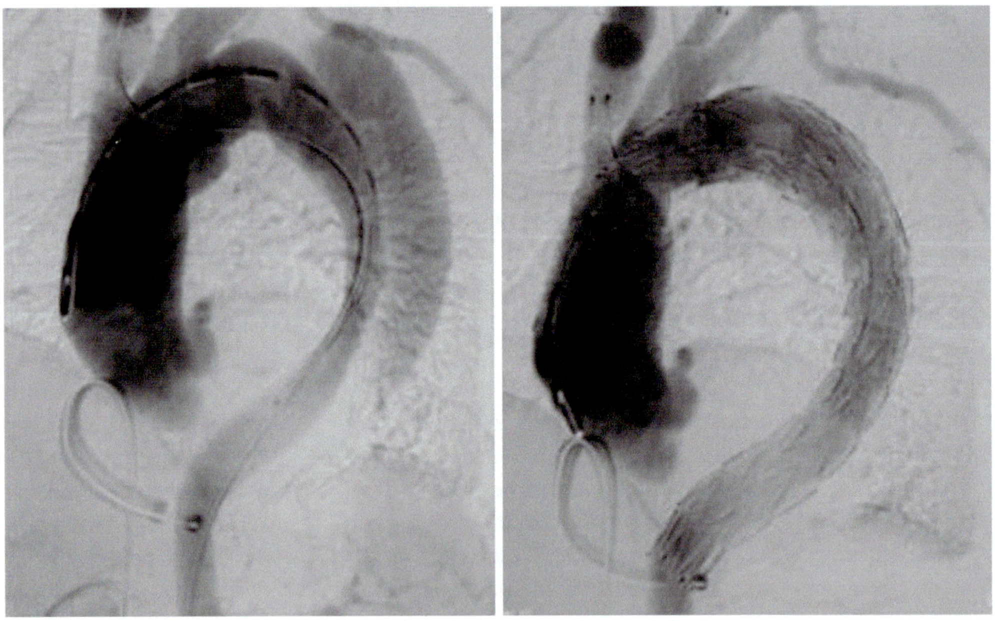

Fig. 13.4 Aortic dissection treatment with triple-chimney endovascular exclusion technique

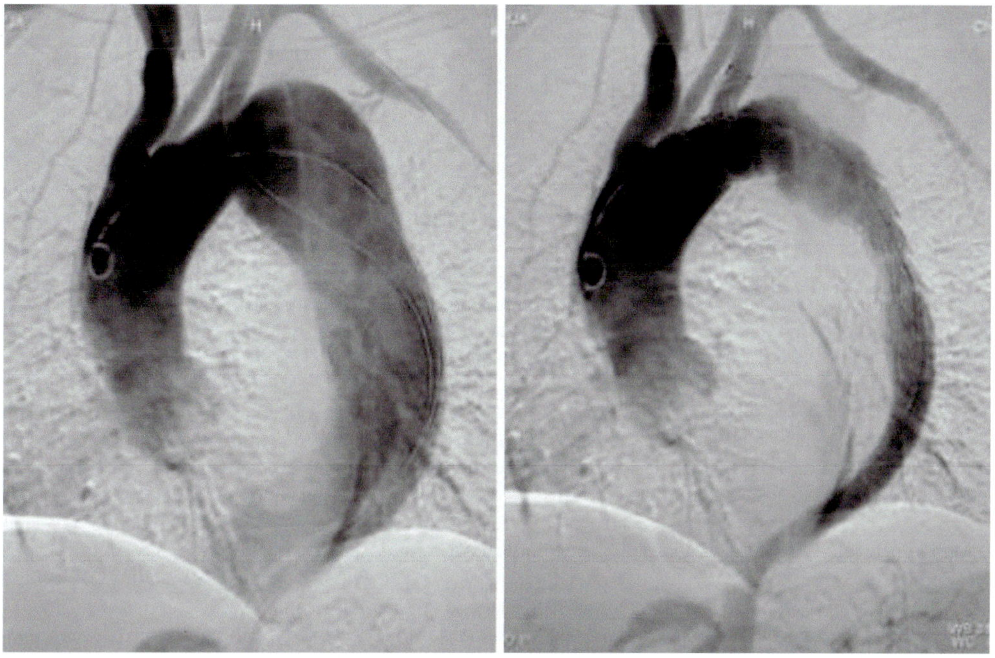

Fig. 13.5 Aortic dissection treatment with endovascular exclusion technique by single-branch TAA stent graft

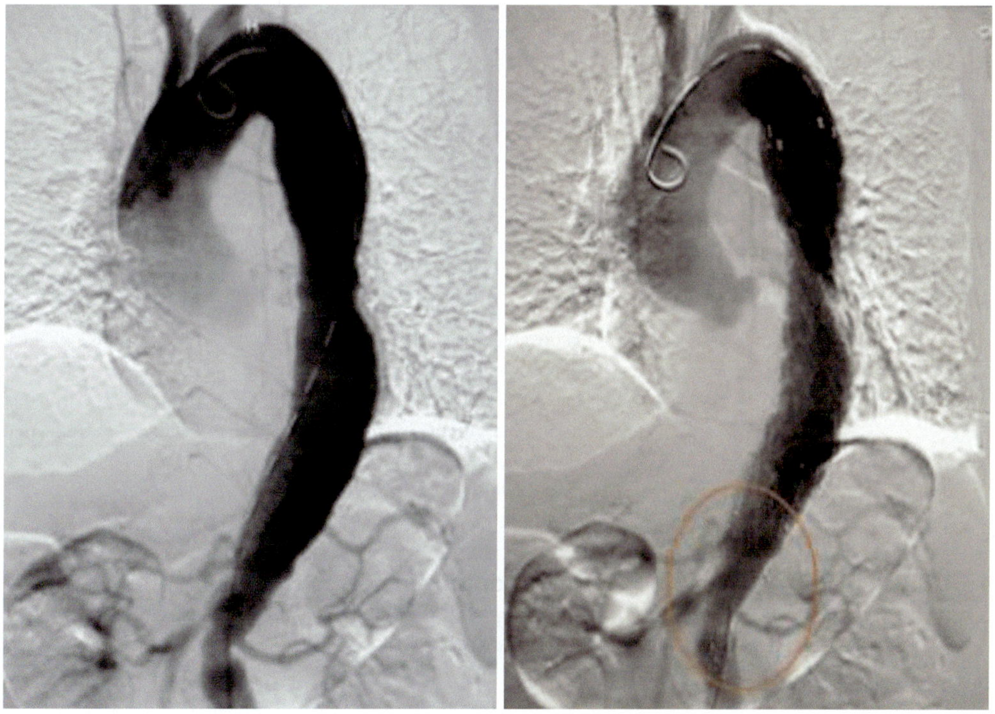

Fig. 13.6 Aortic dissection with endovascular exclusion technique by restrictive bare stent and TAA stent graft

Table 13.3 Procedures and intraoperative coordination process

Procedures	Intraoperative coordination process
1. Patient enters the operation room and receives general anesthesia	(1) Mental nursing; (2) keep the patient warm; (3) take supine position, with two lower limbs slightly at abduction and extorsion position; (4) connect ECG to observe changes in blood pressure, heart rate, and oxygen saturation; (5) establish intravenous infusion, and place indwelling central venous catheter; (6) place the indwelling urinary catheter
2. Routinely sterilize the bilateral groins from the umbilical down to the mid-thigh, exposing the groins	Prepare disinfectant (heated to 98.6 °F with incubator) and assist with draping, deliver iodixanol injection, and prepare heparin diluent (1000 mL normal saline +100 mg heparin sodium injection)
3. Cut a longitudinal or transverse incision of about 3 cm on the common femoral artery of the groin, at the punctum maximum of the pulse, dissociate and expose the unilateral common femoral artery	Deliver the scalpels, large tweezers (flat tweezers or fine tweezers), separating pliers, mosquito pliers, vascular pliers, and 0# silk suture
4. Puncture the unilateral common femoral artery with modified Seldinger technique, insert a 0.035 in common hydrophilic wire 180 cm and a 5F scaled pigtail catheter, conduct thoracic aortic angiography	Deliver the puncture needle, 0.035 in common hydrophilic wire 180 cm, and 5F scaled pigtail catheter; perform systemic heparinization (initial administered dose is 0.67 mg/kg based on body weight, and subsequent dosage is administered according to the actual intraoperative situations); endovascular devices should be flushed with the prepared heparin diluent
5. Evaluate and select an appropriate thoracic aortic stent graft	According to angiography findings, measure aorta profile, and compare it with preoperative CT findings, select appropriate thoracic aortic stent graft
6. Implantation of thoracic aortic stent graft: Exchange via the 5F scaled pigtail catheter to insert the 0.035 in Lunderquist super-stiff wire 260 cm into the ascending aorta; withdraw the 5F scaled pigtail catheter; insert the delivery system of the thoracic aortic stent graft along the super-stiff wire into the aortic lesion, and release it; and then withdraw the delivery system	Deliver the 0.035in Lunderquist super-stiff wire 260 cm and delivery system of the thoracic aortic stent graft
7. Conduct angiography again; check if the aortic dissection is excluded. In case of endoleak, various endovascular technologies can be used	Deliver the 5F scaled pigtail catheter
8. Withdraw the catheter, suture the incision	Deliver the vascular plier and CV suture for vascular incision suturing; deliver round and angled needles and 1# suture to suture the incision layer by layer
9. Anesthesia completed	Safely escort the patient back to the ward

Table 13.4 Preparation of routine items

Name	Qty.	Name	Qty.
Disposable operation kit	1	Disposable venous trocar	1
Disposable 5 mL syringe	1	Disposable syringe	1
Disposable 10 mL syringe	1	T valve	1
Disposable 20 mL syringe	1	100 mL iodixanol injection	1 vials
Disposable gloves	4 pairs	500 mL normal saline	2 bags
100 mg heparin sodium injection	2 vials	Gauze	10 pieces
1% lidocaine injection	2 vials		

13.1.3.2 Intraoperative Coordination for Minimally Invasive Endovascular Surgery of Aortic Dissection with Multilayer Self-Expanding Bare Stent [2]

Anesthesia and Surgical Position

The patient receives local anesthesia and takes supine position (the position to be adjusted according to actual situations during operation).

Preparation of Routine Items

Refer to Table 13.4.

Preparation of Devices

Refer to Table 13.5.

Procedures and Intraoperative Coordination Process

Refer to Table 13.6.

Table 13.5 Preparation of devices

Name	Qty.	Name	Qty.
Puncture needle	1	5F scaled pigtail catheter	1
High-pressure connector	2	5F short sheath	1
0.035 in common hydrophilic wire 180 cm	1	5F Berenstein catheter (if necessary)	1
10F short sheath	1	Coda balloon catheter (if necessary)	1
Visual-XL (16–36 mm)self-expanding bare stent (Optimed)	2–3	0.035 in Lunderquist super-stiff wire 260 cm	1
Vascular closure device (if necessary)	1		

Table 13.6 Procedures and intraoperative coordination process

Procedures	Intraoperative coordination process
1. Patient enters the operation room	(1) Mental nursing; (2) keep the patient warm; (3) take supine position, with two lower limbs slightly at abduction and extorsion position; (4) connect ECG to observe changes in blood pressure, heart rate, and oxygen saturation; (5) establish intravenous infusion
2. Routinely sterilize the bilateral groins from the umbilical down to the mid-thigh, exposing the groins	Prepare disinfectant (heated to 98.6 °F with incubator), and assist with draping; deliver iodixanol injection; prepare heparin diluent (1000 mL normal saline +100 mg heparin sodium injection)
3. Puncture the unilateral common femoral artery with modified Seldinger technique under local anesthesia, insert a 5F short sheath	Deliver 1% lidocaine injection, puncture needle, high-pressure connector, and 5F short sheath; perform systemic heparinization (initial administered dose is 0.67 mg/kg based on body weight, and subsequent dose is administered according to the actual intraoperative situations); endovascular devices should be flushed with the prepared heparin diluent
4. Insert a 0.035in common hydrophilic wire 180 cm and a 5F scaled pigtail catheter, locate the catheter tip at the aortic arch, withdraw the wire, conduct aortic arch angiography	Deliver the 0.035in common hydrophilic wire 180 cm and 5F scaled pigtail catheter
5. Withdraw the 5F short sheath, exchange via the 5F scaled pigtail catheter to insert a 10F short sheath and a 0.035in Lunderquist super-stiff wire 260 cm	Deliver the 10F short sheath and 0.035 in Lunderquist super-stiff wire 260 cm
6. According to angiography findings, measure the aortic diameter, select appropriate self-expanding bare stent, insert the stent into the aortic lesion site, and release it along the 0.035 in Lunderquist super-stiff wire 260 cm	Deliver the Visual-XL (16–36 mm) self-expanding bare stent
7. Conduct angiography again (Fig. 13.7), and observe the blood flow change in the false lumen of the aortic dissection. In case of poor effect, conduct other endovascular techniques, or insert more self-expanding bare stents	Deliver the 5F scaled pigtail catheter
8. Withdraw the catheter and vascular sheath, select appropriate vascular closure device to occlude the puncture site	Deliver the vascular closure device
9. Compression dressing on the puncture site	Deliver the gauze and elastic bandage, and assist with bandaging; safely escort the patient back to the ward

13.1.4 Key for Intraoperative Observation

13.1.4.1 Observe Blood Pressure

Because high requirement is set for the aortic dissection patient regarding blood pressure control during operation, blood pressure should be monitored every 5 min. If necessary, conduct dynamic monitoring of arterial blood pressure. If the blood pressure of the patient is high during operation, calcium ion antagonist and other drugs can be administered to control the blood pressure. Systolic blood pressure should be controlled at 120–130 mmHg and diastolic blood pressure at 70–80 mmHg.

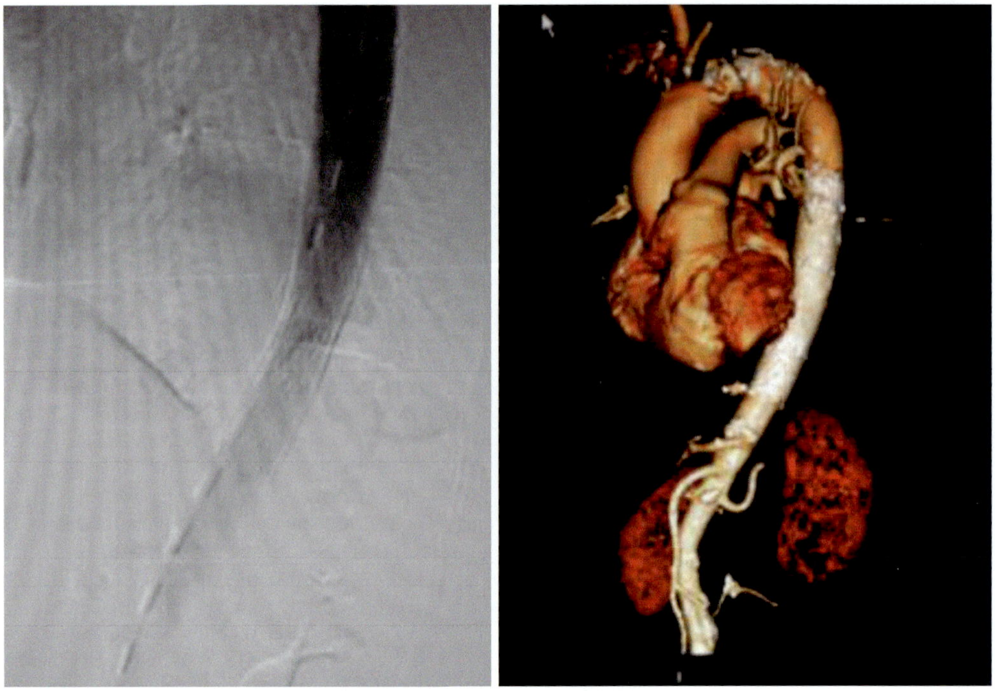

Fig. 13.7 Post-implantation of multilayer bare stent for aortic dissection

13.1.4.2 Observe Renal Function

Sometimes, the aortic dissection patient has his/her unilateral or bilateral renal artery opening in the false lumen. Placing thoracic aortic stent graft will lead to changes in renal blood supply, while 100–200 mL radiocontrast is used during operation. Therefore, the urine output of the patient should be monitored so as to evaluate the renal function of the patient.

13.1.4.3 Observe the Puncture Site

Due to systemic heparinization during operation, the coagulation mechanism of the patient is inhibited, increasing the probability of hematoma formation at the puncture site. Therefore, the puncture site of the patient should be closely observed for bleeding and subcutaneous hematoma and other local symptoms, and the degree of bleeding at the puncture site should be determined according to the status of the vital signs of the patient.

13.1.4.4 Observe Peripheral Artery Blood Supply

Endovascular aortic dissection repair needs to cut open the common femoral artery and even requires for brachial artery puncture in special circumstance. The skin temperature, color, and pulse of four limbs of the patient should be closely observed during operation.

13.2 Abdominal Aortic Aneurysm

13.2.1 Introduction

Abdominal aortic aneurysm (AAA) is a localized enlargement of the abdominal aorta that the diameter is more than 50% larger than its normal diameter (Fig. 13.8). AAA occurs most commonly among aged males, at a male to female ratio of 10:3, especially among smokers, and smoking also significantly increases the risk of aneurysm rupture. The vast majority of abdominal aortic aneurysm occurs below the renal artery level.

13.2.2 Clinical Manifestations

AAA is asymptomatic for most patients and is usually found by accident in physical examination or other kinds of disease examination. Typical abdominal aortic aneurysm is a swelling mass pulsating sidewise or back and forth, accompanied with vascular murmur for most patients, and oppressive symptoms for a few patients, commonly with upper abdominal fullness and discomfort. Symptomatic AAA suggests the need for surgical treatment, the symptoms of which mainly include the following aspects.

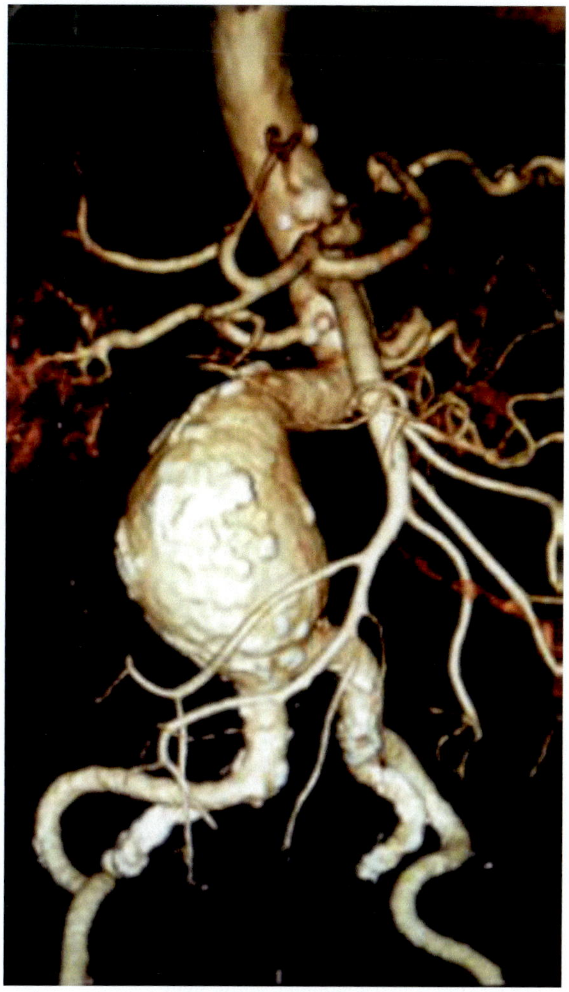

Fig. 13.8 Abdominal aortic aneurysm

13.2.2.1 Pain

Pain is the common symptom occurring before AAA rupture, mostly at periumbilical, upper, and middle abdomen. When AAA involves the lumbar vertebra, lumbosacral pain may occur and in case of sudden onset of sharp abdominal or waist pain, which often indicates that the aneurysm is on the verge of rupture.

13.2.2.2 Shock

The patient with acute AAA rupture shows sudden onset of sharp back and waist pain, accompanied by shock, or even dies before admission. If the ruptured AAA is broken into the retroperitoneum, hemorrhage constraint would lead to the formation of hematoma, abdominal pain, and hemorrhagic shock that can last several hours or days, but hematoma often poses the possibility of causing death because the hematoma may rupture again and flow into the peritoneal cavity. The aneurysm can also break into the inferior vena cava, resulting in aortic vena cava fistula and heart failure symptoms. The aneurysm can occasionally break into the duodenum, causing gastrointestinal bleeding.

13.2.2.3 Other Serious Complications

Formation of mural thrombus in the aneurysmal cavity occurs most frequently, and the falling off of thrombus may lead to artery embolization of lower extremity. Compression on the duodenum may lead to intestinal obstruction; compression and occlusion of the inferior vena cava can cause lower extremity edema.

13.2.3 Intraoperative Coordination

Minimally invasive endovascular therapeutic regime for AAA mainly includes AAA repair with integrated abdominal aortic stent, AAA repair with bifurcated abdominal aortic stent, AAA repair with multilayer self-expanding bare stent [5], etc.

13.2.3.1 Intraoperative Coordination for AAA Repair with Integrated Abdominal Aortic Stent

Anesthesia and Surgical Position

Mainly by lumbar anesthesia or general anesthesia, but with the developing endovascular devices and technologies, local anesthesia has become a new trend. The patient takes a supine position, with two lower limbs being parted and abducted (position to be adjusted according to actual situations of the patient during operation).

Preparation of Routine Items and Instruments

The same as in Table 13.1.

Preparation of Devices

Refer to Table 13.7.

Procedures and Intraoperative Coordination Process

Refer to Table 13.8.

Table 13.7 Preparation of devices

Name	Qty.	Name	Qty.
Puncture needle	1	0.035 in Lunderquist super-stiff wire 260 cm	1
High-pressure connector	2	5F scaled pigtail catheter	1
0.035 in common hydrophilic wire 180 cm	1	5F Berenstein catheter	1
8F short sheath	2	Aegis AAA stent graft (MicroPort)	1
Snare (if necessary)	1	Vascular closure device (if necessary)	1
6F MPA catheter (if necessary)	1	5F Omni Flush catheter (if necessary)	1
Coda balloon catheter (if necessary)	1	0.035 in common hydrophilic wire 260 cm (if necessary)	1

Table 13.8 Procedures and intraoperative coordination process

Procedures	Intraoperative coordination process
1. Patient enters the operation room and receives general anesthesia	(1) Mental nursing; (2) keep the patient warm; (3) help to lie at supine position, with two lower limbs slightly at abduction and extorsion position; (4) connect ECG to observe changes in blood pressure, heart rate, and oxygen saturation; (5) establish intravenous infusion, and place indwelling central venous catheter; (6) place indwelling urinary catheter
2. Routinely sterilize the bilateral groins from the umbilical down to the mid-thigh, exposing the groins	Prepare disinfectant (heated to 98.6 °F with incubator), and assist with draping; deliver iodixanol injection; prepare heparin diluent (1000 mL normal saline +100 mg heparin sodium injection)
3. Cut a longitudinal or transverse incision of about 3 cm on the common femoral artery of the groin, at the punctum maximum of the pulse, dissociate and expose the unilateral common femoral artery	Deliver the scalpels, large tweezers (flat tweezers or fine tweezers), separating pliers, mosquito pliers, vascular pliers, and 0# silk suture
4. Puncture the right (or left) common femoral artery with modified Seldinger technique; insert a 8F short sheath, a 0.035 in common hydrophilic wire 180 cm, and a 5F scaled pigtail catheter; locate the catheter at the same level with the 12th thoracic vertebra; withdraw the common hydrophilic wire; and conduct abdominal aortic angiography (Fig. 13.9)	Deliver the puncture needle, high-pressure connector, the 8F short sheath, 0.035 in common hydrophilic wire 180 cm, and 5F scaled pigtail catheter; perform systemic heparinization (initial administered dose is 0.67 mg/kg based on body weight, and subsequent dose is administered according to the actual intraoperative situations); endovascular devices should be flushed with the prepared heparin diluent
5. According to angiography findings, select an appropriate integrated abdominal aortic stent	
6. Establish crossing catheter: Puncture the left common femoral artery, and insert an 8F short sheath, a 0.035 in common hydrophilic wire 180 cm, and a 5F catheter (Berenstein catheter, Omni Flush catheter, or scaled pigtail catheter). The common hydrophilic wire along with the 5F Berenstein catheter crosses and enters the right iliac artery and draws out the wire and catheter (snare can be used if necessary) from inside the 8F short sheath on the right common femoral artery; withdraw the wire and keep the 5F Berenstein catheter in place	Deliver the puncture needle, 8F short sheath, 0.035 in common hydrophilic wire 180 cm, and 5F Berenstein catheter
7. Draw out the bifurcated wire from inside the 8F short sheath in the left common femoral artery via the 5F crossing catheter, withdraw the 5F crossing catheter, insert a 0.035 in Lunderquist super-stiff wire 260 cm into the distal end of the abdominal aorta via the right common femoral artery, withdraw the 8F short sheath, insert the integrated abdominal aortic stent along the super-stiff wire, and prerelease the stent graft	Deliver the 0.035 in Lunderquist super-stiff wire 260 cm and integrated abdominal aortic stent
8. Locate the integrated abdominal aortic stent: retract the delivery system till the stent bifurcation is located at the patient's aortic bifurcation, release the stent graft main body	
9. Pull the bifurcated wire at the left common femoral artery, release the contralateral wire, withdraw the bifurcated wire (when the assistant helps to pull the bifurcated wire, pull it out compliantly and carefully)	
10. Continuously pull out the delivery system, release the ipsilateral bifurcated wire into the iliac artery	
11. Withdraw the delivery system, insert the 5F scaled pigtail catheter, conduct abdominal aortic angiography again (Fig. 13.10), and check if the AAA is excluded, and if endoleak still exists, various endovascular therapies are available	Deliver the 5F scaled pigtail catheter
12. Withdraw the catheter and vascular sheath, suture the incision of the right common femoral artery, select an appropriate vascular closure device to occlude the puncture site of the left common femoral artery	Deliver the vascular closure device; deliver the vascular pliers and CV suture to suture the vascular incision; deliver small round and angled needles and 1# silk suture to suture the incision layer by layer
13. Anesthesia completed, compression dressing on the puncture site	Deliver the gauze and elastic bandage; assist with dressing; escort the patient back to the ward

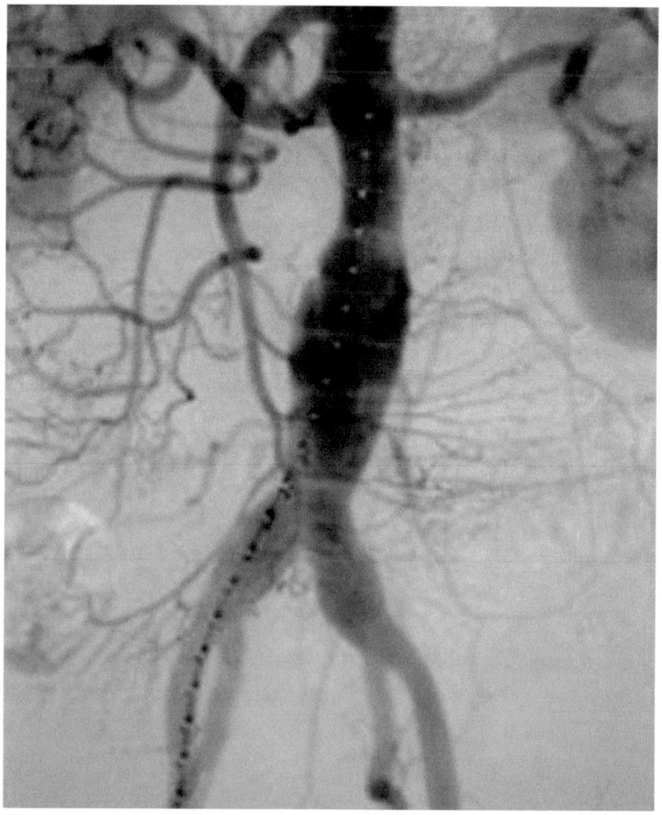

Fig. 13.9 Preoperative abdominal aorta angiography

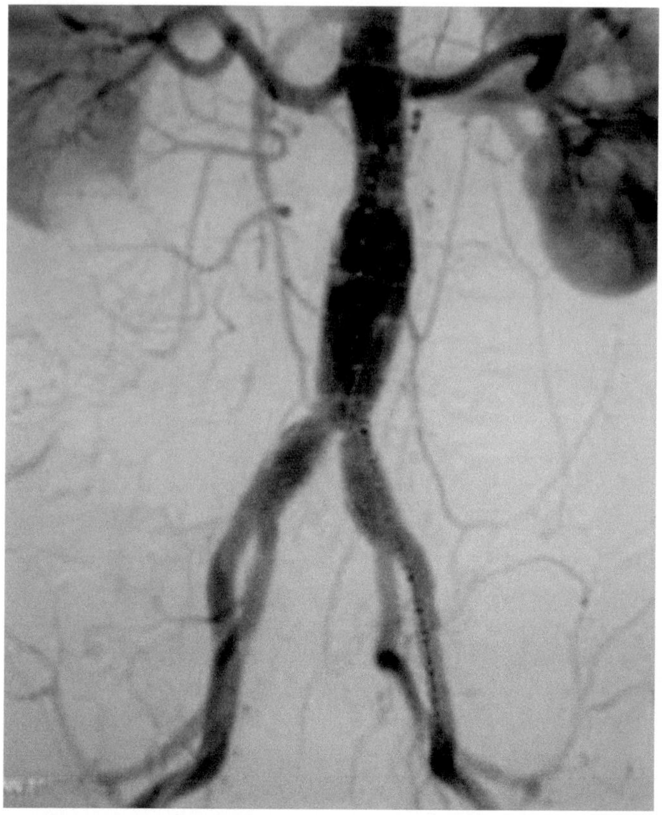

Fig. 13.10 Postoperative abdominal aorta angiography

13.2.3.2 Intraoperative Coordination for AAA Repair with Bifurcated Abdominal Aortic Stent

Anesthesia and Surgical Position

Mainly by lumbar anesthesia or general anesthesia, but with the development of endovascular devices and technologies, percutaneous EVAR technique under local anesthesia has been increasingly becoming a more minimally invasive and more acceptable treatment. This technique requires for no incision to expose the common femoral artery, by which two ProGlide staplers are pre-embedded after percutaneous puncture and upon completion of the endovascular operation, the pre-embedded suture is tightened so as to close the arterial wound and stop bleeding. The patient takes a supine position, with both lower limbs parted and abducted (the position to be adjusted according to the actual situations of the patient during operation).

Preparation of Routine Items and Instruments

The same as in Table 13.1.

Preparation of Devices

Refer to Table 13.9.

Table 13.9 Preparation of devices

Name	Qty.	Name	Qty.
Puncture needle	1	0.035in Lunderquist super-stiff wire 260 cm	2
High-pressure connector	2	5F scaled pigtail catheter	1
0.035 in common hydrophilic wire 180 cm	1	5F Berenstein catheter	1
Abdominal aortic stent body	1	Abdominal aortoiliac stent	Several
Coda balloon catheter (if necessary)	1	5–14 F short sheath (if necessary)	Several
Self-expanding peripheral bare stent (if necessary)	Several	Peripheral stent graft (if necessary)	Several
Balloon expandable peripheral bare stent (if necessary)	Several	Cuff (if necessary)	1
6F long sheath (if necessary)	Several	Embolization (if necessary)	Several
6F Ansel long sheath 45 cm (if necessary)	1	Onyx liquid embolic agent (if necessary)	Several
0.014 in wire (if necessary)	Several	0.035 in Rosen super-stiff wire 260 cm (if necessary)	Several
0.035 in common hydrophilic wire 260 cm (if necessary)	Several	0.035 in hardened hydrophilic wire 260 cm (if necessary)	Several
Vascular closure device (if necessary)	Several		

Selection of Minimally Invasive Endovascular Surgery

Select appropriate minimally invasive endovascular surgery based on the intraoperative AAA morphology and location:

(a) AAA repair with split-type abdominal aortic stent graft: AAA repair with split-type abdominal aortic stent can be used for AAAs involving the iliac artery and complicated with iliac artery aneurysm. The split-type abdominal aortic stents currently commonly used in clinical practice include Hercules (MicroPort), Ankura (LifeTech), Endurant (Medtronic), Excluder (Gore), Zenith Flex (Cook), Incraft (Cordis), etc. If endoleak still exists after release of the split-type abdominal aortic stent during operation, a cuff of extension may be selected for further occlusion or a Coda balloon for expansion or an embolization (Fig. 13.11), a lyophilized human fibrin sealant, or an Onyx liquid embolic agent for embolotherapy.

(b) AAA repair with sandwich technique (Fig. 13.12): Sandwich technique can be used for repair of abdominal aortic aneurysm involving the iliac artery below the renal artery and requiring for retention of the internal iliac artery. That is, insert two peripheral stent grafts at

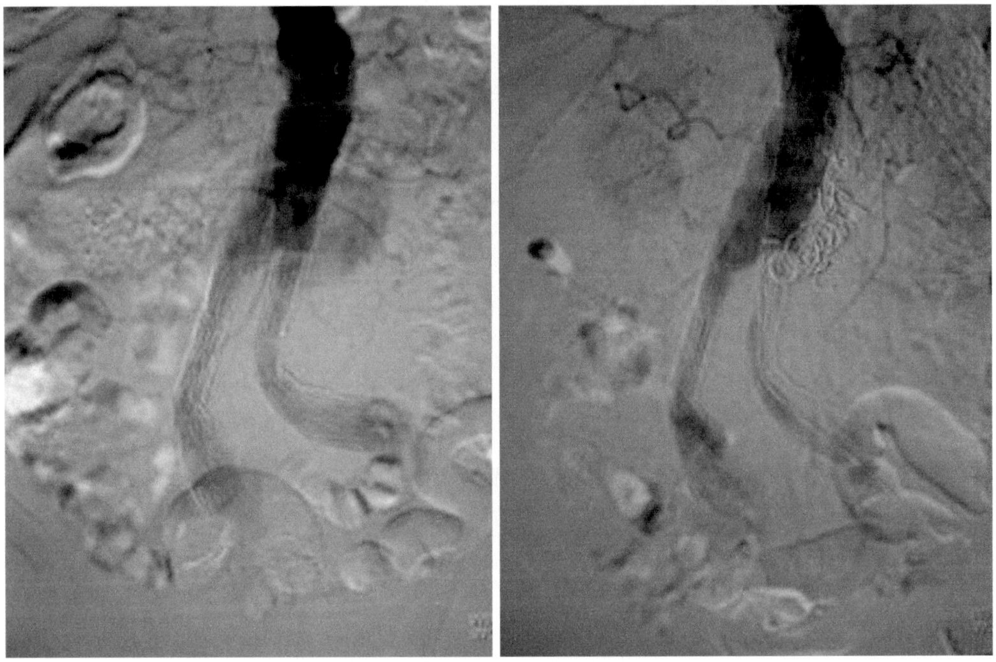

Fig. 13.11 Embolization for endovascular treatment of AAA endoleak

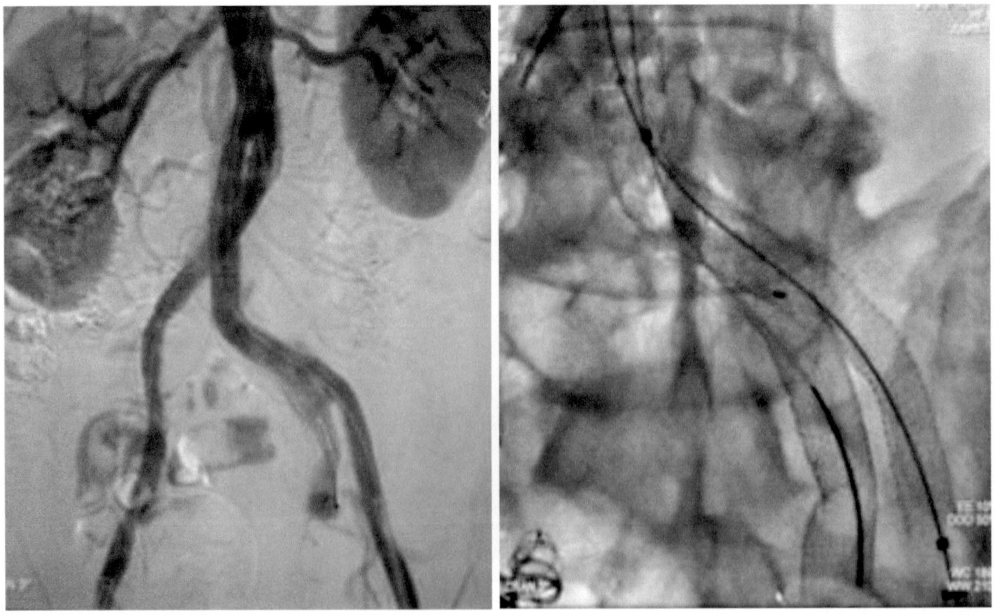

Fig. 13.12 AAA repair with sandwich technique

the distal end of the split-type abdominal aortic stent, one being released outside the iliac artery and the other inside.

(c) AAA repair with chimney or fenestration technique (Fig. 13.13): Chimney technique can be used for AAA with a short aneurysm neck at proximal end. That is, insert a self-expanding peripheral stent graft (or peripheral stent graft or balloon expandable peripheral bare stent) into the renal artery opening. AAA can also be repaired by fenestrated stent graft.

(d) TAA or AAA repair with branching or hybrid technique: (Thoracic) abdominal aortic aneurysm involving visceral artery branches can be treated with branching endovascular graft or hybrid technique of endovascular graft preceded by artificial blood vessel bypass approach for the artery branches.

Procedures and Intraoperative Coordination Process

AAA repair with split-type abdominal aortic stent under general anesthesia is taken as an example, as shown in Table 13.10.

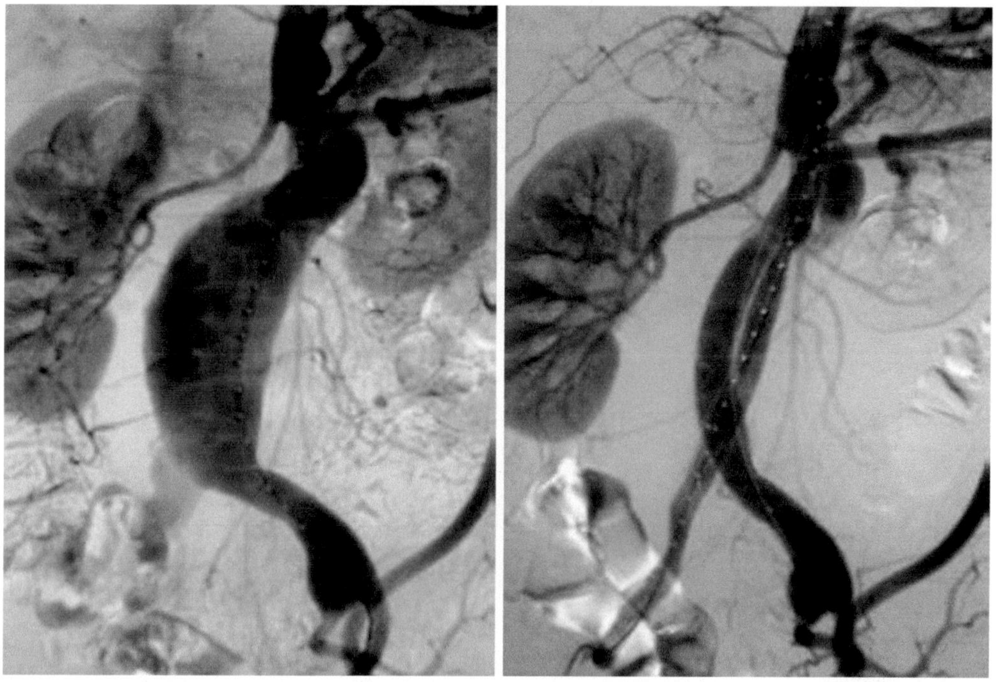

Fig. 13.13 AAA repair with chimney technique

Table 13.10 Procedures and intraoperative coordination process

Procedures	Intraoperative coordination process
1. Patient enters the operation room and receives general anesthesia	(1) Mental nursing; (2) keep the patient warm; (3) help the patient to lie at supine position, with two lower limbs slightly at abduction and extorsion; (4) connect ECG to observe the changes in blood pressure, heart rate, and oxygen saturation; (5) establish intravenous infusion and place the indwelling central venous catheter; (6) place the indwelling catheter
2. Routinely sterilize the bilateral groins from the umbilical down to the mid-thigh, exposing the groins	Prepare disinfectant (heated to 98.6 °F with incubator), and assist with draping; prepare iodixanol injection; prepare heparin diluent (1000 mL normal saline+100 mg heparin sodium injection)
3. Cut a longitudinal or transverse incision of about 3 cm on the common femoral artery of the groin, at the punctum maximum of the pulse, dissociate and expose the unilateral common femoral artery	Deliver the scalpels, large tweezers (flat tweezers or fine tweezers), separating pliers, mosquito pliers, vascular pliers, and 0# silk suture
4. Puncture the right (or left) common femoral artery with modified Seldinger technique, insert a 0.035 in common hydrophilic wire 180 cm and a 5F scaled pigtail catheter, locate the catheter at the same level with the 12th thoracic vertebra, withdraw common hydrophilic wire, and conduct abdominal aortic angiography (Fig. 13.14)	Deliver the puncture needle, high-pressure connector, 0.035 in common hydrophilic wire 180 cm, and 5F scaled pigtail catheter; perform systemic heparinization (initial administered dose is 0.67 mg/kg based on body weight, and subsequent dose is administered according to the actual intraoperative situations); endovascular devices should be flushed with the prepared heparin diluent

(continued)

Table 13.10 (continued)

Procedures	Intraoperative coordination process
5. Select an appropriate split-type abdominal aortic stent	
6. Implantation of abdominal aortic stent: Insert a 0.035 in Lunderquist super-stiff wire 260 cm along the 5F scaled pigtail catheter, withdraw the 5F scaled pigtail catheter, insert the abdominal aortic stent into the abdominal aortic lesion site along the super-stiff wire and release it	Deliver the 0.035in Lunderquist super-stiff wire 260 cm and abdominal aortic main body stent
7. Puncture the left common femoral artery with modified Seldinger technique, insert a 0.035 in common hydrophilic wire 180 cm and a 5F Berenstein catheter, advance the common hydrophilic wire together with the catheter superselectively into the short leg of the abdominal aortic main body stent, withdraw the common hydrophilic wire, and insert the 0.035 in Lunderquist super-stiff wire 260 cm along the catheter	Deliver the 0.035in Lunderquist super-stiff wire 260 cm and 5F Berenstein catheter
8. Implantation of abdominal aortoiliac stent: Withdraw the 5F Berenstein catheter, insert the abdominal aortoiliac stent into the short leg of the abdominal aortic stent via the 260 cm 0.035 in Lunderquist super-stiff wire, and deploy it	Deliver the abdominal aortoiliac stent
9. Withdraw the delivery system, insert the 5F scaled pigtail catheter, conduct abdominal aortic angiography again (Fig. 13.15), observe blood flow change in the aneurysmal cavity, and in case of any endoleak, various endovascular therapies are available	Deliver the 5F scaled pigtail catheter
10. Withdraw the catheter, suture the incisions on bilateral common femoral arteries	Deliver the vascular pliers and CV suture to suture the vascular incisions; deliver small round and angled needles and 1# silk suture to suture the incisions layer by layer
11. Anesthesia completed	Safely escort the patient back to the ward

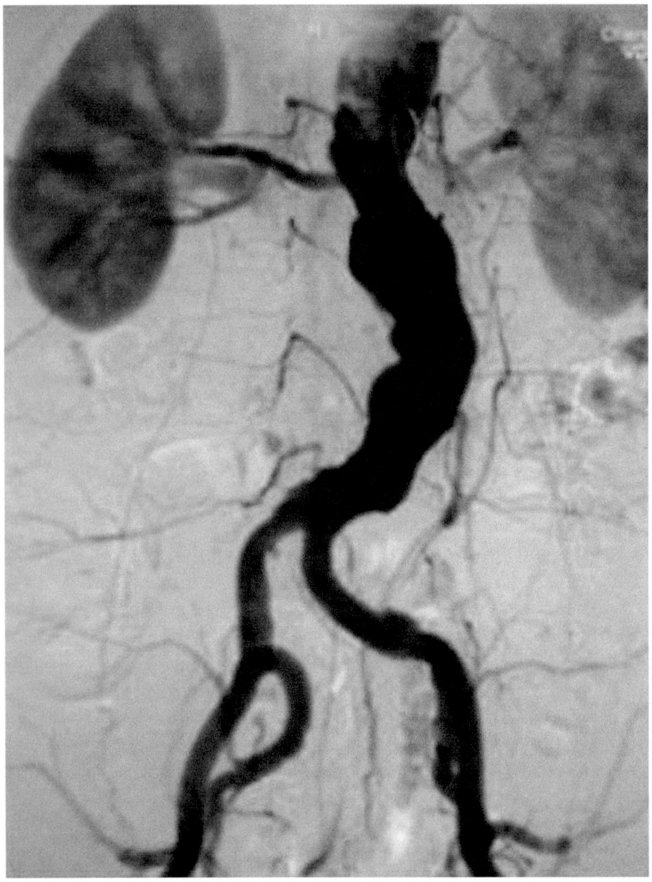

Fig. 13.14 Preoperative abdominal aortic angiography

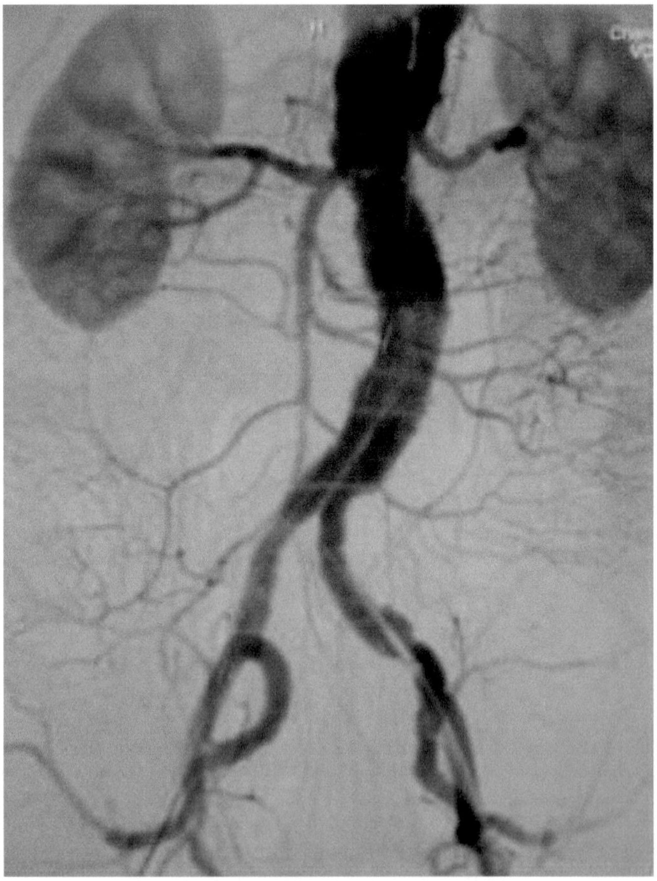

Fig. 13.15 Postoperative abdominal aortic angiography

13.2.3.3 Intraoperative Coordination for AAA Repair with Multilayer Self-Expanding Bare Stent

Anesthesia and Surgical Position

The patient receives local anesthesia and takes a supine position (the position can be adjusted according to the actual situations of the patient during operation).

Preparation Routine Items and Instruments

The same as in Table 13.4.

Preparation of Devices

Refer to Table 13.11.

Procedures and Intraoperative Coordination Process

Refer to Table 13.12.

13.2.4 Key for Intraoperative Observation

13.2.4.1 Observe the Blood Supply of Lower Extremities

As abdominal aortic aneurysm is often accompanied with mural thrombus, the common femoral artery needs to be cut open during operation and then sutured after operation. This may cause the thrombus to fall off or arterial ischemia of lower extremity due to the narrow-down of the sutured common femoral artery. Therefore, blood supply of lower extremity should be closely observed after operation, including skin temperature, color, and dorsalis pedis pulse.

13.2.4.2 Observe Renal Function

In conducting AAA repair, if the location of the AAA stent graft is too high, it can cause renal artery occlusion, and the 100–200 mL contrast medium used during the operation

Table 13.11 Preparation of Devices

Name	Qty.	Name	Qty.
Puncture needle	1	5F scaled pigtail catheter	1
High-pressure connector	2	5F short sheath	1
0.035 in common hydrophilic wire 180 cm	1	5F Berenstein catheter (if necessary)	1
10F short sheath	1	Coda balloon catheter (if necessary)	1
Visual-XL (16–36 mm)self-expanding bare stent (Optimed)	2–3	0.035in Lunderquist super-stiff wire 260 cm	1
Vascular closure device (if necessary)	1		

Table 13.12 Procedures and intraoperative coordination process

Procedures	Intraoperative coordination process
1. Patient enters the operation room	(1) Mental nursing; (2) keep the patient warm, and help the patient to lie at supine position, with two lower limbs slightly at abduction and extorsion; (3) connect ECG to observe changes in blood pressure, heart rate and oxygen saturation; (4) establish intravenous infusion
2. Routinely sterilize the bilateral groins from the umbilical down to the mid-thigh, exposing the groins	Prepare disinfectant (heated to 98.6 °F with incubator), and assist with draping; deliver iodixanol injection; prepare heparin diluent (1000 mL normal saline +100 mg heparin sodium injection)
3. Puncture the unilateral common femoral artery with modified Seldinger technique under local anesthesia, insert a 0.035 in common hydrophilic wire 180 cm and a 5F short sheath	Deliver 1% lidocaine injection, puncture needle, high-pressure connector, 0.035 in common hydrophilic wire 180 cm, and 5F short sheath; perform systemic heparinization (initial administered dose is 0.67 mg/kg based on body weight, and subsequent dose is administered according to the actual intraoperative situations); endovascular devices should be flushed with the prepared heparin diluent
4. Insert a 5F scaled pigtail catheter along the 0.035 in common hydrophilic wire 180 cm, locate the catheter tip at the same level of the 12th thoracic vertebra, withdraw the common hydrophilic wire, and conduct abdominal aortic angiography	Deliver the 5F scaled pigtail catheter
5. Withdraw the 5F short sheath and the 5F scaled pigtail catheter, exchange to insert a 10F short sheath and a 0.035 in Lunderquist super-stiff wire 260 cm	Deliver the 10F short sheath, 5F Berenstein catheter, and 0.035 in Lunderquist super-stiff wire 260 cm
6. Based on the measured diameter of the abdominal aorta, select appropriate self-expanding bare stent, insert the stent into the abdominal aortic lesion site, and deploy it along the 0.035 in Lunderquist super-stiff wire 260 cm	Deliver the Visual-XL (16–36 mm) self-expanding bare stent
7. Withdraw the delivery system, insert the 5F scaled pigtail catheter, conduct angiography again, check if the AAA is excluded, and if endoleak still exists, other endovascular therapies can be performed	Deliver the 5F scaled pigtail catheter
8. Withdraw catheter, vascular sheath, select an appropriate vascular closure device to occlude the puncture site	Deliver the vascular closure device
9. Compression dressing on the puncture site	Deliver the gauze and elastic bandage and assist with dressing; safely escort the patient back to the ward

will also affect the renal function of the patient. Therefore, the urine output, urine color, and creatinine changes of the patient should be closely observed during operation.

13.2.4.3 Observe Intestinal Blood Supply

In conducting AAA repair, the inferior mesenteric artery is isolated, resulting in the insufficiency of sigmoid colon collateral blood supply, which may cause ischemic colitis. Attention should be paid to observing if the patient is with bloating, abdominal pain, peritoneal irritation, and other abdominal signs.

13.3 Extracranial Carotid Artery Aneurysms

13.3.1 Introduction

Extracranial carotid artery aneurysms (ECAA) originate from damaged and thinning arterial wall mostly due to arteriosclerosis degeneration, trauma, tuberculosis infection, syphilis, or congenital arterial cystic medial necrosis, which gradually bulges under the pressure of blood flow and forms artery aneurysm (Fig. 13.16). In addition to aneurysm blockage of blood vessels, or cerebral infarction due to thrombus falling off and subsequent influence on brain blood supply, more serious complication with ECAA is the aneurysm enlargement and rupture, causing fatal bleeding. So once ECAA is diagnosed, surgical treatment must be performed as soon as possible.

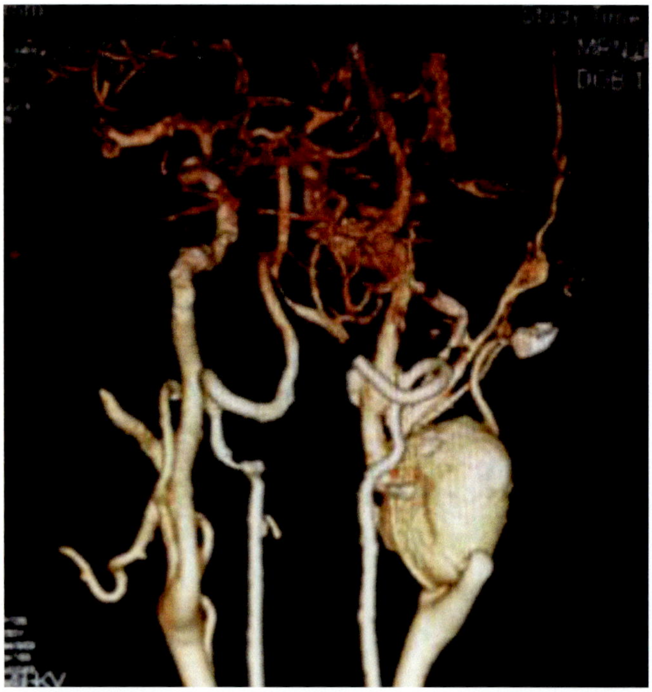

Fig. 13.16 Extracranial carotid artery aneurysms

13.3.2 Clinical Manifestations

The main symptoms are related to the location, size, and cause of ECAA. ECAA's typical clinical manifestation is the pulsatile mass on the neck. Another common manifestation is related to symptoms of the central nervous system caused by the falling off of wall thrombus in the aneurysmal cavity, accounting for about 40% of the cases, and manifested as transient cerebral ischemia (TIA), and even stroke, accompanied with headache, dizziness, amaurosis, hemiplegia, aphasia, and other symptoms. ECAA can also compress the surrounding tissue structures, such as compression of veins leading to local tissue swelling, compression of the esophagus leading to the difficulty in swallowing, compression of the trachea leading to breathing difficulties, compression of cervical sympathetic nerve leading to Horner syndrome, compression of nerves leading to hoarse voice and facial pain, etc.

13.3.3 Intraoperative Coordination

13.3.3.1 Anesthesia and Surgical Position

The patient receives local anesthesia and takes a supine position (the position can be adjusted according to the actual situation of the patient during operation).

13.3.3.2 Preparation of Routine Items and Instruments

Refer to Table 13.13.

13.3.3.3 Preparation of Devices

Refer to Table 13.14.

Table 13.13 Preparation of routine items

Name	Qty.	Name	Qty.
Disposable operation kit	1	Disposable venous trocar	1
Disposable 5 mL syringe	1	Disposable syringe	2
Disposable 10 mL syringe	1	T valve	2
Disposable 20 mL syringe	1	100 mL iodixanol injection	2 vials
Disposable gloves	4 pairs	500 mL normal saline	2 bags
100 mg heparin sodium injection	1 vial	Pressurized infusion bag (if necessary)	1
1% lidocaine injection	2 vials	500 mL sodium lactate Ringer's injection (if necessary)	1 bag
Gauze	10 pieces	Common connector (if necessary)	1

Table 13.14 Preparation of devices

Name	Qty.	Name	Qty.
Puncture needle	1	4F/5F MPA catheter 125 cm	1
High-pressure connector	2	Embolization (Cook) (if necessary)	Several
0.035 in common hydrophilic wire 260 cm	1	Interlock controllable embolization (if necessary)	Several
5F common pigtail catheter	1	Renegade STC 18 microcatheter (if necessary)	1 set
5F short sheath	1	Self-expanding peripheral bare stent (if necessary)	Several
7–12F short sheath (if necessary)	1	Peripheral stent graft (if necessary)	Several
6–10F long sheath (if necessary)	1	Vascular closure device (if necessary)	1
8F guide catheter (if necessary)	1	4F/5F VTK catheter (if necessary)	1
Guide wire accessory kit (if necessary)	1	4F/5F JB2 catheter (if necessary)	1
0.035 in hardened hydrophilic wire 260 cm (if necessary)	1	0.035 in Amplatz super-stiff wire 260 cm (if necessary)	1

13.3.3.4 Selection of Minimally Invasive Endovascular Surgery

Minimally invasive ECAA endovascular surgery mainly includes ECAA repair with peripheral stent graft and ECAA repair with placement of self-expanding peripheral bare stent and embolotherapy.

1. ECAA endovascular repair: Clinically available peripheral stent grafts involve various brands and can be selected in combination with the angiography findings and the features of specific peripheral stent graft. Routinely used peripheral stent grafts are shown in Table 13.15.
2. Placement of self-expanding peripheral bare stent and embolotherapy: This is a minimally invasive endovascular surgery by inserting the self-expanding peripheral bare stent into the carotid lesion site with coil-assisted embolotherapy. In order to prevent the embolization from "floating" to the distal end and leading to normal arterial occlusion, a catheter can be retained in the aneurysm cavity. Embolization is conducted through the retained catheter upon the deployment of the parent artery bare stent, or the retained catheter advances to the aneurysm cavity via superselection through the stent mesh upon the deployment of the self-expanding peripheral bare stent, and then the embolization is implanted via the catheter to fill the aneurysmal cavity. Clinically available embolization brands are multifarious and can be chosen during operation in combination with the angiography findings and the features of embolizations. Routinely used embolizations are shown in Table 13.16.

Table 13.15 Routinely used peripheral stent grafts (for reference only)

Brand	Features
Wallgraft (Boston Scientific)	The stent features excellent compliance and flexibility, and its diameter and length can change with the vascular diameters. The total length of the stent delivery system is 75 cm; selection of vascular sheath is very important, for different peripheral stent graft models are compatible with different vascular sheath models
Fluency (Bard)	The stent features poor compliance but excellent support. Its diameter does not change with the vascular diameters, and the total length of the stent delivery system is 117 cm. Pay attention to the selection of vascular sheath, for different peripheral stent graft models are compatible with different vascular sheath models
Viabahn (Gore)	The stent features excellent compliance but relatively poor support, easy for accessing through tortuous sites, and its diameter does not change with the vascular diameter. The total length of the stent delivery system is 120 cm. Pay attention to the selection of vascular sheath, for different peripheral stent graft models are compatible with different vascular sheath models

Table 13.16 Routinely used embolizations (for reference only)

Brand	Features
Cook	The embolization cannot be retracted once it is deployed. Two systems are available: 0.035 in and 0.018 in, with a length up to 14 cm; the 0.018 in embolization system should be used in combination with the microcatheter and microwire
Interlock (Boston Scientific)	The embolization can be retracted even when not being completely deployed. Two systems are available: 0.035 in and 0.018 in, with a length up to 40 cm; the 0.018 in embolization system should be used in combination with Renegade STC 18 microcatheter; because Interlock controllable embolization has pyknic cilium, pressurized infusion device should be established at the bed end during operation

13.3.3.5 Procedures and Intraoperative Coordination Process

Peripheral stent graft endovascular surgery with common femoral artery puncture technique is taken as an example, as shown in Table 13.17.

13.3.4 Key for Intraoperative Observation

13.3.4.1 Rehemorrhagia Due to Ruptured ECAA

Intraoperative strict control of blood pressure is an important measure to prevent and reduce ECAA rupture and bleeding. Once rupture is found, the following measures should be taken immediately: (1) quickly neutralize the heparin with protamine to restore the coagulation function; (2) complete

Table 13.17 Procedures and intraoperative coordination process

Procedures	Intraoperative coordination process
1. Patient enters the operation room	(1) Mental nursing; (2) keep the patient warm; (3) assist the patient to lie at supine position, with two lower limbs slightly at abduction and extorsion; (4) connect ECG to observe the changes in blood pressure, heart rate, and oxygen saturation; (5) establish intravenous infusion
2. Routinely sterilize the bilateral groins from the umbilical down to the mid-thigh, exposing the groins	Prepare disinfectant (heated to 98.6 °F in incubator), and assist with draping; deliver iodixanol injection; prepare heparin diluent (1000 mL normal saline +100 mg heparin sodium injection)
3. Conduct the retrograde puncture to the unilateral common femoral artery with modified Seldinger technique under local anesthesia, insert a 0.035 in common hydrophilic wire 260 cm and 5F short sheath	Deliver 1% lidocaine injection, puncture needle, high-pressure connector, 0.035 in common hydrophilic wire 260 cm, and 5F short sheath; perform systemic heparinization (initial administered dose is 0.67 mg/kg based on body weight, and subsequent dose is administered according to the actual intraoperative situations); endovascular devices should be flushed with the prepared heparin diluent
4. Insert a 5F common pigtail catheter along the 0.035 in common hydrophilic wire 260 cm, locate the catheter tip at the aortic arch, withdraw the wire, and conduct aortic arch angiography	Deliver the 5F common pigtail catheter
5. Insert the 0.035 in common hydrophilic wire 260 cm along the 5F common pigtail catheter, withdraw the 5F common pigtail catheter and 5F short sheath, exchange to insert a 6F long sheath 90 cm and a 4F/5F MPA catheter 125 cm, superselect the carotid artery for angiography (Fig. 13.17)	Deliver the 6F long sheath 90 cm and 4F/5F MPA catheter 125 cm (catheter replaced according to angiography findings)
6. According to findings of angiography, select and insert an appropriate peripheral stent graft	Deliver the peripheral stent graft (exchange matching vascular sheath according to the selected stent)
7. Withdraw the delivery system, conduct angiography again (Fig. 13.18), and check if the artery aneurysm is isolated. In case of any endoleak, other endovascular therapies can be conducted	
8. Withdraw the long sheath and the common hydrophilic wire, select an appropriate vascular closure device to occlude the puncture site	Deliver the vascular closure device
9. Compression dressing on puncture site	Deliver the gauze and elastic bandage and assist with bandaging; safely escort the patient back to the ward

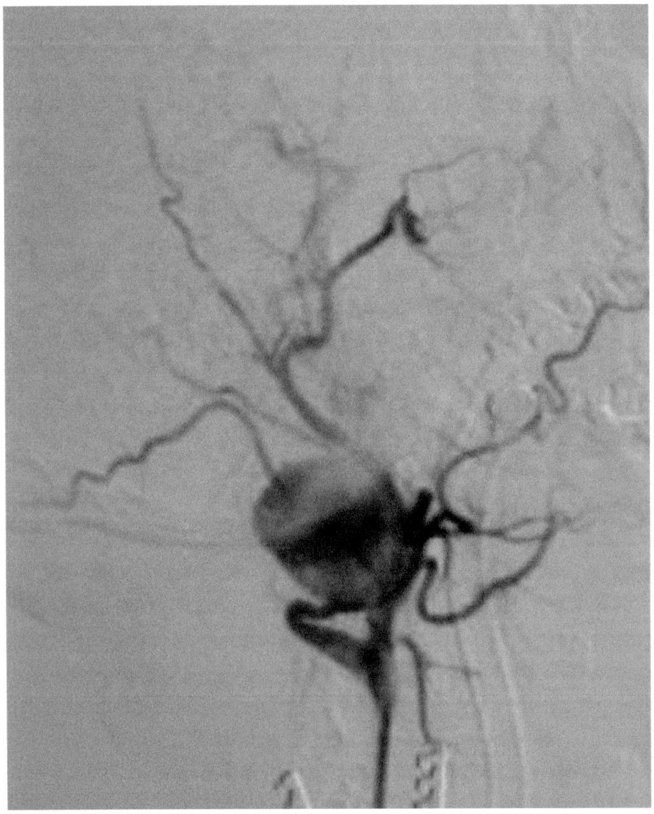

Fig. 13.17 Intraoperative angiography

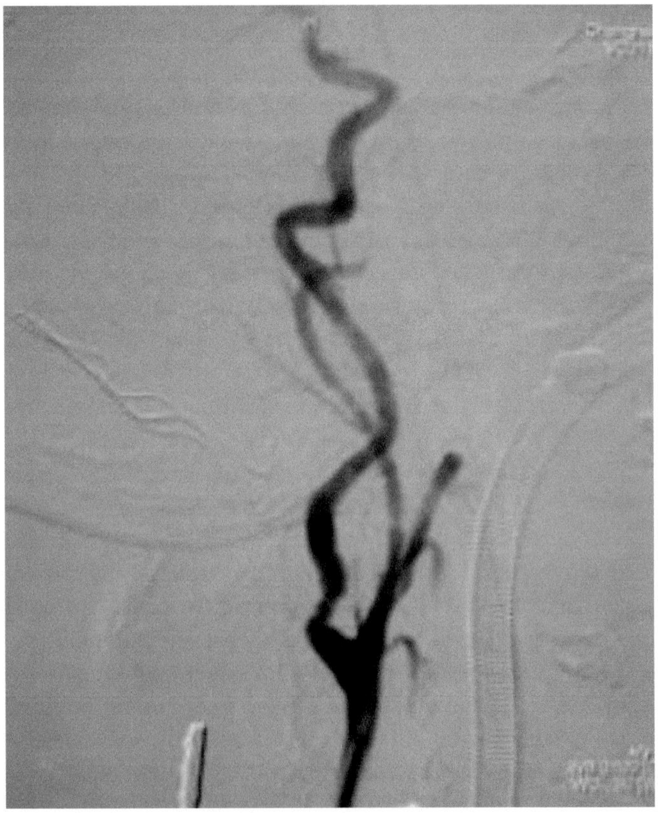

Fig. 13.18 Postoperative angiography

the arterial occlusion and pyknotic aneurysm embolization as soon as possible; (3) bleeding may still exist with incomplete aneurysm embolization—immediately prepare for emergency operation and conduct open surgery; and (4) closely observe the changes of the patient in consciousness, monitor and control blood pressure, and maintain systolic blood pressure at the 130–140 mmHg.

13.3.4.2 Artery Vasospasm

Artery vasospasm is mainly related to the patient's mental stress; improper manipulation; repeated stimulation of the vascular wall by the catheter, wire, and radiocontrast; and vascular wall sensitivity. Once vasospasm is found, the catheter and wire leading to vasospasm should be withdrawn immediately, and trans-arterial injection of papaverine or fasudil should be conducted to expand blood vessels.

13.3.4.3 Thrombogenesis and Intracranial Arterial Embolization

Cerebral infarction resulting from thrombosis and intracranial arterial embolization is the most common complication with interventional embolotherapy, which may be due to the thrombogenesis or the original thrombus falling off into the intracranial artery during the embolization process, falling off of the sclerosis plaque resulting from mechanical stimulation of the vascular wall by the catheter, long-time endovascular operation, insufficient systematic anticoagulation, vasospasm, etc. Once found, urokinase should be prepared immediately, and intra-arterial thrombolysis should be conducted with urokinase or tirofiban via a catheter.

13.3.4.4 Stent and Coil Displacement

Generally, stent displacement occurs very rarely. However, stent may be displaced and fall into the aneurysmal cavity if the stent is insufficiently anchored with the proximal and distal ends of the artery aneurysm, the aneurysmal cavity is very large, or the selected stent profile is smaller than the artery's inner diameter, or the stent is incompletely compatible and cannot be closely attached to blood vessels.

13.4 Renal Artery Aneurysm

13.4.1 Introduction

Renal artery aneurysm (RAA) (Fig. 13.19) is not uncommon, accounting for about 19% of visceral aneurysms, mainly caused by infection, inflammation, atherosclerosis, trauma, muscle fiber dysplasia, and other reasons. Among them, arteriosclerosis is the main reason for the elderly and muscle fiber dysplasia for the young people. 80% RAAs are unilateral, 30% multiple, and 17% intrarenal. Male-to-female incidence rate is roughly the same. RAA can be divided into three types according to its morphology and anatomical location: type I RAA includes saccular aneurysm involving renal arterial trunk and primary branches; type II is fusiform aneurysm; and type III is interlobar aneurysm, among which saccular aneurysm is the most common, accounting for 93%. RAA patients require surgical treatment in the presence of the following symptoms: symptomatic aneurysms, aneurysm rupture, RAA patients with pregnancy, or progressively enlarging aneurysm and dissecting aneurysm.

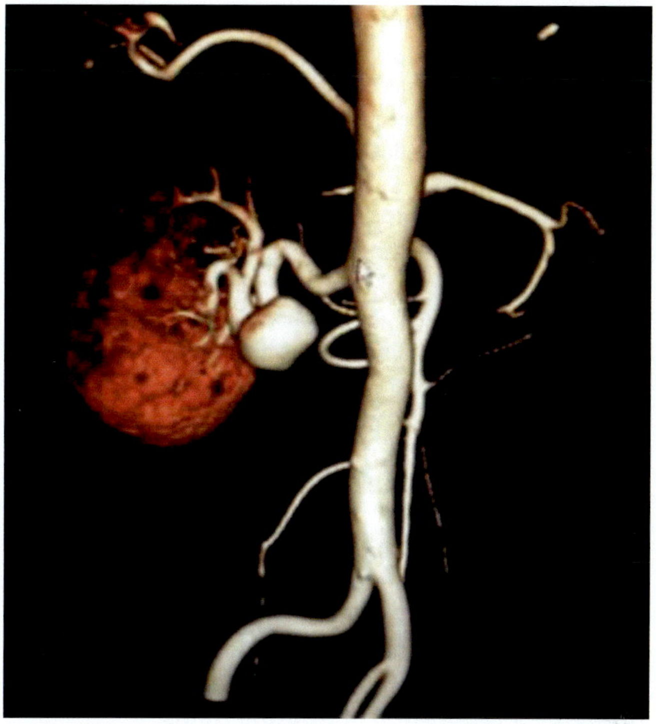

Fig. 13.19 Renal artery aneurysm

13.4.2 Clinical Manifestations

RAA clinical symptoms include hypertension, hematuria, and renal infarction; a considerable number of patients have no significant symptoms. A pulsatile mass can be palpated when the aneurysm grows large, and systolic murmur from the superior abdomen can be heard.

13.4.2.1 Hypertension

Hypertension is the most common presenting symptom of RAA, clinically characterized in continuous elevation of blood pressure, especially the elevation of diastolic blood pressure, difficult to control with common drugs, and often accompanied with such symptoms as dizziness, headache, chest tightness, palpitations, nausea, vomiting, and other symptoms which are related to arterial stenosis, minimal renal infarction, and reduced renal blood perfusion due to compressed branches.

13.4.2.2 Hematuria

Naked eye or microscopic hematuria may occur with some patients, which is associated with hypertension, compression of renal pelvis by artery aneurysm, thrombus falling off, renal arteriovenous fistula, and reflux disorders due to AVF formation.

13.4.2.3 Renal Infarction

The expansion of renal artery aneurysm compresses the surrounding organs, or renal infarction leads to persistent pain. The patient with sudden severe abdominal pain should be alert to the possibility of rupture or impending rupture. At this time, the patient often shows the symptom of hemorrhagic shock.

13.4.3 Intraoperative Coordination

13.4.3.1 Anesthesia and Surgical Position

The patient receives local anesthesia and takes a supine position (the position can be adjusted according to the actual situations of the patient during operation).

13.4.3.2 Preparation of Routine Items and Instruments

The same as in Table 13.13.

13.4.3.3 Preparation of Devices

Refer to Table 13.18.

Table 13.18 Preparation of devices

Name	Qty.	Name	Qty.
Puncture needle	1	4F/5F Sos Omni catheter	1
High-pressure connector	2	6F Ansel long sheath 45 cm	1
0.035 in common hydrophilic wire 260 cm	Several	Embolization (Cook) (if necessary)	Several
5F common pigtail catheter	1	Interlock controllable embolization (if necessary)	Several
5F short sheath	1	Renegade STC 18 microcatheter (if necessary)	1
4F/5F Cobra catheter (if necessary)	1	Self-expanding peripheral bare stent (if necessary)	1
7–12F short sheath (if necessary)	1	Peripheral stent graft (if necessary)	1
7–10F long sheath (if necessary)	1	7–8F guide catheter (if necessary)	1
Y valve three-pieces (if necessary)	1 set	Vascular closure device (if necessary)	1
0.035in Rosen super-stiff wire 260 cm (if necessary)	1	0.014 in spring-head wire 300 cm	Several

13.4.3.4 Selection of Minimally Invasive Endovascular Surgery

RAA minimally invasive endovascular surgery mainly includes RAA repair with peripheral stent graft, embolotherapy, implantation of self-expanding peripheral bare stent, embolotherapy, etc. For RAA repair, peripheral stent grafts available mainly include Wallgraft (Boston Scientific), Fluency (Bard), and Viabahn (Gore) (Table 13.15). Embolization available for RAA embolotherapy mainly includes Cook and Interlock controllable embolization (Boston Scientific) (Fig. 13.16).

13.4.3.5 Procedures and Intraoperative Coordination Process

Take RAA embolotherapy via common femoral artery puncture as an example, as shown in Table 13.19.

13.4.4 Key for Intraoperative Observation

13.4.4.1 Monitor Vital Signs

Blood pressure, heart rate, and oxygen saturation should be continuously monitored during operation, and expectant treatment should be administered with hypertensive patients. The surgeon should be gentle and meticulous during operation, especially in wire superselection, where the wire tip should be visualized throughout the operation, and postoperative delayed renal artery angiography should be conducted to identify any renal perforation and perirenal bleeding so as to avoid harm to the kidney, aneurysm rupture, and other incidences of iatrogenic injury.

13.4.4.2 Observe Puncture Site

In compression dressing on the puncture site, observe if subcutaneous hematoma occurs on the puncture site and if blood oozes out of the dressing, and ask if the patient feels abdominal distension and other kinds of discomfort. If the patient suffers from accelerated heart rate, decline in blood pressure, irritability, and other symptoms, he/she should be treated promptly.

13.4.4.3 Observe Complications

Stent and embolization implantation may cause acute in-stent thrombosis. Therefore, the patient should be monitored for renal area dull pain, nausea, vomiting, and other symptoms during and after operation. Large dosages of radiocontrast agent can also cause harm to renal function, and the patient should be encouraged to drink more water after operation and have his/her renal function reexamined timely.

Table 13.19 Procedures and intraoperative coordination process

Procedures	Intraoperative coordination process
1. Patient enters the operation room	(1) Mental nursing; (2) keep the patient warm, and assist the patient to lie at supine position, with two lower limbs slightly at abduction and extorsion; (3) connect ECG to observe changes in blood pressure, heart rate, and oxygen saturation; (4) establish intravenous infusion
2. Routinely sterilize the bilateral groins from the umbilical down to the mid-thigh, exposing the groins	Prepare disinfectant (heated to 98.6 °F in incubator); assist with draping; deliver iodixanol injection; prepare heparin diluent (1000 mL normal saline +100 mg heparin sodium injection)
3. Perform retrograde puncture to the unilateral common femoral artery with modified Seldinger technique, insert a 0.035in common hydrophilic wire 260 cm and a 5F short sheath	Deliver 1% lidocaine injection, puncture needle, high-pressure connector, 0.035 in common hydrophilic wire 260 cm, and 5F short sheath; perform systemic heparinization (initial administered dose is 0.67 mg/kg based on body weight, and subsequent dose is administered according to the actual intraoperative situations); endovascular devices should be flushed with the prepared heparin diluent
4. Insert a 5F common pigtail catheter along the 0.035 in common hydrophilic wire 260 cm, advance the common hydrophilic wire into the abdominal aorta above the level of the renal artery via the 5F common pigtail catheter, and conduct angiography	Deliver the 5F common pigtail catheter
5. Withdraw the 5F common pigtail catheter and the 5F short sheath, exchange to insert a 6F short sheath 45 cm and a 4F/5F Sos Omni catheter, superselect renal artery for angiography or 3D angiography for complicated lesions (Fig. 13.20)	Deliver the 6F Ansel long sheath 45 cm and 4F/5F Sos Omni catheter (the catheter can be exchanged according to findings of angiography)
6. According to findings of angiography, select an appropriate embolization and insert it into the lesion site (if Interlock controllable embolization is selected, it is recommended to use the 5F catheter) (Fig. 13.21)	Deliver the embolization (if controllable embolization is used, pressurized infusion device should be established at the bed end)
7. Conduct angiography again (Fig. 13.22) and check if the RAA is isolated. In case of poor effect, other endovascular therapies can be used	
8. Withdraw the 6F Ansel long sheath and wire, insert the selected vascular closure device to occlude the puncture site	Deliver the vascular closure device
9. Compression dressing on the puncture site	Deliver the gauze and elastic bandage and assist with dressing; safely escort the patient back to the ward

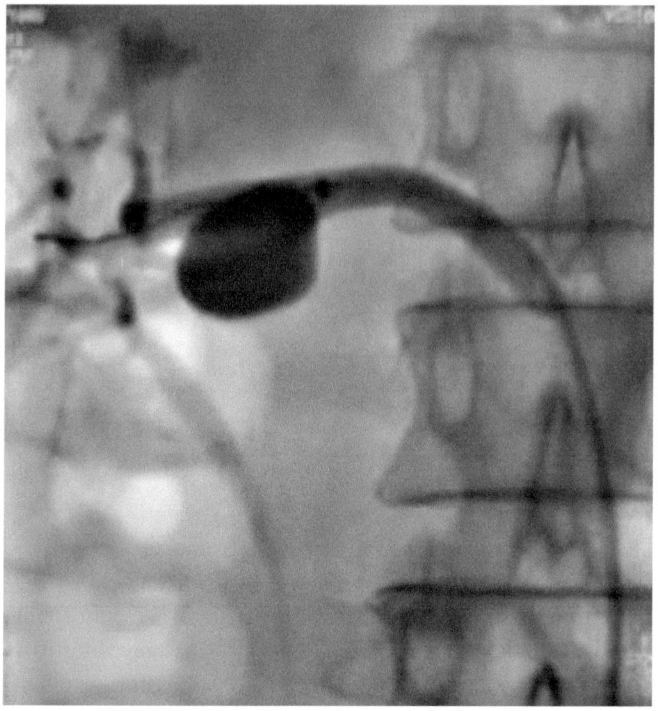

Fig. 13.20 Intraoperative angiography

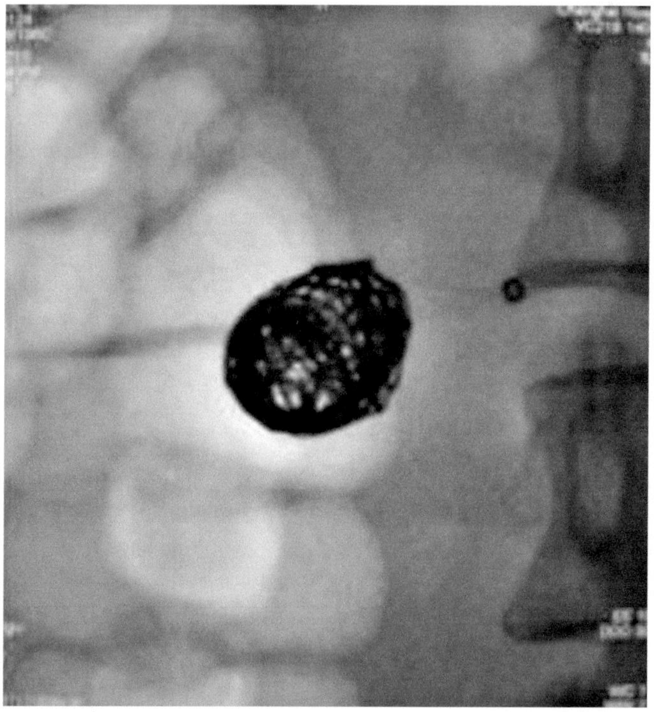

Fig. 13.21 Coil implantation

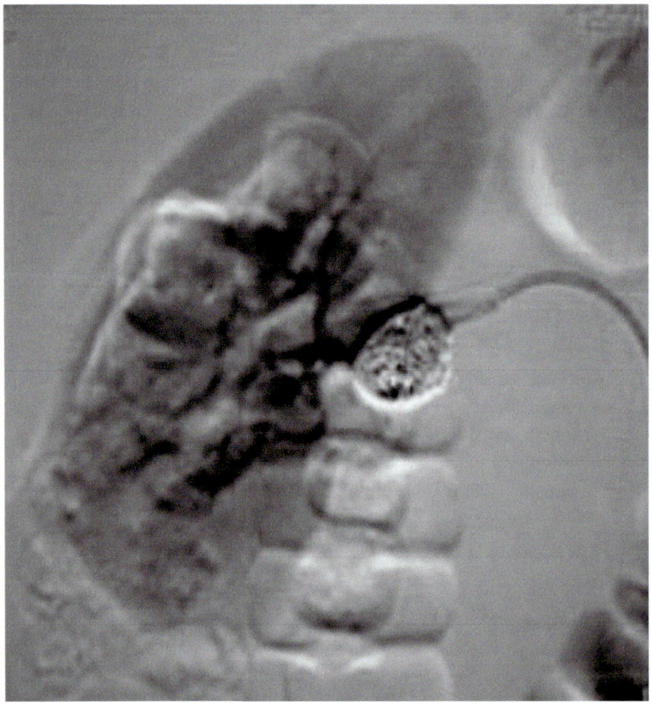

Fig. 13.22 Postoperative angiography

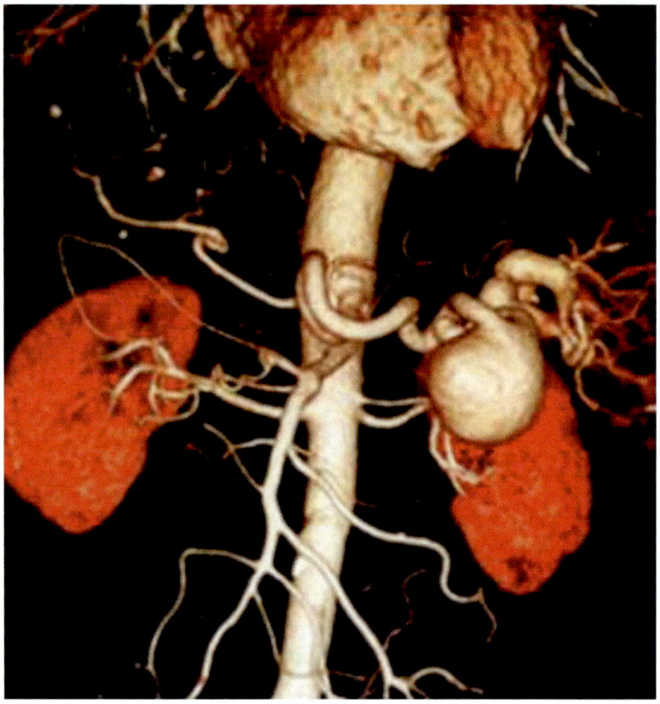

Fig. 13.23 Splenic artery aneurysm

13.5 Splenic Artery Aneurysm

13.5.1 Introduction

Splenic artery aneurysm (SAA) is an aneurysm formed by splenic artery dilation (Fig. 13.23), accounting for 60% of visceral aneurysms at an incidence rate of 0.1–10.4% and male to female incidence rate of about 1:4. Most SAAs occur unilaterally with hidden onset and difficulty in diagnosis, mainly originating from atherosclerosis, splenic artery fibromuscular dysplasia, multiple pregnancies, portal hypertension, acute and chronic pancreatitis, etc. and also uncommonly from iatrogenic injury, trauma, infection, etc. The incidence of true SAA rupture is 3–10%, and the mortality rate of ruptured SAA is 10–25% and even higher in patients complicated with pregnancy or portal hypertension.

13.5.2 Clinical Manifestations

RAA symptoms include upper abdominal pain, paroxysmal colic, nausea, vomiting, splenomegaly, and even intestinal obstruction. Mass can be palpated in about 10% of the patients, and 6% are found with throbbing sensation and bruissement, but most patients may not have significant symptoms and are diagnosed through surgical examination only until the aneurysm ruptures and breaks into the abdominal cavity. Patients that can be definitely diagnosed before SAA rupture are less than 10%. The symptoms after SAA rupture are sharp upper abdominal pain, left shoulder radiating pain (Kehr sign), and left subcostal abdominal haphalgesia, accompanied with nausea, vomiting, and other bleeding performance. Splenic artery aneurysm, if involving the portal system, can also show portal hypertension symptoms such as arteriovenous fistula, AVF, ascites, hepatosplenomegaly, etc.

13.5.3 Intraoperative Coordination

13.5.3.1 Anesthesia and Surgical Position

The patient receives local anesthesia and takes a supine position (to be adjusted according to the actual situations of the patient during operation).

13.5.3.2 Preparation of Routine Items and Instruments

The same as in Table 13.13.

13.5.3.3 Preparation of Devices

Refer to Table 13.20.

13.5.3.4 Selection of Minimally Invasive Endovascular Surgery

According to the anatomic site of the SAA and the morphology of the splenic artery, SAA minimally invasive endovascular surgeries mainly include SAA repair with peripheral stent graft, coil embolotherapy and implantation of self-expanding peripheral stent graft, and embolotherapy.

At present, peripheral stent grafts available for SAA repair mainly include Wallgraft (Boston Scientific), Fluency (Bard), and Viabahn (Gore) (Table 13.15). Embolizations available for SAA embolotherapy mainly include Cook, Interlock controllable (Boston Scientific), and other embolizations (Table 13.16). In case of SAA embolotherapy, please note that radiocontrast injection and embolic material implantation will increase the pressure in aneurysmal cavity, resulting in possible aneurysm rupture. Therefore, the surgeon must be gentle and meticulous in operation. Preferred coil embolotherapy should be free from ectopic embolism, and preoperative preparation of blood and abdominal belt should be conducted so as to get ready for the open surgery.

13.5.3.5 Procedures and Intraoperative Coordination Process

Take SAA embolotherapy via common femoral artery puncture as an example, as shown in Table 13.21.

Table 13.20 Preparation of routine medical supply devices

Name	Qty.	Name	Qty.
Puncture needle	1	6F Ansel long sheath 45 cm (if necessary)	1
High-pressure connector	2	4F/5F Cobra catheter (if necessary)	1
0.035in common hydrophilic wire 260 cm	Several	4F/5F Sos Omni catheter (if necessary)	1
5F common pigtail catheter	1	Renegade STC 18 microcatheter (if necessary)	1
5F short sheath	1	Embolization (Cook) (if necessary)	Several
4F/5F RS splenic artery catheter	1	Interlock controllable embolization (if necessary)	Several
7–12F short sheath (if necessary)	1	Self-expanding peripheral bare stent (if necessary)	1
7–10F long sheath (if necessary)	1	Peripheral stent graft (if necessary)	1
Vascular closure device (if necessary)	1		

Table 13.21 Procedures and intraoperative coordination process

Procedures	Intraoperative coordination process
1. Patient enters the operation room	(1) Mental nursing; (2) keep the patient warm; (3) assist the patient to lie at supine position, with two lower limbs slightly at abduction and extorsion; (4) connect ECG to observe changes in blood pressure, heart rate and oxygen saturation; (5) establish intravenous infusion
2. Routinely sterilize the bilateral groins from the umbilical down to the mid-thigh, exposing the groins	Prepare disinfectant (heated to 98.6 °F in incubator), and assist with draping; deliver iodixanol injection; prepare heparin diluent (1000 mL normal saline +100 mg heparin sodium injection)
3. Conduct retrograde puncture to the unilateral common femoral artery with modified Seldinger technique under local anesthesia, insert a 0.035in common hydrophilic wire 260 cm and a 5F short sheath	Deliver 1% lidocaine injection, puncture needle, high-pressure connector, 0.035 in common hydrophilic wire 260 cm, and 5F short sheath; perform systemic heparinization (initial administered dose is 0.67 mg/kg based on body weight, and subsequent dose is administered according to the actual intraoperative situations); endovascular devices should be flushed with the prepared heparin diluent
4. Insert a 5F common pigtail catheter along the 0.035 in common hydrophilic wire 260 cm, conduct angiography for the splenic artery segment of the abdominal aorta (Fig. 13.24)	Deliver the 5F common pigtail catheter
5. Withdraw the 5F common pigtail catheter and the 5F short sheath, exchange to a 6F Ansel long sheath 45 cm and a 4F/5F RS splenic artery catheter, superselect splenic artery, and conduct angiography or 3D angiography for complicated lesions	Deliver the 6F Ansel long sheath 45 cm and 4F/5F RS splenic artery catheter (catheter to be changed according to angiography findings)
6. According to findings of angiography, select an appropriate embolization and insert it into the lesion (in case of Interlock controllable coil, it is recommended to use 5F catheter)	Deliver the embolization (in case of controllable embolization, the pressurized infusion device should be available at the bed end)
7. Conduct angiography again (Fig. 13.25) and check if SAA is isolated. In case of poor effect, other endovascular therapies can be used	
8. Withdraw the 6F Ansel long sheath and the common hydrophilic wire, select an appropriate vascular closure device to occlude the puncture site	Deliver the vascular closure device
9. Compression dressing on the puncture site	Deliver the gauze and elastic bandage and assist with bandaging; safely escort the patient back to the ward

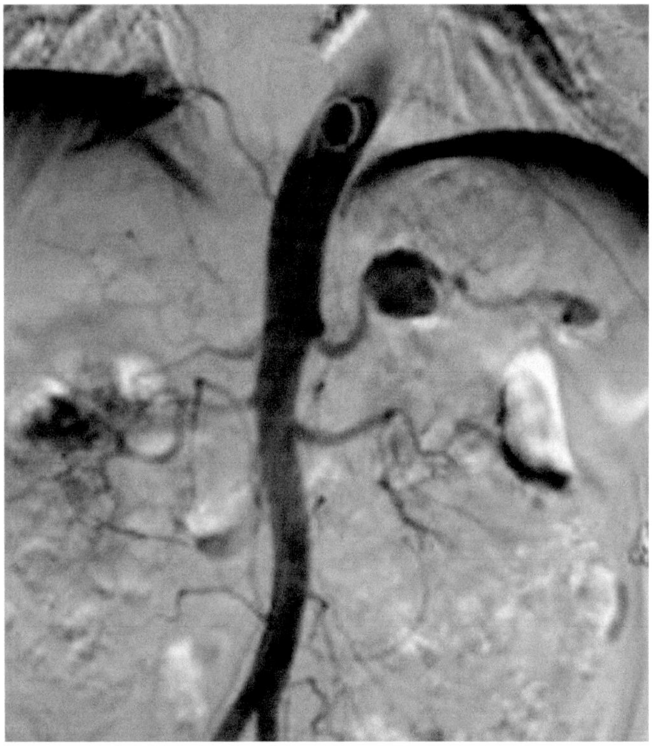

Fig. 13.24 Intraoperative angiography

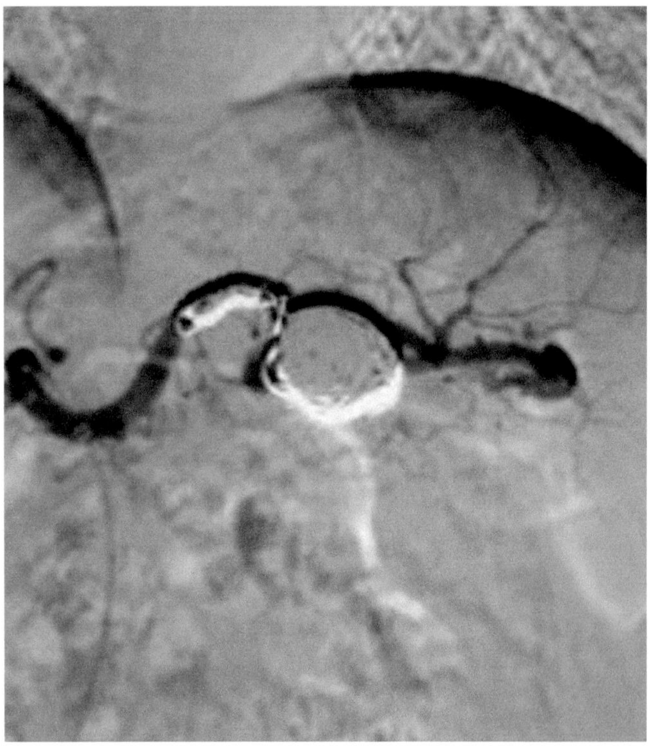

Fig. 13.25 Postoperative angiography

13.5.4 Key for Intraoperative Observation

13.5.4.1 Observation of Vital Signs

During operation, continuously monitor blood pressure, heart rate, and oxygen saturation. Hypertensive patients should be administered with symptomatic treatment. The surgeon should be gentle and meticulous during operation to avoid aneurysm rupture and occurrence of iatrogenic injuries.

13.5.4.2 Observe Abdominal Pain

Stent and coil implantation may cause in-stent acute thrombosis. The surgeon should listen to the complaints of the patient during operation, especially abdominal pain. The patient with embolotherapy is liable of splenic infarction and bleeding. Therefore, abdominal signs of the patient should be closely monitored so as to detect any splenic rupture as early as possible.

13.5.4.3 Observe the Puncture Site

In compression dressing on the puncture site, observe if subcutaneous hematoma occurs on the puncture site and if blood oozes out of the dressing, and ask if the patient feels abdominal distension and other kinds of discomfort. If the patient suffers from accelerated heart rate, decline in blood pressure, irritability, and other symptoms, he/she should be treated promptly.

13.6 Iliac Artery Aneurysm

13.6.1 Introduction

Iliac artery aneurysm (Fig. 13.26) refers to aneurysms involving the common iliac artery and internal and external iliac arteries, but based on the anatomical features, iliac artery aneurysm often stems from abdominal aortic aneurysm involving the iliac artery, and isolated iliac artery aneurysm is uncommon. Iliac artery aneurysm (IAA) with aneurysm cavity diameter > 2.5 cm or 1.5 times larger than normal diameter is considered iliac artery aneurysm, appearing mostly in common iliac artery segment, possibly related to pregnancy, infection, surgical injury, trauma, Marfan's syndrome, and other genetic diseases but mainly due to atherosclerosis.

13.6.2 Clinical Manifestations

Iliac artery aneurysm (IAA) is asymptomatic to most patients and often found in physical examination by accident. Two thirds of the patients can be palpated with pulsatile mass, but due to the deep distribution of the iliac arteries, it is difficult

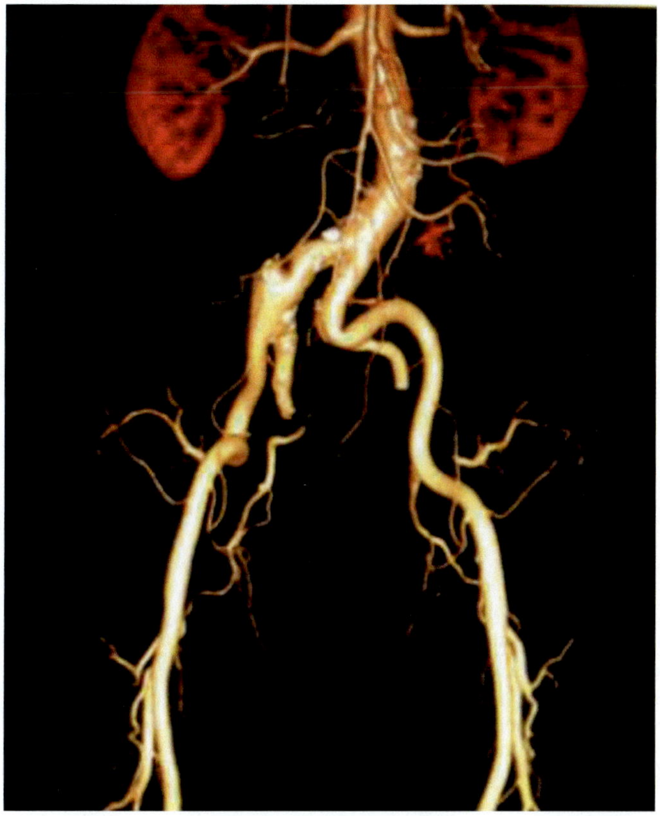

Fig. 13.26 Iliac artery aneurysm

Table 13.22 Preparation of devices

Name	Qty.	Name	Qty.
Puncture needle	1	5F Sos Omni catheter (if necessary)	1
High-pressure connector	2	5F Cobra catheter (if necessary)	1
0.035 in common hydrophilic wire 260 cm	1	5F scaled pigtail catheter (if necessary)	1
5F common pigtail catheter	1	Renegade STC 18 microcatheter (if necessary)	1
5F short sheath	1	Embolization (Cook) (if necessary)	Several
5F Berenstein catheter	1	Interlock controllable embolization (if necessary)	Several
7–16F short sheath (if necessary)	1	Peripheral stent graft (if necessary)	Several
7–10F long sheath (if necessary)	1	Abdominal aortoiliac stent (if necessary)	Several
0.035 in hardened hydrophilic wire 260 cm (if necessary)	1	0.035 in Amplatz super-stiff wire 260 cm (if necessary)	1
Vascular closure device (if necessary)	1		

to detect the aneurysm through physical examination when it is small or the patient is fat. Symptoms of compression relate to the compression of the adjacent anatomical structures, for example, compression of the ureter may lead to hematuria, ureteral dilatation, and even pyelonephritis; compression of rectal bowel may contribute to changes in defecate state and constipation; and compression of the lumbosacral nerve may cause lower limb weakness and numbness. In addition, the breaking off of mural thrombus may result in acute arterial embolization of lower extremity.

13.6.3 Intraoperative Coordination

13.6.3.1 Anesthesia and Surgical Position

The patient receives local anesthesia and takes a supine position (to be adjusted according to the actual situations of the patient during operation).

13.6.3.2 Preparation of Routine Items and Instruments

The same as in Table 13.13.

13.6.3.3 Preparation of Devices

Refer to Table 13.22.

13.6.3.4 Selection of Minimally Invasive Endovascular Surgery

Endovascular therapies for iliac artery aneurysms mainly include IAA repair with peripheral stent graft, coil embolotherapy, IAA repair with stent graft, etc.

1. IAA repair with peripheral stent graft: If there is sufficient “anchoring zone” at the proximal end of the common iliac artery, IAA repair can be performed directly with peripheral stent graft or abdominal aortoiliac stent and, otherwise, with split-type abdominal aortic stent graft or integrated stent graft. If internal iliac artery needs to be retained where the IAA involves the internal and external iliac arteries, the “sandwich” technique can be used for this purpose, that is, to place a peripheral stent graft (alternatively, an abdominal aortoiliac stent) in the common iliac artery, within which two peripheral stent grafts clinically available are nested, one being deployed outside the ilium and the other inside. At present, peripheral stent grafts clinically available mainly include Wallgraft (Boston Scientific), Fluency (Bard), and Viabahn (Gore) (Table 13.15).

2. IAA repair with coil embolization and stent graft: For IAA involving the internal iliac artery, firstly, use the embolization to embolize the internal iliac artery and then implant a stent graft (peripheral stent graft or abdominal aortoiliac stent) in the external iliac artery so as to isolate the aneurysm. At present, embolizations clinically available mainly include Cook, Interlock controllable (Boston Scientific), and other embolizations (Table 13.16).

13.6.3.5 Procedures and Intraoperative Coordination Process

Take IAA repair and internal iliac artery embolotherapy via bilateral common femoral artery puncture as an example, as shown in Table 13.23.

13.6.4 Key for Intraoperative Observation

13.6.4.1 Observe the Puncture Site

Endovascular stent graft implantation is usually conducted via artery puncture, liable of arterial vessel damage and formation of hematoma, which, after being organized, still communicates with the blood flow and forms false aneurysm by circulating out of and into the hematoma cavity through the central arterial holes. Therefore, upon completion of the operation, check the artery pulse on the puncture side and hematoma formation around the puncture site. Meanwhile, attention should also be paid to the patient's vital signs. If the patient happens with dizziness, dry mouth, heart rate increase, and other early-stage shock symptoms, symptomatic treatment should be administered.

Table 13.23 Procedures and intraoperative coordination process

Procedures	Intraoperative coordination process
1. Patient enters the operation room	(1) Mental nursing; (2) keep the patient warm; (3) assist the patient to lie at supine position, with two lower limbs slightly at abduction and extorsion; (4) connect ECG to observe changes in blood pressure, heart rate, and oxygen saturation; (5) establish intravenous infusion
2. Routinely sterilize the bilateral groins from the umbilical down to the mid-thigh, exposing the groins	Prepare disinfectant (heated to 98.6 °F in incubator), and assist with draping; deliver iodixanol injection; prepare heparin diluent (1000 mL normal saline +100 mg heparin sodium injection
3. Puncture the left (or right) common femoral artery with modified Seldinger technique, insert a 0.035 in common hydrophilic wire 260 cm and a 5F short sheath	Deliver 1% lidocaine injection, puncture needle, high-pressure connector, 0.035 in common hydrophilic wire 260 cm, and 5F short sheath; perform systemic heparinization (initially administered dose is 0.67 mg/kg based on body weight, and subsequent dose is administered according to the actual intraoperative situations); endovascular devices should be flushed with the prepared heparin diluent
4. Insert a 5F scaled pigtail catheter along the 0.035 in common hydrophilic wire 260 cm, conduct angiography for bilateral iliac arteries (Fig. 13.27)	Deliver the 5F scaled pigtail catheter
5. Withdraw the 5F scaled pigtail catheter, insert a 5F Berenstein catheter along the 0.035 in common hydrophilic wire 260 cm, superselect the right internal iliac artery, withdraw the common hydrophilic wire, and keep the 5F Berenstein catheter in the right internal iliac artery	Deliver the 5F Berenstein catheter (changed according to findings of angiography)
6. Puncture the right common femoral artery with modified Seldinger technique, insert a 0.035 in hardened wire 260cn and 7–16F short sheath, insert a stent graft into the lesion site of the external iliac artery along the hardened hydrophilic wire, and withdraw the delivery system of the stent graft	Deliver the 0.035 in hardened hydrophilic wire 260 cm and 7–16F stent graft (peripheral stent graft or abdominal aortoiliac stent)
7. Insert an appropriate embolization along the 5F Berenstein catheter retained inside the right internal iliac artery	Deliver the embolization (in case of Interlock controllable embolization, pressurized infusion device shall be available at the bed end because the coil has pyknic cilia)
8. Insert the 5F scaled pigtail catheter along the hardened hydrophilic wire in the right common femoral artery, conduct angiography again (Fig. 13.28), check if IAA is isolated. In case of poor effect, other endovascular therapies can be performed	Deliver the 5F scaled pigtail catheter
9. Withdraw the catheter, wire, and the vascular sheath, select an appropriate vascular closure device to block the puncture site	Deliver the vascular closure device
10. Compression dressing on puncture site	Deliver the gauze and elastic bandage and assist with draping; safely escort the patient back to the ward

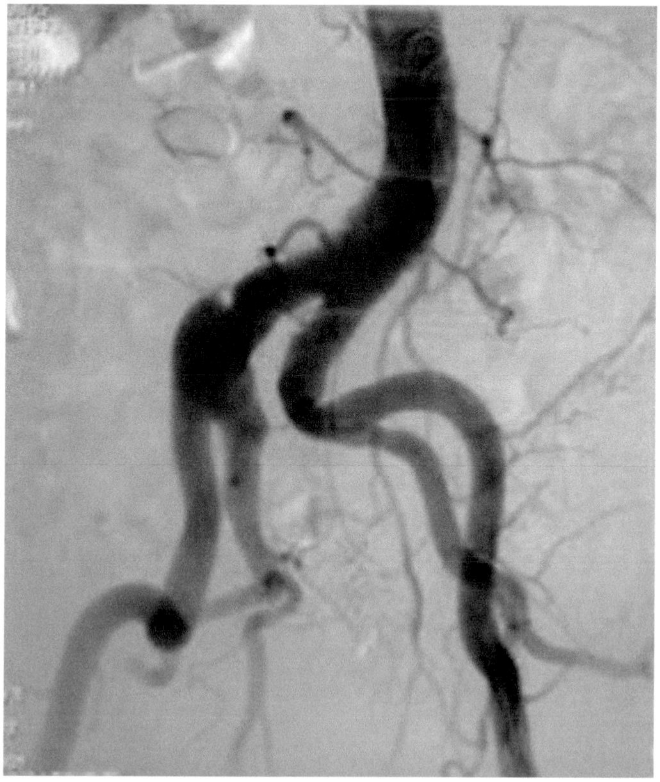

Fig. 13.27 Intraoperative angiography

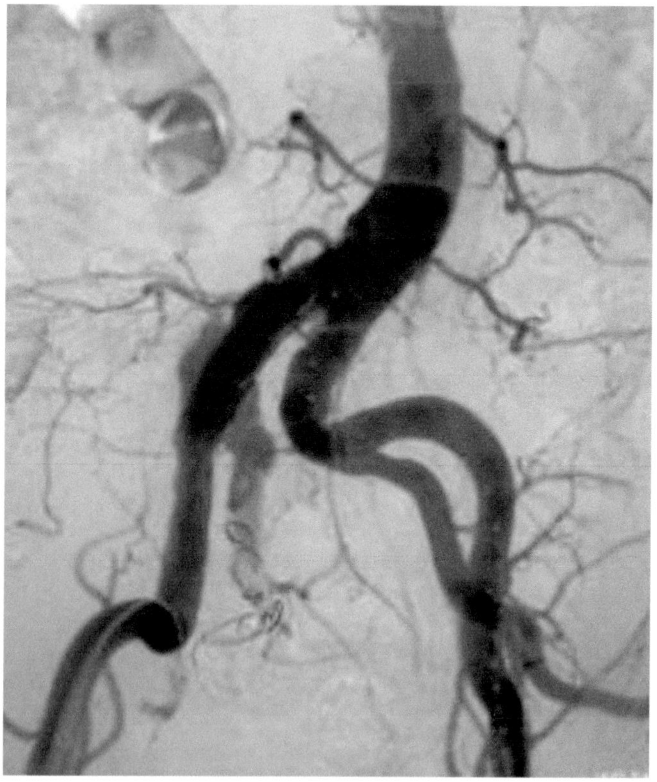

Fig. 13.28 Postoperative angiography

13.6.4.2 Observe the Patient's Blood Supply

Iliac artery aneurysm is often complicated with atherosclerosis. Therefore, attention should be paid to avoiding luminal stenosis or even re-occlusion after using vascular closure devices. In addition, the presence of a cascade of wall thrombus inside the aneurysmal cavity can also lead to breaking off of thrombus during operation, resulting in distal artery stenosis or total occlusion and consequentially acute limb ischemia (ALI) and other symptoms. Therefore, after the operation, closely observe the lower limbs' skin color, temperature, sensation, artery pulse, and any pain complaints. In case of the presence of ischemic pain, pale skin, dysesthesia, loss of arterial pulsation, and other acute artery embolism symptoms, prompt treatment must be performed.

13.6.4.3 Observe Endoleak

Endoleak is the most common complication after endovascular therapies, usually occurring at the proximal end of the stent graft, distal anchorage zone, or damaged site. Maintaining the stability of blood pressure and preventing excessively high arterial pressure are the key to prevent endoleak. Therefore, closely observe the patient's state of consciousness, blood pressure, heart rate, presence of any lower abdominal pain, and pulsatile mass during operation.

References

1. Jing Z. Endovascular therapy. Beijing: People's Medical Publishing House; 2003.
2. Mao H, Zhang L, Mao Y, et al. Intraoperative coordination and nursing for patients undergoing aortic dissection aneurysm repair with multiple self-expanding bare stent. Nurs J Chin People's Liberation Army. 2012;29(18):56–8.
3. Mao Y, Xu X, Li H. Interventional treatment nursing. Beijing: People's Military Medical Press; 2013.
4. Wang Z, Zhang J, Yongquan G. Practical vascular surgery and vascular interventional therapy. Beijing: People's Military Medical Press; 2004.
5. Feng X. Analysis of latest techniques for AAA repair. Beijing: People's Military Medical Press; 2013.
6. Jing Z, Feng X. Aortic dissection endovascular therapy. Beijing: People's Military Medical Press; 2008.

14 Artery Occlusive Diseases

Zaiping Jing, Huajuan Mao, Meiqin Shi, Junmin Bao, Zhiqing Zhao, Xiaolong Wei, and Zhiyong Chen

Abstract

Arterial occlusions refer to a type of diseases mainly characterized by artery stenosis or occlusion. They are frequently seen in peripheral arteries, usually giving rise to the ischemia or necrosis of important distal tissues or organs, etc. With the advent of population aging, arteriosclerosis has become the pathogenesis basis of most occlusive diseases. This chapter mainly introduces clinical manifestations, endovascular surgery process, and intraoperative observation points of carotid artery stenosis, subclavian artery stenosis, renal artery stenosis, and lower extremity atherosclerotic occlusive disease.

Keywords

Arterial occlusion · Carotid artery · Renal artery · Lower extremity artery

14.1 Carotid Artery Stenosis

14.1.1 Introduction

Carotid artery stenosis (Fig. 14.1) is the narrowing in the carotid arterial lumens mainly due to atherosclerotic plaque of the carotid artery, having a high incidence rate and mostly occurring in the bifurcation of the common carotid artery and the starting segment of the internal carotid artery. In particular, the common carotid artery bifurcation lesion is directly related to ischemic stroke. Therefore, its treatment is of paramount importance to prevent the occurrence of stroke [1].

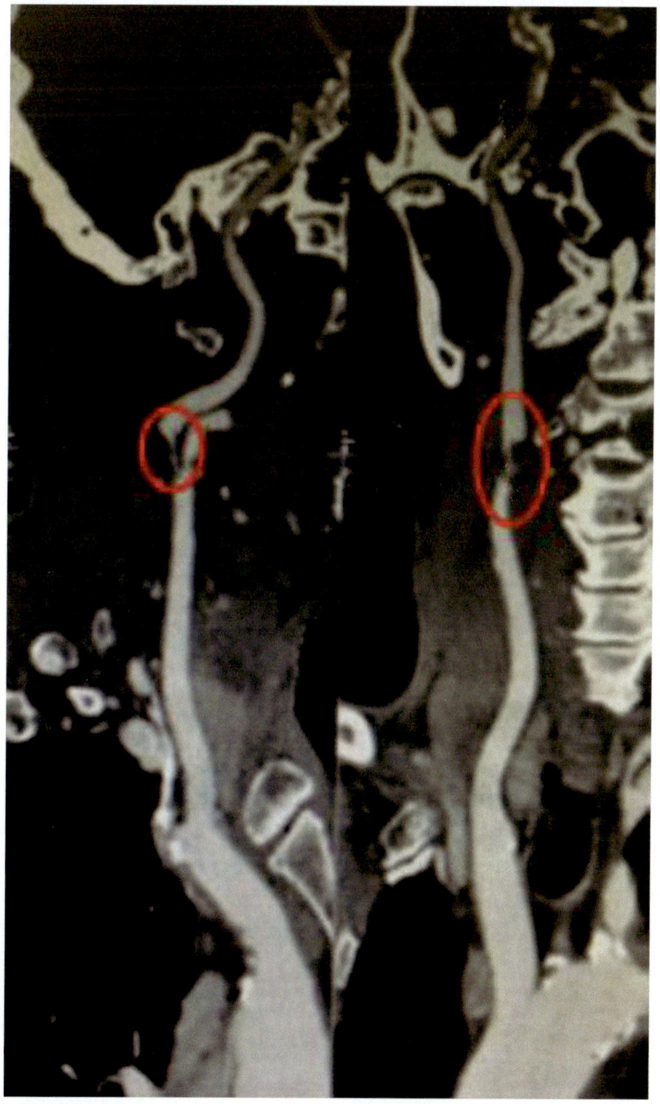

Fig. 14.1 Carotid artery stenosis

Z. Jing (✉) · H. Mao · M. Shi · J. Bao · Z. Zhao · X. Wei
Department of Vascular Surgery, Changhai Hospital, Second Military Medical University, Shanghai, China
e-mail: Jingzp@xueguan.net

Z. Chen
Department of Vascular Surgery, The First Hospital, Anhui Medical University, Hefei, China

Z. Jing et al. (eds.), *Endovascular Surgery and Devices*, https://doi.org/10.1007/978-981-10-8270-2_14

14.1.2 Clinical Manifestations

Atherosclerosis-induced carotid artery stenosis is more common among middle-aged and elderly people, often accompanied by a variety of cardiovascular risk factors. Carotid artery stenosis caused by brachiocephalic Takayasu arteritis (BCTA) is more common among teenagers, especially young women. Clinically carotid artery stenosis is classified as symptomatic and asymptomatic based on the presence of symptoms of cerebral ischemia.

14.1.2.1 Symptomatic Carotid Artery Stenosis

1. Cerebral ischemic symptoms: possible tinnitus, vertigo, amaurosis, blurred vision, dizziness, headache, insomnia, memory loss, lethargy, dreaminess, and other symptoms. Ocular ischemia manifests as vision loss, hemianopia, diplopia, etc.
2. Transient ischemic attack (TIA): a transient loss of focal neurological function, clinically manifested by transient sensory disorder or dyskinesia of the unilateral limbs, a transient monocular blindness, or aphasia, usually lasting for only several minutes and being completely recovered within 24 h after onset. No focal lesion is found under imaging examination.
3. Ischemic stroke: Common clinical symptoms include unilateral limb sensory disturbance, hemiplegia, aphasia, cranial nerve injury, coma, etc., showing corresponding signs of the nervous system and imaging findings.

14.1.2.2 Asymptomatic Carotid Artery Stenosis

Many patients with carotid artery stenosis show no clinical symptoms and signs of the nervous system and are sometimes found only in physical examination to have weakened or disappeared carotid artery pulsation with the presence of vascular murmur at the root of the neck or places where the carotid artery accesses through. Asymptomatic carotid artery stenosis, especially severe stenosis or plaque ulcer lesions, is recognized as "high-risk lesions" and is increasingly taken seriously.

14.1.3 Intraoperative Coordination

14.1.3.1 Anesthesia and Surgical Position

The patient receives local anesthesia and takes a supine position (to be adjusted according to the actual situation of the patient during operation).

14.1.3.2 Preparation of Items

The same as in Table 13.13.

14.1.3.3 Preparation of Devices

Refer to Table 14.1.

These listed above are the routine devices for minimally invasive endovascular treatment of carotid artery stenosis. During actual operation, different kinds of vascular sheath, protective umbrella, RX balloon catheter, carotid stent graft, and other devices can be changed according to the degree of stenosis and vascular shape of the carotid artery [1, 2].

1. Long sheath and guide catheter: Long sheath and guide catheter can all be used for endovascular treatment of carotid artery stenosis. During actual operation, long sheath and guide catheter of different lengths can be chosen according to the actual situation of the patient, the difference of which is shown in Table 14.2.
2. Selection of protective umbrella: The protective umbrella should be chosen according to angiography findings and the characteristics of the umbrella during operation. Protective umbrella brands mainly include Angioguard (Cordis), FilterWire EZ (Boston Scientific), Embolished

Table 14.1 Preparation of devices

Name	Qty.	Name	Qty.
Puncture needle	1	6F long sheath 90 cm	1
High-pressure connector	2	Inflation device	1
0.035 in. common hydrophilic wire 260 cm	1	Protective umbrella	1 set
5F common pigtail catheter	1	RX balloon catheter	Several
5F short sheath 125 cm	1	Carotid artery stent	Several
4F/5F MPA catheter	1	Guide wire accessory kit (if necessary)	1 set
8–9F short sheath (if necessary)	1	4F/5F JB2 catheter (if necessary)	1
8F guide catheter (if necessary)	1	Vascular closure device (if necessary)	1
5F VTK catheter 120 cm (if necessary)	1		

Table 14.2 Differences of long sheath and guide catheter (for reference only)

Name	Difference
Long sheath	Long sheath includes straight and curved-tip sheath, having strong support and protecting the blood vessels. Routinely used long sheath is with 6F inner diameter. Long sheath brands include Cook, Terumo, Arrow, etc.
Guide catheter	Guide catheter has a curved tip, having common support and protecting the blood vessels. Routinely used guide catheter is with 8F outer diameter. If 8F guide catheter is used, 8F short sheath, Y valve, and T valve should be prepared additionally

NAV6 (Abbott), SpiderFX (Medtronic), Mo.Ma (Medtronic), etc.

3. Selection of RX balloon catheter: RX balloon catheter can be chosen during operation according to the angiography findings and the actual characteristics of the balloon, and its brands mainly include Submarine (Medtronic), LitePAC (Bard), Sterling Monorail (Boston Scientific), etc.
4. Selection of the carotid artery stent: Carotid artery stent can be chosen during operation according to angiography findings and the features of the stent, and its brands mainly include Acculink (Abbott), Cristallo Ideale (Medtronic), Wallstent (Boston Scientific), Precise (Cordis), etc.

14.1.3.4 Selection of Minimally Invasive Endovascular Surgery

At present, the minimally invasive endovascular surgeries for carotid artery stenosis mainly include carotid artery balloon dilatation and stent implantation; for patients with severe occlusive carotid arteries, hybrid surgery (carotid endarterectomy and minimally invasive endovascular surgery) can be performed under general anesthesia.

14.1.3.5 Procedures and Intraoperative Coordination Process

Take carotid balloon dilatation plus stent implantation with common femoral artery puncture as an example. Refer to Table 14.3.

Table 14.3 Procedures and intraoperative coordination process

Procedures	Intraoperative coordination process
1. Patient enters the operation room	(1) Mental nursing; (2) keep the patient warm; (3) help to lie at supine position, with two lower limbs slightly at abduction and extorsion position; (4) connect ECG to observe changes in blood pressure, heart rate, and oxygen saturation; (5) establish intravenous infusion
2. Routinely sterilize the bilateral groins from the umbilical down to the mid-thigh, exposing the groins	Prepare disinfectant (heated to 98.6 °F in incubator), and assist with draping; deliver iodixanol injection; prepare heparin diluent (1000 mL normal saline +100 mg heparin sodium injection)
3. Puncture the common femoral artery with modified Seldinger technique under local anesthesia, insert a 5F short sheath and a 0.035 in. common hydrophilic wire 260 cm	Deliver 1% lidocaine injection, puncture needle, high-pressure connector, 0.035 in. common hydrophilic wire 260 cm, and 5F short sheath; perform systemic heparinization (initial administered dose is 0.67 mg/kg based on body weight, and subsequent dosage is administered according to the actual intraoperative situations); endovascular devices should be flushed with the prepared heparin diluent
4. Insert a 5F common pigtail catheter along the 0.035 in. common hydrophilic wire 260 cm, locate the catheter tip at the aortic arch, withdraw the wire, and conduct aortic arch angiography	Deliver the 5F common pigtail catheter
5. Withdraw the 5F common pigtail catheter and the 5F short sheath, exchange to insert a 6F long sheath 90 cm and 4F/5F MPA catheter 125 cm, superselect carotid artery to conduct angiography (Fig. 14.2)	Deliver the 6F long sheath 90 cm and the 4F/5F MPA catheter 125 cm (catheter to be changed according to angiography findings)
6. According to angiography findings, select appropriate protective umbrella, exhaust air by heparin diluent (air in the umbrella must be completely exhausted), withdraw the 4F/5F MPA catheter, insert the umbrella into the relatively straight vessel 2 cm above the distal end of the carotid artery lesion site via the 6F long sheath	Deliver the protective umbrella
7. Select an appropriate RX balloon catheter, insert it to the stenotic site along the wire of the umbrella and inflate the balloon (pre-dilatation or post-dilatation is determined according to actual intraoperative situations)	Connect the pressurized infusion device; deliver the inflation device and the RX balloon catheter
8. Withdraw the balloon along the wire of the umbrella, select appropriate carotid artery stent, and insert it to the stenotic site along the wire of the umbrella; locate and deploy it	Deliver the carotid artery stent (matching vascular sheath needs to be changed according to the selected stent diameter)
9. Withdraw the delivery system of carotid artery stent, conduct angiography again, and if necessary, conduct balloon post-dilatation; insert the retraction sheath along the wire of the umbrella, retract the umbrella into the sheath, and conduct carotid artery angiography again (Fig. 14.3)	Deliver the retraction sheath
10. Withdraw the long sheath, select an appropriate vascular closure device to block the puncture site	Deliver the vascular closure device
11. Compression dressing on puncture site	Deliver the gauze and the elastic bandage and assist with draping; safely escort the patient back to ward

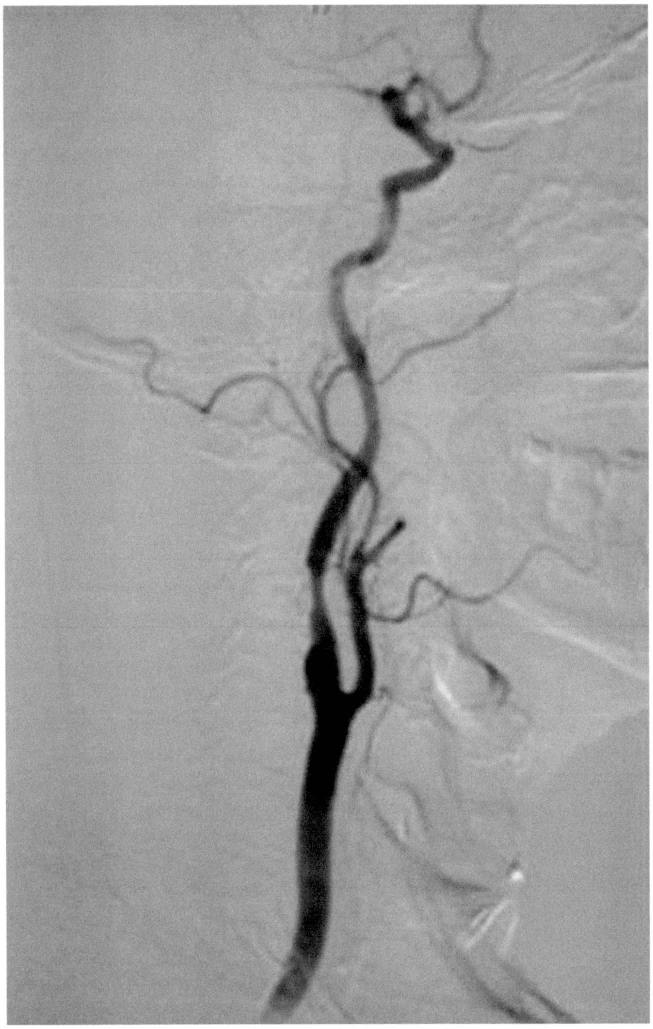

Fig. 14.2 Preoperative carotid angiography

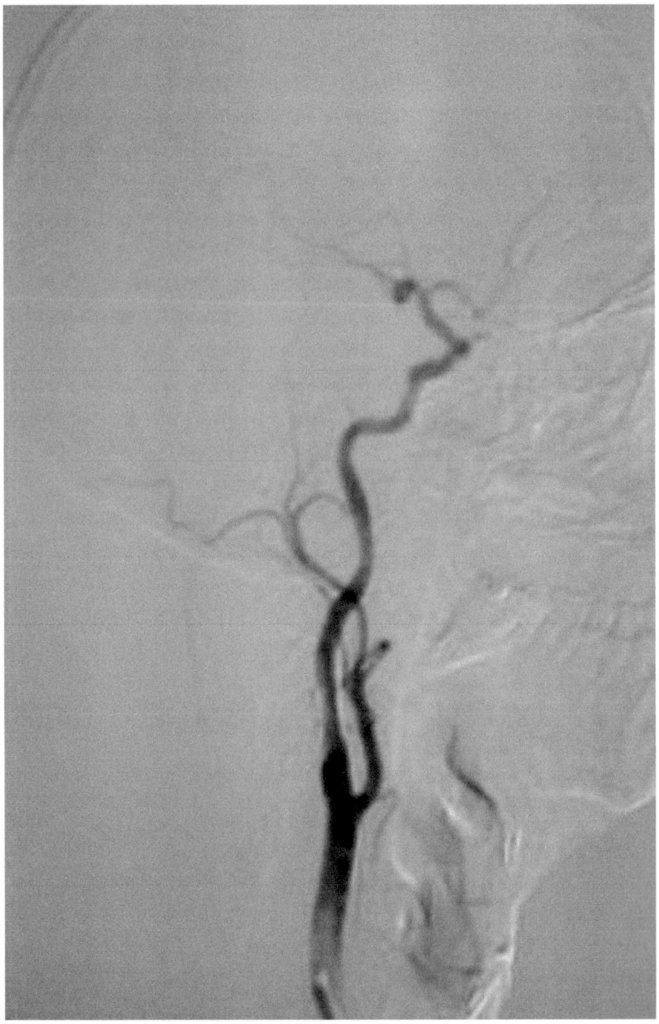

Fig. 14.3 Postoperative carotid artery angiography

14.1.4 Essentials for Intraoperative Observation

14.1.4.1 Observe Carotid Sinus Reaction

Intraoperative balloon dilatation and stent deployment stimulate carotid baroreceptor, possibly resulting in vagal reflex and causing decreased blood pressure and heart rate or even serious cardiac arrest or cerebral hypoperfusion. The heart rate and blood pressure changes of the patient should be closely monitored during operation, and if necessary, atropine or dopamine is used to regulate the heart rate and blood pressure and ensure stable blood circulation.

14.1.4.2 Observe Hyperperfusion Syndrome

Hyperperfusion syndrome is one of the common complications after stent implantation, manifested as headache, local and/or systemic epilepsy, or even life-threatening intracranial hemorrhage. The patient should be closely monitored during operation for any presence of such intracranial hemorrhage and cranial hypertension symptoms as headache, vomiting, elevated blood pressure, and breathing and pulse becoming lower, with the systolic blood pressure controlled at 20 mmHg below the basal blood pressure. When the patient suffers from headache, discomfort, elevated blood pressure, changes in consciousness, or pupil abnormalities, the possibility of hyperperfusion syndrome should be considered and be treated promptly [3].

14.2 Subclavian Artery Stenosis

14.2.1 Introduction

Subclavian artery stenosis (Fig. 14.4) is the partial or total occlusion occurring from the ostium of the subclavian artery to the origin of the vertebral artery, which, due to the siphoning effect, causes the blood in the involved vertebral artery to flow back to reversely provide blood supply to the ischemic

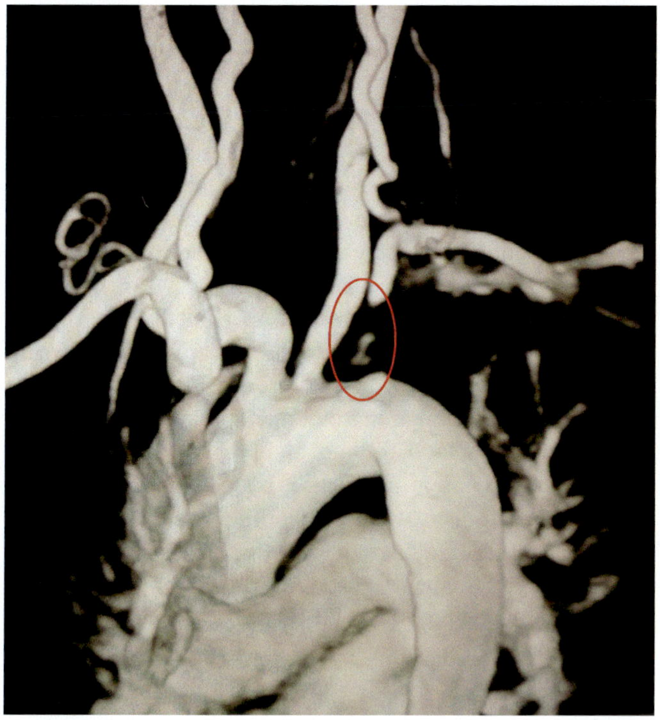

Fig. 14.4 Subclavian artery stenosis

involved upper limbs, resulting in vertebro-basilar artery ischemic attack and ischemic symptoms of the affected upper limbs, mostly originating from atherosclerosis or Takayasu arteritis.

14.2.2 Clinical Manifestations

Subclavian artery stenosis is the common disease of the vascular surgery, clinically manifested as the following:

14.2.2.1 Blood Pressure

The blood pressure of the affected upper limbs decreases, with the systolic blood pressure difference of the two upper limbs ranging from 20 to 150 mmHg, mostly between 20 and 70 mmHg. Viewed from angiography, symptoms, and frequency of attack, the difference of blood pressure has no connection with the degree of subclavian artery stenosis.

14.2.2.2 Pulse

Pulse sluggishness may happen to the affected limbs, which is because the pulse wave transmits from the contralateral vertebral artery to the affected vertebral artery and then to the wrist, resulting in long distance of transmission. The radial artery pulsation of the affected side may also weaken or disappear, which, sometimes, even happens to the brachial artery or the subclavian artery.

14.2.2.3 Limb Hypofunction and Neurological Symptoms

Due to insufficient blood supply to the upper extremities and consequential post-activity fatigue, the patient with severe ischemia may even have upper limb numbness, fingertip cyanosis, and other symptoms. Most patients with stenosis have audible systolic murmur heard in the supraclavicular area, which may be aggravated due to the activity of the affected limbs. The affected limb movement may cause paroxysmal vertigo, blurred vision, diplopia, ataxia, dysarthria, syncope, and other posterior circulation (brain stem, occipital, and cerebellum) problems, and in more serious cases, the internal carotid blood flows back via the posterior communicating artery, resulting in ischemic symptoms happening to the internal carotid artery, such as hemiplegia, hemidysesthesia, and aphasia.

14.2.3 Intraoperative Coordination

14.2.3.1 Anesthesia and Surgical Position

The patient receives local anesthesia and takes a supine position (to be adjusted according to the actual situation of the patient during operation).

14.2.3.2 Preparation of Items

The same as in Table 13.13.

14.2.3.3 Preparation of Devices

Refer to Table 14.4.

Table 14.4 Preparation of devices

Name	Qty.	Name	Qty.
Puncture needle	1	5F common pigtail catheter	1
High-pressure connector	2	5–6F short sheath	Several
0.035 in. common hydrophilic wire 260 cm	Several	6F–7F long sheath 90 cm	1
4F/5F MPA catheter 125 cm	1	Inflation device (if necessary)	1
4F/5F Berenstein catheter (if necessary)	1	Balloon catheter (if necessary)	1
Guide wire accessory kits (if necessary)	1 set	Self-expanding peripheral bare stent (if necessary)	1
4F/5F Mariner Berenstein catheter 130 cm (if necessary)	1	OTW balloon-expandable peripheral bare stent (if necessary)	1
Vascular closure device (if necessary)	1	0.035 in. Amplatz super-stiff wire 260 cm (if necessary)	1

14.2.3.4 Selection of Minimally Invasive Endovascular Surgery

Endovascular therapies for subclavian artery stenosis give priority to balloon dilatation and stent implantation technique, during which appropriate self-expanding peripheral bare stent or OTW balloon-expandable peripheral bare stent can be selected according to angiography findings and stent-specific characteristics. In treatment of subclavian artery occlusive lesions, if the occluded segment cannot be recanalized via the femoral artery approach in the direction of blood flow, the brachial artery approach can be chosen to perform retrograde puncture for recanalization in combination with wire and catheter [3].

14.2.3.5 Procedures and Intraoperative Coordination Process

OTW balloon-expandable peripheral bare stent implantation of the subclavian artery via common femoral artery puncture is here taken as an example, as shown in Table 14.5 [2].

14.2.4 Essentials for Intraoperative Observation

14.2.4.1 Observe Vital Signs

When the balloon dilates, the blood vessels are propped open, possibly resulting in the coming off of the arterial plaques that will form emboli and cause cerebral infarction. Therefore, the patient should be closely observed for their consciousness and any signs of headache, dizziness, blurred vision, and limb movement disorders. Also, it may cause blood vessel rupture and bleeding. If the patient is found with persistent sharp pain complicated with declined blood pressure, accelerated heart rate, difficult breathing, and other symptoms, increase infusion speed, raise blood volume, and prepare peripheral stent graft. During operation, stimulation by radiocontrast and wire catheter can cause vasospasm, and, therefore, vasodilator can be administered. Intraoperative feeling of tension, pain, and other factors by the patient can lead to higher blood pressure than normal blood pressure, and antihypertensive therapy can be administered, if necessary.

Table 14.5 Procedures and intraoperative coordination process

Procedures	Intraoperative coordination process
1. Patient enters the operation room	(1) Mental nursing; (2) keep the patient warm; (3) help to lie at supine position, with two lower limbs slightly at abduction and extorsion position; (4) connect ECG to observe changes in blood pressure, heart rate, and oxygen saturation; (5) establish intravenous infusion
2. Routinely sterilize the bilateral groins from the umbilical down to the mid-thigh, exposing the groins	Prepare disinfectant (heated to 98.6 °F in incubator), and assist with draping; deliver iodixanol injection; prepare heparin diluent (1000 mL normal saline +100 mg heparin sodium injection)
3. Puncture the unilateral common femoral artery with modified Seldinger technique under local anesthesia, locate catheter tip at aortic arch, withdraw the hydrophilic wire, and conduct aortic arch angiography	Deliver 1% lidocaine injection, puncture needle, high-pressure connector, 0.035 in. common hydrophilic wire 260 cm, and 5F short sheath; perform systemic heparinization (initial administered dose is 0.67 mg/kg based on body weight, and subsequent dose is administered according to the actual intraoperative situations); endovascular devices should be flushed with the prepared heparin diluent
4. Insert a 5F common pigtail catheter along the 0.035 in. common hydrophilic wire 260 cm, locate the catheter tip at the aortic arch, withdraw the hydrophilic wire, and conduct aortic arch angiography	Deliver the 5F common pigtail catheter
5. Withdraw the 5F common pigtail catheter and 5F short sheath, exchange to insert a 6F long sheath 90 cm and a 4F/5F MPA catheter 125 cm, superselect subclavian artery, and conduct angiography (Fig. 14.5)	Deliver the 6F long sheath 90 cm and the 4F/5F MPA catheter 125 cm (exchange the catheter according to angiography findings)
6. Withdraw the 4F/5F MPA catheter 125 cm, select an appropriate OTW balloon-expandable peripheral bare stent and insert it into the lesion site along the 0.035 in. common hydrophilic wire 260 cm, inflate the balloon after positioning, and deploy the stent	Deliver the inflation device and the balloon-expandable peripheral bare stent (the matching vascular sheath needs to be changed according to the selected stent diameter)
7. Withdraw the delivery system, conduct subclavian artery angiography again (Fig. 14.6)	
8. Withdraw the long sheath and wire, select an appropriate vascular device to block the puncture site	Deliver the vascular closure device
9. Compression dressing on puncture site	Deliver gauze and elastic bandage and assist with draping; safely escort the patient back to ward

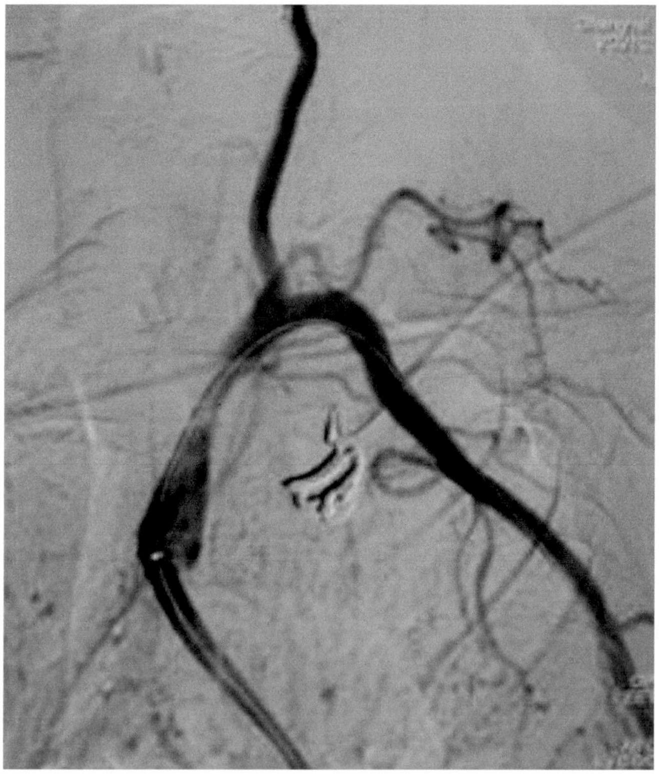

Fig. 14.5 Subclavian artery angiography

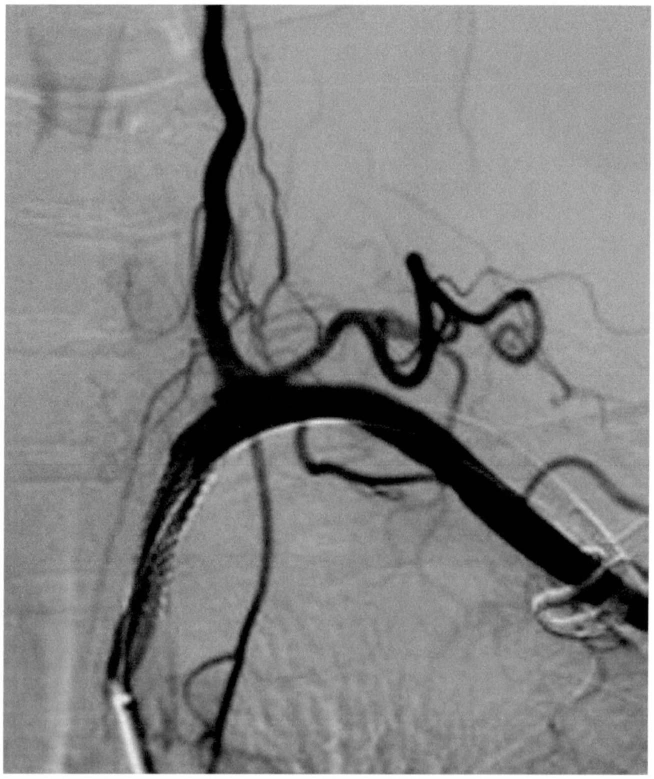

Fig. 14.6 Postoperative subclavian artery angiography

14.2.4.2 Observe Neurological Symptoms

After subclavian artery stenosis or occlusion is relieved, steal phenomenon disappears, blood circulation returns normal, and cerebral blood flow (CBF) increases. At this time, cerebral autoregulation function is insufficient, possibly leading to cerebral hyperemia, brain edema, and bleeding, manifested as headache, nausea, projectile vomiting, optic disk edema, and other symptoms. Once such signs are present, the patient should be promptly treated with dehydration and reduction in intracranial pressure, with his blood pressure being controlled at 20–30 mmHg lower than the basal blood pressure.

14.3 Renal Artery Stenosis

14.3.1 Introduction

Renal artery stenosis (RAS) significantly contributes to inter alia secondary hypertension and/or renal insufficiency, accounting for 5–10% of the patients with secondary hypertension, and it is hard to control secondary hypertension. Renal artery stenosis leads to insufficient renal perfusion and ultimately results in ischemic nephropathy or even renal failure (Fig. 14.7), originating most commonly from atherosclerosis, fibromuscular dysplasia, and Takayasu arteritis.

14.3.2 Clinical Manifestations

14.3.2.1 Characteristics of Case History

- No family history of primary hypertension.
- Age and gender: Moderate and severe hypertension occurs before 20 years of age or after 50 years of age. Takayasu arteritis is more common among women, while atherosclerosis-induced hypertension is mostly seen among men.
- A relatively short history but quick development, unexplainable malignant hypertension.
- Poor response to common hypotensive drugs, being relatively sensitive to angiotensin-converting enzyme (ACE) inhibitor.

14.3.2.2 Symptoms and Signs

- Hypertension, usually over 200/120 mmHg, more evident with the increase in diastolic blood pressure.
- Asymmetrical limb blood pressure happens to patients with Takayasu arteritis.
- Audible abdominal or waist vascular murmur of some RAA patients.

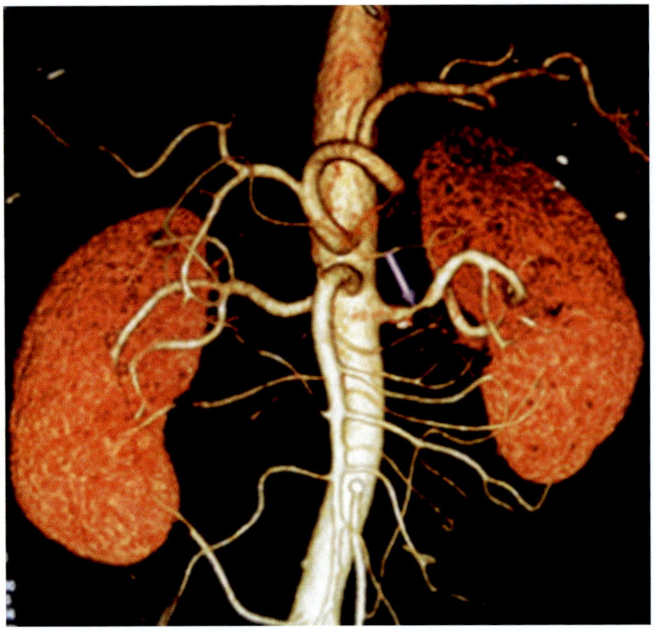

Fig. 14.7 Renal artery stenosis

Table 14.6 Preparation of devices

Name	Qty.	Name	Qty.
Puncture needle	1	5F common pigtail catheter	1
High-pressure connector	2	5F short sheath	1
0.035 in. common hydrophilic wire 180 cm	1	6F Ansel long sheath 45 cm	1
4F/5F Sos Omni catheter	1	0.014 in. spring-head wire 300 cm	1
Inflation device (if necessary)	1	RX balloon-expandable peripheral bare stent	1
4F/5F Cobra catheter (if necessary)	1	7F guide catheter (if necessary)	1
4F/5F Berenstein catheter (if necessary)	1	7F short sheath (if necessary)	1
0.035 in. Rosen super-stiff wire 260 cm (if necessary)	1	Guide wire accessory kits (if necessary)	1 set
Vascular closure device (if necessary)	1	RX balloon catheter (if necessary)	Several

14.3.3 Intraoperative Coordination

14.3.3.1 Anesthesia and Surgical Position

The patient receives local anesthesia and takes a supine position (to be adjusted according to the actual situation of the patient during operation).

14.3.3.2 Preparation of Items

The same as in Table 13.13.

14.3.3.3 Preparation of Devices

Refer to Table 14.6.

14.3.3.4 Selection of Minimally Invasive Endovascular Surgery

At present, endovascular surgery for renal artery stenosis gives priority to balloon dilatation and stent implantation technique, during which appropriate RX balloon-expandable peripheral bare stent can be selected according to angiography findings and stent-specific characteristics. The brands available at present include Express SD (Boston Scientific), PALMAZ Blue (Cordis), Hippocampus (Medtronic), etc.

14.3.3.5 Procedures and Intraoperative Coordination Process

Renal artery balloon dilatation and stent implantation via common femoral artery puncture are here taken as an example, as shown in Table 14.7.

14.3.4 Essentials for Intraoperative Observation

14.3.4.1 Monitor Blood Pressure

Change in blood pressure is an important indicator in observing efficacy. Refractory high blood pressure in patients is mainly attributed to severe renal artery stenosis, causing increased release of renin and persistent increase in blood pressure. Postoperative blood pressure change may be a relatively slow process due to renin metabolism.

14.3.4.2 Observe Complications

During operation, ask the patients of any symptoms such as waist and back pain, closely observe urine output, and strictly control the blood pressure to avoid excessive blood pressure fluctuation. Long-term hypertension can also impair the

Table 14.7 Procedures and intraoperative coordination process

Procedures	Intraoperative coordination process
1. Patient enters the operation room	(1) Mental nursing; (2) keep the patient warm; (3) help to lie at supine position, with two lower limbs slightly at abduction and extorsion position; (4) connect ECG to observe changes in blood pressure, heart rate, and oxygen saturation; (5) establish intravenous infusion
2. Routinely sterilize the bilateral groins from the umbilical down to the mid-thigh, exposing the groins	Prepare disinfectant (heated to 98.6 °F in incubator) and assist with draping; deliver iodixanol injection; prepare heparin diluent (1000 mL normal saline +100 mg heparin injection)
3. Conduct retrograde puncture to the unilateral common femoral artery with modified Seldinger technique under local anesthesia, insert a 0.035 in. common hydrophilic wire 180 cm and a 5F short sheath	Deliver 1% lidocaine injection, the puncture needle, the high-pressure connector, 0.035 in. common hydrophilic wire 260 cm, and 5F short sheath; systemic heparinization (initial administered dose is 0.67 mg/kg based on body weight, and subsequent dose is administered according to the actual intraoperative situations); endovascular devices should be flushed with the prepared heparin sodium diluent
4. Insert a 5F common pigtail catheter along the 0.035 in. common hydrophilic wire 180 cm, locate the catheter tip at above the renal artery, withdraw the hydrophilic wire, and conduct abdominal aortic angiography (Fig. 14.8)	Deliver the 5F common pigtail catheter
5. Withdraw the 5F common pigtail catheter and 5F short sheath, exchange to insert a 6F Ansel long sheath 45 cm and 4F/5F Sos Omni catheter, superselect renal artery, and conduct angiography	Deliver 6F Ansel long sheath 45 cm and 4F/5F SOS Omni catheter (catheter to be changed according to angiography findings)
6. Withdraw the 0.035 in. common hydrophilic wire 260 cm, insert the 0.014 in. spring-head wire to the distal end of the renal artery along the 4F/5F Sos Omni catheter, withdraw the 4F/5F Sos Omni catheter, insert the RX balloon-expandable peripheral bare stent into the lesion site along the 0.014 in. spring-head wire, locate and then inflate the balloon, deploy the stent	Deliver the 0.014 in. spring-head wire, the inflation device, the RX balloon-expandable peripheral bare stent (matching vascular sheath needs to be changed according to the selected stent diameter)
7. Withdraw the delivery system and conduct renal angiography again (Fig. 14.9)	
8. Withdraw the 6F Ansel long sheath and wire, select an appropriate vascular closure device to block the puncture site	Deliver the vascular closure device
9. Compression dressing on puncture site	Deliver the gauze and the elastic bandage and assist with draping; safely escort the patient back to ward

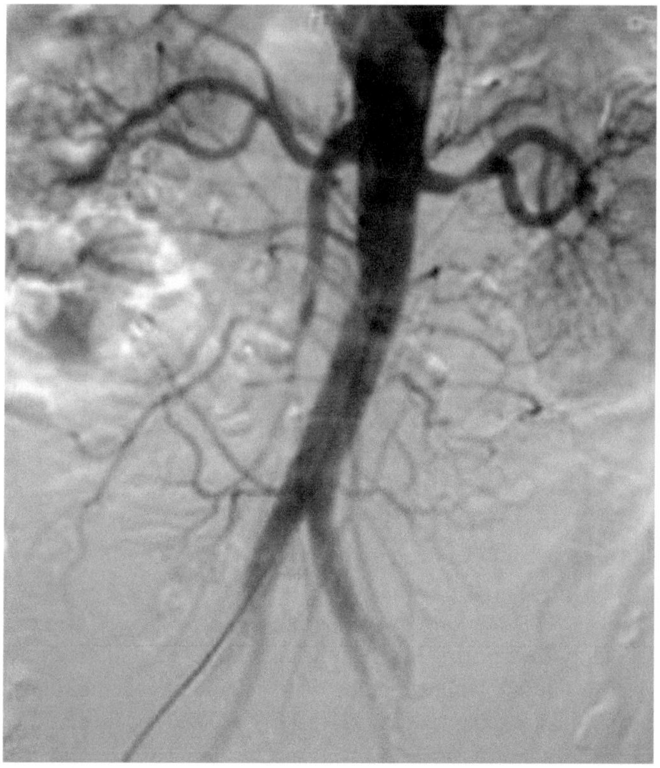

Fig. 14.8 Intraoperative angiography

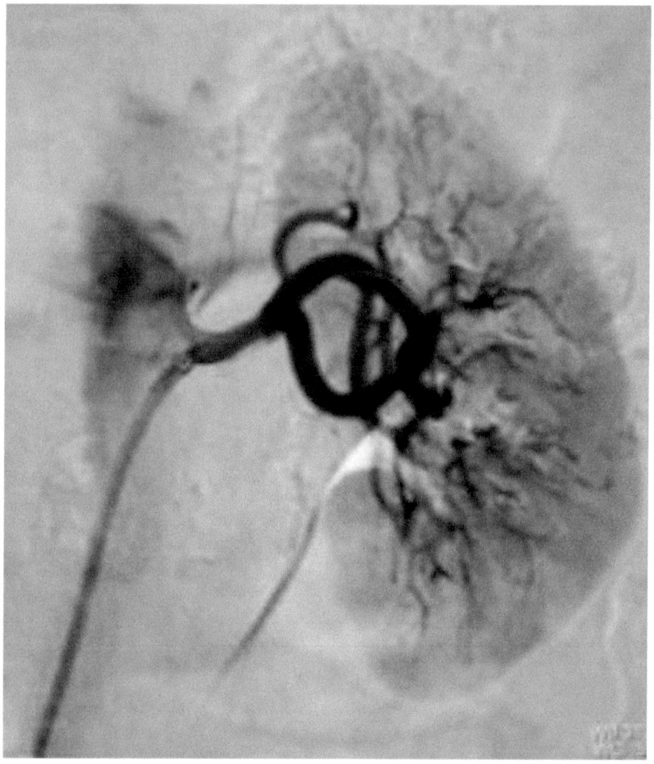

Fig. 14.9 Postoperative angiography

heart, brain, and other target organs, and postoperative use of anticoagulant and antiplatelet drugs should continue, reducing heart and cerebrovascular complications. In addition, attention should be paid to blood pressure decrease and even shock caused by bleeding due to accidental perforation of renal parenchyma during operation.

14.4 Lower Extremity Arteriosclerosis Obliterans

14.4.1 Introduction

Lower extremity arteriosclerosis obliterans (LEASO) is an ischemic lesion due to lower extremity artery stenosis and occlusion caused by continual enlargement of atherosclerotic plaque with secondary thrombosis (Fig. 14.10). LEASO is commonly seen among the middle-aged and elderly people, often accompanied by smoking, diabetes, hypertension, hyperlipidemia, and other risk factors, among which smoking and diabetes contribute the most and can increase the incidence of peripheral arterial diseases, and the two, if existing simultaneously, will pose a higher risk. Then there comes hyperlipidemia, especially elevated low-density lipoprotein cholesterol (LDL-CH), which is closely related to the occurrence of systemic multiple atherosclerosis. Prompt detection and control of risk factors leading to atherosclerosis can delay the process of arteriosclerosis and reduce the risk of LEASO occurrence.

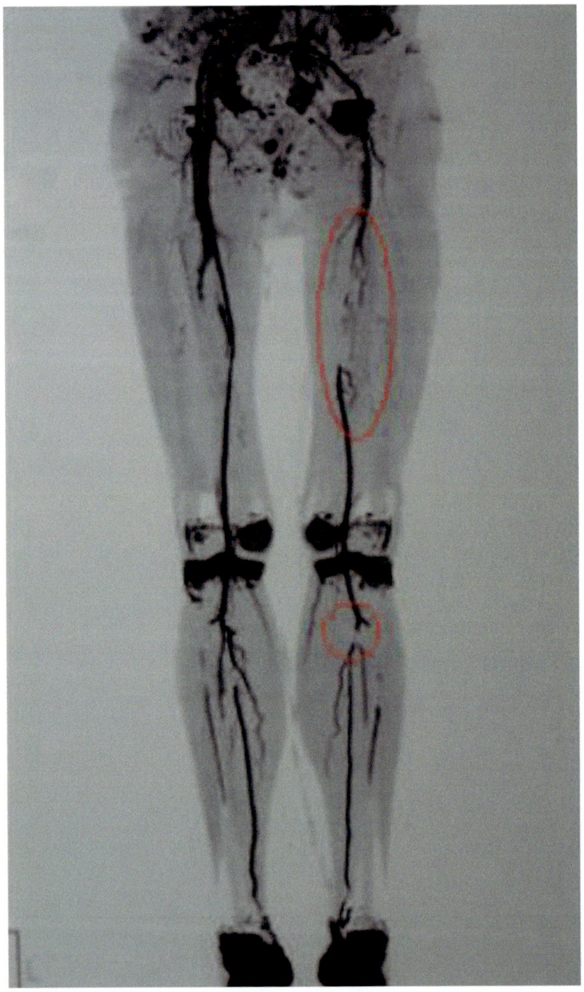

Fig. 14.10 LEASO

14.4.2 Clinical Manifestations

14.4.2.1 Fontaine Staging System

According to the severity of the patient, clinical manifestations are generally divided into four stages under Fontaine staging system:

1. Stage I: mild complaint stage, where most patients show no symptoms or minor symptoms, such as sensation of chill by the affected limbs, easy fatigue in walking, etc. In this case, ask the patient to walk some distance before examination, usually finding that the pulsation of the patient's lower extremity arteries weakens or even disappears.
2. Stage II: intermittent claudication stage—intermittent claudication is a characteristic manifestation of LEASO. The longer the claudication exists, the shorter the walking distance is and the more severe the arterial disease. Clinically, claudication distance of 200 m is often used to classify the stage of intermittent claudication. Stage II is often divided into stage IIa (absolute claudication distance > 200 m) and stage IIb (absolute claudication distance ≤ 200 m).
3. Stage III: rest pain stage, where collateral circulation of the affected limb is insufficiently established as the disease progresses and consequently the affected limb is in such a very serious ischemic state that it still feels pain, numbness, and sensory abnormalities even at rest, most with acral pains.
4. Stage IV: tissue necrosis stage, where the lesion progresses and reaches the occlusion stage with very limited collateral circulation and presence of symptoms of nutritional disorders. Before the presence of ulcers or gangrene, skin temperature decreases, and skin color becomes dark purple. Early gangrene and ulcers often occur in the toes, and with the progress of the disease, infection and gangrene can gradually develop upward to the feet, ankle, or calf or even lead to severe systemic symptoms of poisoning.

14.4.2.2 Rutherford Classification

Clinical manifestations are generally classified into 0–6 stages according to Rutherford staging system:

1. LEASO Stage 0: asymptomatic—showing no clinical symptoms, normal in treadmill test or reactive hyperemia test, and showing no signs of arterial occlusive hemodynamics (standard treadmill test at 15° of slope, at 2 miles per hour for 5 min)

2. LEASO Stage 1: mild intermittent claudication—completion of treadmill test, with post-exercise ankle artery pressure (AP) >50 mmHg but about 20 mmHg lower than that at rest
3. LEASO Stage 2: moderate intermittent claudication—manifestations between Stages 1 and 3
4. LEASO Stage 3: severe intermittent claudication—fail to complete treadmill test with post-exercise ankle artery pressure <50 mmHg
5. LEASO Stage 4: ischemic rest pain, ankle artery pressure at rest <40 mmHg, almost no blood pressure palpated on the dorsalis pedis artery and posterior tibial artery, and toe artery pressure <30 mmHg
6. LEASO Stage 5: minor tissue defect—focal gangrene with diffused foot ischemic change, ankle artery pressure at rest <60 mmHg, almost no blood pressure palpated on the dorsalis pedis artery and posterior tibial artery, and toe artery pressure <40 mmHg
7. LEASO Stage 6: tissue ulcers and gangrene

14.4.3 Intraoperative Coordination

14.4.3.1 Anesthesia and Surgical Position

The patient receives local anesthesia and takes a supine position (to be adjusted according to the actual situation of the patient during operation).

14.4.3.2 Preparation of Items

Same as in Table 13.13.

14.4.3.3 Preparation of Devices

Refer to Table 14.8.

14.4.3.4 Selection of Minimally Invasive Endovascular Surgery

Minimally invasive LEASO endovascular therapies mainly include balloon dilation, stent implantation, catheter-directed thrombolysis, aspiration thrombectomy, atherectomy, etc. [4–8]:

1. Lower extremity balloon dilatation: Balloon dilatation is indicated for dilatation of lower extremity stenosis caused by various reasons. The balloons currently available for this treatment are multifarious and can be selected during operation according to the angiography findings and balloon-specific characteristics.
2. Lower extremity stent implantation: For LEASO patients after receiving lower extremity balloon dilatation therapy, if severe elastic retraction or blood flow-limited dissection occurs, stent implantation technique can be selected for treatment of lower extremity lesions. Currently, clinically used conventional stent brands for LEASO treatment are diversified, mainly divided into three categories: self-expanding peripheral bare stent, balloon-expandable bare stent (containing balloon-expandable drug-eluting stent), and peripheral stent graft, which can be selected during operation according to angiography findings and stent-specific characteristics [6–8].
3. Lower extremity catheter-directed thrombolysis: For patients with acute lower extremity artery embolism or lower extremity thrombosis, Uni-Fuse infusion catheter can be used to insert into the lower extremity lesion with injection of thrombolytic drugs (such as urokinase) for local thrombolysis, which should last for about 30 min before conducting lower extremity angiography. If the lower extremity artery shows no obvious thrombus

Table 14.8 Preparation of devices

Name	Qty.	Name	Qty.
Puncture needle	1	5F Omni Flush catheter	1
High-pressure connector	2	4F/5F MPA catheter 125 cm	1
0.035 in. common hydrophilic wire 260 cm	1	4–6F short sheath (if necessary)	1
6–8F crossing sheath 40 cm	1	4–6F long sheath (if necessary)	1
4F/5F Mariner Bernstein catheter (if necessary)	1	Inflation device (if necessary)	1
Support catheter (if necessary)	1	Common balloon catheter (if necessary)	Several
4F/5F Berenstein catheter (if necessary)	1	Drug-eluting balloon catheter (if necessary)	Several
5F rim catheter (if necessary)	1	Cutting balloon catheter (if necessary)	Several
4F/5F aqua catheter (if necessary)	1	Balloon-expandable drug-eluting stent (if necessary)	Several
5F common pigtail catheter (if necessary)	1	Self-expanding peripheral bare stent (if necessary)	Several
3–5F thrombolytic catheter (if necessary)	Several	Peripheral stent graft (if necessary)	Several
0.014 in. wire 300 cm (if necessary)	1	AngioJet aspiration thrombectomy system (if necessary)	1 set
0.018 in. wire 300 cm (if necessary)	1	Straub mechanical thrombectomy system (if necessary)	1 set
0.035 in. hardened hydrophilic wire 260 cm (if necessary)	1	SilverHawk peripheral plaque excision system (if necessary)	1 set
Guide wire accessory kit (if necessary)	1 set	Vascular closure device (if necessary)	1

according to angiography findings, endovascular therapies such as balloon dilatation and stent implantation can be chosen; if thrombus is still present, indwelling infusion catheter or other endovascular therapies can be conducted. There are two techniques used for arterial catheter-directed thrombolysis: continuous micropump infusion and pulse jet, among which pulse jet technique is commonly used in operation (Fig. 14.11) [9].

4. Lower extremity aspiration thrombectomy: For acute or subacute lower extremity embolism or thrombosis, AngioJet aspiration thrombectomy system (Boston Scientific) can be selected; for acute, subacute, and chronic occlusive thrombus of the lower extremity arteries and mechanical removal of atherosclerotic material, Rotarex mechanical thrombectomy system (Straub) can be selected [10].
5. Lower extremity atherectomy: For primary and restenotic atherosclerotic lesions of the lower extremity, SilverHawk/TurboHawk peripheral plaque excision system (Medtronic) or Turbo Elite laser fiber-optic catheter system (Spectranetics) can be used [4].

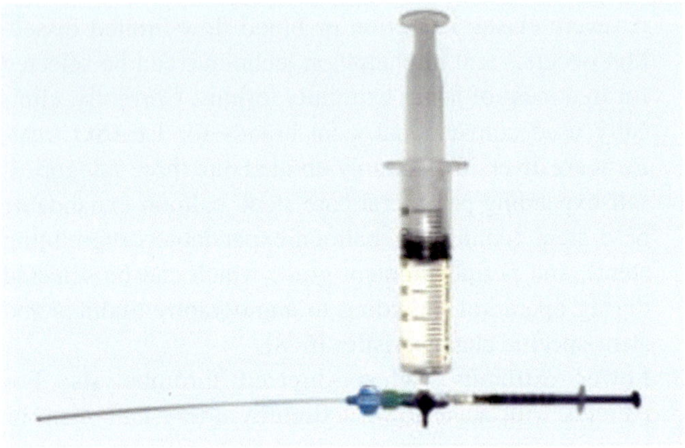

Fig. 14.11 Pulse jet technique

14.4.3.5 Procedures and Intraoperative Coordination Process

With arteriosclerosis obliterans of superficial femoral artery of the left lower extremity as an example, left lower extremity artery balloon dilatation plus self-expanding bare stent implantation by crossing over the right common femoral artery is performed, as shown in Table 14.9.

14.4.4 Essentials for Intraoperative Observation

14.4.4.1 Observe Vital Signs

Closely observe the vital signs, especially blood pressure and heart rate changes. Excessive large balloon expansion pressure may cause life-threatening arterial rupture and bleeding. Once it occurs, the extent of vascular rupture can be determined according to the radiocontrast extravasation visualized under angiography. Angioplasty-induced distal vascular rupture of the inguinal is rarely life-threatening, but

Table 14.9 Procedures and intraoperative coordination process

Procedures	Intraoperative coordination process
1. Patient enters the operation room	(1) Mental nursing; (2) keep the patient warm; (3) help to lie at supine position, with two lower limbs slightly at abduction and extorsion position; (4) connect ECG to observe changes in blood pressure, heart rate, and oxygen saturation; (5) establish intravenous infusion
2. Routinely sterilize the bilateral groins from the umbilical down to the mid-thigh, exposing the groins	Prepare disinfectant (heated to 98.6 °F in incubator) and assist with draping; deliver iodixanol injection; prepare heparin diluent (1000 mL normal saline +100 mg heparin sodium injection)
3. Conduct retrograde puncture to the right common femoral artery with modified Seldinger technique	Deliver 1% lidocaine injection, puncture needle, high-pressure connector; perform systemic heparinization (initial administered dose is 0.67 mg/kg based on body weight, and subsequent dose is administered according to the actual intraoperative situations); endovascular devices should be flushed with the prepared heparin diluent
4. Insert a 6F crossing sheath 40 cm and a 0.035 in. common hydrophilic wire 260 cm, insert a 5F Omni Flush catheter into the abdominal aorta along the hydrophilic wire, withdraw the wire, conduct angiography to the iliac artery, superficial femoral artery, popliteal artery, and infrapopliteal artery, respectively (Fig. 14.12)	Deliver the 6F Balkin sheath 40 cm, the 0.035 in. common hydrophilic wire 260 cm, and the 5F Omni Flush catheter (catheter changed according to actual situation)
5. Insert a 0.035 in. common hydrophilic wire 260 cm along the 5F Omni Flush catheter and coordinate to cross over to the left lower extremity artery, withdraw the 5F Omni Flush catheter and exchange to a 4F MPA catheter 125 cm, coordinate the hydrophilic wire with the 4F MPA catheter to revascularize the occlusive segment of the left superficial artery, measure its length and diameter, and select appropriate balloon catheter	Deliver the 4F MPA catheter 125 cm (catheter changed according to angiography findings)

Table 14.9 (continued)

Procedures	Intraoperative coordination process
6. Upon successful revascularization of the occlusive segment, withdraw the 125 cm 4F MPA catheter, insert the balloon catheter into the lesion site along the 0.035 in. common hydrophilic wire 260 cm, aspire iodixanol diluent by the inflation device, and quickly inject it into the balloon catheter to inflate the balloon and expand the stenotic segment	Deliver the inflation device and the balloon catheter
7. Withdraw the balloon catheter, select appropriate self-expanding peripheral bare stent system, and insert it into the lesion site of the left superficial artery along the 260 cm 0.035 in. common hydrophilic wire, locate and deploy the stent	Deliver the self-expanding peripheral bare stent
8. Withdraw the stent delivery system, conduct angiography to the affected limb artery again, check if the distal blood flow of the affected limb is smooth (Fig. 14.13)	
9. Withdraw the Balkin sheath and wire, select appropriate vascular closure device to block the puncture site	Deliver the vascular closure device
10. Compression dressing on puncture site	Deliver the gauze and the elastic bandage and assist with draping; safely escort the patient back to ward

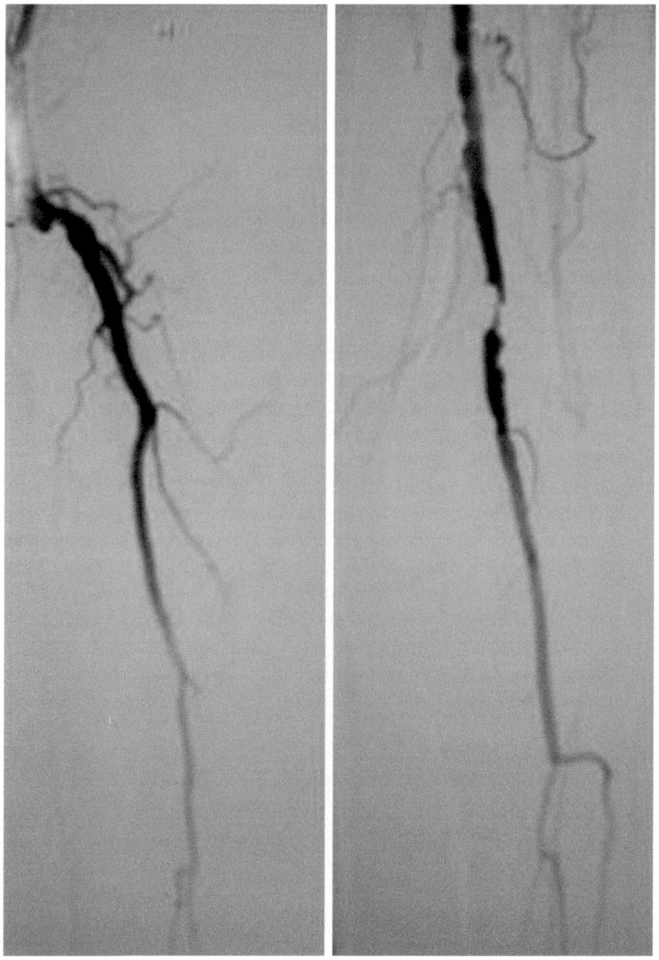

Fig. 14.12 Intraoperative angiography of the affected limb

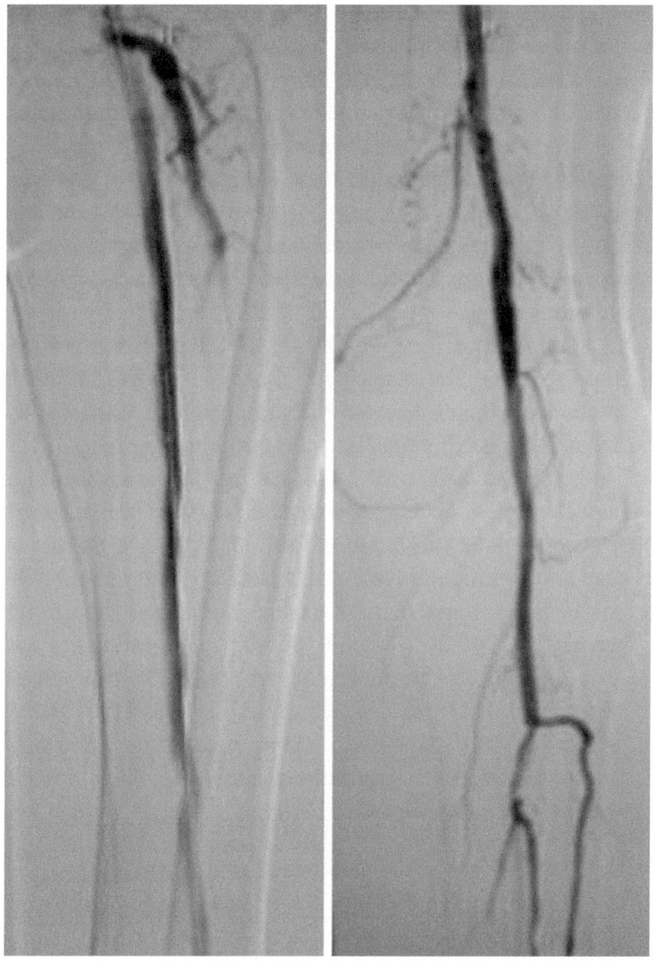

Fig. 14.13 Postoperative lower extremity artery angiography

it can cause formation of pseudoaneurysm or arterial occlusion. Most inferior inguinal vascular perforation cases take conservative treatment. Auxiliary endovascular therapies include balloon compression, peripheral stent graft implantation, or coil embolization due to continuous radiocontrast extravasation or hematoma.

14.4.4.2 Observe Pains

1. Arterial spasm and lateral obliterans: a common complication in the treatment of lower extremity arterial angioplasty, mainly manifested as severe pain and unbearable lower extremity pain. This is because, during the lower extremity arterial angioplasty treatment, excessive and extensive stimulation of the blood vessels can easily lead to arterial spasm. Once arterial spasm occurs, inject 10 μg nitroglycerin or 30–60 mg papaverine via a catheter, and if necessary, administer the same dosage half an hour later.
2. Acute limb arterial thrombosis: one of the complications of lower extremity arterial angioplasty, mainly manifested as lower limb pain, skin color change, and weakened or disappeared distal arterial pulsation. In the course of endovascular treatment, anticoagulant and/or antiplatelet drugs are not administered in time when the dilated balloon causes damage to local arterial intima or catheter (wire) stimulation of the arteries results in arterial spasms and when endovascular treatment fails; or although anticoagulant drugs are administered, intraventricular intervention time is too long, and no additional anticoagulant is administered in time. Once it is found, thrombolytic therapy should be conducted immediately. Thrombolysis includes catheter-directed thrombolysis and intravenous thrombolysis. Catheter-directed thrombolysis is to inject 200,000-1MM units of urokinase into the artery via the catheter, and if necessary, indwelling catheter can be used for continuous thrombolysis at 200,000-1MM units per day and continually for 3–5 days. Intravenous thrombolysis is to administer drugs via the peripheral superficial vein, at 500,000-1MM units per day and continually for 3–5 days. In the thrombolytic process, activated partial thromboplastin time (ATPP) should be monitored daily, generally maintained at about two times normal. Intraoperative arterial thrombosis should be timely treated with thrombolytic therapy. When important lateral branches are occluded, endovascular treatment can be conducted, such as balloon dilatation and stent implantation, and also surgical revascularization.
3. Reperfusion injury: mostly occurred in PTA (percutaneous transluminal angioplasty) patients with severe limb ischemia, mainly manifested as muscle and intermuscular tissue edema, which results in increased osteofascial compartment tension, affected limb edema, and consequential compression of blood vessels and nerves and severe pain. When becoming serious, distal arterial pulsation weakens or disappears, leading to limb avascular necrosis, renal failure, etc., which is called osteofascial compartment syndrome. With this syndrome diagnosed, decompression fasciotomy should be conducted to save the affected limbs. Delay in diagnosis may result in muscle necrosis and even limb necrosis, loss of limbs, kidney failure, and other serious consequences.

References

1. Jing Z. Endovascular therapy. Beijing: People's Medical Publishing House; 2003.
2. Mao Y, Xu X, Li H. Interventional treatment nursing. Beijing: People's Military Medical Press; 2013.
3. Wang Z, Zhang J, Yongquan G. Practical vascular surgery and vascular interventional therapy. Beijing: People's Military Medical Press; 2004.
4. Zhang R, Shii G, Zhou S, et al. Interventional therapy for in-stent restenosis. Chin Med J. 2001;114:67.
5. Jiang W, Wu Z, Liu W, et al. Application of percutaneous and transluminal therapies in artery stenosis diseases. Chin J Radiol. 2000;34:528–30.
6. Yuan L, Bao J, Zhao Z, et al. Endovascular therapy for long- segment atherosclerotic aortoiliac occlusion. J Vasc Surg. 2014;59:663–8.
7. Tunesen KH, Sager P, Karle A, et al. Percutaneous transluminal angioplasty of the superficial artery by retrograde catheterization via the popliteal artery. Cardiovasc Intervent Radiol. 1988;1:127.
8. Liu C. Guidelines for treatment of lower extremity arteriosclerotic occlusive disease. Chin J Pract Surgy. 2008;28(11):923–4.
9. Bao J, Mei Z. How to standardize catheter-directed thrombolysis for treatment of arterial occlusive disease. Clin Misdiag Misther. 2014;27:42–5.
10. Jiang W, Li X, Ren A, et al. Popliteal artery embolotherapy with pulse-jet thrombolysis. Chin J Radiol. 1996;30:301–5.

Superficial Varicosis of Lower Extremity

15

Wen Tian, Zhijun Mei, and Zaiping Jing

Abstract

Lower extremity superficial varicosis is the most common vascular disease. Strictly speaking, lower extremity varicose vein is not an independent disease but a clinical manifestation of lower extremity venous disease. Its treatment can be classified into conservative treatment and surgical treatment. Depending on the principles followed, surgical treatment can be further classified into the removal of diseased vein and in situ destruction of diseased vein. At the Vascular Surgery Department of Changhai Hospital, the surgical treatment for lower extremity varicose vein no longer requires hospitalization, as it can be entirely completed at the outpatient department, without delaying one's normal routines. This chapter introduces clinical manifestations, minimally invasive surgery process, and intraoperative observation points of lower extremity varicose vein.

Keywords

Lower extremity varicose vein · Minimally invasive

15.1 Introduction

Superficial varicosis of lower extremity is the most common in vascular diseases, mostly belonging to lesions of the great saphenous vein (GSV) and its branches (Fig. 15.1). Lower extremity venous valve insufficiency, lower extremity deep venous postthrombotic syndrome (PTS), K-T syndrome, and other diseases can all cause varicose veins, which is not an isolated disease but a clinical manifestation of the lower extremity venous disease. Treatment of varicose veins includes conservative treatment and surgical treatment. Conservative treatment covers the entire course of varicose vein treatment, while surgical treatment is usually conducted in the presence of complications or esthetic affection or when the patient is willing for operation. Currently, surgical treatment has various approaches available, classified into two categories according to surgical principle: removal of the diseased vein and in situ destruction of the diseased vein. The way for the removal of the diseased vein is called vein stripping technique; the traditional long-incision vein stripping technique has been basically abandoned, and instead, small-incision punctate stripping is currently available. The way for destruction of the diseased vein includes sclerotherapy, laser ablation, radiofrequency endovenous, and other options for treatment. No matter what kind of surgery it is, the purpose is to eliminate the poor hemodynamic state of varicose veins [1].

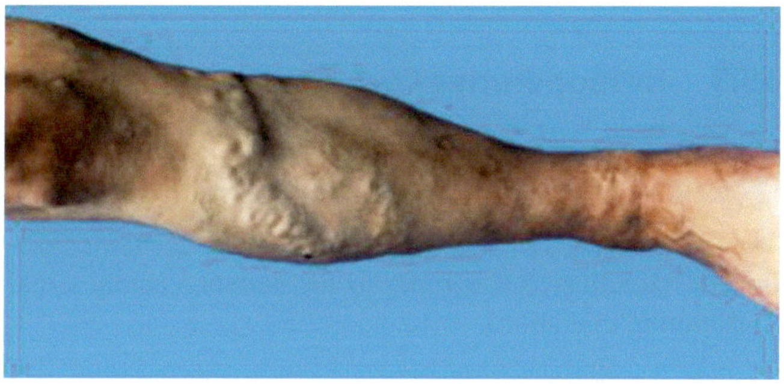

Fig. 15.1 Varicose veins (source: Changhai Hospital)

15.2 Clinical Manifestations

In clinical practice, patients with varicose veins have diversified clinical manifestations, requiring for case-specific identification and judgment. The most common leg symptoms include the following: irregular pain in the lower limbs, tingling, paresthesia, fatigue, leg and foot burning sensation, nocturnal muscle spasms, restless legs, burning sensation

W. Tian · Z. Mei · Z. Jing (✉)
Department of Vascular Surgery, Changhai Hospital, Second Military Medical University, Shanghai, China
e-mail: Jingzp@xueguan.net

Z. Jing et al. (eds.), *Endovascular Surgery and Devices*, https://doi.org/10.1007/978-981-10-8270-2_15

and cold feeling, tractional pain, etc. Its physical signs include spider veins, telangiectasia, lower extremity edema, venous lumbrical protrusions, skin pigmentation, lipid sclerosis, eczema, ulcers, etc. [2].

Varicose veins have diversified manifestations, some with obvious varicose but no obvious leg symptoms and some just the opposite. Different patients should be consulted in detail to understand their specific conditions and work out the best program for treatment. Vascular color Doppler ultrasound can be used to ascertain the lower extremity hemodynamic state, venous diameter, and valve function, which is very helpful for the diagnosis and treatment of the diseases [3].

15.3 Intraoperative Coordination

15.3.1 Anesthesia and Surgical Position

The patient receives local anesthesia and takes a supine position (to be adjusted according to the patient's actual situations during operation).

15.3.2 Preparation of Items

Refer to Table 15.1.

Table 15.1 Preparation of items

Name	Qty.	Name	Qty.
Disposable operation kit	1	Needle holder	1
Disposable 1 mL, 2 mL, 5 mL syringes	1 each	Suture scissors, surgical scissors	1 each
Disposable gloves	2 pairs	Medium curved pliers	2
Large gauze	1 bags	Mill's pliers	1
T valve	1	Small curved pliers	6
1% lidocaine injection	4 vials	Mosquito pliers	6
Silk suture (1#)	1 bag	Shank, blade	1 each
Atraumatic suture(4–0)	1	5F Berenstein catheter	1
Toothed forceps	2	1% polidocanol injection	1~2 vials
Histoacryl	1	Therapeutic varicose socks	1 pairs
Muller hook	1	Mepore self-adhesive aseptic dressing	Several
Elastic bandage	2 coils	500 mL normal saline	1 bag
Skin retractor	2		

15.3.3 Selection of Minimally Invasive Endovascular Surgery

At present, the endovascular therapies of venous varicose mainly include endovenous laser treatment (EVLT), radiofrequency ablation (RT), and sclerotherapy. The Department of Vascular Surgery of Changhai Hospital affiliated to the Second Military Medical University mainly uses high ligation of great saphenous vein and endovenous occlusion and punctate stripping for varicose veins surgery (Fig. 15.2). This is a minimally invasive technique for treatment of venous varicose by integrating the advantages of surgical stripping with the currently prevailing endovascular occlusion therapy, featuring fewer complications, quick recovery, same-day discharge, etc. [4].

15.3.4 Procedures and Intraoperative Coordination Process

Refer to Table 15.2.

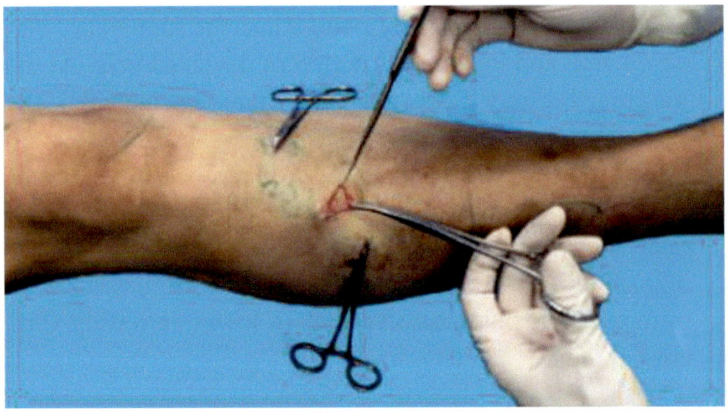

Fig. 15.2 High ligation of great saphenous vein and endovenous occlusion and punctate stripping technique (source: Changhai Hospital)

Table 15.2 Procedures and intraoperative coordination process

Procedures	Intraoperative coordination process
1. Patient enters the operation room, mark the great saphenous vein and its varicose branches	(1) Mental nursing; (2) keep the patient warm; (3) help to lie at supine position; (4) connect ECG to observe changes in blood pressure, heart rate, and oxygen saturation
2. Conduct routine sterilization up to the navel and down to the entire affected limbs and one-third upper part of the contralateral thigh	Prepare disinfectant (heated to 98.6 °F in incubator); assist with draping; deliver iodixanol injection; tidy up the surgical table; and prepare surgical devices

Table 15.2 (continued)

Procedures	Intraoperative coordination process
3. Conduct local anesthesia at the root of the thigh where the saphenofemoral junction is and along the superficial varicose veins	Deliver 1% lidocaine injection
4. Conduct high ligation of great saphenous vein: start from the pulsatile point of the common femoral artery; cut a 3 cm incision on the medial of the inguinal; cut open the skin, subcutaneous fat, and scape fascia, in turn, to dissociate the trunk of the great saphenous vein. Devascularize the root branches of the great saphenous vein, and conduct ligation, respectively. Dissociate to the oval fossa toward the proximal end, and devascularize the great saphenous vein at 0.5 cm from the point where the great saphenous vein converges with the common femoral vein; conduct ligation and clamp the distal end	Deliver the surgical devices
5. Dissociate the trunk of the great saphenous vein at the knee joint, devascularize it, insert 5F Berenstein catheter from the proximal end to the root of the great saphenous vein, prepare sclerosing foam of 1% polidocanol injection and air at a proportion of 1:4, inject the foam via the 5F Berenstein catheter into the superior knee segment of the trunk of the great saphenous vein, withdraw the catheter while injecting. Ligate both ends of the superior knee segment of the great saphenous vein, find out the site with obvious great saphenous dilation at the mid-piece of the thigh, sever the great saphenous vein, strip off part of the vein, and ligate	Deliver the 5F Berenstein catheter, 1% polidocanol injection
6. Make about 0.5 cm incision at the marked site, and pull out the superficial varicose vein with Muller hook, and strip off. During stripping, try to reduce damage to the peripheral tissues; ligate large lacerated ends of the veins to reduce bleeding. Ligation should perforate through branch veins	Deliver the devices, and clean up the table promptly
7. Close the inguinal incision, glue the incision with Histoacryl, and bandage the wound with Mepore self-adhesive aseptic dressing (Fig. 15.3)	Deliver the Mepore self-adhesive aseptic dressing and Histoacryl; assist with bandaging

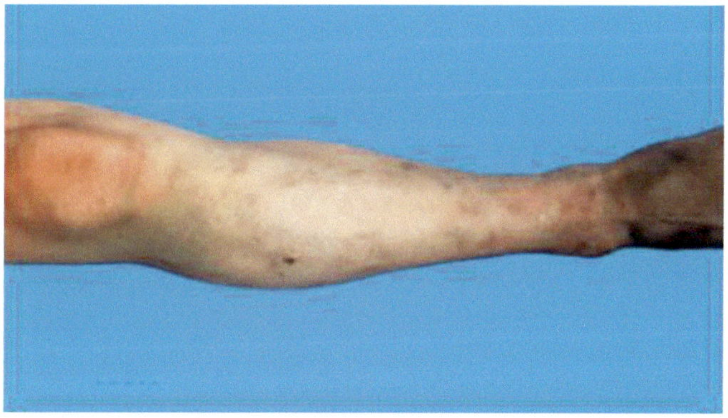

Fig. 15.3 Postoperative effect (source: Changhai Hospital)

15.4 Essentials for Intraoperative Observation

15.4.1 Observe Vital Signs

For patients with primary cerebrovascular diseases, their blood pressure and heart rate changes should be closely monitored during operation, especially under local anesthesia; the patient must be closely monitored for any local anesthetic allergies or toxic reactions.

15.4.2 Observe Bleeding

In venous stripping, sometimes the lacerated end of the vein may be pulled apart, leading to continuously bleeding incision. At this time, compression hemostasis should be conducted immediately. The corresponding sites of the pulled-apart perforated branch veins should be compression dressed with thickened cotton pad after operation to prevent bleeding [5].

Reference

1. Jing Z. Endovascular therapy. Beijing: People's Medical Publishing House; 2003.
2. Nuo P. Clinical diagnosis and treatment of varicose veins. Shanghai: The Second Military University Press; 2012.
3. Raju S, Neglen P. Chronic venous insufficiency and varicose veins. N Engl J Med. 2009;360:2319–27.
4. Partsch H. Varicose veins and chronic venous insufficiency. Vasa. 2009;38:293–301.
5. Cassina PC, Brunner U, Kessler W. Surgical management of varicose veins in advanced chronic venous insufficiency. Curr Probl Dermatol. 1999;27:174–81.

Veno-occlusive Disease

16

Zaiping Jing, Huajuan Mao, Meiqin Shi, Junmin Bao,
Xiaolong Wei, and Hongfei Wang

Abstract

Vein occlusion refers to a type of diseases characterized by venous stenosis or occlusion. Its main clinical manifestations include poor distal venous return, swelling, and aching pain. To be specific, lower extremity deep venous thrombosis is relatively common. As soon as the thrombus drops, it can easily give rise to pulmonary embolism and other acute diseases. This chapter introduces the formation of lower extremity deep venous thrombosis as well as clinical manifestations, surgical process, and intraoperative observation points of Budd-Chiari syndrome.

Keywords

Vein occlusion · Deep venous thrombosis · Budd-Chiari syndrome

16.1 Deep Venous Thrombosis of Lower Extremity

16.1.1 Introduction

Deep venous thrombosis of lower extremity (DVT) is the abnormal coagulation of venous blood in the lower extremity deep venous vessels (Fig. 16.1), often involving iliac, common femoral, deep femoral, popliteal and calf veins, and about 1/5 pelvic vein. Most thrombi happen with the calf and spread upward and can also happen at multiple sites. DVT risk factors include obesity, thromboembolic history, varicose veins, potential malignancies, oral contraceptives, immobilization, post-operation and postpartum, and heart disorders. In addition, thromboangiitis obliterans, lupus erythematosus, and ulcerative colitis can also cause DVT; thrombosis among some young people may attribute to the lack of innate anticoagulant factor or acquired hypercoagulable state that leads to venous thrombosis [1, 2].

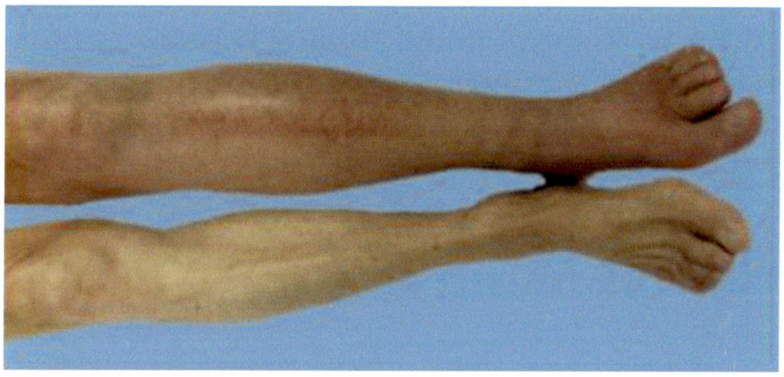

Fig. 16.1 Deep vein thrombosis, DVT (source: Changhai Hospital)

16.1.2 Clinical Manifestations

DVT is mainly manifested as sudden swelling and pain of the affected limbs, increased soft tissue tension, post-activity exacerbation, ease with the affected limb being raised, and tenderness at the venous thrombosis site. One to two weeks after the onset, the affected limbs can have exposed or expanded superficial veins. When the thrombus lies in the muscular veniplex of the calf, Homans sign and Neuhof sign appear positive.

Patients with severe DVT may have leukophlegmasia or even phlegmasia cerulea dolens. Leukophlegmasia (white leg) refers to highly swollen limbs and high tension and persistent spasm of the femoral artery after acute thrombosis of the lower extremity deep vein, accompanied with total limb swelling, pale skin, and subcutaneous reticular vein expansion. Phlegmasia cerulea dolens (blue leg) is the most serious situation for the lower extremity DVT, clinically manifested as sharp pain of the affected limbs, shiny and indigo-colored skin, low-temperature skin with blisters, disappeared pulsation of dorsalis pedis artery, strong systematic reaction, and

Z. Jing (✉) · H. Mao · M. Shi · J. Bao · X. Wei · H. Wang
Department of Vascular Surgery, Changhai Hospital, Second Military Medical University, Shanghai, China
e-mail: Jingzp@xueguan.net

Z. Jing et al. (eds.), *Endovascular Surgery and Devices*, https://doi.org/10.1007/978-981-10-8270-2_16

decreased skin temperature. If not treated promptly, phlegmasia cerulean dolens may lead to shock and venous gangrene.

Once the phlebothrombosis breaks off, it can enter and occlude the pulmonary artery along the blood flow and result in pulmonary artery embolism.

Postthrombotic syndrome (PTS) may occur during DVT chronic phase, mainly manifested as swollen lower extremity and mainly showing signs of lower extremity edema, pigmentation, eczema, varicose veins, and, more seriously, fatty scleroderma and ulcers that occur in the boot area of the foot.

16.1.3 Intraoperative Coordination

16.1.3.1 Anesthesia and Surgical Position

The patient receives local anesthesia and takes a supine position (to be adjusted according to the actual situations of the patient during operation).

16.1.3.2 Preparation of Items

The same as in Table 13.13.

16.1.3.3 Preparation of Devices

Refer to Table 16.1.

16.1.3.4 Selection of Minimally Invasive Endovascular Surgery

Minimally invasive endovascular surgery for lower extremity deep vein thrombosis, LDVT, mainly includes vena cava filter implantation (removal) technique, catheter-directed thrombolysis, balloon dilatation, stent implantation, aspiration thrombectomy, etc. LDVT patients can choose indwelling dorsal vein needle before operation to conduct anterograde angiography of the lower extremity veins (Fig. 16.2), and the surgeon can choose appropriate surgical operation according to the angiography findings.

1. Inferior vena cava filter (VCF) implantation (Fig. 16.3): VCF implantation aims to block and capture the larger free thrombosis from the lower extremities and reduce the probability of fatal pulmonary embolism caused by emboli flowing into the pulmonary artery along the blood flow. In conducting inferior VCF implantation, the filter is routinely placed at about 1 cm from below

Table 16.1 Preparation of devices

Name	Qty.	Name	Qty.
Puncture needle	1	5F short sheath	1
High-pressure connector	2	5F common pigtail catheter	1
0.035 in. common hydrophilic wire 260 cm	1	4F/5F Berenstein catheter	1
3-5F infusion catheter (if necessary)	Several	Vena cava filter (if necessary)	1
Inflation device (if necessary)	1	Single-loop/three-loop snare (if necessary)	1
OTW balloon catheter (if necessary)	Several	6F MPA catheter (if necessary)	1
Self-expanding peripheral bare stent (if necessary)	Several	10Fguide catheter (if necessary)	1
AngioJet aspiration thrombectomy system	1 set	8-10F short sheath (if necessary)	1
Aspirex mechanical thrombectomy system	1 set	0.035 in. hardened hydrophilic wire 260 cm (if necessary)	1

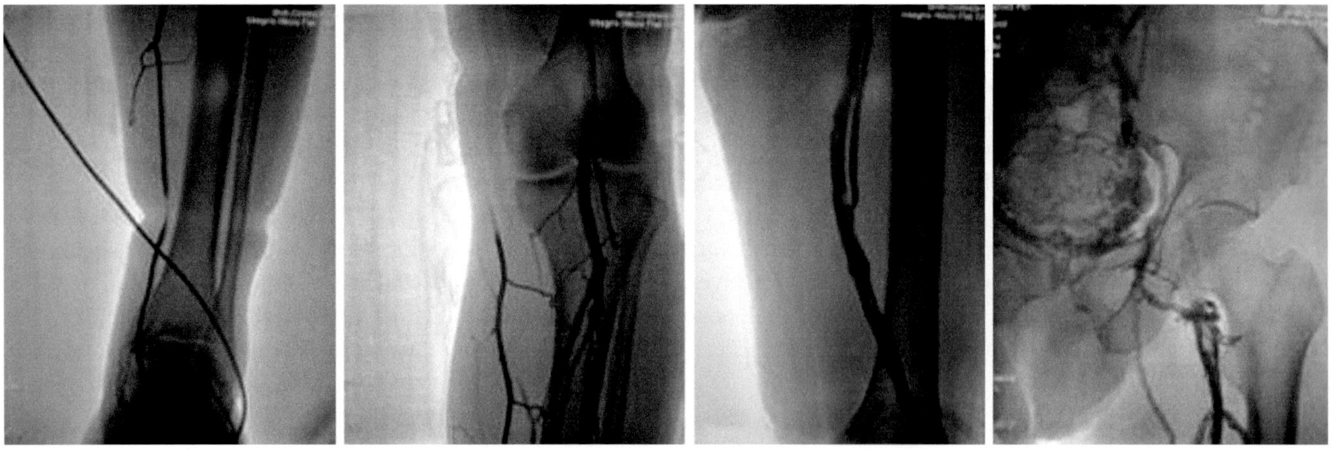

Fig. 16.2 Lower extremity anterograde angiography

the kidney vein level. The time to remove the filter is decided by the surgeon according to the actual situation of the patient or angiography findings and the filter implanted.

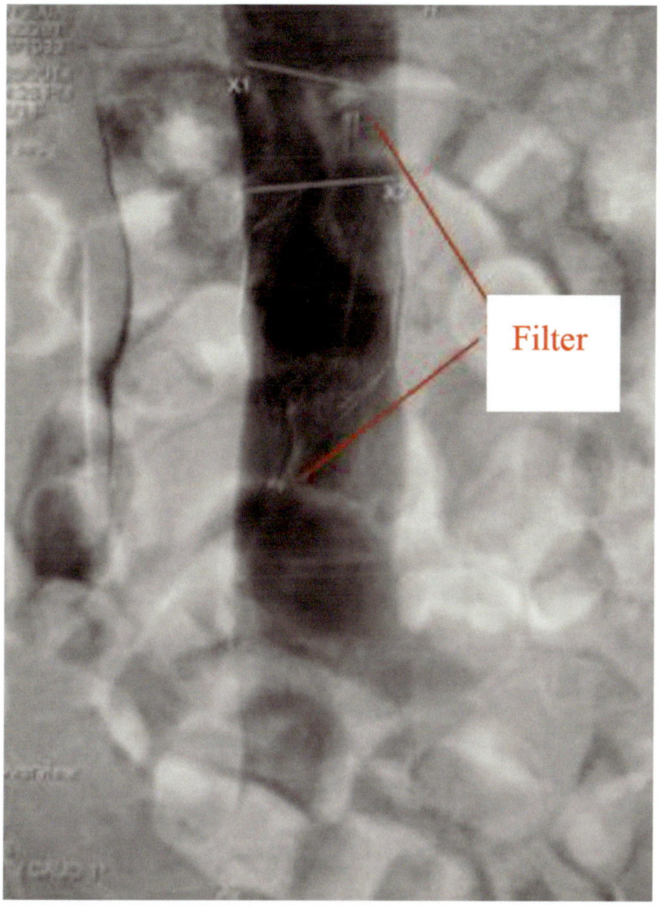

Fig. 16.3 Inferior VCF implantation

2. Catheter-directed thrombolysis: for acute LDVT patients, after the filter placement, insert Uni Fuse infusion catheter to the lesion site via the femoral artery (or puncture the popliteal vein, posterior tibial vein, great saphenous vein, small saphenous vein, etc.), and use urokinase micropump to continually administer drugs for thrombolysis. Subsequently conduct angiography again and select relevant therapies according to the thrombolytic situation of the affected limbs.
3. Balloon dilatation and stent implantation (Fig. 16.4): for DVT due to iliac vein compression, and after the removal of thrombosis by catheter-directed thrombolysis, the residual iliac venous lesion can be pre-dilated or post-dilated by balloon dilatation catheter according to the intraoperative angiography findings, and meanwhile, stent angioplasty should be conducted at the lesion site to ensure smooth blood flow. At present, clinically used iliac venous stents include Wallstent (Boston Scientific), E-Luminexx (Bard), etc.
4. Aspiration thrombectomy of lower extremity deep veins: AngioJet aspiration thrombectomy system (Boston Scientific) or Aspirex mechanical thrombectomy system (Straub) can be used for acute or sub-acute lower extremity deep vein thrombosis. The shorter the course of disease is, the better the aspiration effect will be.

16.1.3.5 Conventional Procedures and Intraoperative Coordination Process

Vena cava filter implantation via femoral vein puncture and catheter-directed thrombolysis via popliteal vein puncture are taken here as an example. Refer to Table 16.2.

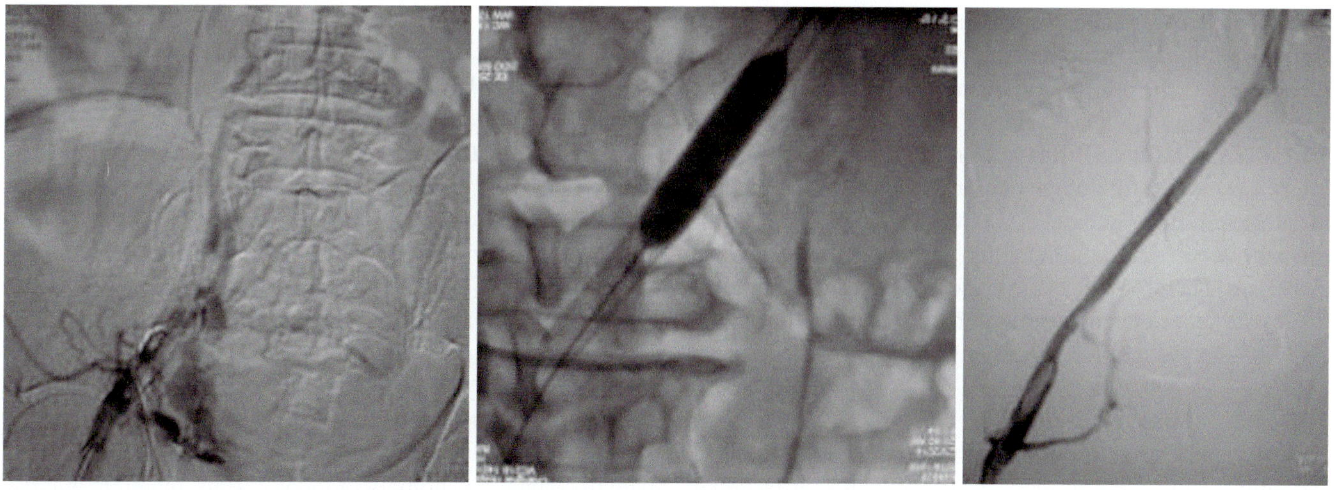

Fig. 16.4 Iliac vein balloon dilatation and stent implantation

Table 16.2 Procedures and intraoperative coordination process

Procedures	Intraoperative coordination process
1. Patient enters the operation room	(1) Mental nursing; (2) keep the patient warm; (3) help to lie at supine position, with two lower limbs slightly at abduction and extorsion position; (4) connect ECG to observe changes in blood pressure, heart rate and oxygen saturation; (5) establish intravenous infusion
2. Sterilize bilateral groins and knee joint of the affected limb	Prepare disinfectant (heated to 98.6 °F in incubator); assist with draping; deliver iodixanol injection; prepare heparin diluent (1000 mL normal saline +100 mg heparin sodium injection)
3. Puncture the common femoral vein of the normal side under local anesthesia with modified Seldinger technique, insert a 0.035 in. common hydrophilic wire 260 cm and a 5F common sheath, insert a 5F common pigtail catheter along the hydrophilic wire, and conduct angiography for inferior vena cava and iliofemoral vein	Deliver 1% lidocaine injection, puncture needle, high-pressure connector, 0.035 in. common hydrophilic wire 260 cm, 5F short sheath, and 5F common pigtail catheter; perform systemic heparinization (initial administered dose is 0.67 mg/kg based on body weight, subsequent dose is administered according to the actual intraoperative situations); endovascular devices should be flushed with the prepared heparin diluent
4. According to inferior vena cava angiography, select appropriate vena cava filter, withdraw 5F shorter sheath and 5F common pigtail catheter, exchange to the long sheath matching with the vena cava filter, and insert the vena cava filter into the inferior vena cava along the long sheath	Deliver the vena cava filter
5. Withdraw the delivery system of the vena cava filter, insert 5F common pigtail catheter, conduct angiography to the inferior vena cava again, and check the position of the vena cava filter	Deliver the 5F common pigtail catheter
6. Withdraw the catheter and long sheath, apply pressure to bind up the puncture site of the common femoral vein, puncture the vena cava of the affected side, insert a 5F short sheath and 0.035 in. common hydrophilic wire 260 cm, and insert an infusion catheter along the wire to the lesion site	Deliver the infusion catheter
7. If necessary, conduct thrombolysis during operation or continue thrombolytic therapy after back to the ward	Prepare and deliver thrombolytic drugs
8. Properly secure the indwelling infusion catheter	Deliver T valve, gauze, paste, and elastic bandage, assist the surgeon to secure the infusion catheter, and safely escort the patient back to ward

16.1.4 Essentials for Intraoperative Observation

16.1.4.1 Observe Vital Signs

Intraoperative patients are always in a state of being conscious, mostly feeling nervous. Therefore, establish frequent communication with the patient, and closely observe their consciousness, breathing, and other changes in vital signs.

16.1.4.2 Observe Pulmonary Embolism

Inferior vena cava filter implantation can reduce the incidence of fatal pulmonary embolism, but thrombus less than 3 mm can still access through the filter and result in pulmonary embolism. Therefore, the patient should be closely monitored for any presence of cough, chest tightness, chest pain, hemoptysis, tachypnea, and other symptoms during operation.

16.1.4.3 Observe Bleeding

The first and foremost complication occurred during lower extremity venous catheter-directed thrombolysis is bleeding, most frequently accompanied with hematoma at the injection site or puncture site. Therefore, closely observe the puncture site, and monitor the presence of any hemorrhagic spots on body skin and mucous membrane, as well as the presence of any hematuria, hematochezia, bleeding gums, nasal bleeding, etc. The most serious complication is cerebral hemorrhage. Closely observe the changes in vital signs, such as headache, projectile vomiting, changes in limb activities, consciousness, etc.

16.2 Budd-Chiari Syndrome

16.2.1 Introduction

Budd-Chiari syndrome (BCS) is a posthepatic portal hypertension resulting from the occlusive disease of the inferior vena cava of the superior segment of the hepatic vein or its opening due to various reasons, often accompanied by inferior vena cava hypertension (Fig. 16.5). The disease presents itself most with young people, at a male to female ratio of (1.2–2):1, aged between 2.5 and 75 years old but more common with 20–40 years of age. The disease is mainly attributed to congenital anomaly of great vessels, hypercoagulable and hyperviscous state, toxins, intracavitary non-thrombotic obstruction, exogenous compression, vascular wall lesions, diaphragm factors, abdominal trauma, etc. [1–3].

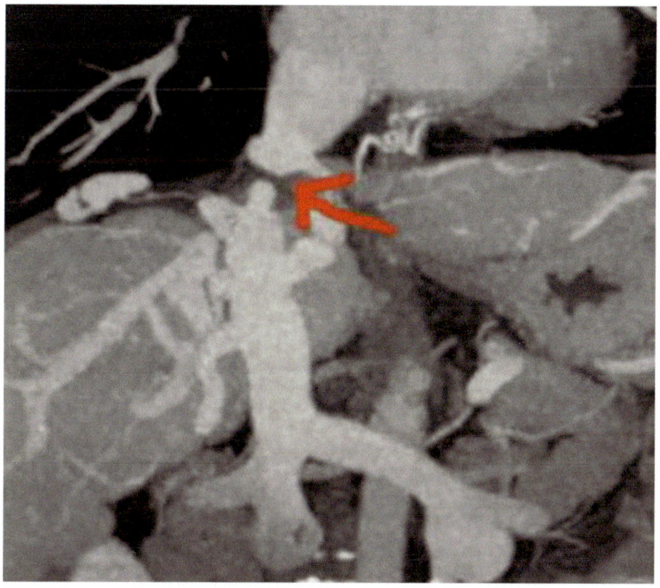

Fig. 16.5 Budd-Chiari syndrome

16.2.2 Clinical Manifestations

The clinical manifestations of BCS patients are related to the number and extent of vascular involvement and the nature and status of obstructive lesions. Patients in acute phase of simple hepatic venous thrombosis often present with fever, right upper abdominal pain, rapid presence of massive ascites, jaundice and liver enlargement, liver area tenderness, and oliguria and die of circulatory failure, liver function failure, or gastrointestinal bleeding in several days or weeks. Patients in chronic phase (CP) of simple hepatic venous thrombosis present with portal hypertension, hepatosplenomegaly, refractory ascites, and esophagogastric varices. Patients with simple inferior vena cava obstruction present with thoracoepigastric, back superficial, and lower extremity varicose veins, edema, pigmentation, and ulcers. Some patients may be marked by post-activity tachypnea due to reduced venous return resulting from hepatic vein and inferior vena cava obstruction.

16.2.3 Intraoperative Coordination

16.2.3.1 Anesthesia and Surgical Position

The patient receives local anesthesia and takes a supine position (to be adjusted according to the actual situations of the patient during operation).

16.2.3.2 Preparation of Items

The same as in Table 13.4.

Table 16.3 Preparation of devices

Name	Qty.	Name	Qty.
Puncture needle	1	5F common pigtail catheter	1
High-pressure connector	3	5F short sheath	1
0.035 in. common hydrophilic wire 260 cm	1	Triple T valve	1
5F Berenstein catheter	1	5F straight-tip catheter (if necessary)	1
Inflation device (if necessary)	1	7-12F short sheath (if necessary)	Several
Balloon catheter (if necessary)	Several	Self-expanding bare stent (if necessary)	1

16.2.3.3 Preparation of Devices

Refer to Table 16.3.

16.2.3.4 Selection of Minimally Invasive Endovascular Surgery

Endovascular therapy, as a safe and effective minimally invasive technique, has become the preferred method for treating Budd-Chiari syndrome. Endovascular therapy includes balloon dilatation, self-expanding bare stent implantation (if necessary), or TIPS (transjugular intrahepatic portosystemic shunt) for extensive hepatic vein occlusion. For membranous obstruction of inferior vena cava (MOVC) and/or short segment obstruction, balloon dilatation is generally used, instead of self-expanding bare stent implantation. If obvious stenosis still presents after dilatation, or occurrence of restenosis after multiple dilatations, self-expanding bare stent implantation can be considered, but the hepatic vein opening should not be blocked so as to avoid more severe hepatic vein BCS. BCS therapies for membranous obstruction of inferior vena cava with thrombosis mainly include aspiration thrombectomy combined with balloon dilatation, pre-vascularization technique, recyclable stent implantation, etc., or the combination thereof. BCS with segmental or total occlusion of the inferior vena cava is still available for opening up. Some patients are easy for opening and provided with balloon dilatation after opening, followed by implantation of Z-type self-expanding bare stent, but braided stent should be avoided [1]:

1. Balloon dilatation technique for inferior vena cava: Considering the large diameter of the inferior vena cava, routinely use balloons of 10–25 mm diameter for operation. At present, clinically available balloon catheters for the inferior vena cava include Maxi LD (Cordis), XXL (Boston Scientific), and others.
2. Stent implantation technique for the inferior vena cava: At present, the self-expanding bare stents for inferior vena cava stent implantation are mainly Gianturco Z-type stent,

a cylindrical structure enclosed with Z-type bends twined with 0.25–0.5 mm stainless steel wire at different lengths and in different diameters, and convenient for delivery, characterized in large stent meshes, rare occurrence of obstruction in the vascular bifurcation, strong radial support, and no shortening. It is mainly indicated for venous system lesions, especially for the inferior vena cava lesions at the hepatic vein opening of Budd-Chiari syndrome, not liable to the occurrence of obstruction at the openings of the hepatic vein and accessory hepatic veins. Its disadvantage is forward-jump upon deployment. To increase its stability and prevent stent displacement due to forward-jump, three Z-type stents should be routinely used. For its strong support, it can be used for tough, fibrosis, calcified lesions or lesions with highly elastic retraction [1–4].

16.2.3.5 Procedures and Intraoperative Coordination Process

Minimally invasive endovascular surgery with femoral vein puncture is here taken as an example. Refer to Table 16.4.

16.2.4 Essentials for Intraoperative Observation

16.2.4.1 Cardiac Failure

The blood is clogged below the abdomen before operation, and venous return decreases significantly. However, the venous return suddenly increases after revascularization of the blood vessels during operation; the workload of the originally dysfunctional heart increases, prone to heart failure. During operation, the heart rate and blood pressure change of the patient should be closely observed. In case of any abnormality, promptly administer the patient with cardiotonic, inject diuretics, expand blood vessels with sodium nitroprusside, reduce cardiac workload, and carry out other treatment. Also in infusion, limit the volume and speed of liquid infusion. In case of no contraindications after operation, urge the patient to lie at a head-up tilt position to reduce blood reflux of the lower extremities and prevent heart failure and embolism.

Table 16.4 Procedures and intraoperative coordination process

Procedures	Intraoperative coordination process
1. Patient enters the operation room	(1) Mental nursing; (2) keep the patient warm; (3) help to lie at supine position, with two lower limbs slightly at abduction and extorsion position; (4) connect ECG to observe changes in blood pressure, heart rate, and oxygen saturation; (5) establish intravenous infusion and control liquid infusion rate
2. Routinely sterilize bilateral groins up to the naval and down to the mid-thigh, exposing the groin (if necessary, sterilize the neck)	Prepare disinfectant (heated to 37 degrees in incubator) and assist with draping; deliver iodixanol injection; prepare heparin diluent (1000 mL normal saline +100 mg heparin sodium injection)
3. Puncture femoral vein with modified Seldinger technique under local anesthesia, insert a 5F short sheath and a 0.035 in. common hydrophilic wire 260 cm, insert a 5F common pigtail catheter along the hydrophilic wire, and conduct angiography for the inferior vena cava (Fig. 16.6)	Deliver 1% lidocaine injection, puncture needle, high-pressure connector, 5F short sheath, 5F common pigtail catheter, and 0.035 in. common hydrophilic wire 260 cm; perform systematic heparinization (initial administered dose is 0.67 mg/kg based on body weight and subsequent dose according to the intraoperative situation); endovascular devices should be flushed with prepared heparin diluent
4. Withdraw the 5F common pigtail catheter, insert a 5F Berenstein catheter to the lesion site along the 0.035 in. common hydrophilic wire 260 cm; connect the 5F Berenstein catheter with the high-pressure connector by the triple T valve (note: air should be exhausted); then connect the high-pressure connector with the pressure measurement device and measure the inferior vena cava pressure (note: reset the invasive pressure to 0 in. measurement)	Prepare pressure measurement device, and deliver the 5F Berenstein catheter, the triple T valve, and the high-pressure connector
5. According to angiography findings, determine type of lesion, insert the balloon to the lesion site through the stenotic segment or by breaking open the membrane (if necessary, by the hard tip of the wire) with the hydrophilic wire for patients with inferior vena cava stenosis or membranous obstruction, repeatedly conduct dilatation several times till the lumens in the lesion area become normal, and withdraw balloon expandable catheter	Deliver the inflation device and the balloon catheter (matching vascular sheath should be changed according to the diameter of the selected balloon)
6. According to angiography findings, and if necessary, select an appropriate self-expanding Z-type bare stent to implant into the lesion site, withdraw its delivery system, conduct inferior vena cava angiography again, and measure the pressure (Fig. 16.7)	Deliver the self-expanding Z-type bare stent (matching vascular sheath should be changed according to the diameter of the selected balloon)
7. Withdraw the catheter and short sheath, and locally compress the puncture site for 5 min to stop bleeding before compression dressing	Deliver the gauze and the elastic bandage, assist with binding, and safely escort the patient back to ward

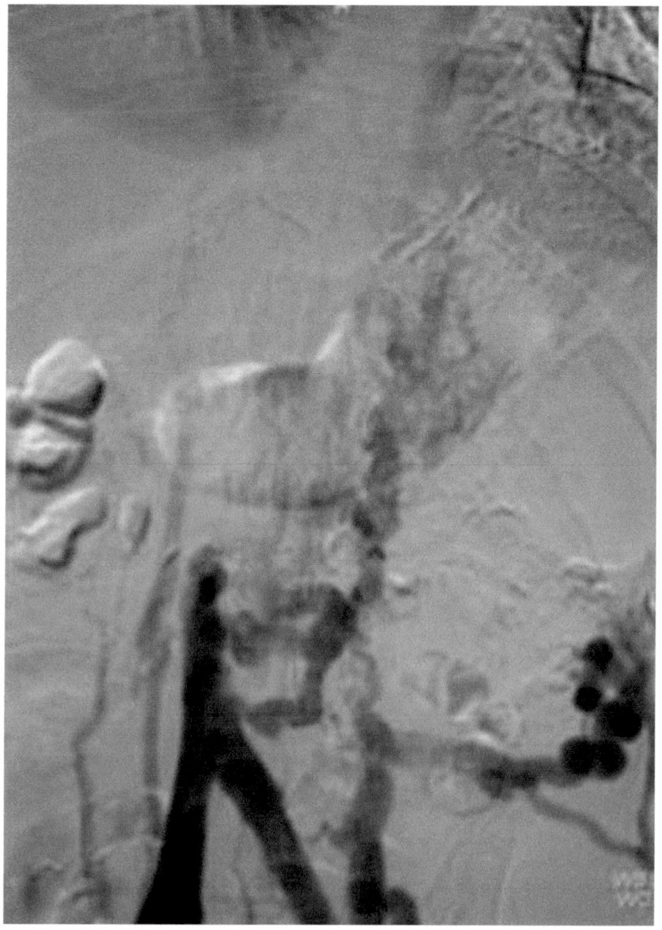

Fig. 16.6 Inferior vena cava angiography

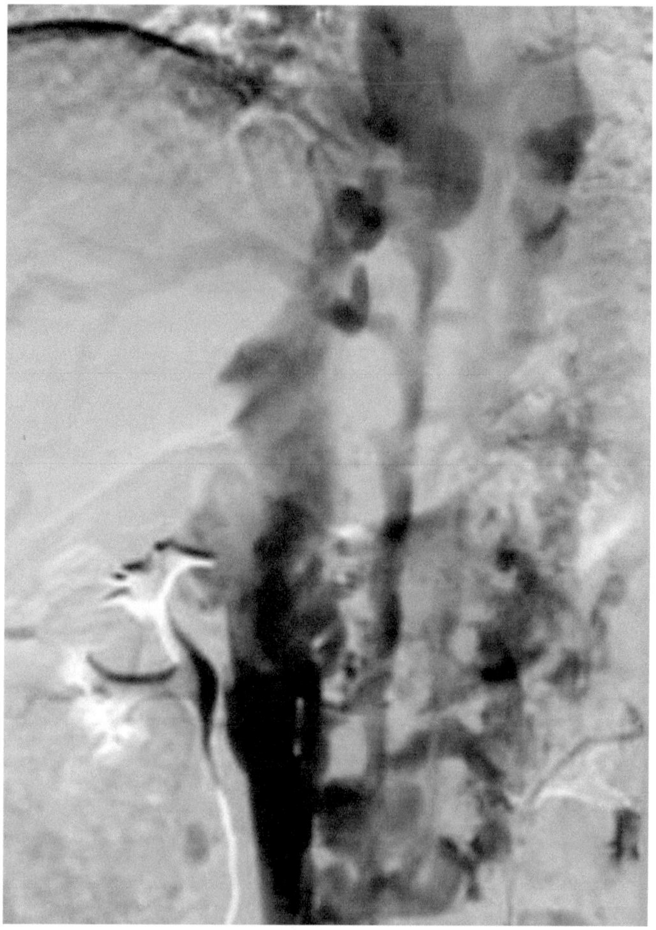

Fig. 16.7 Postoperative inferior vena cava angiography

16.2.4.2 Hemorrhage

When the membrane is broken open during operation for the patient with membranous occlusion, the blood vessels are prone to be damaged. Incorrect puncture direction may perforate blood vessels and cause damage to the inferior vena cava, resulting in hemorrhage or, more seriously, pericardial tamponade. Injury to the inferior vena cava is related to the surgeon's technical proficiency, mainly including wire-induced perforation and bleeding of the inferior vena cava. In this case, generally no analgetic and sedative are given to the patient during operation. Strictly and continually record the patient symptoms and vital signs, and listen to his complaint of abdominal pain and distension. In case of any abnormalities, get ready for rescue immediately.

16.2.4.3 Pulmonary Embolism

For some patients with inferior vena cava occlusion, thrombosis occurs in the inferior vena cava, or wall thrombus forms on the vascular wall, which, after opening of the vena cava, breaks off and results in pulmonary embolism. The catheter should be flushed with heparin diluent at specified time, and systematic heparinization should be ensured throughout the operation to prevent thrombosis. Patients with definitely diagnosed vena cava thrombosis can be treated with local thrombolysis or thrombectomy to remove thrombus before revascularization therapy. Pay attention to the patient's changes in respiratory rate and depth and monitor oxygen saturation. Small embolism generally presents with no symptoms, but large embolism should be treated as acute pulmonary embolism. In case the patient presents with chest pain, chest distress, tachypnea, cough, hemoptysis, and other symptoms, immediately urge the patient to lie at Fowler's position and inhale oxygen and get ready for emergency treatment.

References

1. Jing Z. Endovascular therapy. Beijing: People's Medical Publishing House; 2003.
2. Mao Y, Xu X, Li H. Interventional treatment nursing. Beijing: People's Military Medical Press; 2013.
3. Wang Z, Zhang J, Yongquan G. Practical vascular surgery and vascular interventional therapy. Beijing: People's Military Medical Press; 2004.
4. Ying D, Xiaoling W, Zeng Y, et al. Observation and nursing of Budd-Chiari syndrome and complications with interventional treatment. J Qilu Nurs. 2011;17(26):74–5.

17 Arteriovenous Fistula

Zaiping Jing, Huajuan Mao, Meiqin Shi, Xiang Feng, and Chao Song

Abstract

Arteriovenous fistula refers to an abnormal passage between arteries and veins. Based on pathogenesis, it can be classified into congenital and acquired arteriovenous fistula. If the fistula orifice is relatively large, the long-term abnormal passage may result in distal organ ischemia and cardiac insufficiency. The aim of endovascular treatment is to block the fistula orifice and restore normal blood flow. This chapter introduces clinical manifestations, minimally invasive endovascular surgery process, and intraoperative observation points of common arteriovenous fistula.

Keywords

Arteriovenous fistula · Endovascular treatment

17.1 Introduction

Arteriovenous fistula (AVF) is an abnormal passageway between an artery and a vein, which can be congenital or acquired due to pathologic process, such as trauma (Fig. 17.1). The congenital arteriovenous fistula is caused by the residual abnormal passage between the artery and the vein during the developmental evolution of the embryonic. The acquired AVF is mainly caused by trauma, including perforating wound, crush injury (such as various puncture

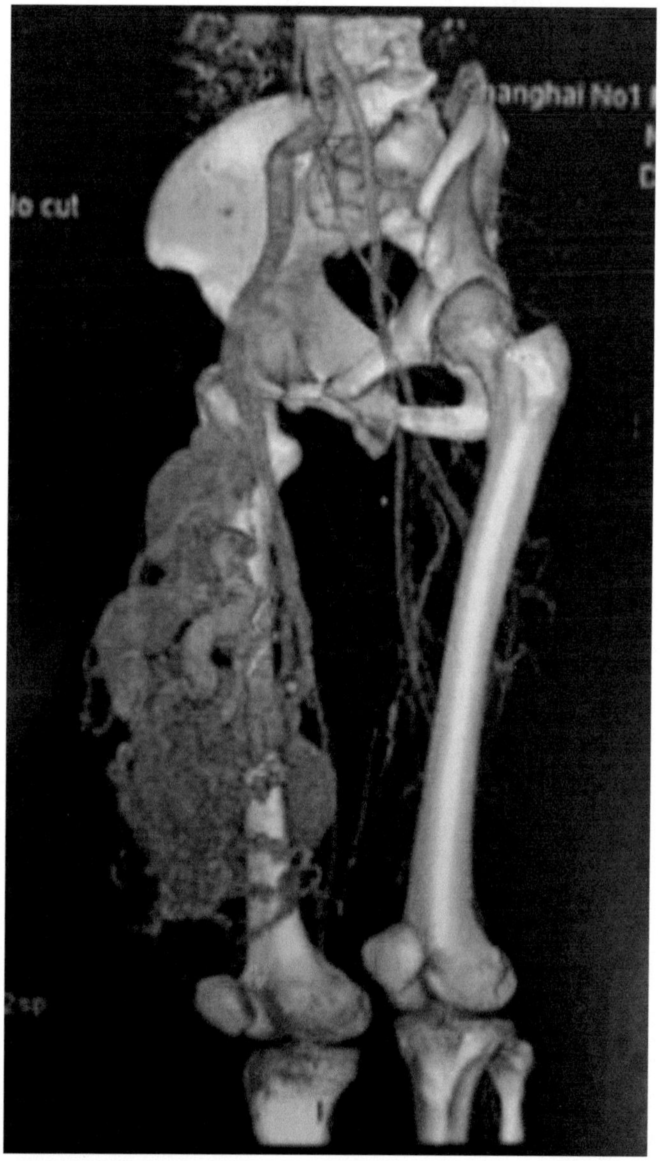

Fig. 17.1 Arteriovenous fistula (AVF)

Z. Jing (✉) · H. Mao · M. Shi · C. Song
Department of Vascular Surgery, Changhai Hospital, Second Military Medical University, Shanghai, China
e-mail: Jingzp@xueguan.net

X. Feng
Department of Urology, Changhai Hospital, Second Military Medical University, Shanghai, China

Z. Jing et al. (eds.), *Endovascular Surgery and Devices*, https://doi.org/10.1007/978-981-10-8270-2_17

injury, gunshot wounds, wounds caused by steel and glass debris, etc.), local hematoma forms with the wounds and the hematoma, after being organized, corms the AVF wall. The fistula between the artery and the vein is simple and rarely seen. Most traumatic aneurysms are located at the artery side or the venous side or between the artery and the vein, some accompanied with arterial aneurysm or venous aneurysm. Therefore, the artery blood flows into the accompanied vein via the abnormal passage, resulting in local vascular lesion of the fistula and hemodynamic changes of local fistula, surrounding circulation and the entire body system [1].

17.2 Clinical Manifestations

Acute acquired arteriovenous fistula (AVF) can occur immediately after injury or after clot dissolution outside the arteriovenous communication, mostly accompanied with tremor and murmur. The affected limbs of the chronic arteriovenous fistula patients are manifested as swelling, numbness, pain, and fatigue symptoms, with "buzzing" sound heard in local pulsatile mass. Patients with heart failure may have chest tightness, palpitations, tachypnea, and other symptoms. AVF common signs include the following aspects.

17.2.1 Murmur and Tremor Present in Fistula Area

Apart from tiny arteriovenous fistula, typically rough and continuous "rumbling" sound can often be heard at AVF site, called "machine-like" noise, which goes up during the systolic phase of the heart and transmits along the proximal and distal ends of the trunk blood vessels. This noise should be distinguished from the weak diastolic murmur caused by pseudoaneurysm and the systolic murmur caused by arterial stenosis.

17.2.2 Pulse Rate Increased

This results from the Bainbridge reflex due to increased venous return or increased cardiac workload owing to the decrease in average arterial pressure.

17.2.3 Cardiac Enlargement and Heart Failure

As a large number of blood flow quickly into the vein through the fistula, venous pressure increases, and blood return to the heart also increases, resulting in heart enlargement, and progressive heart enlargement can lead to heart failure. The extent of cardiac enlargement and heart failure is closely related to the size, location, and duration of the fistula. The fistula closer to the heart, such as AVF formed with the direct branches (carotid artery, anonymous artery, subclavian artery) of the aortic arch and the accompanying veins, will result in earlier and more serious symptoms of heart failure.

17.2.4 Local Temperature Rise

The skin temperature of the affected limbs at the AVF site increases, with a high flow rate, but that far from the AVF site may be normal or lower than normal.

17.2.5 Venous Insufficiency

Direct arteriovenous communication increases the venous pressure, and most patients manifest AVF proximal or distal superficial varicose veins, skin pigmentation, and toe or finger ulcers and present with similar symptoms after deep vein thrombosis.

17.3 Intraoperative Coordination

17.3.1 Anesthesia and Surgical Position

The patient receives local anesthesia and lies in a supine position (to be adjusted according to the actual situations of the patient during operation).

17.3.2 Preparation of Items

The same as in Table 13.13.

17.3.3 Preparation of Devices

Refer to Table 17.1 (taking lower extremities arteriovenous fistula as an example).

Table 17.1 Preparation of devices

Name	Qty.	Name	Qty.
Puncture needle	1	5F common pigtail catheter	1
High-pressure connector	2	5F short sheath	1
0.035 in. common hydrophilic wire 260 cm	1	4F Berenstein catheter	1
6-8F Balkin sheath 40 cm	1	7-12F short sheath (if necessary)	1
0.035 in. hardened hydrophilic wire 260 cm (if necessary)	1	Renegade STC 18 micro-catheter (if necessary)	1
Peripheral stent graft (if necessary)	Several	Echelon micro-catheter (if necessary)	1
Embolization (Cook) (if necessary)	Several	Onyx liquid embolic agent (if necessary)	Several
Interlock controllable embolization (if necessary)	Several	Vascular closure device (if necessary)	1

17.3.4 Selection of Minimally Invasive Endovascular Surgery

Currently arteriovenous fistula (AVF) happens most frequently in the lower extremities. The endovascular therapies for the lower extremities AVF mainly include AVF embolization (Fig. 17.2), endovascular exclusion with peripheral stent graft, peripheral stent graft exclusion and embolization, and others. AVF with hiatal communication that occurred in the non-trunk arteries (such as deep femoral artery) is often treated with arterial embolization. Available embolization materials mainly include spring coil Onyx liquid embolic agent (Medtronic). However, if AVF occurs with such trunk arteries as superficial artery, the fistula must be excluded by peripheral stent graft. Stent graft exclusion has better effect for acquired arteriovenous fistula with relatively small opening but has limited therapeutic effect for congenital AVF. Peripheral stent grafts in clinical use mainly include Viabahn (Gore), Fluency (Bard), and Wallgraft (Boston Scientific) (Table 13.15) [1–3].

17.3.5 Procedures and Intraoperative Coordination Process

Take endovascular exclusion of right lower limb AVF with peripheral stent graft via the left common femoral artery as an example, as shown in Table 17.2.

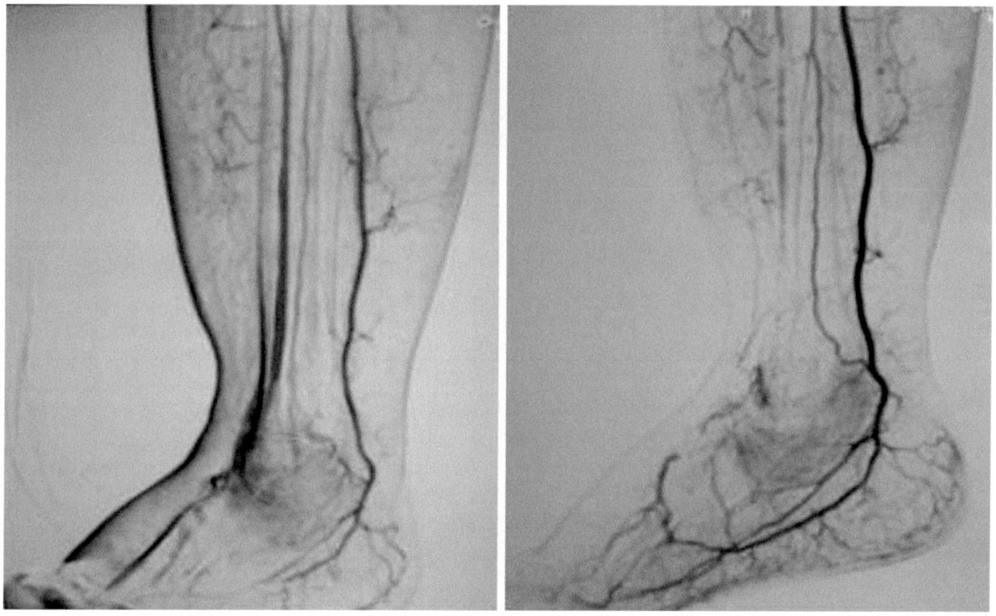

Fig. 17.2 Lower extremity AVF embolization with Onyx liquid embolic agent + controllable spring coil

Table 17.2 Procedures and intraoperative coordination process

Procedures	Intraoperative coordination process
1. Patient enters the operation room	(1) Mental nursing; (2) keep the patient warm; (3) help to lie at supine position, with two lower limbs slightly at abduction and extorsion position; (4) connect ECG to observe changes in blood pressure, heart rate, and oxygen saturation; (5) establish intravenous infusion
2. Routinely sterilize the bilateral groins from the umbilical down to mid-thigh, exposing the groins	Prepare disinfectant (heated to 98.6 °F in incubator) and assist with draping; deliver iodixanol injection; prepare heparin diluent (1000 mL normal saline +100 mg heparin sodium injection)
3. Puncture left common femoral artery with modified Seldinger technique under local anesthesia, insert a 0.035 in. common hydrophilic wire 260 cm and a 5F short sheath	Deliver 1% lidocaine injection, puncture needle, high-pressure connector, 0.035 in. common hydrophilic wire 260 cm, and 5F short sheath; perform systematic heparinization (initial administered dose is 0.67 mg/kg based on body weight, and subsequent dose according to the intraoperative situation); endovascular devices should be flushed with prepared heparin diluent
4. Insert a 5F common pigtail catheter to the abdominal aorta along the hydrophilic wire, withdraw the hydrophilic wire and conduct arteriography of the right lower limb (Fig. 17.3)	Deliver the 5F common pigtail catheter

(continued)

Table 17.2 (continued)

Procedures	Intraoperative coordination process
5. According to angiography findings, use 5F common pigtail catheter to cross to the contralateral limb, insert the hydrophilic wire, withdraw the 5F common pigtail catheter and 5F short sheath, exchange to insert a 7-8F Balkin sheath 40 cm and 4F elbowed catheter to the lesion site along the hydrophilic wire	Deliver the 7-8F Balkin sheath and the 4F Berenstein catheter
6. Withdraw the 4F Berenstein catheter, select an appropriate peripheral stent graft, and insert it to the lesion site along the 0.035 in. common hydrophilic wire 260 cm	Deliver the peripheral stent graft (the matching vascular sheath to be changed according to the selected stent)
7. Withdraw the delivery system, conduct angiography to the affected limb again (Fig. 17.4), and check if the lower extremity AVF is excluded	
8. Withdraw the Balkin sheath and wire, select appropriate vascular closure device to block the puncture site	Deliver the vascular closure device
9. Compression dressing on puncture site	Deliver the gauze and the elastic bandage, assist with draping, safely escort the patient back to ward

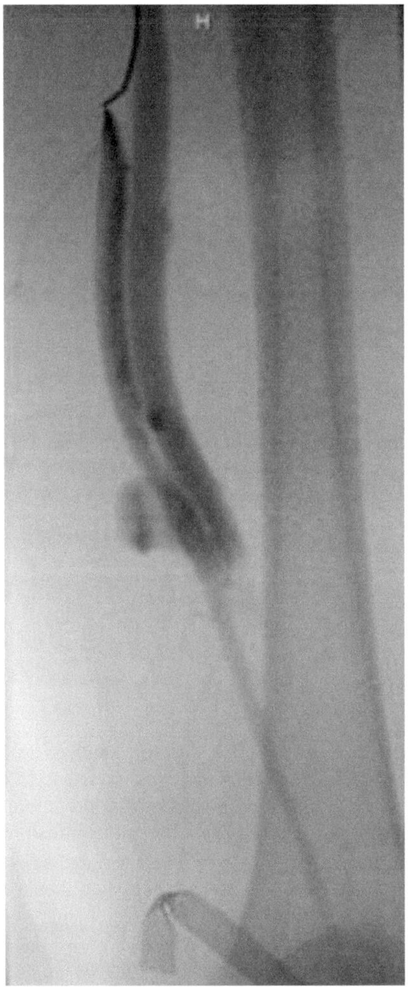

Fig. 17.3 Intraoperative angiography

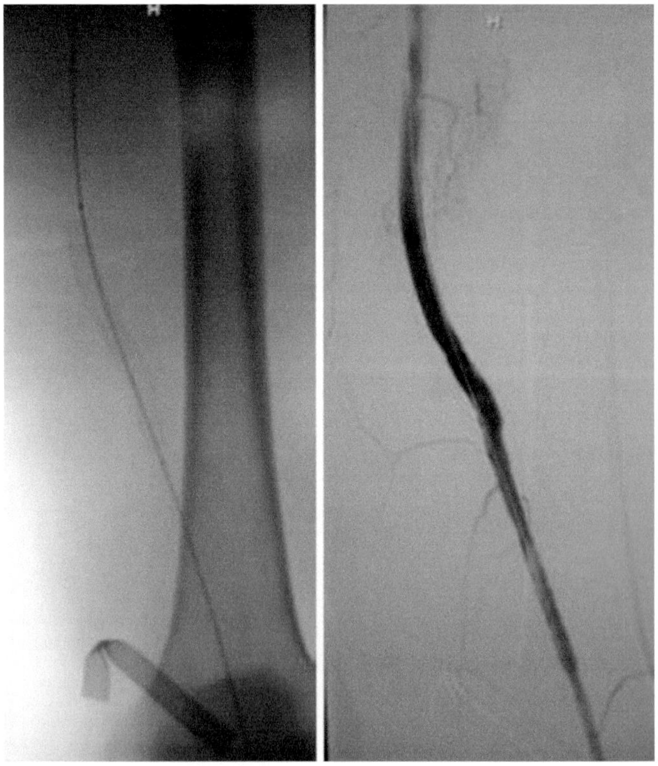

Fig. 17.4 Postoperative angiography

17.4 Essentials for Intraoperative Observation

17.4.1 Pulmonary Embolism

Due to short-circuited passage by AVF, the blood flow at the venous side decreases after exclusion of the arterial side, with declined flow rate, resulting in increased local thrombosis and, consequently, higher probability of occurrence of pulmonary embolism when the thrombus falls off or the embolus moves to the pulmonary artery. Therefore, attention should be paid to observing the consciousness and breathing changes of the patient. If the patient presents with dyspnea, chest pain, chest tightness, cough, hemoptysis, anxiety, syncope, and other symptoms, high flow oxygen should be immediately administered, venous access established, and ECG monitored; and the patient should also be prepared for emergency rescue.

17.4.2 Post-embolization Distal Ischemia and Venous Thrombosis

During the operation, the patient should be asked for any presence of calf and foot skin paresthesia or numbness and other abnormal embolisms that lead to distal ischemia. After the operation, the patient should be observed for any occurrence of limb swelling, and occurrence of deep vein thrombosis should be avoided. If any, immobilize and raise the affected limb so as to promote blood reflux. Meanwhile, ask the patient not to hot compress and massage the affected limb so as to prevent the emboli from falling off and receive treatment according to the treatment program for deep vein thrombosis [1].

References

1. Jing Z. Endovascular therapy. Beijing: People's Medical Publishing House; 2003.
2. Mao Y, Xu X, Li H. Interventional treatment nursing. Beijing: People's Military Medical Press; 2013.
3. Wang Z, Zhang J, Yongquan G. Practical vascular surgery and vascular interventional therapy. Beijing: People's Military Medical Press; 2004.

18 Endovascular Operation-Related Complications and Treatment

Zaiping Jing and Liangxi Yuan

Abstract

With the development of intravascular technology, endovascular treatment has become the first choice for the patients with cardiovascular disease. However, endovascular operation-related complications may cause potential threats to the patient in the process of puncturing the blood vessels. For vascular puncture-related complications, such as puncture site bleeding and hematoma, treatment measures including close observation and correction of potential coagulation disorders should be taken to maintain appropriate hemoglobin levels. Artery anterior wall puncture technique should be used to avoid multiple puncture at the same site, and arteriovenous fistula could be avoided consequently. For artery perforation and artery dissection caused by wire and catheter, surgical repair or stents should be used to restore the patency of the vascular lumens. For balloon- and stent-related complications, distal arterial embolism could be prevented by color Doppler ultrasound and CT before endovascular treatment. Operation should be carried out strictly in accordance with the instructions of the endovascular devices to prevent the occurrence of arteriorrhexis. The incidence of complications can be reduced by identifying the patients with risk factors, including large-sized vascular sheath, unmatched stent with vascular diameter, excessive balloon dilatation in normal vessels, careless and rough operation by the surgeon, and so on.

Keywords

Endovascular treatment · Complications · Treatment

Z. Jing (✉) · L. Yuan
Department of Vascular Surgery, Changhai Hospital, Second Military Medical University, Shanghai, China
e-mail: Jingzp@xueguan.net

Endovascular surgery is a minimally invasive treatment through Seldinger's vascular puncture technique by using wire, catheter, vascular sheath, balloon, stent, and other endovascular devices [1–3]. In the process of puncturing the blood vessels and manipulating the endovascular devices, complications that may cause potential threats to the patient's limbs or life may occur consequentially. In order to safely and successfully perform endovascular treatment, it must identify whether the involved blood vessels are of high risk or not before preoperative imaging examination or before angiography. This can suggest early anticoagulation, application of protective devices, or the use of the finer catheter and vascular sheath to avoid the occurrence of complications. This chapter focuses on complications associated with manipulating the vascular puncture, wire, catheter, and balloon stent.

18.1 Vascular Puncture-Related Complications and Treatment

The main risk factors for the puncture site complications include large-sized vascular sheath, minimally invasive endovascular surgery, arterial incision site, inflammatory arterial properties such as Behcet's syndrome, previous history of intubation, slight of figure, female, uncontrolled hypertension, excessive anticoagulation therapy, the use of glycoprotein II b/III a inhibitors, aging, etc. The incidence of complications can be reduced by identifying high-risk patients and using strategies of risk reduction.

18.1.1 Puncture Site Bleeding and Hematoma

This is the most common complication occurred with endovascular minimally invasive treatment, accounting for 1–2%, a majority of which presents with the puncture sites and a few with retroperitoneal space due to high position of the puncture site or bleeding resulting from damaged small

Z. Jing et al. (eds.), *Endovascular Surgery and Devices*, https://doi.org/10.1007/978-981-10-8270-2_18

arteries, mainly manifested as puncture site swelling, subcutaneous congestion, and sometimes local mass accompanied by tenderness [4–7]. The most common symptoms of retroperitoneal hemorrhage are abdominal pain (60%), followed by the back pain and lateral abdominal pain (25%), and a mass of different nature can be touched sometimes in physical examination sometimes, and diagnosis should be ascertained by CT scanning or abdominal B ultrasound.

18.1.1.1 Causes

This is mainly attributed to rough operation, long-time operation, the use of larger vascular sheath, excessive dose of heparin, and thrombolysis. It can also occur after multiple vascular punctures, because hematoma can conceal the pulsation of the common femoral artery itself. Therefore, multiple punctures can further lead to difficult arterial puncture. Puncture needle damage to the posterior wall of the blood vessels can also cause intraoperative angiorrhea, especially in patients using anticoagulant drugs. Blood leak around the vascular sheath during operation can also lead to blood clot and, finally, hematoma. This kind of complication attributes to arterial anterior wall calcification and asymmetric or stellate tearing caused to the arterial wall by puncture. In this situation, round sheath cannot play the role of hemostasis, and moreover, the manipulation of the wire and the catheter inside the sheath can aggravate the bleeding. Inguinal hematoma can have a variety of clinical manifestations, mainly including postoperative inguinal swelling, in addition to other common signs and symptoms such as pain, skin ecchymosis, puncture site bleeding, neuropathy secondary to nerve compression, anemia, low blood pressure, and, more seriously, possible occurrence of intraoperative and postoperative shock. Peritoneal hemorrhage and hematoma mostly occur in inguinal ligament artery puncture, difficult for immediate discovery and having minor or less significant early clinical manifestations. However, if there are hematocrit decline, hypotension, and oliguria, all active bleeding signs must be subject to timely and rapid imaging examination so as to rule out retroperitoneal hematoma.

18.1.1.2 Prevention

The high-risk factors prone to inguinal hematoma include female, old age (over 65 years old), and the use of aspirin and glycoprotein II b/III a inhibitors; the above factors have been shown to moderately increase the possibility of bleeding complications. Puncture site bleeding should be treated with the correct method of hemostasis by compression at the vascular puncture site, rather than the entry point of the skin and right on the femoral head. Compression lasts till the bleeding basically stops before compression bandage. Bandaging time can accord to the size of the sheath. But attention should be paid to the pulsation situation of the distal artery of the punctured limb. Occurrence, if any, should be dealt with promptly. Correct use of various vascular closure devices is helpful for reducing the incidence of such complications.

18.1.1.3 Treatment

Treatment strategies for inguinal hematoma include close observation and correction of potential coagulation disorders, discontinuation of anticoagulant therapy, and transfusion to maintain appropriate hemoglobin levels. Hand compression or other similar mechanical compressions of the hematoma may be used in acute conditions. In addition, computed tomography (CT) can be used to determine the extent of hematoma, identifying whether it is active bleeding according to the leakage of the radiocontrast agent and clearly understanding if the hematoma has spread to the retroperitoneum. Hemoglobin laboratory tests must be carried out every 4–6 h till it becomes stable. In addition, ultrasound must also be carried out to exclude the formation of pseudoaneurysm. Once pseudoaneurysm is diagnosed, choices should be made according to the patient's conditions: reduce or discontinue anticoagulation or antiplatelet therapy, perform long-term local compression, or, if necessary, conduct minimally invasive endovascular treatment or surgical treatment.

Retroperitoneal hemorrhage may stop by self-filling; most patients can maintain hemodynamic stability, requiring for only close observation. The patient with suspected peritoneal hemorrhage should be measured with hematocrit and hemoglobin. If the patient presents with hematocrit decline, blood transfusion should be administered, if necessary, according to the actual situations of the patient. In the case of hemodynamic instability, continued anemia even with continued blood transfusion, local skin necrosis after compression, neurological compression symptoms, severe pain, etc., inguinal exploration can be performed to remove hematoma. Hematoma formed around the puncture site is difficult for open surgery, and therefore, the key is prevention. In case of open surgery, the complete common femoral artery should be dissected and exposed to check if there is active bleeding. And during operation, the posterior wall of the common femoral artery should be examined to determine whether the posterior wall is injured or not. Most patients with retroperitoneal hematoma can have their disease controlled by continually detecting hematocrit changes, correcting coagulation abnormalities, and timely receiving blood transfusion. Indications for surgical treatment include neurological abnormalities of the affected limbs, hemodynamic instability, progressive blood loss, and severe pain. In retroperitoneal hematoma decompression technique, the iliac blood vessels can be exposed through the inguinal incision or by directly accessing the peritoneum through the incision above the inguinal ligament.

18.1.2 Pseudoaneurysm

Pseudoaneurysm occurs after withdrawal of the vascular sheath upon completion of endovascular treatment. At that time, the arterial puncture hole is not completely closed, and the blood leaks into the surrounding soft tissues, forming lumens connected with the arterial lumens that are usually manifested as pulsatile mass with tenderness, at an incidence rate between 0.05 and 8.0% [8, 9]. Ultrasound examination can indicate the size and location of the pseudoaneuryms at common femoral artery bifurcation, deep femoral artery, and superficial femoral artery and can identify hematoma and pseudoaneurysm. In ultrasound detection, pseudoaneurysm can show that blood flows out from the arterial lumens. Typical ultrasound manifestation of pseudoaneurysm is a pulsatile anechoic bladder, and color Doppler ultrasonography shows the presence of eddy current signal in the bladder. In the spectral waveform analysis, pseudoaneurysm shows distinctive "back and forth" flow characteristics. The sensitivity of ultrasonography in the diagnosis of pseudoaneurysm is 94% and the specificity 97%. If the pseudoaneurysm is significantly extended to the retroperitoneal, then the abdominal pelvic enhanced CT or arterial CTA examination may help assess the size and the site of vascular injury.

18.1.2.1 Causes

The formation of pseudoaneurysm is often associated with the failure of properly compressing the arterial vascular puncture site after withdrawal of the vascular sheath, mostly occurring at superficial femoral artery or lower common femoral artery, which is because the femoral head faces headward so that the artery is incompletely compressed when under compression. Pseudoaneurysm is manifested as pulsatile mass at the puncture site, usually occurring within 24–48 h after operation, accompanied with groin tenderness, and possibly difficult to distinguish it from hematoma. Large pseudoaneurysm can result in neurological signs due to compression of the femoral nerves, or venous thrombosis due to compression of the femoral veins, and also local skin ischemia, or even necrosis. In physical examination, systolic murmur can be heard, and pulsatile mass at the groin can be palpated.

18.1.2.2 Prevention

Postoperative compression dressing position must be appropriate. The compression should be applied above the vascular puncture site, avoiding compression only at the puncture site and on the femoral head. Compression bandaging should last for 24 h, while the pulsating situation of the distal artery of the punctured limb should be closely observed. The use of vascular closure device greatly reduces the occurrence of such complications.

18.1.2.3 Treatment

Pseudoaneurysm in a diameter <3 cm can be subject to clinically follow-up observation, usually experiencing self-thrombosis and requiring for no surgical repair; ≥3 cm is not easy for self-thrombosis, and the rather simple and minimally invasive treatment is ultrasound-guided compression treatment and thrombin injection, and if necessary, it can be treated with direct surgical repair and endovascular surgery. Endovascular therapies include stent graft implantation and spring coil embolization.

18.1.3 Arteriovenous Fistula

Inguinal AVF is a rare complication after percutaneous puncture. It involves the communication between the common femoral artery and the vein, at an incidence rate of 0.1–1% [10, 11]. Inguinal AVF is usually asymptomatic and can be diagnosed by palpating tremor or auscultating continuous murmur in physical examination of the inguinal area. Because of this type of AVF, shunt volume (average 160–510 mL/min), is much lower than the threshold that can cause heart insufficiency, most AVF patients present with no signs of heart insufficiency. Duplex ultrasound is an optional imaging examination that shows the signal characteristics of the arterialized venous blood flow during the systole and the diastole.

18.1.3.1 Causes

AVF usually occurs after improper lower puncture of the femoral artery bifurcation or femoral deep artery and vein. These positions are close to the superficial femoral artery; however, AVF can also occur after the perforation between the common or superficial femoral artery and the femoral vein. The risk factors leading to AVF include female, hypertension, and operation-related factors such as left inguinal puncture and high-dose anticoagulant use. The reason why left inguinal puncture is prone to AVF is the angle of the puncture; this is because most surgeons perform the left common femoral artery puncture by standing at the contralateral side.

18.1.3.2 Prevention

Use artery anterior wall puncture technique, try to avoid multiple punctures at the same site, and avoid inserting the vascular sheath into veins via artery puncture.

18.1.3.3 Treatment

As the incidence of AVF is low, its natural course of disease is not fully understood, so the relevant treatment principles are still controversial. Therapeutic approaches mainly include conservative treatment (follow-up observation), surgical repair, and endovascular therapy. About 2/3 fistula can close by themselves in the follow-up process, requiring no surgical treatment. If conservative treatment is used, the patient should go through intensive ultrasound monitoring and regular physical examination. If the symptoms aggravate or the fistula range increases, surgical treatment is required.

18.1.4 Acute Arterial Thrombosis in Limbs

Common femoral arterial thrombosis is one of the complications of minimally invasive endovascular surgery, usually more obvious after sheath removal and manipulated compression [12, 13]. The blood flow in the common femoral artery slows down, and the accompanied superficial femoral artery lesion or the endometrial injury in percutaneous puncture can cause thrombosis. Thrombus can extend to the deep femoral or iliac arteries, causing deep femoral artery ischemia. In contrast, thrombus may be formed around the sheath or at the arterial puncture site during endovascular treatment. Thrombus can rush toward the distal blood vessels and cause arterial embolization after the manipulated compression stops.

18.1.4.1 Causes

Simple compression of the common femoral artery after sheath removal can lead to thrombosis, particularly among patients with severe atherosclerotic disease of the common femoral artery or experiencing previous inguinal reconstruction. The use of vascular closure device at the puncture site increases the risk of potential thrombosis.

18.1.4.2 Prevention

Upon completion of endovascular operation, proper force should be applied in compressing the puncture site, ensuring smooth blood flow at the compression location under the premise of no bleeding. Frequently check the peripheral arterial pulsation and the skin temperature of the puncture side, which helps to find the situation of lower limb ischemia.

18.1.4.3 Treatment

Acute ischemia requires urgent intervention; otherwise, the patient may present with new intermittent claudication or rest pain. At present, the main clinical therapies include surgical treatment and minimally invasive endovascular treatment. Surgical treatment includes inguinal exploration, embolectomy by lower extremity arteriotomy, common femoral endarterectomy, patch repair, etc.; minimally invasive endovascular treatment includes mechanical thrombectomy, thrombolytic therapy, or atherectomy.

18.1.5 Osteofascial Compartment Syndrome

Osteofascial compartment syndrome is a less common complication in vascular puncture, often caused by improper compression of limb puncture site, mostly occurring in the lower extremities in vascular surgery. For example, if the anterograde approach in femoropopliteal endovascular therapy fails to access through the diseased blood vessel, retrograde puncture of the distal artery may be used. In particular, if no effective compression methods are taken after popliteal artery or calf artery puncture, it may lead to osteofascial compartment hematoma. If bleeding continues, it may lead to osteofascial compartment muscle and nerve compression, acute ischemia, hypoxia, muscle necrosis, and even secondary renal insufficiency that threatens the life of the patient.

18.1.5.1 Causes

Improper compression after popliteal artery or calf artery puncture may result in osteofascial compartment hemorrhage and subsequently hematoma squeezing on other tissues, causing a sudden increase in compartment volume.

18.1.5.2 Prevention

Appropriate balloon can be used to inflate the inner compression passage at the puncture site for 5 min after popliteal artery retrograde puncture, with compression bandage applied to the popliteal fossa. Continuous bleeding can stop for the calf artery generally by appropriate compression. Operation-related vascular rupture can be treated with appropriate compression, stent graft, coil embolization, and other methods.

18.1.5.3 Treatment

The patient with suspected osteofascial compartment syndrome should be closely observed, going through angiography again to confirm no recurrence of active bleeding. If bleeding still exists, balloon compression can be repeated to stop bleeding. If the tension increases continually, osteofascial compartment incision decompression technique should be performed immediately. Early incision decompression of osteofascial compartment is the only effective method to prevent muscle and nerve ischemic necrosis and should not wait till the presence of the "5P" signs leading to irreversible ischemic muscle contracture.

18.1.6 Puncture Site Infection

Puncture site infection takes place more common among patients with inguinal puncture and arterial catheterization, often manifested as local redness, swelling, heat, pain, fever, chills, and other bacteremia signs. If handled improperly, it may lead to local infectious aneurysm, soft tissue necrosis, femoral artery erosion and rupture resulting in massive hemorrhage, and ultimately death.

18.1.6.1 Causes

As the puncture is performed repeatedly at the same position of the femoral artery, accompanied by improper puncture technique, arterial vascular wall is damaged and ruptured, and blood extravasates, which is not timely stopped and forms hematoma, or local hematoma forms due to bleeding around the indwelling sheath, and the wound is polluted by urine or improperly treated after operation, resulting in local infection, or excessive compression of local skin leads to skin necrosis and secondary infection.

18.1.6.2 Prevention

Aseptic technique should be strictly followed during operation. For high-risk groups, intraoperative operation should be gentle, avoiding formation of local hematoma at the puncture site. For patients incompletely self-reliant in life, indwelling urinary catheter should be placed, if necessary, avoiding pollution of the wound or puncture site by urine, and intensive dressing change should be ensured to keep the dressing dry. For patients with low immunity and diabetes and experiencing multiple operations and indwelling catheter in a short time, preventive use of antibiotics is allowed for preventing infection.

18.1.6.3 Treatment

For simple local infection, use antibiotics for anti-infectious treatment according to experience. Abscess formation can be cut open for drainage, and local dressing change can be intensified. Generally it can recover via early treatment, but for patient with secondary pseudoaneurysm after infection, reasonable treatment program should be selected according to the length of the patient's course. In resection of infectious pseudoaneurysm, if the blood vessels are available for repair, angiorrhaphy is still recommended.

18.2 Wire- and Catheter-Related Complications and Treatment

18.2.1 Arterial Perforation

Arterial perforation is a less common complication [14, 15]. Wire-related arterial perforation can be determined by identifying if the wire route deviates itself from the normal arterial anatomy route under X-ray. If the wire accesses into the surrounding soft tissues, its tip shows abnormal bending. Once the wire is removed, radiocontrast leakage can be found in angiography.

18.2.1.1 Causes

Careless and rough operation by the surgeon may lead to arterial perforation. In addition, use of rigid wire may also lead to arterial perforation. Therefore, rigid wire should not be used as the preferred wire for angiography or used for superselection of severely diseased fine arteries. Risk factors leading to vascular perforation include old age, diabetes, and endometrial angioplasty.

18.2.1.2 Prevention

In operating the wire, the surgeon should ensure the wire tip always falls within the X-ray scanning screen. In case of any resistance, stop further insertion of the wire. Before the catheter or other endovascular devices enter into the blood vessels, it must ascertain that no perforation exists. In case of any doubt, retract the wire and attempt to find new endovascular or subintimal approaches to access through the lesion vessels. Type J wire with very flexible tip can be chosen in operation.

18.2.1.3 Treatment

Isolated wire-related perforation requires no special treatment. Those with obvious small artery bleeding can be embolized by spring coil and other embolus to stop bleeding. If bleeding continues, endovascular repair by balloon compression or stent grafts, such as peripheral stent graft, can be performed, and if necessary, surgical repair can be used.

18.2.2 Artery Dissection

Vascular dissection is one of the frequently encountered problems in the process of percutaneous endovascular surgery, caused due to entry into normal or diseased arterial vascular intima by wire, catheter, or other endovascular devices. The positions under the vascular intima show radiocontrast retained at the vascular dissection under angiography.

18.2.2.1 Causes

The surgeon mistakenly inserts the wire or catheter under the arterial intima. Any resistance or coiled tip of any endovascular devices indicates possible entry into the arterial intima. Small dissection may occur in normal and lesion-free vascular segments, especially in high-profile arteries, such as iliac artery.

18.2.2.2 Prevention

Operation should be meticulous, while needle and wire should be advanced under X-ray fluoroscopy, radiocontrast being injected at any time. Wire, catheter, or other endovascular devices can continue advancing only until the blood vessel accessed is confirmed to be true lumen. If it is not sure if the wire, catheter, or other endovascular devices are under the vascular intima, suspend any operation and use low-profile catheter to access through the resistance site. If blood cannot be retracted through the catheter, then the catheter is possible under the vascular intima; retract the catheter till blood can be retracted, and then confirm it by hand injection of radiocontrast under lower pressure. Avoid rough action and blind advance of the wire and catheter into the blood vessels.

18.2.2.3 Treatment

If thrombosis occurs in vascular lumen without stenosis, especially in the direction reverse to the blood flow of the tear of the dissection, only follow-up observation is required. In contrast, iatrogenic large dissection is most likely to cause vascular lumen occlusion or thrombosis; then, intervention treatment is required. This type of vascular dissection can be treated by additional angioplasty (e.g., balloon dilatation for 5 min) with the aim of fixing the vascular intima again. The intima can also be secured by implanting self-expanding stent so as to restore the patency of the vascular lumens.

18.2.3 Device Rupture or Embolism

In the complex percutaneous endovascular treatment, a variety of complex endovascular devices are required. Device failure is not uncommon, for example, broken wire or catheter is left in the arterial lumen and becomes a free floating object. To avoid embolization or thrombosis of the distal arteries, the above devices must be captured. The most common technique for capturing foreign matter in the vessel is to use the endovascular snare, biopsy forceps, etc. If the broken wire is left in the sheath, the balloon can be inserted along the wire, and the wire is pulled out to the entrance of the sheath after dilatation [16–18].

18.3 Balloon- and Stent-Related Complications and Treatment

18.3.1 Arterial Embolism

Arterial embolism is a serious complication in the course of endovascular treatment, which can translate relatively simple treatment into complex therapeutic procedures. In the lower limb, for example, arterial embolism is a common complication in femoral and popliteal atherosclerotic occlusive lesions accompanied with thrombosis, and it can occur in the process of angioplasty, stent implantation, antherectomy, and other endovascular treatment. In endovascular treatment, the incidence of embolism of the distal vessel is 3–5%, and a very small number of patients may even present themselves with outflow tract (OT) vascular occlusion, leading to amputation and other serious consequences. The main clinical manifestations depend on the site of the embolization and the size of the emboli, mainly manifested as sudden onset of severe pain. The pain begins at the arterial embolization, and after a period of time, the pain plane moves slightly down and involves the entire limb below the embolic level; the arterial pulse of the limb below the embolic level disappears, showing pale skin. Plane below the limb arterial pulse disappeared, the skin becomes pale and gradually graniphyric with decreased skin temperature. When embolism occurs for some time, the affected limb may feel numb, manifested as hand or foot drop [19–22].

18.3.1.1 Causes

Most frequently, arterial embolism occurs when arterial wall thrombus breaks off and moves to the distal vessel or when atherosclerotic plaque breaks off due to damage to the vascular intima. A few many may be due to unmatched stent with vascular diameter or broken stent, causing vascular embolism.

18.3.1.2 Prevention

During operation, anticoagulation should be performed, operation meticulous, action gentle, measurement accurate, and stent selection appropriate, and particular care should be taken when performing transluminal angioplasty of the wall thrombus.

18.3.1.3 Treatment

The best way to prevent distal arterial embolism is to identify high-risk vessels by color Doppler ultrasound, CT, and X-ray images before endovascular treatment. In combination with the case history, imaging, and hand feeling of the patient during operation, any suspected sclerosis-related thrombus should be first treated with catheter-directed thrombolysis or mechanical thrombectomy technique, rather than rashly with balloon dilatation and stent implantation, preventing thrombus from breaking off and causing distal vascular embolism. In addition, some treatment groups, by learning from carotid endovascular angioplasty and stent implantation experience, use embolic protection device in the lower extremity endovascular treatment, especially for those high-risk embolism cases having massive plaques or having only outflow tract. If an arterial embolism occurs, a sufficient amount of systemic heparinization may be given to the patient according to the activated clotting time (ACT), and appropriate endovascular treatment may be selected according to the patient's condition, such as thrombus aspiration (using aspiration catheter,

AngioJet thrombus aspiration system, Straub mechanical thrombectomy system), catheter-directed thrombolysis, etc. If the above treatment is not successful, and the patient presents with acute ischemic symptoms, surgical open surgery can be taken into consideration.

18.3.2 Arteriorrhexis

Arteriorrhexis is a rare complication, especially for blood vessels with severe atherosclerosis, and improper angioplasty can cause arterial rupture, and iliac artery rupture can be life-threatening.

18.3.2.1 Causes

Excessive balloon dilatation or the use of balloon and stent exceeding the vascular size can lead to arterial rupture. For the calcified blood vessels having no elastic compliance, a very slightly excessive dilatation may lead to full-thickness rupture of the arterial wall.

18.3.2.2 Prevention

In the course of endovascular treatment, operation should be carried out strictly in accordance with the instructions of the endovascular devices. Each operation procedure must be standard and meticulous so as to avoid occurrence of vascular rupture. In addition, before choosing endovascular devices, angiography should be performed and the diameter and length of the blood vessels should be accurately measured so as to select matching balloon, stent, and other endovascular devices accordingly. Selection of excessively large or small devices should be avoided.

18.3.2.3 Treatment

Endovascular angioplasty-induced inguinal distal vascular rupture is less life-threatening; however, it may cause pseudoaneurysm formation or arterial occlusion. Most inferior inguinal vascular perforation cases adopt conservative treatment, and auxiliary endovascular treatment methods include balloon compression, stent graft exclusion, or spring coil embolization therapy.

18.3.3 Arteriospasm and Lateral Branch Occlusion

Arteriospasm and lateral branch occlusion is a more common complication, which is not taken seriously in the past, but in fact, the consequences of which are very serious. Arteriospasm tends to cause acute thrombosis of the arteries, resulting in distal limb ischemia and other complications.

18.3.3.1 Causes

In transcutaneous transluminal angioplasty treatment, limb arteries may present with spasm, often involving major lateral branches and resulting in occlusion. The risk of occlusion taking place with major lateral branches depends on whether the primary lesion involves in the lateral branch or whether the lateral branch has a stenosis and other lesions.

18.3.3.2 Prevention

In the treatment of limb angioplasty, try to avoid excessively and frequently stimulating the blood vessels. If necessary, 10 μg nitroglycerin or 30–60 mg papaverine can be injected via the catheter for prevention purpose. In performing stent, especially stent graft implantation, try to avoid covering major lateral branches.

18.3.3.3 Treatment

In the event of arterial spasm, inject 10 μg nitroglycerin or 30–60 mg papaverine via the catheter, and administer with the same dose half an hour later. In case of arterial embolism, thrombolytic therapy should be performed promptly. When major lateral branch occlusion occurs, endovascular treatment (such as balloon dilatation, stent implantation, etc.) or surgical operation to revascularize the blood vessels is available.

18.3.4 Arterial Dissection

Atherosclerotic blood vessels are prone to endometrial detachment complication after balloon angioplasty, where the balloon, after dilatation, will extrude and damage the vascular intima, causing endometrial tear or dissection. If the lesion further aggravates on this basis, pulsatile arterial blood flow will tear off the vascular dissection and move it to arterial distal end, causing flow-restricting occlusion or arterial occlusion and further resulting in serious complications.

18.3.4.1 Causes

In angioplasty, the high-risk lesion prone to the formation of dissection is seriously calcified plaques, especially at the proximal superficial femoral artery. Excessive balloon dilatation in normal vessels may lead to arterial dissection.

18.3.4.2 Prevention

In performing balloon dilatation angioplasty, appropriate balloon should be selected according to the vascular diameter. Dilatation and deployment should be performed slowly.

18.3.4.3 Treatment

Any dissection taking place after angioplasty is preferably treated by continuous dilatation of the low-pressure balloon so that the protruding intimal flap attaches to the vascular wall. If the low-pressure balloon angioplasty fails and obvious dissection (restricted blood flow) still exists, self-expanding stent or balloon-expandable stent should be implanted to repair the vascular dissection. The stent can secure the vascular intima, enlarge vascular lumen, and effectively prevent further spreading of the intimal flap of the dissection. In addition, the localized arterial dissection at the inguinal can also be excised with a guided plaque resection device (e.g., SilverHawk/TurboHawk Peripheral Plaque Excision System).

References

1. Feng Y. Vascular surgery. Ver. 2. Shanghai: Shanghai Science and Technology Press; 1985.
2. Zhang R, Shi G, Zhou S, et al. Interventional therapy for in-stent restenosis. Chin Med J. 2001;114:67.
3. Jiang W, Li X, Ren W, Li X, Ren A, et al. Treatment of popliteal artery embolism by pulse spray thrombolytic technique. Chin J Radioact. 1996;30:301–5.
4. Bao J. Progress in endovascular therapies for lower extremity occlusive diseases. Chin J Bases Clin Gen Surg. 2010;17:645–8.
5. Li X, Jiang W, Zhu J, et al. Application of Strecker stent in treatment of peripheral artery stenosis or occlusive diseases. Chin J Radioact. 1996;30:296–300.
6. Jiang W, Wu C, Liu W, et al. Application of percutaneous and transluminal intervention technique in treatment of arterial stenosis diseases. Chin J Radioact. 2000;34:528–30.
7. Bao J, Mei Z. How to standardize catheter-directed thrombolysis for treatment of arterial occlusive disease. Clin Misdiag Misther. 2014;27:42–5.
8. Allaire E, Melliere D, Poussier B, et al. Iliac artery rupture during balloon dilatation: what treatment? Ann Vasc Surg. 2003;17:306–14.
9. Dauerman HL, Applegate RJ, Cohen DJ. Vascular closure devices: the second decade. J Am Coll Cardiol. 2007;50:1617–26.
10. Kelm M, Perings SM, Jax T, et al. Incidence and clinical outcome of iatrogenic femoral arteriovenous fistulas: implications for risk stratifiation and treatment. J Am Coll Cardiol. 2002;40:291–7.
11. Koreny M, Riedmüller E, Nikfardjam M, et al. Arterial puncture closing devices compared with standard manual compression after cardiac catheterization: systematic review and meta-analysis. JAMA. 2004;291:350–7.
12. Piper WD, Malenka DJ, Jr RTJ, et al. Predicting vascular complications in percutaneous coronary interventions. Am Heart J. 2003;145:1022–9.
13. Streiff MB. Vena caval filters: a review for intensive care specialists. J Intensive Care Med. 2003;18:59–79.
14. Tavris DR, Gallauresi BA, Lin B, et al. Risk of local adverse events following cardiaccatheterization by hemostasis device use and gender. J Invasive Cardiol. 2004;16:459–64.
15. Webber GW, Jang J, Gustavson S, et al. Contemporary management of postcatheterization pseudoaneurysms. Circulation. 2007;115:2666–74.
16. Tunesen KH, Sager P, Karle A, et al. Percutaneous transluminal angioplasty of the superficial artery by retrograde catheteration via the poplitealartery. Cardiovasc Interv Radiol. 1988;1:127.
17. Yuan L, Bao J, Zhao Z, et al. Endovascular therapy for long-segment atherosclerotic aortoiliac occlusion. J Vasc Surg. 2014;59:663–8.
18. Yuan L, Bao J, Zhao Z, et al. Transbrachial and femoral artery approach endovascular therapy for flush infrarenal aortic occlusion. Eur J Vasc Endovasc Surg. 2014;48:46–52.
19. Bonelli FC, McKusick MA, Textor SC, et al. Renal artery angioplasty: technical results and clinical outcome in 320 patients. Mayo Clin Proc. 1995;70(11):1041–7.
20. Plouin PF, Dame B, Chatellier G, et al. Restenosis after a first percutaneous transluminal renal angioplasty. Hypertension. 1993;21(1):89–93.
21. Dotter CT, Judkins MP. Transluminal treatment of arteriosclerotic obstructions: description of a new technique and a preliminary report of its applications. Circulation. 1964;30:654.
22. Katzen BT, Chang J, Knox WG. Percutaneous transluminal angioplasty with the Grüntzig balloon catheter: a review of 70 cases. Arch Surg. 1979;114:1389.

Case Studies

19

Zaiping Jing, Huajuan Mao, Meiqin Shi, Junmin Bao, Zhiyong Chen, Yifei Pei, Xiaolong Wei, Chao Song, Liangxi Yuan, Hongfei Wang, Lei Zhang, Wen Tian, and Lei Zhang

Abstract

Starting with cutting-edge clinical techniques, this chapter introduces 20 special and complicated cases of minimally invasive endovascular treatment. Based on a combination of endovascular devices and clinical cases, it performs detailed elaboration and analysis from the aspects of the surgical planning, device preparation, operating steps, intraoperative cooperation, technical essentials, intraoperative precautions, etc.

Keywords

Endovascular treatment · Surgical case

19.1 Case 1 Chimney Graft Technique for Aortic Arch Pseudoaneurysm Repair

19.1.1 Patient Data

The male patient, aged 56, felt a sudden surge of chest, back, and abdominal pain in 2013 but paid no attention to it. After that, he presented himself repeatedly with symptomatic hoarseness and coughing after drinking water. Aorta CTA examination by local hospital indicated aortic arch pseudoaneurysm, which significantly enlarged in the CTA reexamination in 2015, and the patient was admitted for "aortic arch pseudoaneurysm" in May.

19.1.2 Surgical Operation

CTA examination indicated the lesser curvature of the aortic arch presented with pseudoaneurysm, which was planned to be excluded by chimney technique, that is, to insert a TAA stent graft into the aortic lesion site of the patient and a self-expanding peripheral bare stent into the left subclavian artery. The chimney technique can fully ensure smooth blood flow of the branch arteries, exclusion of the pseudoaneurysm, and prevention of endoleak. The subject gave informed consent for the procedure.

19.1.3 Device Preparation

Refer to Table 19.1.

19.1.4 Procedures and Intraoperative Coordination Process

Refer to Table 19.2.

Z. Jing (✉) · H. Mao · M. Shi · J. Bao · Y. Pei · X. Wei · C. Song
L. Yuan · H. Wang · L. Zhang · W. Tian · L. Zhang
Department of Vascular Surgery, Changhai Hospital, Second Military Medical University, Shanghai, China
e-mail: Jingzp@xueguan.net

Z. Chen
Department of Vascular Surgery, The First Hospital, Anhui Medical University, Hefei, China

Z. Jing et al. (eds.), *Endovascular Surgery and Devices*, https://doi.org/10.1007/978-981-10-8270-2_19

Table 19.1 Device preparation

Name	Qty.	Name	Qty.
Puncture needle (Cook)	1	0.035 in. Lunderquist super-stiff wire 260 cm (Terumo)	1
High-pressure connector (SCW Medicath)	2	5F scaled pigtail catheter (Optimed)	1
0.035 in. common hydrophilic wire 180 cm (Terumo)	1	5F Berenstein catheter (AngioDynamics)	1
0.035 in. common hydrophilic wire 260 cm (Terumo)	1	6F short sheath (Terumo)	1
Zenith TX2 TAA stent graft 32 mm × 200 mm (Cook)	1	Self-expanding peripheral bare stent 10 mm × 60 mm (Optimed)	1

Note: The devices listed above (*A* mm × *B* mm), wherein *A* is the diameter of the device and *B* the length

Table 19.2 Procedures and intraoperative coordination process

Procedures	Intraoperative coordination process
1. Patient enters the operation room, general anesthesia	(1) Mental nursing; (2) keep the patient warm; (3) help to lie at supine position, with two lower limbs slightly at abduction and extorsion position and the left upper limb stretching at extorsion position; (4) connect ECG to observe changes in blood pressure, heart rate, and oxygen saturation; (5) establish intravenous infusion and place indwelling central venous catheter; (6) place indwelling urinary catheter
2. Sterilize bilateral inguen and left upper limb	Prepare disinfectant (heated to 98.6 °F with incubator), and assist with draping; deliver iodixanol injection; prepare heparin diluent (1000 mL normal saline +100 mg heparin sodium injection)
3. Cut a longitudinal incision of about 3 cm on the common femoral artery of the right groin, at the punctum maximum of the pulse, dissociate and expose the common femoral artery	Deliver the scalpels, large tweezers (flat tweezers or fine tweezers), separating pliers, mosquito pliers, vascular pliers, and 0# silk suture
4. Puncture the right common femoral artery with modified Seldinger technique, insert a 0.035 in. common hydrophilic wire 180 cm and a 5F scaled pigtail catheter, conduct thoracic aortic angiography (Fig. 19.1), and mark the positions of the left subclavian artery ostium and the aneurysm body	Deliver the puncture needle, high-pressure connector, 0.035 in. common hydrophilic wire 180 cm, 5F scaled pigtail catheter; perform systematic heparinization; intraoperative endovascular devices should be flushed with the prepared heparin diluent
5. Puncture the left femoral artery with modified Seldinger technique, insert 6F short sheath, 260 cm 0.035 in. common hydrophilic wire, and 5F elbowed catheter to the ascending aorta	Deliver the puncture needle, 6F short sheath,0.035 in. common hydrophilic wire 260 cm, and 5F Berenstein catheter
6. Implantation of Zenith TX2 thoracic aortic stent graft (Fig. 19.2): insert the 0.035 in. Lunderquist super-stiff wire 260 cm into the ascending aorta via the 5F scaled pigtail catheter; insert a Zenith TX2 thoracic aortic stent graft 32 mm × 200 mm into the lesion site along the super-stiff wire; meanwhile, insert a self-expanding peripheral bare stent 10 mm × 60 mm into left subclavian artery via the left femoral artery (the delivery system of the bare stent can be first placed at the left subclavian artery opening, and after the stent graft is deployed, deploy the chimney stent)	Deliver the 0.035 in. Lunderquist super-stiff wire 260 cm, Zenith TX2 thoracic aortic stent graft 32 mm × 200 mm, self-expanding peripheral bare stent 10 mm × 60 mm
7. Withdraw the delivery system of the thoracic aortic stent graft, insert the 5F scaled pigtail catheter again, and conduct thoracic aortic angiography, showing exclusion of thoracic aortic pseudoaneurysm, no endoleak, and smooth blood flow of bifurcated arteries	Deliver the 5F scaled pigtail catheter
8. Withdraw the catheter, wire, and short sheath, suture the right common femoral artery incision, and apply compression bandage at the puncture site of the left femoral artery	Deliver the vascular plier and CV suture for vascular incision suturing; deliver small round and angled needles and 1# suture to suture the incision layer by layer; deliver gauze and elastic bandage for compression dressing on puncture site
9. Anesthesia completed	Safely escort the patient back to ward

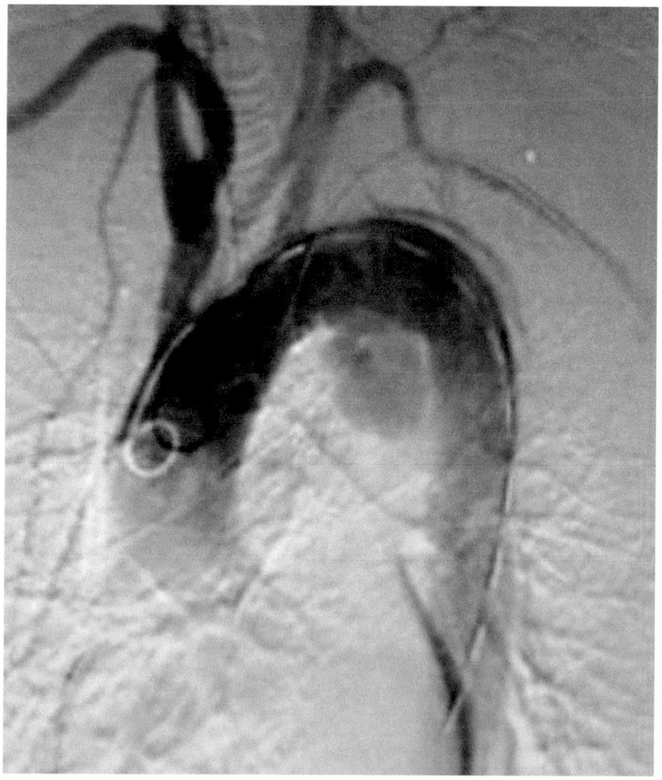

Fig. 19.1 Aortic arch angiography

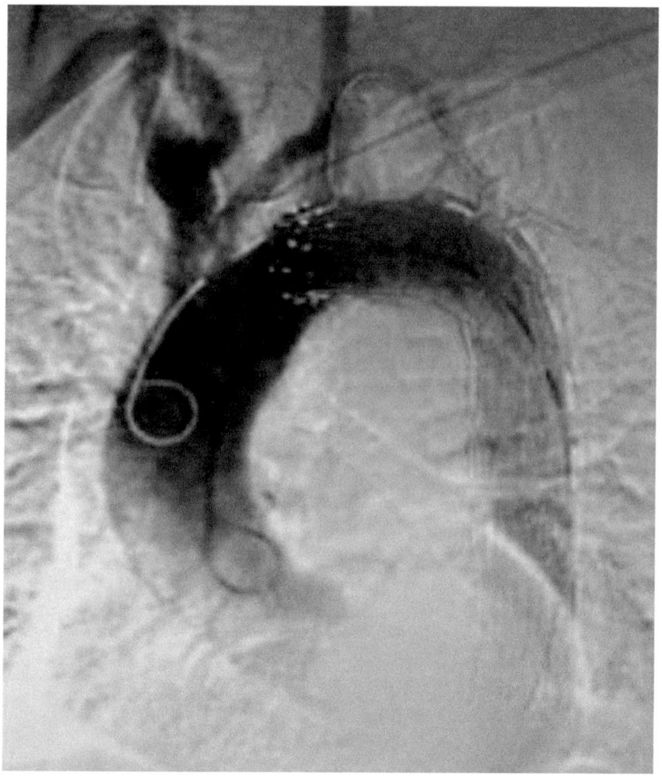

Fig. 19.2 Postoperative angiography

19.1.5 Technical Essentials and Precautions

- The aneurysm in this case is located at the lesser curvature of the aortic arch and near to the opening of the left subclavian artery. If the stent is deployed at the distal end of the left subclavian artery, it is prone to endoleak. Therefore, the surgeon adopts the chimney technique for the left subclavian artery.
- The aortic arch in this case is Type III arch; excessively short arch-crossing distance of the body stent will lead to increased stress of the stent and the aortic wall, thus increasing the risk of reverse tear at the proximal end of the aorta.
- The patient manifested recurrent laryngeal nerve compression symptoms, and the key to improve the symptoms is to promote aneurysm thrombosis during operation. Therefore an indwelling catheter can be placed in the aneurysm cavity for catheter-directed embolization treatment.

19.2 Case 2 Single-Branched Stent and Fenestration Technique for Treatment of Aortic Dissection

19.2.1 Patient Data

The female patient, aged 66, was diagnosed with aortic dissection in a physical examination in 2011 and was given conservative treatment. In April 2013, she felt a sudden onset of sharp back pain, accompanied by nausea and vomiting symptoms, and was diagnosed with aortic dissection acute tear by local hospital and was admitted for aortic dissection in May.

19.2.2 Surgical Operation

As shown by intraoperative angiography, the patient's aortic dissection was torn from the innominate artery to the left renal artery opening, and the proximal and distal ends of the aortic dissection are the "restricted area" for endovascular therapy. If TAA stent graft is used for exclusion of the aortic dissection, the innominate artery (brachiocephalic trunk), left common carotid artery, left subclavian artery, and visceral artery will be excluded together, causing ischemic complications. After repeated assessment, it intended to adopt "single-branched stent and fenestration" technique for endovascular repair of the aortic dissection. The subject gave informed consent for the procedure.

19.2.3 Device Preparation

Refer to Table 19.3.

19.2.4 Procedures and Intraoperative Coordination Process

Refer to Table 19.4.

Table 19.3 Device preparation

Name	Qty.	Name	Qty.
Puncture needle (Cook)	1	6F short sheath (Terumo)	2
High-pressure connector (SCW Medicath)	2	Self-expanding peripheral bare stent 10 mm × 60 mm (Optimed)	2
0.035 in. common hydrophilic wire 180 cm (Terumo)	1	Self-expanding peripheral bare stent 12 mm × 60 mm (Optimed)	1
0.035 in. common hydrophilic wire 260 cm (Terumo)	3	0.035 in. Lunderquist super-stiff wire 260 cm (Cook)	1
5F scaled pigtail catheter (Optimed)	1	Valiant TAA stent graft 30 mm × 200 mm (Medtronic)	1
5F MPA catheter 125 cm (Cordis)	1	Castor bifurcated fenestration-type TAA stent graft (MicroPort)	1
8F short sheath (Terumo)	1		

Note: The devices listed above (*A* mm × *B* mm), wherein *A* is the diameter of the device and *B* the length

Table 19.4 Procedures and intraoperative coordination process

Procedures	Intraoperative coordination process
1. Patient enters the operation room, general anesthesia	(1) Mental nursing; (2) keep the patient warm; (3) help to lie at supine position, with both lower and upper limbs slightly at abduction and extorsion position and turning the head right; (4) connect ECG to observe changes in blood pressure, heart rate, and oxygen saturation; (5) establish intravenous infusion; (6) place indwelling urinary catheter
2. Sterilize bilateral groins, two upper limbs, and left neck	Prepare disinfectant (heated to 98.6 °F with incubator), and assist with draping; deliver iodixanol injection; prepare heparin diluent (1000 mL normal saline +100 mg heparin sodium injection)
3. Cut a longitudinal incision of about 3 cm on the common femoral artery of the right groin, at the punctum maximum of the pulse, dissociate and expose the common femoral artery	Deliver the scalpels, large tweezers (flat tweezers or fine tweezers), separating pliers, mosquito pliers, vascular pliers, and 0# silk suture
4. Puncture right common femoral artery with modified Seldinger technique, insert a 0.035 in. common hydrophilic wire 180 cm and a 5F scaled pigtail catheter to the ascending aorta, withdraw the hydrophilic wire, and conduct angiography, showing that the proximal fissure of the dissection lies at the ascending aorta and involves the innominate artery, and the distal fissure lies at the descending aorta (Fig. 19.3). Measure the diameter and length of the aortic proximal end, distal end, and branch artery	Deliver the puncture needle, high-pressure connector, 0.035 in. common hydrophilic wire 180 cm, 5F scaled pigtail catheter; perform systematic heparinization; intraoperative endovascular devices should be flushed with the prepared heparin diluent
5. Puncture the left femoral artery with Seldinger technique under fluoroscopy, and insert a 6F short sheath and the first 0.035 in. common hydrophilic wire 260 cm; puncture the left carotid artery, and insert another 6F short sheath and the second 0.035 in. common hydrophilic wire 260 cm; puncture the right brachial artery, insert an 8F short sheath and the third 0.035 in. common hydrophilic wire 260 cm, insert a 5F MPA catheter 125 cm to the right common femoral artery along the third common hydrophilic wire, and pull out the catheter from the right common femoral artery; withdraw the third common hydrophilic wire	Deliver the puncture needle, two 6F short sheaths, a 8F short sheath, three 0.035 in. common hydrophilic wire 260 cm, and a 5F MPA catheter 125 cm
6. Lead out the branched wire on the delivery system of the Castor single-branch fenestrated thoracic aortic stent graft from within the 8F short sheath of the right brachial artery via the tip of the 5F MPA catheter 125 cm, withdraw the 5F MPA catheter 125 cm	Deliver the Castor single-branch fenestrated thoracic aortic stent graft
7. Implantation of Castor single-branch fenestrated thoracic aortic stent graft: insert a 0.035 in. Lunderquist super-stiff wire 260 cm to the ascending aorta via the right common femoral artery; implant the delivery system of the Castor stent graft (the stent proximal diameter is 44 mm, distal 28 mm, the diameter of the innominate artery branch stent is 14 mm, left common carotid artery and left subclavian artery are fenestrated) into the lesion site along the super-stiff wire, and deploy it; pull the branch wire of the right brachial artery; and deploy the branch stent to the innominate artery	Deliver the 0.035 in. Lunderquist super-stiff wire 260 cm

Table 19.4 (continued)

Procedures	Intraoperative coordination process
8. Implantation of fenestrated bare stent: implant one self-expanding peripheral bare stent 10 mm × 60 mm into the left subclavian artery and left common carotid artery, respectively, along the hydrophilic wire on the left brachial artery and the left carotid artery, respectively; implant the 0.035 in. common hydrophilic wire 260 cm to the right subclavian artery along the right brachial artery; insert one self-expanding peripheral bare stent 12 mm × 60 mm into the branch stent of the innominate artery along the hydrophilic wire	Deliver two self-expanding peripheral bare stents 10 mm × 60 mm and one self-expanding peripheral bare stent 12 mm × 60 mm
9. Implantation of Valiant thoracic aortic stent graft: withdraw the Castor single-branch fenestrated stent graft delivery system, insert a thoracic aortic stent graft 30 mm × 200 mm, and overlap it to the distal end of the Castor single-branch fenestrated stent graft before deployment	Deliver the Valiant thoracic aortic stent graft 30 mm × 200 mm
10. Withdraw the Valiant thoracic aortic stent graft delivery system, insert the 5F common pigtail catheter, and conduct ascending aorta angiography again, showing no endoleak at the proximal end of the aortic dissection and vascular patency of the branch arteries (Fig. 19.4)	Deliver the 5F scaled pigtail catheter
11. Withdraw the catheter, wire, and short sheath, suture the incision on the right common femoral artery, apply compression bandaging to the puncture sites on the bilateral brachial arteries and left carotid artery	Deliver the vascular plier and CV suture for vascular incision suturing; deliver small round and angled needles and 1# suture to suture the incision layer by layer; deliver gauze and elastic bandage for compression dressing on puncture site
12. Anesthesia completed	Safely escort the patient back to ward

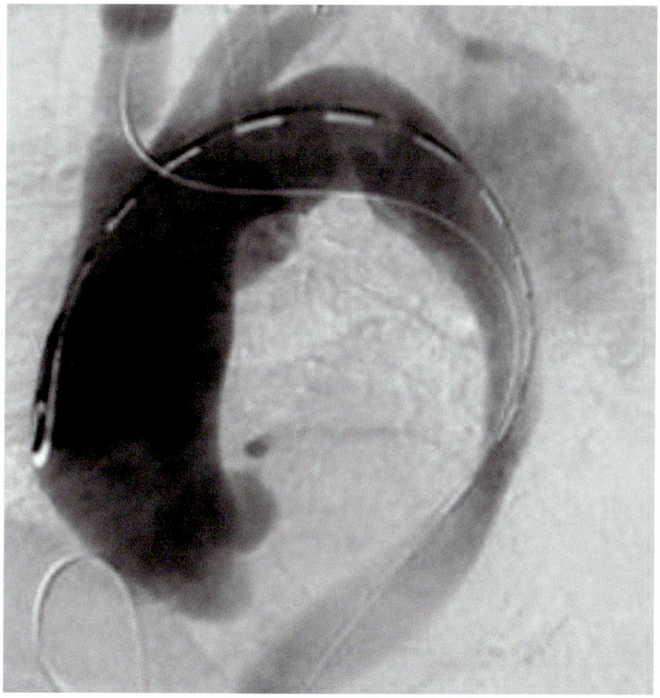

Fig. 19.3 Preoperative angiography

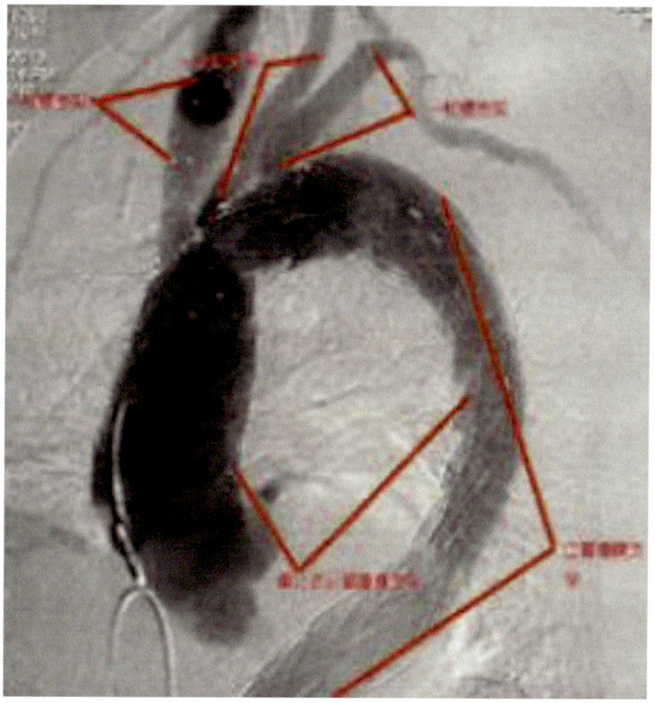

Fig. 19.4 Post-stent implantation angiography

19.2.5 Technical Essentials and Precautions

- The aortic dissection for the patient in this case is complex, and the "single-branched and fenestration" technique is an individually customized scheme. Preoperative CTA measurement and intraoperative accurate positioning are the key to ensure successful treatment, which can be assessed through Mark criteria and reduce the interference to stereotaxis by DSA 2D imaging.
- In this case, the aorta is Type III arch, and it is difficult to superselect brachiocephalic arteries by the branch artery wire, and if necessary, snare can be selected for coordination purpose. Because the cephalic trifurcated blood vessels are operated together, quick and highly efficient

deployment of the branched artery stent should be ensured so as to reduce the occurrence of cerebral infarction caused by cephalic ischemia [1].

19.3 Case 3 Double-Chimney + Guglialmi Detachable Coil Embolotherapy for Endovascular Aortic Aneurysm Repair

19.3.1 Patient Data

The female patient, aged 22, was found with pulmonary mass via X-ray examination in January 2014 in local hospital, showing no cough, chest tightness chest pain and other symptoms. In May 2015, chest radiography examination again indicated pulmonary mass, and in June, color Doppler and aortic CTA examination in other hospital showed presence of stenosis at the proximal segment of the descending aorta and multiple aneurysms at the descending part of the aortic arch. In July the patient was admitted for "thoracic aortic aneurysm."

19.3.2 Surgical Operation

According to the aortic CTA findings provided by the patient, "double chimney and Guglialmi detachable coil embolization" technique is used for endovascular repair of thoracic aortic aneurysm, that is, to implant TAA stent graft into the thoracic aortic lesion site and, at the same time, implant chimney stent into the subclavian artery and left common carotid artery. In case of any endoleak, Guglialmi detachable coil can be inserted to avoid the endoleak while ensuring vascular patency of branch arteries. The subject gave informed consent for the procedure.

19.3.3 Device Preparation

Refer to Table 19.5.

19.3.4 Procedures and Intraoperative Coordination Process

Refer to Table 19.6.

Table 19.5 Device preparation

Name	Qty.	Name	Qty.
Puncture needle (Cook)	1	5F Berenstein catheter (AngioDynamics)	1
High-pressure connector (SCW Medicath)	2	5F scaled pigtail catheter (Optimed)	1
0.035 in. common hydrophilic wire 260 cm (Terumo)	3	5F short sheath (Terumo)	3
2.2F microcatheter (Cook)	1	9F short sheath (Terumo)	1
0.018 in. microwire 180 cm (Cook)	1	Guide wire accessory kit (Abbott)	1 set
Fluency peripheral stent graft 8 mm × 60 mm (Bard)	1	Fluency peripheral stent graft 6 mm × 80 mm (Bard)	1
Fluency peripheral stent graft 6 mm × 100 mm (Bard)	1	Jasper Guglialmi detachable embolization 20 mm × 300 mm (Achieva Medical)	2
Endurant abdominal aortoiliac stent 16 mm × 28 mm × 120 mm (Medtronic)	1	Jasper standard Guglialmi detachable controller (Achieva Medical)	1 set
Endurant abdominal aortoiliac stent 16 mm × 24 mm × 120 mm (Medtronic)	1	Jasper standard electrode wire (Achieva Medical)	1

Note: The devices listed above (*A* mm × *B* mm), wherein *A* is the diameter of the device, *B* the length; abdominal aortoiliac stent (*A* mm × *B* mm × *C* mm), wherein *A* is the proximal diameter of the stent, *B* the distal diameter, and *C* its length

Table 19.6 Procedures and intraoperative coordination process

Procedures	Intraoperative coordination process
1. Patient enters the operation room, general anesthesia	(1) Mental nursing; (2) keep the patient warm; (3) help to lie at supine position, with lower limbs slightly at abduction and extorsion position and upper limbs at abduction position and turning the head right; (4) connect ECG to observe changes in blood pressure, heart rate, and oxygen saturation; (5) establish intravenous infusion; (6) place indwelling urinary catheter
2. Sterilize bilateral groins, bilateral upper limbs, and left neck	Prepare disinfectant (heated to 98.6 °F with incubator), and assist with draping; deliver iodixanol injection; prepare heparin diluent (1000 mL normal saline +100 mg heparin sodium injection)
3. Cut a longitudinal incision of about 3 cm on the common femoral artery of the left groin, at the punctum maximum of the pulse, dissociate and expose the common femoral artery	Deliver the scalpels, large tweezers (flat tweezers or fine tweezers), separating pliers, mosquito pliers, vascular pliers, and 0# silk suture
4. Puncture the left common femoral artery, left brachial artery, and right brachial artery with modified Seldinger technique, and insert 5F short sheath, respectively; meanwhile, puncture the left carotid artery, and insert a 9F short sheath	Deliver three 5F short sheath and one 9F short sheath; systematic heparinization; intraoperative endovascular devices should be flushed with the prepared heparin diluent

Table 19.6 (continued)

Procedures	Intraoperative coordination process
5. Advance a 0.035 in. common hydrophilic wire 260 cm and a 5F scaled pigtail catheter to the ascending aorta along the 5F short sheath of the left common femoral artery, withdraw the hydrophilic wire, and conduct angiography, showing thoracic aortic aneurysm complicated with stenosis at the beginning segment of the descending aorta (Fig. 19.5)	Deliver 260 cm 0.035 in. common hydrophilic wire and 5F scaled common pigtail catheter
6. Advance from the right brachial artery a 0.035 in. common hydrophilic wire 260 cm and a 5F Berenstein catheter to establish the stretching wire with the left common femoral artery, and retain the 5F Berenstein catheter in the aneurysm cavity; advance the 0.035 in. common hydrophilic wire 260 cm to the ascending aorta via the left carotid artery; advance the 0.035 in. common hydrophilic wire 260 cm to the abdominal aorta via the left brachial artery	Deliver two 0.035 in. common hydrophilic wires 260 cm and one 5F Berenstein catheter
7. Reverse the placement of the abdominal aortoiliac stent: reversely place an Endurant stent 28 mm × 16 mm × 120 mm after in vitro deployment, use the suture to compress the Endurant stent, and remount it into the delivery system	Deliver the Endurant abdominal aortoiliac stent 16 mm × 28 mm × 120 mm
8. Implantation of abdominal aortoiliac stent (1): implant a reversely placed Endurant stent 28 mm × 16 mm × 120 mm into the thoracic aortic aneurysm segment along the stretching wire of the left common femoral artery; meanwhile, implant the Fluency peripheral stent graft 8 mm × 60 mm into the left common carotid artery along the hydrophilic wire; upon completion of stent positioning, first deploy the Endurant stent and then the Fluency stent graft; withdraw Endurant stent delivery system and Fluency stent graft delivery system	Deliver the Fluency peripheral stent graft 8 mm × 60 mm
9. Implantation of abdominal aortoiliac stent (2): implant an Endurant stent 16 mm × 24 mm × 120 mm into the distal end of the previous Endurant stent 28 mm × 16 mm × 120 mm along the stretching wire, and deploy it; meanwhile, implant a Fluency peripheral stent graft 6 mm × 80 mm and a Fluency peripheral stent graft 6 mm × 100 mm into the subclavian artery along the hydrophilic wire of the left brachial artery, and form the artery "periscope" of the left subclavian artery	Deliver the Endurant abdominal aortoiliac stent 16 mm × 24 mm × 120 mm, Fluency peripheral stent graft 6 mm × 80 mm, and Fluency peripheral stent graft 6 mm × 100 mm
10. Withdraw the Endurant stent delivery system, insert the 5F scaled pigtail catheter, and conduct ascending aorta angiography again, showing endoleak at the proximal end of the thoracic aortic aneurysm	
11. Implantation of Guglialmi detachable coil: implant a 2.2F microcatheter and 0.018 in. microwire 180 cm into the endoleak site along the 5F Berenstein catheter pre-retained in the aneurysm cavity, withdraw the microwire, connect a Y valve at the end of the microcatheter, connect the side hole of the Y valve with high-pressure drip; connect a guide sheath of the Jasper Guglialmi detachable coil 20 mm × 300 mm straightly with the Y valve and the tip of the microcatheter, tighten the Y valve, and withdraw the locking sheath; advance the delivery wire of the coil, loosen the Y valve, withdraw the guide sheath, and advance the Jasper coil to the endoleak site along the microcatheter under fluoroscopy	Connect pressure transfusion unit; deliver the 0.018 in. microwire, 2.2F microcatheter, guide wire accessory kit, Guglialmi detachable coil 20 mm × 300 mm; self-check Guglialmi detachable controller in advance (press the switch button, showing 9.8–11.2 mV voltage, current flashes three times and shows 1 mA, and returns to 0 mA 10 s later
12. Connection of electrode wire: puncture into the subcutaneous muscle of the inguinal puncture site on the left common femoral artery with a 20# stainless steel needle, clap the stainless steel needle with one end of the hook of the red electrode wire, and connect the other end with the positive pole of the Guglialmi detachable controller	Deliver the standard Jasper electrode wire
13. Electrolytic detachment of coil: start the Guglialmi detachable controller under DSA fluoroscopy, and perform electrolytic detachment twice (30 s for each detachment at 0.3–0.5 mA current and 3–6 mA voltage); confirm if the coil is electrolytically detached, and slowly withdraw the delivery wire of the coil; implant again one Jasper Guglialmi detachable coil 20 mm × 300 mm to the endoleak site following the above procedures	Deliver the Jasper Guglialmi detachable coil 20 mm × 300 mm
14. Again connect the tip of the 5F scaled pigtail catheter to the high-pressure syringe, and conduct ascending aorta angiography, showing thoracic aortic aneurysm has to be excluded and no obvious endoleak presents and the superior arch trifurcated artery blood flows smoothly (Fig. 19.6)	
15. Withdraw the microcatheter, catheter, wire, and vascular sheath, suture the incision of the left common femoral artery, apply compression bandaging on the puncture sites of the bilateral brachial arteries and left carotid artery	Deliver the vascular plier and CV suture for vascular incision suturing; deliver the small round and angled needles and 1# suture to suture the incision layer by layer; deliver gauze and elastic bandage for compression dressing on puncture site
16. Anesthesia completed	Safely escort the patient back to ward

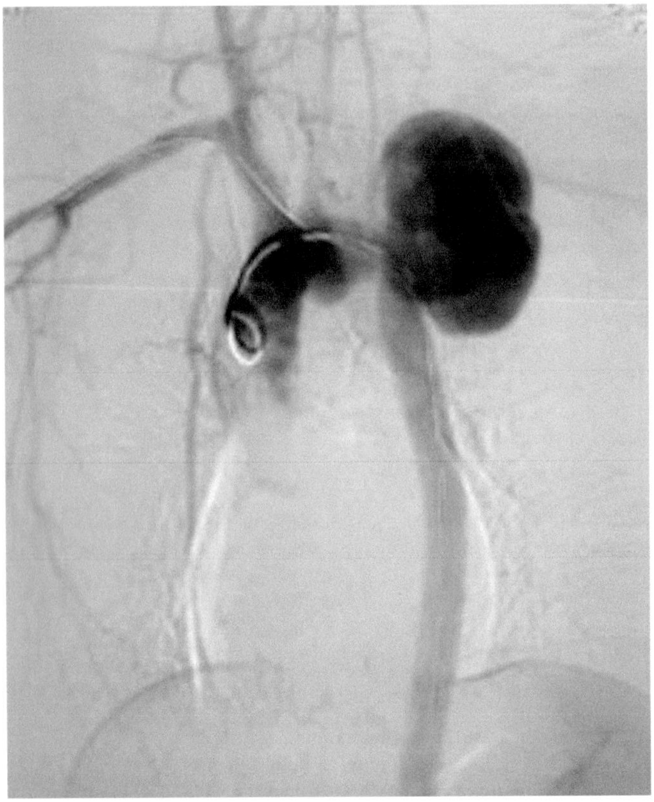

Fig. 19.5 Preoperative angiography

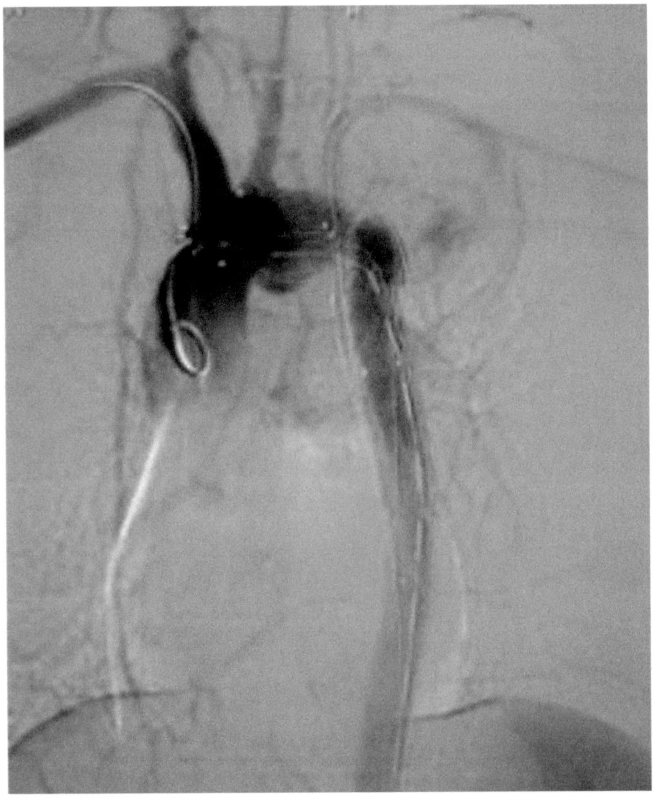

Fig. 19.6 Postoperative angiography

19.3.5 Technical Essentials and Precautions

- The patient also presents himself/herself with descending aortic stenosis, and due to the problem of profile matching, it is difficult to achieve excellent proximal and distal anchoring at the same time, because the narrowest part of the stenosis is only 14 mm. It is very difficult to adopt traditional endovascular therapies, so overlapping deployment of two abdominal aortoiliac stents (one is reversely placed) is carried out to the proximal and the distal end, so as to ensure excellent anchoring to both the proximal and the distal end and ultimately achieve complete exclusion. The highlight in this case is the flexible reverse placement of the abdominal aortoiliac stent during operation [1–3].
- There is a high risk of endoleak in the giant tumor cavity of the patient, the use of spring coil embolization can increase the probability of complete exclusion and reduce the risk of postoperative rupture, but it needs to retain a catheter in advance in the tumor cavity prior to the deployment of the body stent. During operation, it requires for close observation of the lower limb blood pressure so as to avoid occurrence of poor perfusion at the distal end of the aortic stenotic segment, resulting in paraplegia, lower limb ischemia, abdominal organ ischemia, and other complications [4].
- The operation uses left subclavian artery "periscope" technique for revascularization, but attention should be paid to the oversize relationship between the branch artery stent graft and the body stent graft and influence among different stent materials so as to avoid occurrence of branch artery occlusion.

19.4 Case 4 Cuff Graft Technique for Endovascular Repair of Ascending Aortic Dissection Artery Aneurysm

19.4.1 Patient Data

The female patient, aged 68, presented herself with sudden severe tear-like chest pain in November 2015 and was CT examined in local hospital, indicating "ascending aortic dissection aneurysm" (Fig. 19.7). The patient still showed poor therapeutic effect after conservative treatment, with intermittent attack of chest pain. And in December, the patient was admitted for "ascending aortic dissection aneurysm."

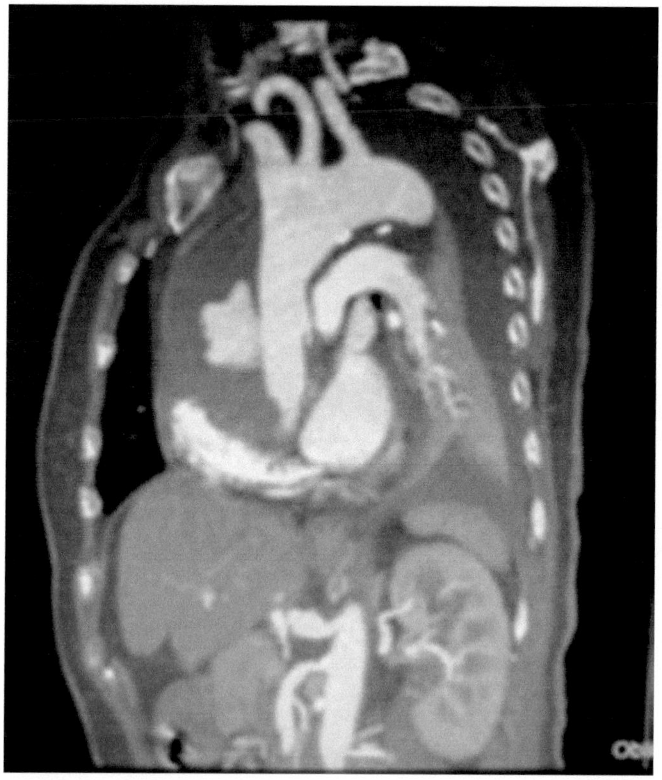

Fig. 19.7 Preoperative CT

19.4.2 Surgical Operation

Because the ascending aorta of the patient is very close to the heart, heart beat and blood pumping will affect the positioning of TAA stent graft. Therefore, it intended to use temporary pacemaker in placing the cuff so as to pace the heart rate to 180/200 beats per minute and reduce the cardiac output to the lowest level and ensure accurate placement of the cuff. The subject gave informed consent for the procedure.

19.4.3 Device Preparation

Refer to Table 19.7.

19.4.4 Procedures and Intraoperative Coordination Process

Refer to Table 19.8.

Table 19.7 Device preparation

Name	Qty.	Name	Qty.
Puncture needle (Cook)	1	5F Berenstein catheter (AngioDynamics)	1
High-pressure connector (SCW Medicath)	2	6F short sheath (Terumo)	1
0.035 in. common hydrophilic wire 260 cm (Terumo)	2	5F scaled pigtail catheter (Optimed)	1
0.035 in. Lunderquist super-stiff wire 260 cm (Cook)	1	Temporary pacing electrode catheter (St. Jude)	1
Cuff 42 mm × 81 mm (Cook)	1	Temporary pacemaker (Biotronik)	1

Note: The devices listed above (*A* mm × *B* mm), wherein *A* is the diameter of the device and *B* its length

Table 19.8 Procedures and intraoperative coordination process

Procedures	Intraoperative coordination process
1. Patient enters the operation room, general anesthesia	(1) Mental nursing; (2) keep the patient warm; (3) help to lie at supine position, with two lower limbs slightly at abduction and extorsion position; (4) connect ECG to observe changes in blood pressure, heart rate, and oxygen saturation; (5) establish intravenous infusion and place indwelling central venous catheter; (6) place indwelling urinary catheter
2. Routinely sterilize bilateral groins up to the navel and down to the middle of the leg, expose the groin	Prepare disinfectant (heated to 98.6 °F in incubator), and assist with draping; deliver iodixanol injection; prepare heparin diluent (1000 mL normal saline +100 mg heparin sodium injection)
3. Cut a longitudinal incision of about 3 cm on the common femoral artery of the right groin, at the punctum maximum of the pulse, dissociate and expose the common femoral artery	Deliver the scalpels, large tweezers (flat tweezers or fine tweezers), separating pliers, mosquito pliers, vascular pliers, and #0 silk suture
4. Puncture the left femoral vein with Seldinger technique under fluoroscopy, insert a 6F short sheath and a 0.035 in. common hydrophilic wire 260 cm, insert a temporary pacing electrode catheter to the right ventricle along the hydrophilic wire, withdraw the hydrophilic wire, and connect the temporary pacemaker	Deliver the 6F short sheath, 0.035 in. common hydrophilic wire 260 cm, and temporary pacing electrode catheter, connect the pacemaker and pacing electrode catheter, check if the parameters and functions of the temporary pacemaker are normal

(continued)

Table 19.8 (continued)

Procedures	Intraoperative coordination process
5. Puncture the right common femoral artery with a modified Seldinger technique, insert a 0.035 in. common hydrophilic wire 260 cm and a 5F scaled pigtail catheter to the ascending aorta, withdraw the hydrophilic wire, and conduct angiography, showing ascending aortic dissection aneurysm (Fig. 19.8)	Deliver the puncture needle, high-pressure connector, 0.035 in. common hydrophilic wire 260 cm, 5F scaled pigtail catheter; perform systematic heparinization; intraoperative endovascular devices should be flushed with the prepared heparin diluent
6. Shape a straight-tip 0.035 in. Lunderquist super-stiff wire 260 cm, and then insert it to the distal end of ascending aorta along the 5F scaled pigtail catheter; withdraw the catheter	Deliver the 0.035 in. Lunderquist super-stiff wire 260 cm
7. Cuff implantation: insert a cuff 42 mm × 81 mm into the ascending aortic lesion site along the shaped 0.035 in. Lunderquist super-stiff wire 260 cm, and position it; when artificially paced heart rate reaches 180–200 beats per minute, deploy the cuff 42 mm × 81 mm	Deliver the cuff 42 mm × 81 mm; start or stop pacing; and adjust pacing frequency according to the physician's instructions
8. Withdraw the cuff delivery system, again insert the 5F scaled pigtail catheter along the super-stiff wire to the ascending aorta, withdraw the super-stiff wire, and conduct angiography, showing the ascending aortic dissection aneurysm has been completely excluded, without endoleak (Fig. 19.9)	Deliver the 5F scaled pigtail catheter
9. Withdraw the 5F scaled pigtail catheter, 6F short sheath, and temporary pacing electrode catheter, and suture the incision on the right common femoral artery; apply compression bandaging on the puncture site of the left femoral vein	Deliver the vascular plier and CV suture for vascular incision suturing; deliver small round and angled needles and 1# suture to suture the incision layer by layer; deliver gauze and elastic bandage for compression dressing on puncture site
10. Anesthesia completed	Safely escort the patient back to ward

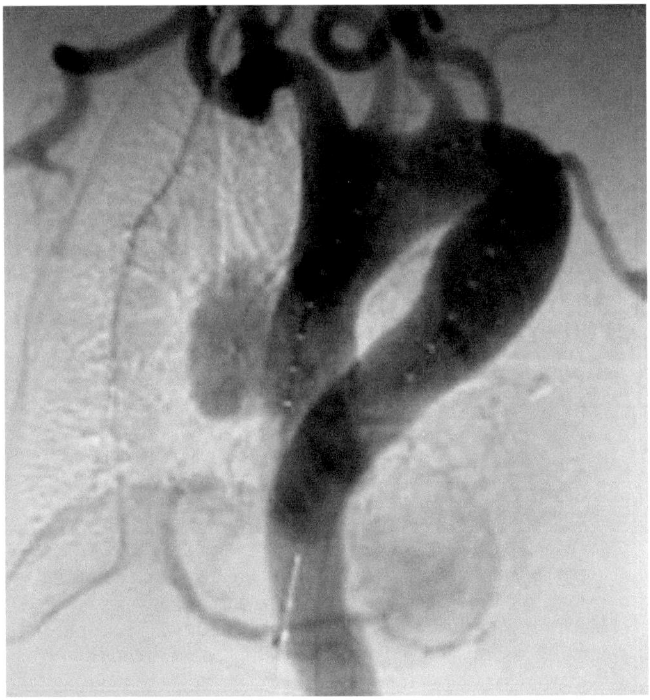

Fig. 19.8 Intraoperative angiography

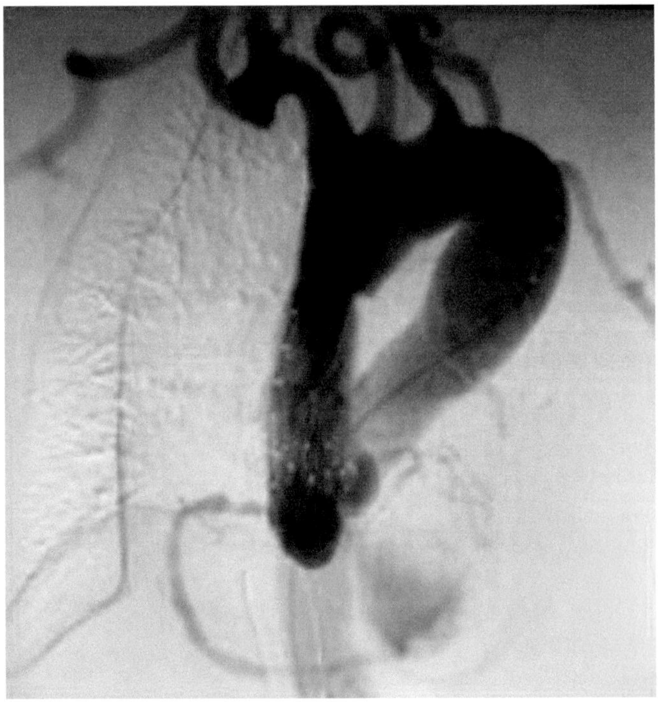

Fig. 19.9 Postoperative angiography

19.4.5 Technical Essentials and Precautions

- In this operation, the conical tips of the catheter, wire, and delivery system need to access into the left ventricle. Therefore, attention should be paid to prevent the occurrence of malignant arrhythmia, and so it is necessary to retain in advance a temporary pacemaker in the common femoral veins, which ensures quick cardioversion in the event of malignant arrhythmia. The placement accuracy of the TAA stent graft is closely related to whether quick cardiac pacing can effectively reduce cardiac output or not. Before actual deployment, rapid ventricular rate should be simulated before actual deployment so as to ensure matching accuracy and efficiency and reduce stent displacement and other complications due to heart beat.

- Before operation in this case, the position relation between the dissection fissure and the coronary opening should be carefully evaluated. The operation in this case for lesions with fissure being too close to the coronary opening should be selected carefully so as to avoid the occurrence of coronary opening occlusion and other malignant complications during the operation.
- The cuff 42 × 81 mm (Cook) used in this case features short length, high profile, and excellent performance of the delivery system crossing the aortic arch. Therefore, this device is used in this operation.

19.5 Case 5 Balloon Occlusion and Endovascular Accelerated Blood Coagulation Technique for Ruptured Abdominal Aortic Aneurysm Repair

19.5.1 Patient Data

The female patient, aged 83, was given conservative treatment for "right limb asthenia" at local hospital and presented with left lower abdominal pain without obvious cause in the evening on July 18, 2016, which was ignored. But in the next morning, abdominal pain still existed, and no improvement was shown after purgative treatment. In the evening of July 19, abdominal pain aggravated, and abdominal CT suggested "abdominal aortic aneurysm" (Fig. 19.10), and the patient was admitted for "abdominal aortic aneurysm rupture."

19.5.2 Surgical Operation

According to the clinical manifestations and abdominal CT imaging of the patient, it was clear that the abdominal aortic aneurysm has been ruptured. Considering that the patient presented with acute bleeding due to giant abdominal aortic aneurysm rupture and was older and in general has poor condition, so the patient could not tolerate open surgery. It intended to conduct endovascular aneurysm repair by "balloon occlusion and intracavitary coagulation" technique with general anesthesia under emergency treatment. The subject gave informed consent for the procedure.

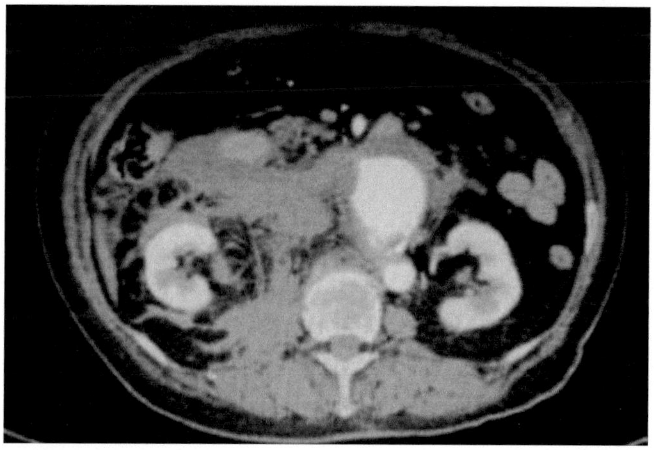

Fig. 19.10 Preoperative abdominal CT

Table 19.9 Device preparation

Name	Qty.	Name	Qty.
Puncture needle (Cook)	1	5F scaled pigtail catheter (Optimed)	1
High-pressure connector (SCW Medicath)	2	5F Berenstein catheter (AngioDynamics)	2
0.035 in. common hydrophilic wire 260 cm	1	0.035 in. Lunderquist super-stiff wire 260 cm (Cook)	2
Endurant abdominal aortic body stent 25 mm × 13 mm × 170 mm (Medtronic)	1	Coda balloon catheter (Cook)	1
Endurant abdominal aortoiliac stent 16 mm × 13 mm × 95 mm (Medtronic)	2	Fibrin Sealant, Human (RAAS)	3

Note: The devices listed above (*A* mm × *B* mm), wherein *A* is the diameter of the device and *B* the length; abdominal aortic body (aortoiliac) stent (*A* mm × *B* mm × *C* mm), wherein *A* is the diameter of the proximal end of the stent, *B* the distal end, and *C* its length

19.5.3 Device Preparation

Refer to Table 19.9.

19.5.4 Procedures and Intraoperative Coordination Process

Refer to Table 19.10.

Table 19.10 Procedures and intraoperative coordination process

Procedures	Intraoperative coordination process
1. Patient enters the operation room, local anesthesia, prepared for general anesthesia	(1) Mental nursing; (2) keep the patient warm; (3) help to lie at supine position, with two lower limbs slightly at abduction and extorsion position; (4) connect ECG to observe changes in blood pressure, heart rate, and oxygen saturation; (5) establish intravenous infusion; (6) place indwelling urinary catheter
2. Routinely sterilize the bilateral groins from the umbilical down to the midthigh, exposing the groins	Prepare disinfectant (heated to 98.6 °F in incubator), and assist with draping; deliver Iodixanol injection; prepare heparin diluent (1000 mL normal saline +100 mg heparin sodium injection)
3. The "balloon occlusion" technique: cut a longitudinal incision of about 3 cm on the right common femoral artery under local anesthesia, at the punctum maximum of the pulse; dissociate and expose the right common femoral artery: puncture the right common femoral artery and insert a 0.035 in. Lunderquist super-stiff wire 260 cm, insert a Coda balloon catheter to the arterial level of the superior mesentery of the abdominal aorta along the super-stiff wire, inflate the balloon, and block the proximal blood flow of the abdominal aortic aneurysm	Deliver the puncture needle, Coda balloon catheter, 0.035 in. Lunderquist super-stiff wire 260 cm, scalpels, large tweezers (flat tweezers or fine tweezers), separating pliers, mosquito pliers, vascular pliers, and 0# silk suture
4. Cut a longitudinal incision of about 3 cm on the left common femoral artery under local anesthesia, at the punctum maximum of the pulse, dissociate and expose the left common femoral artery	Deliver the scalpels, large tweezers (flat tweezers or fine tweezers), separating pliers, mosquito pliers, vascular pliers, and 0# silk suture; prepare three vials of Fibrin Sealant (Human) in advance
5. Wait till the blood pressure gets stable, puncture the left common femoral artery with modified Seldinger technique, insert a 0.035 in. common hydrophilic wire 260 cm, insert a 5F scaled pigtail catheter along the hydrophilic wire, withdraw the wire, loosen the occlusive balloon, insert the pigtail catheter into the renal artery level, and conduct quick angiography, showing proximal rupture of the abdominal aortic aneurysm (Fig. 19.11)	Deliver the puncture needle, high-pressure connector, 0.035 in. common hydrophilic wire 260 cm, 5F scaled pigtail catheter; perform systematic heparinization; intraoperative endovascular devices should be flushed with the prepared heparin diluent
6. Rapidly withdraw the occlusive balloon on the right common femoral artery; rapidly insert the abdominal aortic body stent; insert an Endurant abdominal aortic main body stent 25 mm × 13 mm × 170 mm to the abdominal aortic lesion site, and deploy it along the 0.035 in. Lunderquist super-stiff wire 260 cm; withdraw the abdominal aortic main body stent delivery system; insert the Coda balloon to the proximal end of the abdominal aortic main body stent along the super-stiff wire on the right common femoral artery; conduct balloon occlusion again	Deliver the 0.035 in. Lunderquist super-stiff wire 260 cm and Endurant abdominal aortic main body stent 25 mm × 13 mm × 170 mm
7. Withdraw the 5F scaled pigtail catheter, exchange to insert a 5F Berenstein catheter, and retain it in advance in the aneurysm cavity; puncture via the left common femoral artery (not at the same position as the previous puncture site of the left common femoral artery), and insert the 260 cm 0.035 in. common hydrophilic wire and 5F Berenstein catheter; superselect with matched wire and catheter to insert into the short leg of the abdominal aortic main body stent; exchange to insert a 0.035 in. Lunderquist super-stiff wire 260 cm; adequately loosen the occlusive balloon; insert the super-stiff wire to a level above coeliac trunk; rapidly implant two Endurant abdominal aortoiliac stents 16 mm × 13 mm × 95 mm to the short leg of the abdominal aortic main body stent, and deploy it so as to reach distal end to left external iliac level; withdraw the Endurant abdominal aortoiliac stent delivery system; and conduct balloon occlusion to the proximal end of the abdominal aorta	Deliver the 5F Berenstein catheter, 0.035 in. Lunderquist super-stiff wire 260 cm and two Endurant abdominal aortoiliac stents 16 mm × 13 mm × 95 mm
8. Insert a 5F scaled pigtail catheter to the abdominal aorta via the left 0.035 in. Lunderquist super-stiff wire 260 cm, retract the occlusive balloon, and conduct abdominal aortic angiography, showing incomplete exclusion of the abdominal aortic aneurysm, present with proximal endoleak and m-type endoleak	Deliver the 5F scaled pigtail catheter
9. Inflate the Coda balloon catheter again, inject the fibrin sealants (human) into the aneurysm cavity via the retained 5F Berenstein catheter with the help of the balloon occlusion	Deliver three fibrin sealants (human)
10. Withdraw the occlusive balloon, and conduct abdominal aortic angiography via the 5F scaled pigtail catheter again, showing complete exclusion of the abdominal aortic aneurysm, present with no endoleak (Fig. 19.12)	Deliver the 5F scaled pigtail catheter
11. Withdraw the catheter and wire, and suture the incisions on the bilateral common femoral arteries	Deliver the vascular plier and CV suture for vascular incision suturing; deliver the small round and angled needle and 1# suture to suture the incision layer by layer; deliver the gauze and elastic bandage; and assist with dressing
12. Anesthesia completed	Safely escort the patient back to ward

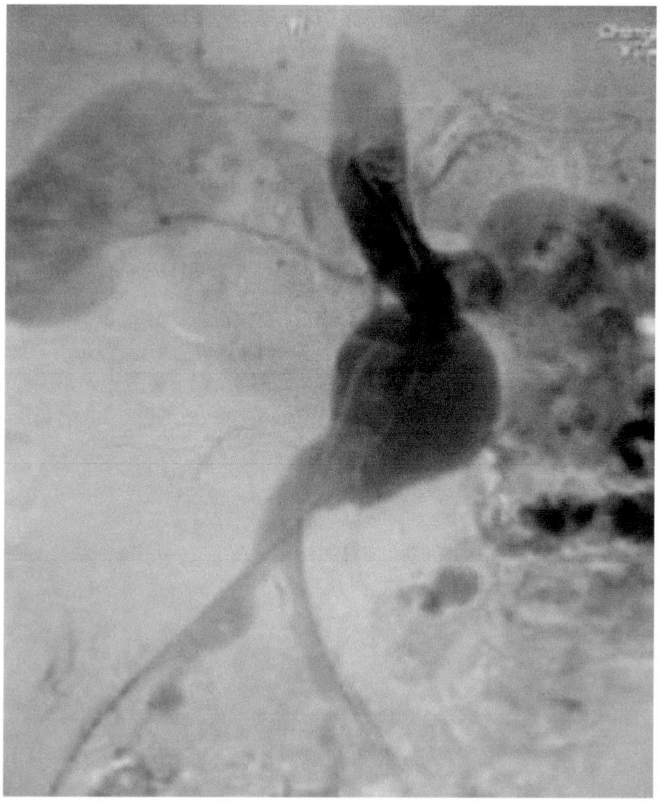

Fig. 19.11 Intraoperative angiography

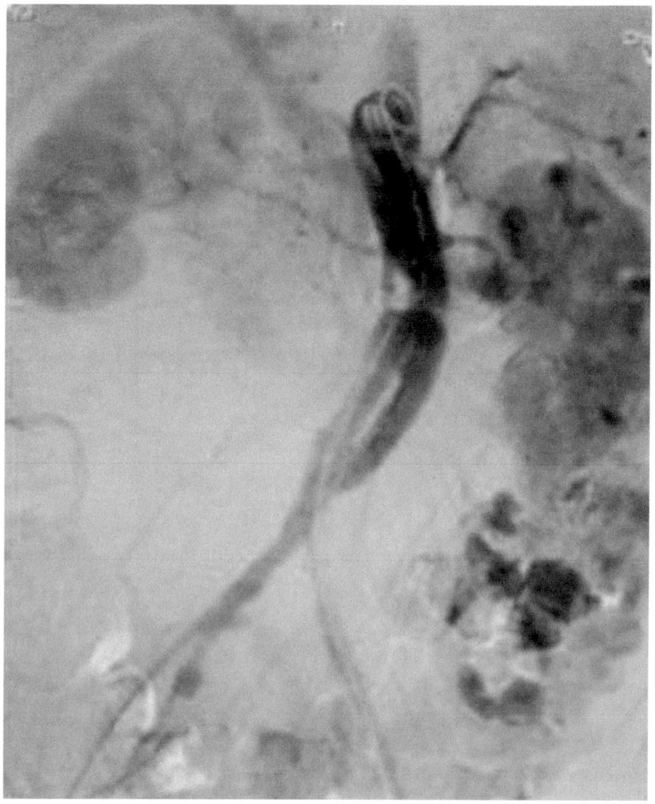

Fig. 19.12 Postoperative angiography

19.5.5 Technical Essentials and Precautions

- The patient in this case was of old age and presented with acute aneurysm rupture and bleeding. Due to the significant influence to the circulation by general anesthesia, the unilateral common femoral artery was cut open under local anesthesia before the operation, and after bleeding was stopped by inflated balloon, general anesthesia was conducted, and then endovascular aneurysm repair was performed.
- The patient presented with a huge abdominal aortic aneurysm. Considering possible endoleak after endovascular aneurysm repair, a catheter was retained in the AAA cavity upon completion of the first angiography, for the purpose of injection of Fibrin Sealant (Human). To accelerate coagulation in the aneurysm cavity and to avoid the access of Fibrin Sealant (Human) into major branch arteries, the proximal abdominal aorta should be occluded during injection.
- In this case, the balloon occlusion technique was used throughout the operation, but the following key points should be noticed during operation:
- (1) In conducting angiography, the occlusive balloon should be retracted; otherwise, the radiocontrast will refuse to flow, resulting in angiography missing.
- (2) AAA stent graft deployment is not allowed when the occlusive balloon operates; otherwise, the balloon cannot be retracted later on, and therefore, the stent should be kept away from the balloon.
- (3) Similar to conventional AAA repair, but act quickly to avoid aggravated bleeding and try to reduce the occurrence of endoleak.

19.6 Case 6 Sandwich Technique for Endovascular Repair of Abdominal Aortic Aneurysm with Iliac Artery Aneurysm

19.6.1 Patient Data

The male patient, aged 75, was found with abdominal aortic aneurysm in physical examination in April 2013, and abdominal aortic CTA showed "abdominal aortic aneurysm accompanied with bilateral internal iliac aneurysm" (Fig. 19.13), and he was admitted to the hospital in May.

19.6.2 Surgical Operation

As shown by the abdominal aorta CTA, the abdominal aortic aneurysm of the patient has been involved in bilateral internal iliac artery. If the AAA stent graft was directly covered onto the external iliac artery, it could achieve the purpose of aneurysm exclusion, but it would lead to inter-

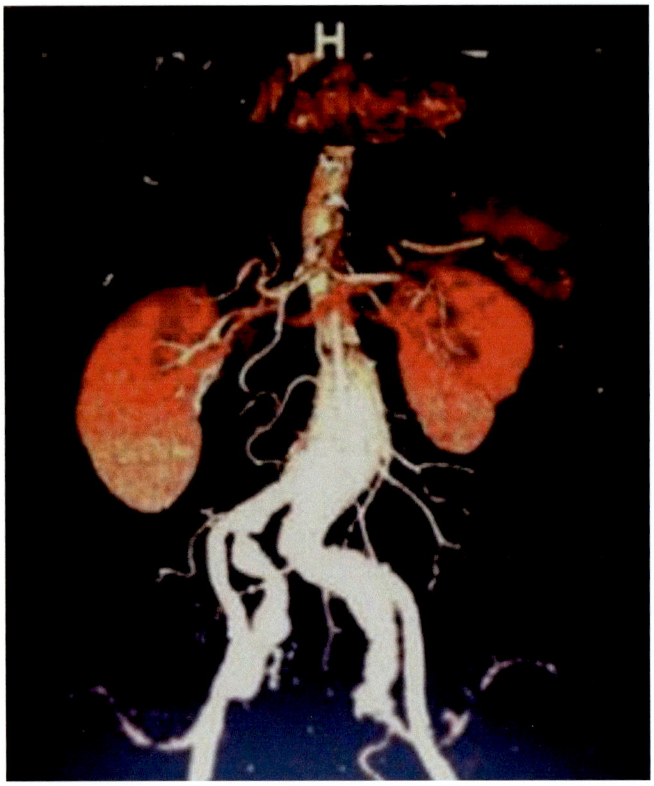

Fig. 19.13 Preoperative CTA

nal iliac artery occlusion and pelvic ischemia, resulting in gluteus limping, sexual dysfunction, and even tissue necrosis and other risks. In order to completely exclude the aneurysm and maintain the flow patency of the patient's internal iliac artery and considering the old age of the patient, it intended to use the sandwich technique to retain the left internal iliac artery (insert abdominal aortic body stent via the right common femoral artery, insert two peripheral stent grafts inside the distal end of the left abdominal aortoiliac stent, one of which being deployed outside the left iliac artery and one inside). And the right internal iliac artery was treated with spring coil embolization. The subject gave informed consent for the procedure.

19.6.3 Device Preparation

Refer to Table 19.11.

19.6.4 Procedures and Intraoperative Coordination Process

Refer to Table 19.12.

Table 19.11 Device preparation

Name	Qty.	Name	Qty.
Puncture needle (Cook)	1	5F scaled pigtail catheter (Optimed)	1
High-pressure connector (SCW Medicath)	2	5F Berenstein catheter (AngioDynamics)	1
0.035 in. common hydrophilic wire 260 cm (Terumo)	1	5F short sheath (Terumo)	2
0.035 in. hardened hydrophilic wire 260 cm (Terumo)	1	12F short sheath (Cook)	1
0.035 in. Lunderquist super-stiff wire 260 cm (Cook)	2	Viabahn peripheral stent graft 13 mm × 100 mm (Gore)	2
Coda balloon catheter (Cook)	1	Embolization 12 mm × 50 mm (Cook)	1
18F DrySeal vascular sheath (Gore)	1	Embolization 10 mm × 80 mm (Cook)	3
12F DrySeal vascular sheath (Gore)	1	Embolization 8 mm × 50 mm (Cook)	1
Excluder abdominal aortic body stent 23 mm × 12 mm × 180 mm (Gore)	1	Excluder abdominal aortoiliac stent 16 mm × 14 mm × 140 mm (Gore)	1

Note: The devices listed above (*A* mm × *B* mm), wherein *A* is the diameter of the device and *B* the length; abdominal aortic body (aortoiliac) stent (*A* mm × *B* mm × *C* mm),
wherein *A* is the diameter of the proximal end of the stent, *B* the distal end, and *C* the length

Table 19.12 Procedures and intraoperative coordination process

Procedures	Intraoperative coordination process
1. Patient enters the operation room, general anesthesia	(1) Mental nursing; (2) keep the patient warm; (3) help to lie at supine position, with two lower limbs slightly at abduction and extorsion position and the left upper limb stretching at abduction position; (4) connect ECG to observe changes in blood pressure, heart rate, and oxygen saturation; (5) establish intravenous infusion; (6) place indwelling urinary catheter
2. Sterilize bilateral groins and the left upper limb	Prepare disinfectant (heated to 98.6 °F in incubator), and assist with draping; deliver iodixanol injection; prepare heparin diluent (1000 mL normal saline +100 mg heparin sodium injection)

Table 19.12 (continued)

Procedures	Intraoperative coordination process
3. Cut a longitudinal incision of about 3 cm on bilateral common femoral arteries and the left brachial artery, at the punctum maximum of the pulse, dissociate and expose bilateral common femoral arteries and the left brachial artery	Deliver the scalpels, large tweezers (flat tweezers or fine tweezers), separating pliers, mosquito pliers, vascular pliers, and 0# silk suture
4. Puncture the right common femoral artery with modified Seldinger technique, insert a 5F short sheath and 0.035 in. common hydrophilic wire 260 cm, and insert a 5F scaled pigtail catheter along the hydrophilic wire, position the catheter tip at the 12th lumbar level, withdraw the hydrophilic wire, and conduct abdominal aortic angiography, showing abdominal aortic aneurysm accompanied with bilateral internal iliac aneurysm	Deliver the puncture needle, high-pressure connector, 0.035 in. common hydrophilic wire 260 cm, and 5F scaled pigtail catheter; perform systematic heparinization; intraoperative endovascular devices should be flushed with the prepared heparin diluent
5. Puncture the left common femoral artery with modified Seldinger technique; insert a 5F short sheath, 0.035 in. common hydrophilic wire 260 cm, and a 5F Berenstein catheter; superselect the hydrophilic wire in combination with the Berenstein catheter to access into the right iliac artery; withdraw the hydrophilic wire	Deliver the 5F short sheath, 0.035 in. common hydrophilic wire 180 cm, and 5F Berenstein catheter
6. Implantation of spring coil: insert five embolization inside the right internal iliac artery along the Berenstein catheter in sequence, manually push the 5F Berenstein catheter, and conduct angiography, showing no image of the distal end of the right internal artery	Deliver one embolization 12 mm × 50 mm, three embolizations 10 mm × 80 mm, and one embolization 8 mm × 50 mm
7. Implantation of abdominal aortic split-type stent: exchange to insert an 18F DrySeal vascular sheath and a 0.035 in. Lunderquist super-stiff wire 260 cm via the right common femoral artery; insert an Excluder abdominal aortic main body stent 23 mm × 12 mm × 180 mm to the abdominal aortic lesion site along the super-stiff wire, and deploy it; insert a 12F DrySeal vascular sheath and a 0.035 in. Lunderquist super-stiff wire 260 cm via the left common femoral artery; insert a Excluder abdominal aortoiliac stent 16 mm × 14 mm × 140 mm inside the short leg of the abdominal aortic main body stent, and deploy it	Deliver two 0.035 in. Lunderquist super-stiff wires 260 cm, 18F DrySeal vascular sheath, 12F DrySeal vascular sheath, Excluder abdominal aortic main body stent 23 mm × 12 mm × 180 mm, and Excluder abdominal aortoiliac stent 16 mm × 14 mm × 140 mm
8. Withdraw the Excluder abdominal aortic split-type stent delivery system, insert a 5F scaled pigtail catheter along the 0.035 in. Lunderquist super-stiff wire 260 cm, and conduct angiography, showing endoleak at the proximal end of the abdominal aorta	Deliver the 5F scaled pigtail catheter
9. Insert Coda balloon catheter into the proximal end of the abdominal aortic main body stent along the 0.035 in. Lunderquist super-stiff wire 260 cm on the left common femoral artery, and inflate it; withdraw the balloon catheter; conduct angiography again, showing significant reduction of endoleak at the proximal end of the abdominal aorta	Deliver the Coda balloon catheter
10. "Sandwich" technique: implant a 12F short sheath and a 0.035 in. hardened hydrophilic wire 260 cm via the left brachial artery; insert one Viabahn peripheral stent graft 13 mm × 100 mm to the left internal iliac artery along the hardened hydrophilic wire; insert one Viabahn peripheral stent graft 13 mm × 100 mm to the left external iliac artery via the super-hard wire on the left common femoral artery; meanwhile, deploy both the Viabahn peripheral stent grafts of the internal and external iliac arteries (the proximal ends of two Viabahn peripheral stent grafts are required to be partially overlapped with the distal ends of the abdominal aortoiliac stent)	Deliver the 12F short sheath, 0.035 in. hardened hydrophilic wire 260 cm, and two Viabahn peripheral stent grafts 13 mm × 100 mm
11. Withdraw the Viabahn peripheral stent graft delivery system, and conduct abdominal aorta and iliac artery angiography, showing excluded abdominal aortic aneurysm and flow patency of the left internal and external iliac arteries (Fig. 19.14)	
12. Withdraw the catheter, wire, and vascular sheath, and suture the incisions on bilateral common femoral arteries and left brachial artery	Deliver the vascular plier and CV suture for vascular incision suturing; deliver small round and angled needles and 1# suture to suture the incision layer by layer; deliver gauze and elastic bandage
13. Anesthesia completed	Safely escort the patient back to ward

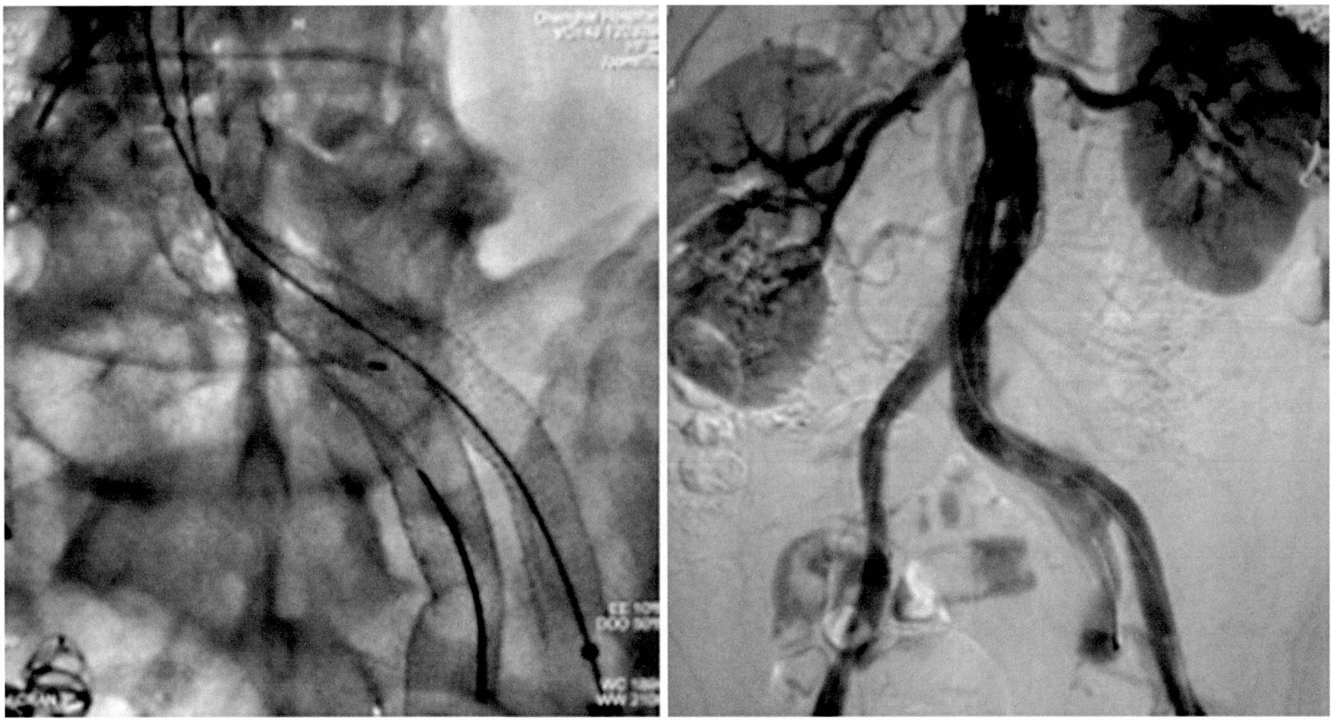

Fig. 19.14 Postoperative AAA angiography

19.6.5 Technical Essentials and Precautions

- Endovascular abdominal aortic aneurysm and iliac artery aneurysm repair has become a routine clinical treatment, but for patients with abdominal aortic aneurysm combined with iliac aneurysm, most scholars still tend to revascularize at least one side of the internal iliac artery, so as to avoid gluteal muscle ischemia and other complications. There are many techniques to retain the internal iliac artery at present, such as revascularization of the internal iliac artery by artificial vascular bypass, branch AAA stent graft, or fenestrated AAA stent graft technique. Although the former can retain the internal iliac artery, this technique exists with huge trauma and high operation risk, while the latter is more complex, and furthermore, there is no suitable product in China. Therefore, sandwich technique is more clinically practical, easily available with operation devices, rather simple in technology, and easy to master.
- The branch approach should be selected according to the type of AAA stent graft. If the abdominal aorta-integrated stent is selected, the internal iliac artery peripheral stent graft system can be accomplished through the contralateral femoral artery approach or brachial artery approach; if the abdominal aorta split-type stent is selected, the internal iliac artery peripheral stent graft system can only be advanced via the brachial artery approach. In this case, it is suggested to cut open and expose the left brachial artery to reduce the incidence of complications.
- How to choose the right type of peripheral stent graft is the key to successful surgery. According to the current clinical experience and internationally popular technology, $\pi D + 2D = \pi d1 + \pi d2$ is generally used, where D is the diameter of the trunk artery (common iliac artery) and $d1$ and $d2$ are the diameters of the two branch vessels. According to the total diameter of the iliac artery of the patient, the sum of the diameters of $d1$ and $d2$ is figured out, and then the peripheral stent graft with appropriate size is implanted into the internal and the external iliac arteries, respectively, according to the internal and the external iliac arteries, thus ensuring vascular patency for both the internal and the external iliac arteries.
- When sandwich technique is used for implanting the peripheral stent graft for the internal and the external iliac arteries, the stent graft of the internal iliac artery should be slightly lower than that of the external iliac artery, preventing the two stent grafts from being entangled and twined together when being deployed simultaneously. The patient in this case should be administered with oral antiplatelet drugs after operation so as to ensure long-term patency rate.

19.7 Case 7 Self-Expanding Bare Stent-Assisted Spring Coil Embolotherapy for Endovascular Repair of Visceral Abdominal Aortic Pseudoaneurysm

19.7.1 Patient Data

The male patient, aged 35, felt a sudden burst of chest-back pain in 2013 and was treated with endovascular abdominal aortic aneurysm repair at another hospital. In April 2015, abdominal aorta CTA examination showed "visceral abdominal aortic pseudoaneurysm," and the patient was admitted in May.

19.7.2 Surgical Operation

Preoperative abdominal aorta CTA showed the presence of eccentric enlargement of the abdominal aorta stretching from the proximal end of the AAA stent graft to the inferior coeliac trunk and abdominal aortic pseudoaneurysm formation in the visceral area. After careful evaluation, it intended to use "self-expanding bare stent plus spring coil embolization" technique to repair the visceral abdominal aortic pseudoaneurysm, that is, to implant the self-expanding bare stent into the abdominal aortic lesion site and embolize the aneurysm cavity by spring coil. The technique can not only exclude the visceral abdominal aortic pseudoaneurysm but also ensure vascular patency of the coeliac trunk artery, mesenteric artery, renal artery, and other collateral arteries. The subject gave informed consent for the procedure.

19.7.3 Device Preparation

Refer to Table 19.13.

19.7.4 Procedures and Intraoperative Coordination Process

Refer to Table 19.14.

Table 19.13 Device preparation

Name	Qty.	Name	Qty.
Puncture needle (Cook)	1	5F Cobra catheter (AngioDynamics)	1
High-pressure connector (SCW Medicath)	2	5F scaled pigtail catheter (Optimed)	1
0.035 in. common hydrophilic wire 260 cm (Terumo)	1	5F short sheath (Terumo)	
10F short sheath (St. Jude)	1	6F Ansel long sheath 45 cm (Cook)	1
0.035 in. Lunderquist super-stiff wire 260 cm (Cook)	1	Interlock-35 controllable embolization 15 mm × 400 mm (Boston Scientific)	4
Visual-XL self-expanding bare stent 20 mm × 80 mm (Optimed)	1	Interlock-35 controllable embolization 18 mm × 400 mm (Boston Scientific)	5
6F ProGlide vascular closure device (Abbott)	2		

Note: The devices listed above (*A* mm × *B* mm), wherein *A* is the diameter of the device and *B* the length

Table 19.14 Procedures and intraoperative coordination process

Procedures	Intraoperative coordination process
1. Patient enters the operation room	(1) Mental nursing; (2) keep the patient warm; (3) help to lie at supine position, with two lower limbs slightly at abduction and extorsion position; (4) connect ECG to observe changes in blood pressure, heart rate, and oxygen saturation; (5) establish intravenous infusion
2. Routinely sterilize the bilateral groins from the umbilical down to midthigh, exposing the groins	Prepare disinfectant (heated to 98.6 °F with incubator) and assist with draping; deliver iodixanol injection; prepare heparin diluent (1000 mL normal saline + 100 mg heparin sodium injection)
3. Puncture the right common femoral artery with modified Seldinger technique under local anaesthesia, insert a 5F short sheath, a 0.035 in. common hydrophilic wire 260 cm, insert a 5F scaled pigtail catheter to the superior coeliac trunk artery along the common hydrophilic wire and conduct angiography, showing abdominal aortic pseudoaneurysm in the visceral area (Fig. 19.15)	Deliver 1% lidocaine injection, puncture needle, high-pressure connector, 5F short sheath, 0.035 in. common hydrophilic wire 260 cm, 5F scaled pigtail catheter; systematic heparinization; intraoperative endovascular devices should be flushed with the prepared heparin diluent
4. Conduct retrograde puncture of the left common femoral artery with modified Seldinger technique, insert a 6F Ansel long sheath 45 cm, the 0.035 in. common hydrophilic wire 260 cm, and a 5F Cobra catheter, superslect to access into the abdominal aortic pseudoaneurysm cavity, withdraw the common hydrophilic wire, and retain the 5F Cobra catheter in place	Deliver 6F Ansel long sheath 45 cm and 5F Cobra catheter

Table 19.14 (continued)

Procedures	Intraoperative coordination process
5. Implantation of self-expanding bare stent: withdraw the 5F scaled pigtail catheter and 5F short sheath, exchange to a 10F short sheath and a 0.035 in. Lunderquist super-stiff wire 260 cm, insert one Visual-XL Self-Expanding bare stent 20 mm × 80 mm along the super-stiff wire to the abdominal aortic lesion site, withdraw the Visual-XL self-expanding bare stent delivery system	Deliver 10F short sheath, 0.035 in. Lunderquist super-stiff wire 260 cm, and Visual-XL Self-Expanding bare stent 20 mm × 80 mm
6. Implantation of controllable embolization: insert nine Interlock-35 controllable embolization along the Cobra catheter retained in the aneurysm cavity	Deliver five Interlock-35 controllable embolization 15 mm × 400 mm and four Interlock-35 controllable embolization 18 mm × 400 mm
7. Insert the 5F scaled pigtail catheter to the abdominal aorta via the super-stiff wire on the right common femoral artery, withdraw the super-stiff wire and conduct angiography, showing complete exclusion of the abdominal aortic pseudoaneursym, and vascular patency of coeliac trunk artery, mesenteric artery, renal artery, and other collateral arteries (Fig. 19.16)	Deliver the 5F scaled pigtail catheter
8. Withdraw the catheter, vascular sheath, use two 6F Proglide vascular closure devices to suture the puncture sites on bilateral common femoral arteries	Deliver two 6F Proglide vascular closure devices
9. Compression dressing on the puncture sites of the bilateral common femoral arteries	Deliver gauze and elsatic bandage, assist with dressing; escort the patient safely back to ward

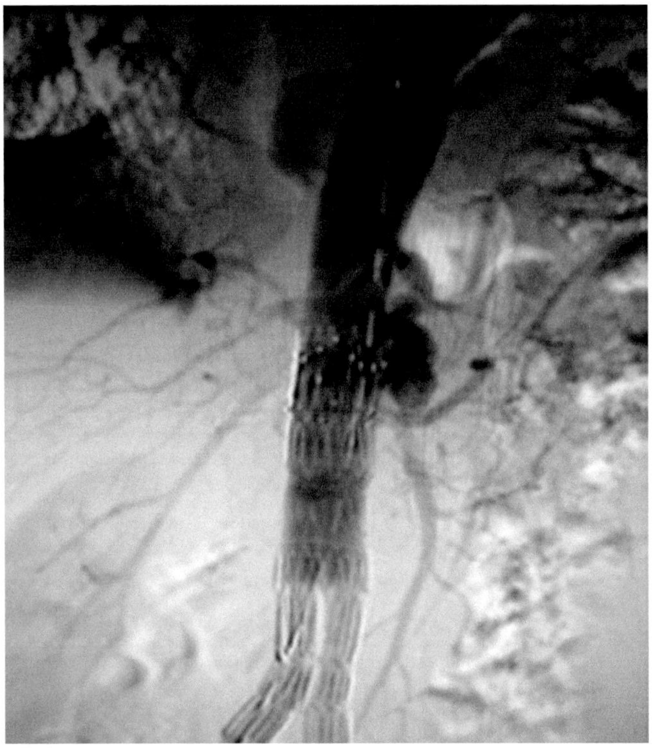

Fig. 19.15 Preoperative angiography

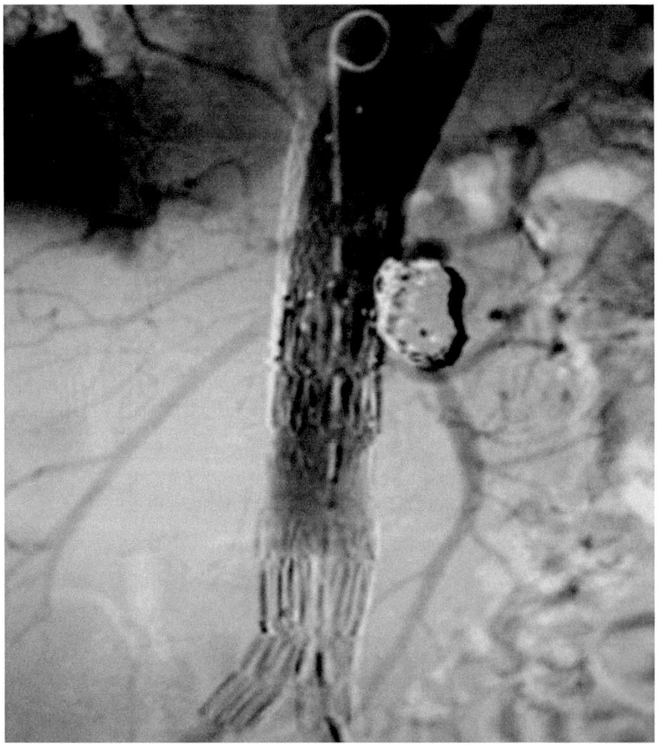

Fig. 19.16 Postoperative angiography

19.7.5 Technical Essentials and Precautions

- The principle of using self-expanding bare stent for aneurysm repair in this case is to reduce the flow rate of the blood entering the tumor cavity after passing through the self-expanding bare stent mesh, forming local eddy that leads to intracavitary thrombosis and ultimately excluding the aneurysm. Using multiple self-expanding bare stent can have similar function, but if the multiple bare stent has excessive meshes, it may lead to distal stenosis and occlusion of the branch vessels in the visceral area. For this kind of patients, it is suggested to use single self-expanding bare stent accompanied by spring coil embolization.
- Considering the particularity of the lesion site, common spring coil used in the tumor cavity may displace or break off into the distal end of the aorta when using self-

expanding bare stent plus coil embolization for aneurysm repair, leading to distal occlusion of the aorta. Therefore, controllable spring coil was used in this case, and the embolic catheter was retained before the implantation of the self-expanding bare stent (or superselected via the meshes after the self-expanding bare stent is deployed in place).

19.8 Case 8 Hybrid Technique for Repair of Vertebral Artery Pseudoaneurysm Complicated with Brachial Plexus Compression

19.8.1 Patient Data

The female patient, aged 52, presented herself with the right upper limb weakness and numbness for 5 months, which was aggravated with pain for 3 weeks, and carotid artery CT showed a 5.0 cm × 4.5 cm × 5.4 cm slightly high-density shadow at the root of the right neck and patchy enhancement after contrast-enhanced CT imaging that wrapped around the proximal segment of the right vertebral artery, which was considered as the pseudoaneurysm formation of the proximal segment of the right vertebral artery (Fig. 19.17). The patient was admitted for "Vertebral artery pseudoaneurysm complicated with brachial plexus compression" in March 2016.

19.8.2 Surgical Operation

Considering the clinical symptoms and preoperative CT examination of the patient, if extracranial vertebral artery pseudoaneurysm repair and artery ligation technique were used, its distal outflow tract has entered the intervertebral foramen, the vertebral artery is difficult to be exposed, and palliative suture would achieve less effect. After repeated assessment, it intended to use "hybrid" technique to the right vertebral artery embolization and pseudoaneurysectomy and brachial plexus release technique under general anesthesia. The subject gave informed consent for the procedure.

19.8.3 Device Preparation

Refer to Table 19.15.

19.8.4 Procedures and Intraoperative Coordination Process

Refer to Table 19.16.

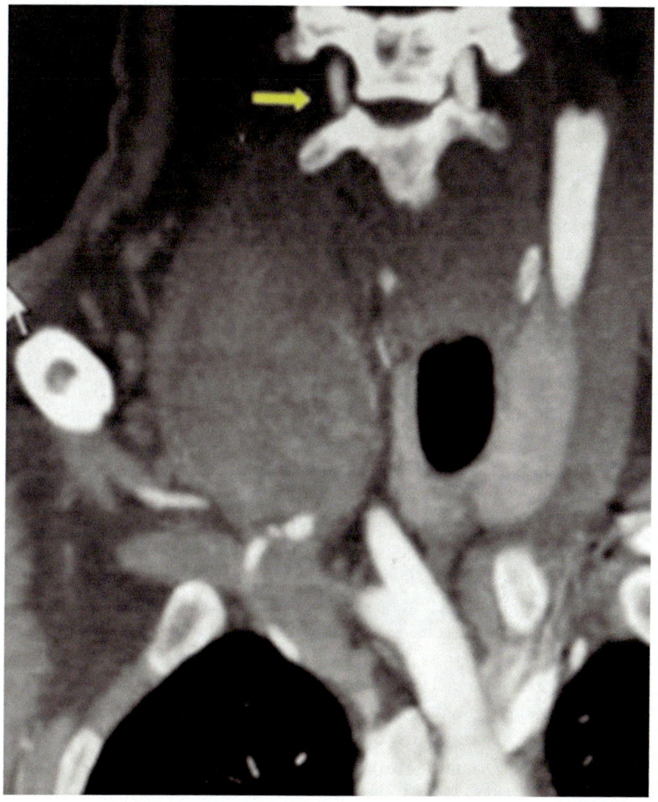

Fig. 19.17 Contrast-enhanced carotid artery CT

Table 19.15 Device preparation

Name	Qty.	Name	Qty.
Puncture needle (Cook)	1	5F Berenstein catheter (AngioDynamics)	1
High-pressure connector (SCW Medicath)	2	5F common pigtail catheter (Optimed)	1
0.035 in. common hydrophilic wire 260 cm (Terumo)	1	6F short sheath (Terumo)	1
6F Raabe long sheath 90 cm (Cook)	1	Echelon-10 microcatheter (Medtronic)	1
0.014 in. Traxcess wire 200 cm (MicroVention)	1	Axium detachable embolization 3.5 mm × 12 mm (Medtronic)	1
Reliever (Medtronic)	1	Helical-Soft Guglialmi detachable micro-embolization 3 mm × 10 mm (Terumo)	3
6F ProGlide vascular closure device (Abbott)	1		

Note: The devices listed above (*A* mm × *B* mm), wherein *A* is the diameter of the device and *B* the length

Table 19.16 Procedures and intraoperative coordination process

Procedures	Intraoperative coordination process
1. Patient enters the operation room, general anesthesia	(1) Mental nursing; (2) keep the patient warm; (3) help to lie at supine position, with two lower limbs slightly at abduction and extorsion position the head turning left; (4) connect ECG to observe changes in blood pressure, heart rate, and oxygen saturation; (5) establish intravenous infusion, and place indwelling central venous catheter; (6) place indwelling urinary catheter
2. Sterilize bilateral groins and right supraclavicular fossa	Prepare disinfectant (heated to 98.6 °F°F with incubator), and assist with draping; deliver iodixanol injection; prepare heparin diluent (1000 mL normal saline +100 mg heparin sodium injection)
3. Puncture the right common femoral artery with modified Seldinger technique; insert a 6F short sheath and a 0.035 in. common hydrophilic wire 260 cm; insert a 5F common pigtail catheter to the aortic arch along the common hydrophilic wire; withdraw the hydrophilic wire; conduct angiography for the brachiocephalic artery, the left common carotid and the left subclavian arteries, and left and right vertebral arteries, respectively, showing good images of the brachiocephalic artery, the left common carotid and the left subclavian arteries, and the left vertebral artery, but no image of the proximal end of the right vertebral artery and pseudoaneurysm formation presented after retrograde imaging of the intracranial blood flow	Deliver the puncture needle, high-pressure connector, 6F short sheath, 0.035 in. common hydrophilic wire 260 cm, and 5F common pigtail catheter; perform systematic heparinization; intraoperative endovascular devices should be flushed by the prepared heparin diluent
4. Withdraw the 5F common pigtail catheter, exchange to insert a 6F Raabe long sheath 90 cm and a 5F Berenstein catheter to the left vertebral artery, and conduct angiography, showing left vertebral artery patency, intact connection of the vertebrobasilar artery, and retrograde blood flow of the right vertebral artery with visible rupture at the proximal end (Fig. 19.18)	Deliver the 6F Raabe long sheath 90 cm and 5F Berenstein catheter
5. Withdraw the 0.035 in. common hydrophilic wire 260 cm, insert a 0.014 in. Traxcess wire 200 cm and the Echelon-10 microcatheter via the 5F Berenstein catheter, superselect the Traxcess wire in combination with the microcatheter and access to the distal end of the right vertebral artery rupture, withdraw the wire, insert an Axium detachable embolization 3.5 mm × 12 mm to the distal end of the rupture via the microcatheter	Deliver the 0.014 in. Traxcess wire 200 cm and Axium detachable embolization 3.5 mm × 12 mm
6. Insert a Helical-Soft Guglialmi detachable micro-embolization 3 mm × 10 mm via the microcatheter, insert the shaft of the spring coil into the reliever for detachment (if the reliever shows green, indicating the coil can be detached), confirm successful detachment, insert two Helical-Soft Guglialmi detachable micro-embolizations 3 mm × 10 mm to the distal end of the rupture in sequence, manually advance the coil via the microcatheter, and conduct angiography, showing significant reduction of blood flow of the right vertebral artery	Deliver the reliever, three Helical-Soft Guglialmi detachable micro-embolization 3 mm × 10 mm
7. Make a horizontal incision at the right supraclavicular fossa, and explore it (Fig. 19.19), showing deep hematoma formation on the anterior scalene muscle, significant increase in compression tension of the right brachial plexus and phrenic nerves, lower subclavian artery compression, and no visible adhesion between the medial margin and the carotid sheath	Deliver the scalpel and vascular pliers
8. Remove most of the hematoma, showing return blood flow of the vertebral artery. Partially suture to stop bleeding, and check no visible active bleeding on the wound and significant reduction of the brachial plexus tension	Deliver the suturing hemostat and gauze, and assist with local suturing hemostasis
9. Withdraw the microcatheter and 5F Berenstein catheter, and conduct right vertebral artery angiography via the 6F Raabe long sheath, showing right vertebral pseudoaneurysm disappeared, without visible regurgitant blood flow (Fig. 19.20)	
10. Suture the incision on the right supraclavicular fossa, withdraw the 6F Raabe long sheath and wire, and suture the puncture site on the right common femoral artery by 6F ProGlide vascular closure device	Deliver the vascular plier and CV suture for vascular incision suturing; deliver the small round and angled needles and 1# suture to suture the incision layer by layer; deliver the 6F ProGlide vascular closure device
11. Anesthesia completed	Deliver the gauze and elastic bandage, apply compression dressing on the puncture site, safely escort the patient back to ward

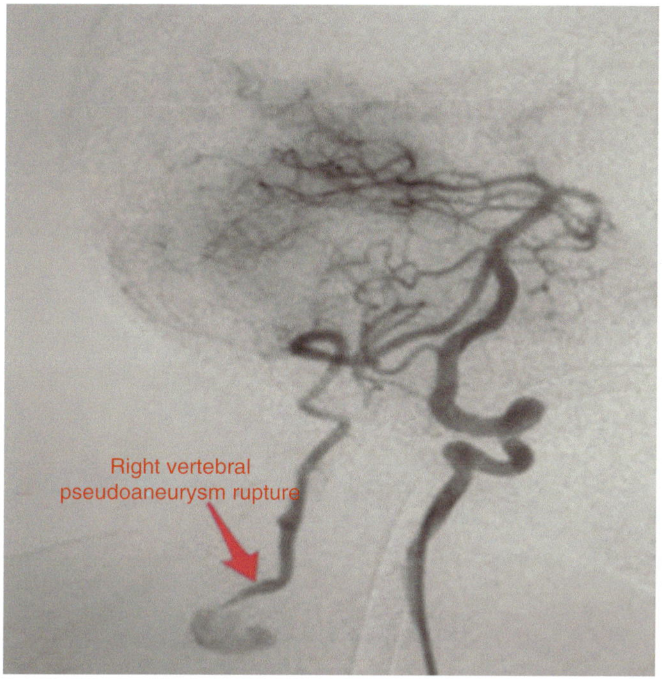

Fig. 19.18 Right vertebral artery pseudoaneurysm rupture

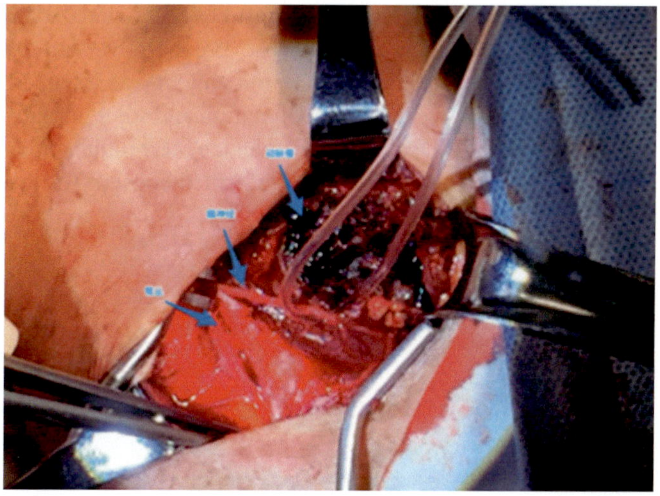

Fig. 19.19 Explore right supraclavicular fossa

19.8.5 Technical Essentials and Precautions

- The treatment in this case adopted "hybrid technique of endovascular repair combined with open surgery," indicated for cases where the symptoms of oppression are obvious, the aneurysm is difficult to be exposed, proximal and distal control is difficult, and the risk of intraoperative bleeding is high, which reduce the risk of intraoperative

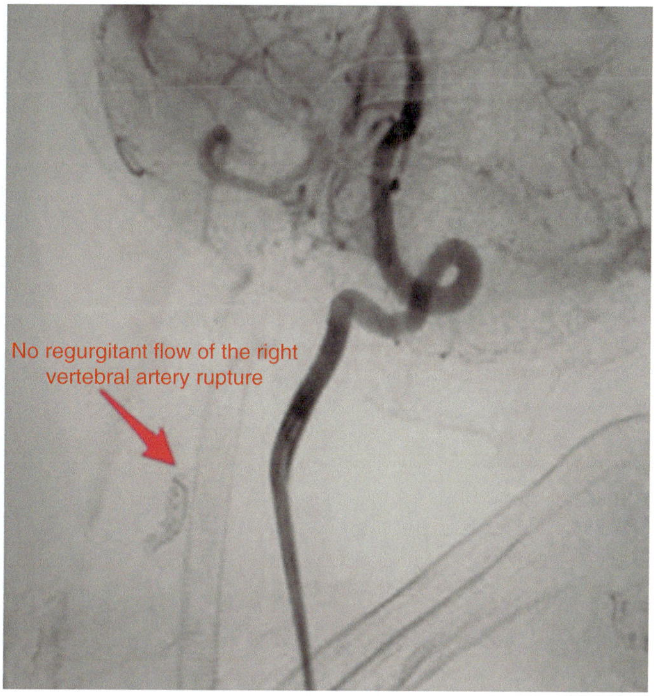

Fig. 19.20 No regurgitant flow of the right vertebral artery under angiography

bleeding and quickly relieve the symptoms of oppression, so as to achieve the effect of improving the prognosis of patients.
- The right upper limb numbness of the patient progressed to pain complicated with decreased muscle strength due to the brachial plexus compression, which, if not relieved promptly, may lead to difficult recovery of the patient's limb functions. Therefore, simple endovascular therapy is not suitable for the treatment of the patient.

19.9 Case 9 Double-Protection Device Technique for Minimally Invasive Endovascular Repair of Left Carotid Subtotal Occlusive Lesion

19.9.1 Patient Data

The male patient, aged 66, presented himself with dizziness with intermittent irregular attack in October 2016, having blood pressure at 160/85 mmHg, and on November 9, a head MRA examination in local hospital showed "lacunar infarction," and further cardiac color Doppler ultrasound examination showed "severe aortic valve regurgitation." The patient was treated with "aortic valve replacement" on

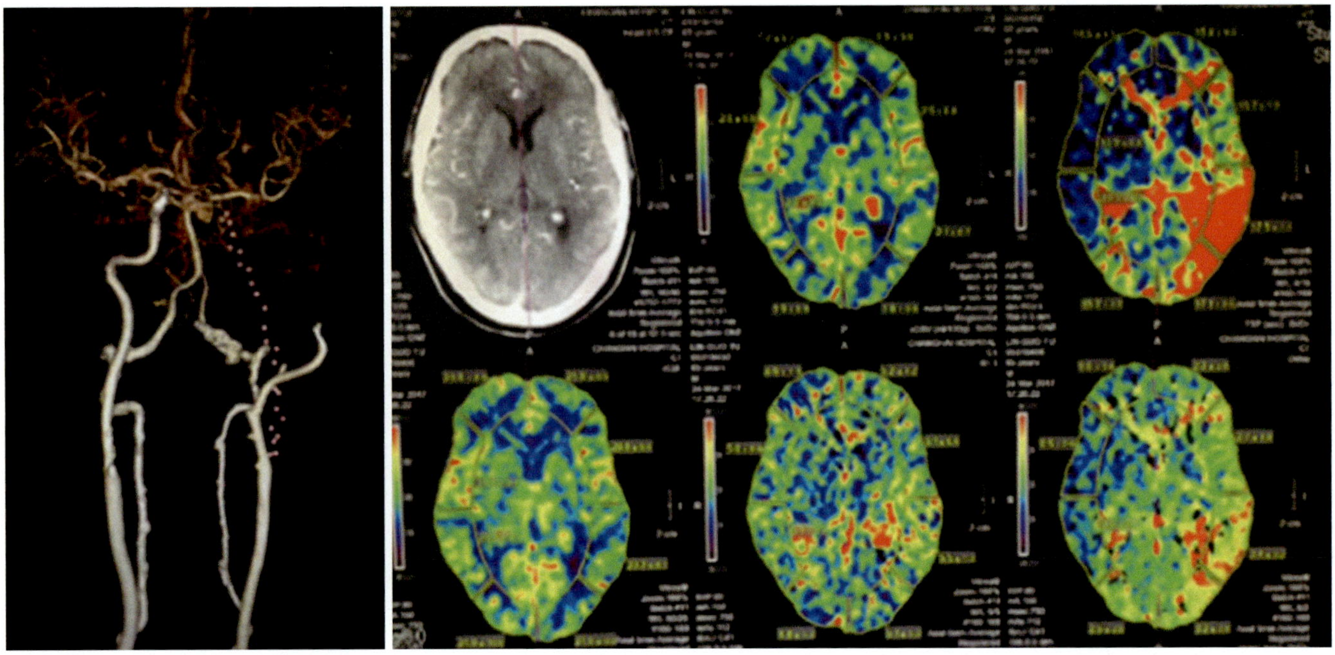

Fig. 19.21 Preoperative CTA and CTP examination

November 16, having a good recovery after operation, but still with dizziness and occasional right limb weakness. On February 27, 2017, a cervical artery angiography for the patient in local hospital showed "severe stenosis of the proximal left internal carotid artery." For further treatment, the patient was admitted for "left internal carotid stenosis complicated with cardiac dysfunction after aortic valve replacement surgery" in March 2017.

19.9.2 Surgical Operation

The patient was diagnosed with severe left carotid artery stenosis before admission, but carotid artery CTA after admission showed left internal carotid artery occlusion, and head CT perfusion (CTP) showed hypoperfusion in the blood supply area of the left middle cerebral artery (Fig. 19.21). In combination with the patient's past symptoms of right limb weakness, it was considered meaningful to revascularize the occluded left carotid artery. Because preoperative carotid artery CTA showed an extensive lesion area, it was intended to perform carotid artery balloon dilatation and stent implantation by using the "Dual protective device" technique under local anesthesia. The subject gave informed consent for the procedure.

19.9.3 Device Preparation

Refer to Table 19.17.

19.9.4 Procedures and Intraoperative Coordination Process

Refer to Table 19.18.

Table 19.17 Device preparation

Name	Qty.	Name	Qty.
Puncture needle (Cook)	1	8F short sheath (Terumo)	1
High-pressure connector (SCW Medicath)	3	6F long sheath 90 cm (Cook)	1
0.035 in. common hydrophilic wire 260 cm (Terumo)	2	8F Mo.Ma embolic protection device (Medtronic)	1
5F short sheath (Terumo)	1	SpiderFX (5 mm) protective umbrella (Medtronic)	1
5F MPA catheter 125 cm (Cordis)	1	0.014 in. PT2 wire 300 cm (Boston Scientific)	1
5F common pigtail catheter (Cordis)	1	Inflation device (Boston Scientific)	1
V-18 control wire 300 cm (Boston Scientific)	1	LitePAC balloon catheter 4 mm × 30 mm (Bard)	1
Renegade STC 18 microcatheter (Boston Scientific)	1	Deep balloon catheter 2.5 mm × 40 mm (Medtronic)	1
Wallstent self-expanding carotid artery stent 7 mm × 40 mm (Boston Scientific)	1	Deep balloon catheter 3 mm × 80 mm (Medtronic)	1

Note: The devices listed above (A mm × B mm), wherein A is the diameter of the device and B the length

Table 19.18 Procedures and intraoperative coordination process

Procedures	Intraoperative coordination process
1. Patient enters the operation room	(1) Mental nursing; (2) keep the patient warm; (3) help to lie at supine position, with two lower limbs slightly at abduction and extorsion position; (4) connect ECG to observe changes in blood pressure, heart rate, and oxygen saturation; (5) establish intravenous infusion
2. Sterilize bilateral groins up to the navel and down to the midthigh	Prepare disinfectant (heated to 98.6 °F with incubator), and assist with draping; deliver iodixanol injection; prepare heparin diluent (1000 mL normal saline +100 mg heparin sodium injection)
3. Puncture the right common femoral artery with modified Seldinger technique under local anesthesia, insert a 5F short sheath and a 0.035 in. common hydrophilic wire 260 cm, insert a 5F common pigtail catheter to the aortic arch along the hydrophilic wire, withdraw the wire, and conduct aortic arch angiography	Deliver 1% lidocaine injection, puncture needle, high-pressure connector, 5F short sheath, 0.035 in. common hydrophilic wire 260 cm, and 5F common pigtail catheter; perform systematic heparinization; intraoperative endovascular devices should be flushed with the prepared heparin diluent
4. Exchange to implant a 0.035 in. common hydrophilic wire 260 cm and a 5F MPA catheter 125 cm via the 5F common pigtail catheter, superselect left carotid artery, and conduct angiography, showing minor stenosis of the left common carotid artery and full-range thin internal carotid artery (Fig. 19.22)	Deliver the 5F MPA catheter 125 cm
5. Withdraw the 5F short sheath, insert a 6F long sheath along the hydrophilic wire, insert Renegade STC 18 microcatheter along the 5F MPA catheter 125 cm, and combine with a 0.014 in. PT2 wire 300 cm to superselect access through the occlusive segment of the carotid artery and enter into the carotid artery of the distal intracranial segment	Deliver the 6F long sheath 90 cm, Renegade STC 18 microcatheter, and 0.014 in. PT2 wire 300 cm
6. Insert a V-18 control wire 300 cm into the left external carotid artery via the 6F long sheath, withdraw the long sheath, exchange to insert a 8F short sheath supported by dual wires, and then insert the 8F Mo.Ma embolic protection device (Fig. 19.23)	Deliver the V-18 control wire 300 cm, 8F short sheath, and 8F Mo.Ma embolic protection device
7. When the 8F Mo.Ma embolic protection device is advanced in place and the blood flow of the common and external carotid arteries is occluded, inject radiocontrast via the operation cavity, but no radiocontrast is retained. Considering the regurgitant superior thyroid artery and incomplete proximal protection, insert the SpiderFX protective umbrella via the 0.014 in. PT2 wire on the internal carotid artery for distal protection	Deliver the SpiderFX protective umbrella 5 mm
8. When the SpiderFX protective umbrella is advanced in place, insert Deep balloon catheters 2.5 mm × 40 mm and 3.0 mm × 80 mm along the protective umbrella wire to dilate the occluded stenotic segment in sequence, and conduct angiography, showing image of the left carotid artery and formation of local small dissection	Deliver inflation device and Deep balloon catheters 2.5 mm × 40 mm and 3 mm × 80 mm
9. Insert a Wallstent self-expanding carotid artery stent 7 mm × 40 mm via the SpiderFX protective umbrella, and deploy it at the original stenotic occlusion lesion site of the carotid artery. Conduct angiography via the operating passage of the Mo.Ma embolic protective device, and when carotid artery patency is achieved, withdraw the distal SpiderFX protective umbrella, and conduct angiography again, showing thin right carotid artery lumen, vascular patency, visible image of the distal middle cerebral artery, and no intracranial embolism (Fig. 19.24)	Deliver the Wallstent self-expanding carotid artery stent 7 mm × 40 mm
10. Withdraw the Mo.Ma embolic protective device and the 8F short sheath, and compress the right common femoral artery for 20 min till no bleeding	Deliver the gauze and elastic bandage
11. Compression dressing on the puncture site of the right common femoral artery	Assist with dressing

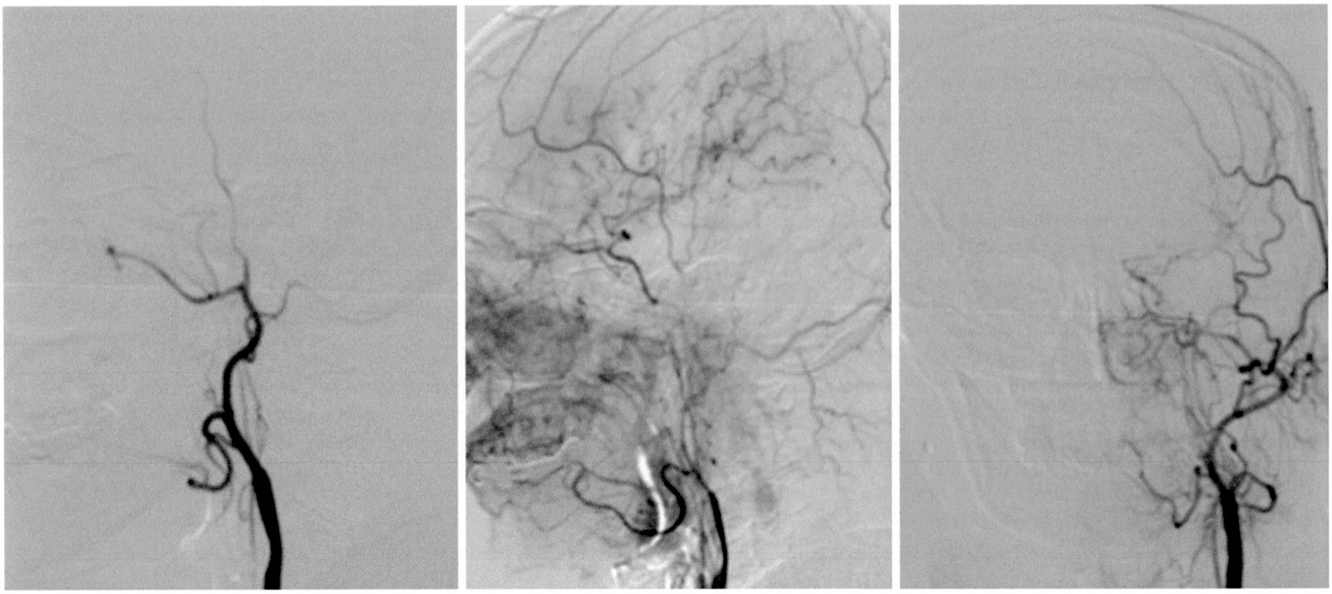

Fig. 19.22 Left internal carotid artery proximal occlusion, delayed distal imaging via lateral artery, imaging of carotid intracranial segment and the middle cerebral artery

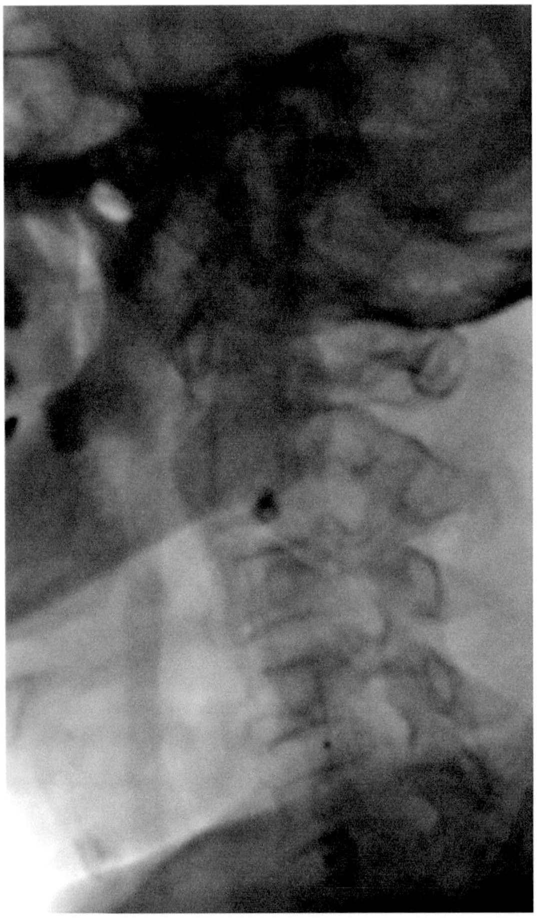

Fig. 19.23 Implant Mo.Ma embolic protection device

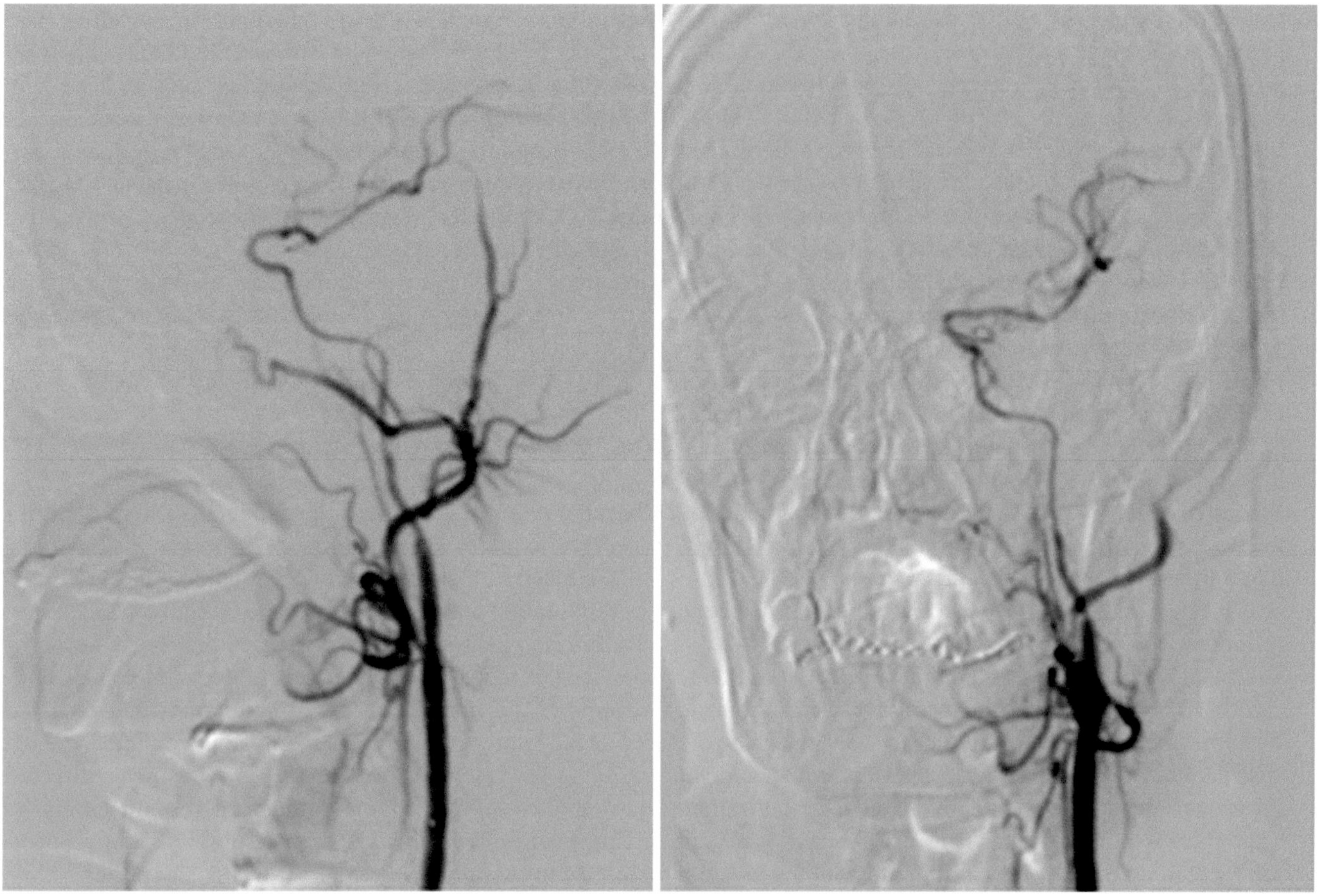

Fig. 19.24 Postoperative angiography

19.9.5 Technical Essentials and Precautions

- The patient presented with symptomatic left internal carotid artery subocclusion cerebral infarction, which was considered to be caused by low perfusion, indicated for the left internal carotid artery stent angioplasty. The occlusive causes were considered to be chronic atherosclerotic lesions, the left middle cerebral artery was not compensated by the right internal carotid artery through the anterior communicating artery, the primary lateral branches were fair, external carotid artery was compensatory for the carotid artery of the intracranial segment, distal secondary thrombosis of the occlusive segment of the internal carotid artery was unlikely, and intraoperative intracranial embolism risk was low. However, the distal blood vessel of the patient significantly collapsed, with a slow flow rate but with fair primary branch vessels. Therefore, primary stent implantation was conducted, and to avoid high perfusion, blood pressure should be controlled strictly after operation, accompanied with double-antiplatelet and enhanced statin treatment.
- Symptomatic carotid occlusion or secondary occlusion lesions are often accompanied with insufficient cerebrovascular reserve capacity (CVRC) or vascular reactivity. Therefore, preoperative DSA should be conducted to assess the situations of the distal outflow tract and collateral circulation compensation. Primary stent implantation can be conducted for patient without carotid artery collapse and collateral circulation compensation. Staging treatment should be conducted for the patient with obvious distal vascular collapse and slow flow rate so as to avoid high perfusion and difficulty in stent implantation: first-stage balloon dilatation and second-stage stent implantation.
- In revascularizing occlusive or subocclusion lesions, it is suggested to choose proximal protection device—Mo.Ma embolic protection device. If there is operation space for distal embolic protection device in the carotid artery of the intracranial segment, SpiderFX protective umbrella can also be selected, for it has better crossability by accessing to the umbrella via the wire and, at the same time, retracting the sheath, resulting in low risk of embolus breaking off. Usually only one protection device is selected for intraoperative protection, but if Mo. Ma embolic protection device is used during operation and when the patient appears intolerable to occlusion, try to exchange to the distal protection device for embolic pro-

tection as soon as possible as the condition permits and pump out the occlusive balloon of the Mo. Ma embolic protection device so as to restore the forward blood flow of the carotid artery.

- In this case, the superior thyroid artery of the patient stems out from the initial part of the external carotid artery, and if proximal protective device is used to occlude the common and the external carotid arteries, the blood flows reversely into the occluded carotid artery area via the superior thyroid artery, which can offer no embolic protection. Therefore, the T valve of the operation lumen for the angiography of Mo.Ma embolic protection device is opened, making the reverse flow into the carotid artery to flow out of the body via the Mo.Ma embolic protection device, and then after the wire is exchanged into the distal SpiderFX protective umbrella and starts functioning via the occlusive segment of the carotid artery, retract 40 mL blood from the occluded lumen, and pump out the occlusive balloon of the Mo. Ma embolic protection device to restore the forward blood flow of the carotid artery.
- Stent selection: the patient presented with left internal carotid artery lesion, with heavy atherosclerotic plaque load; the plaque may be cut into pieces and enter into the vascular lumens via the stent meshes after implantation of open-loop stent, resulting in intracranial embolization. Therefore, it is more suitable to use braided Wallstent self-expanding carotid artery stent to fit with the vascular wall, which, to a certain extent, can reduce the risk of postoperative intracranial embolization.

19.10 Case 10 Catheter-Directed Thrombolysis and Rotarex Mechanical Aspiration Thrombectomy Technique for Treatment of Acute Superior Mesenteric Artery Embolization

19.10.1 Patient Data

The male patient, aged 81, presented himself with abdominal discomfort having no obvious causes on March 25 of 2017, mainly manifested as persistent periomphalic swelling pain with a little bloody excrement and diarrhea with watery stool after bloody excrement disappeared and accompanied with nausea but without vomiting. The abdominal CT imaging at a local hospital on the same day showed "superior mesenteric artery embolization with incomplete intestinal obstruction." After water fasting and symptomatic supportive treatment, the pain symptoms eased somewhat. For further treatment, the patient was admitted for "superior mesenteric artery embolization with incomplete intestinal obstruction" on March 28.

19.10.2 Surgical Operation

The abdominal CT of the patient suggested acute superior mesenteric artery embolization, presented with hemafecia at the onset but disappeared later, abdominal tenderness, no abdominal muscle tension, and rebound tenderness. Therefore, intestinal necrosis-induced peritoneal peritonitis was not taken into consideration. Hemafecia was considered to be mucosal necrosis after intestinal mucosal acute ischemic attack. It was intended to conduct superior mesenteric artery angiography and catheter-directed thrombolysis and Rotarex mechanical thrombectomy so as to restore blood flow as soon as possible, but reperfusion injury should be prevented during the perioperative period. The subject gave informed consent for the procedure.

19.10.3 Device Preparation

Refer to Table 19.19.

19.10.4 Procedures and Intraoperative Coordination Process

Refer to Table 19.20.

Table 19.19 Device preparation

Name	Qty.	Name	Qty.
Puncture needle (Cook)	1	4F Cobra catheter (Cordis)	1
High-pressure connector (SCW Medicath)	3	6F Ansel long sheath 45 cm (Cook)	1
0.035 in. common hydrophilic wire 260 cm (Terumo)	1	6F short sheath (Terumo)	1
5F short sheath (Terumo)	1	6F Exoseal vascular closure device (Cordis)	1
5F common pigtail catheter (Cordis)	1	6F Rotarex mechanical thrombectomy system 110 cm (Straub)	1 set
4F thrombolytic catheter135 × m (5 cm perfusion segment length) (AngioDynamics)	1		

Note: The devices listed above (*A* mm × *B* mm), wherein *A* is the diameter of the device and *B* the length

Table 19.20 Procedures and intraoperative coordination process

Procedures	Intraoperative coordination process
1. Patient enters the operation room	(1) Mental nursing; (2) keep the patient warm; (3) help to lie at supine position, with two lower limbs slightly at abduction and extorsion position; (4) connect ECG to observe changes in blood pressure, heart rate, and oxygen saturation; (5) establish intravenous infusion
2. Routinely sterilize the bilateral groins from the umbilical down to the midthigh, exposing the groins	Prepare disinfectant (heated to 98.6 °F with incubator), and assist with draping; deliver iodixanol injection; prepare heparin diluent (1000 mL normal saline +100 mg heparin sodium injection)
3. Puncture the right common femoral artery with modified Seldinger technique under local anesthesia, implant a 5F short sheath and a 0.035 in. common hydrophilic wire 260 cm, implant a 5F common pigtail catheter to the 12th thoracic vertebra level along the hydrophilic wire, withdraw the hydrophilic wire, and conduct angiography, showing normal renal arteries and no obvious imaging of the distal end of superior mesenteric trunk artery	Deliver the puncture needle, high-pressure connector, 0.035 in. common hydrophilic wire 260 cm, and 5F common pigtail catheter; perform systematic heparinization; intraoperative endovascular devices should be flushed with the prepared heparin diluent
4. Withdraw the 5F short sheath and 5F common pigtail catheter, exchange to implant q 6F Ansel long sheath 45 cm and a 4F Cobra catheter, use the hydrophilic wire and the 4F Cobra catheter for superselective access into the superior mesenteric artery, withdraw the hydrophilic wire, and conduct angiography by manual push via the 4F Cobra catheter, showing distal occlusion of the superior mesenteric trunk artery and delayed imaging of the peripheral vessels via the collateral branch (Fig. 19.25)	Deliver the 6F Ansel long sheath 45 cm and 4F Cobra catheter
5. Catheter-directed thrombolysis: implant the common hydrophilic wire via the 4F Cobra catheter, withdraw the catheter, implant a 4F infusion catheter (perfusion segment is 5 cm long) 135 cm to the distal end of the superior mesenteric artery via the hydrophilic wire, conduct partial pulsed urokinase thrombolysis for 30 min, withdraw the infusion catheter, and conduct angiography via the 6F Ansel long sheath, showing no obvious improvement in the superior mesenteric artery imaging	Deliver the 4F infusion catheter (perfusion segment is 5 cm long) 135 cm; prepare and deliver urokinase (200 mL normal saline +250,000 units of urokinase)
6. Again implant the 4F Cobra catheter via the 6F Ansel long sheath, exchange to implant the supporting 0.018 in. wire of the 6F Rotarex mechanical thrombectomy system via the 4F Cobra catheter to the distal end of the superior mesenteric artery	Connect the power cord and motor for the Straub medical power system; open the 6F Rotarex mechanical thrombectomy system; deliver the 6F Rotarex catheter, supporting 0.018 in. wire, sterilizing covering cloth, and fluid collection bag
7. Cover the unsterilized motor with the sterilizing covering cloth, connect the sterilized motor with the 6F Rotarex catheter and the fluid collection bag with the infusion catheter	Assist with covering the motor
8. Thrombus aspiration: implant a 6F Rotarex catheter along the 0.018 in. supporting wire, initiate hand or foot control model, advance the 6F Rotarex catheter to the superior mesenteric artery for thrombus aspiration via the 0.018 in. supporting wire	Initiate the hand or foot control model according to the physician's habit (in case of foot control, connect the foot pedal with the Straub medical power system in advance)
9. Upon completion of thrombus aspiration, withdraw the 6F Rotarex catheter, insert the 4F Cobra catheter along the 0.018 in. wire, and conduct angiography via the 4F Cobra catheter, showing significant improvement in the imaging of the superior mesenteric artery and normal imaging of the peripheral vessels	Deliver the 4F Cobra catheter
10. Withdraw the catheter and 6F Ansel long sheath, exchange to insert the 6F short sheath, occlude the puncture site on the right common femoral artery by 6F Exoseal vascular closure device (Fig. 19.26)	Deliver the 6F short sheath and 6F Exoseal vascular closure device
11. Compression dressing at the puncture site	Deliver the gauze and elastic bandage, assist with dressing, escort the patient safely back to ward

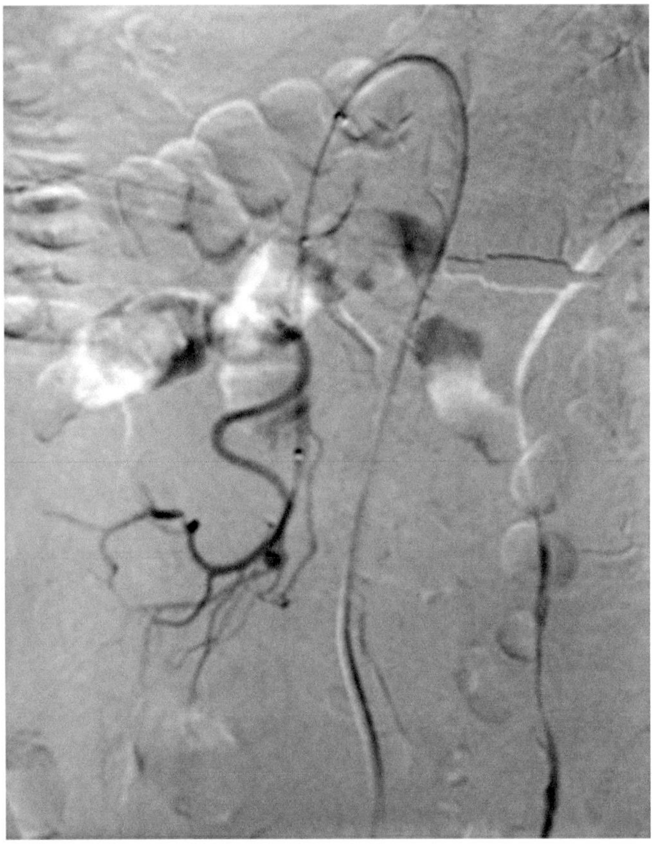

Fig. 19.25 Preoperative angiography

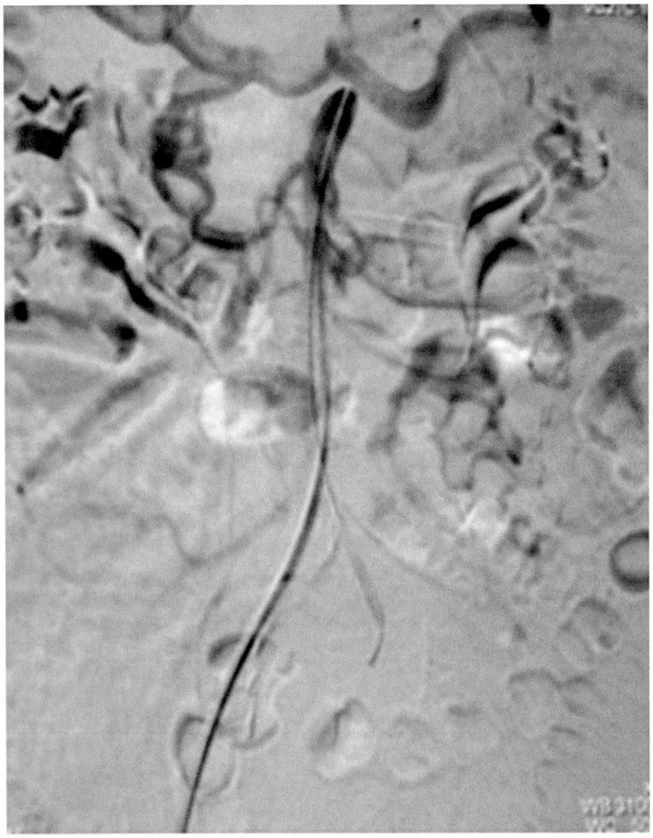

Fig. 19.26 Postoperative angiography

19.10.5 Technical Essentials and Precautions

- The patient had a previous history of atrial fibrillation and received no formal anticoagulation therapy. The acute mesenteric artery embolization was considered to be related to the breaking off of the intra-atrial emboli, the time from the onset to diagnosis exceeded 72 h, and the fact that embolic occlusion of the superior mesenteric artery resulted in secondary distal thrombolysis by the emboli could not be ruled out. Therefore, the patient was first treated with the superior mesenteric artery catheter-directed pulse thrombolysis for 30 min, which alleviated the thrombus burden in the superior mesenteric artery lesion. However, emboli thrombolytic effect was not obvious. To quickly remove the emboli and revascularize blood flow, Rotarex catheter was used for thrombus aspiration, which eliminated the secondary fresh thrombus and also cut the old thrombotic lesions into pieces with its rotary blade within the catheter, thus recanalizing blood flow.
- Acute superior mesenteric artery embolization is a life-threatening symptom for the vascular surgery, which, if not treated promptly, has high mortality. Patients of this kind should be treated with revascularization as soon as possible so as to restore their intestinal blood flow. Furthermore, considering the large number of bacteria in the intestine, it is a thorny problem to prevent intestinal reperfusion injury after revascularization. Fasting of drinking water should be required after revascularization and patient's situations closely observed, and diet could be taken only after no abdominal signs were seen.
- Anticoagulant therapy is very important for secondary thrombosis after superior mesenteric artery embolization, reducing intestinal ischemia symptoms and the scope of necrotic intestines and improving the prognosis of patients. Once the superior mesenteric artery embolization is confirmed, start anticoagulation treatment as soon as possible, and if necessary, conduct intravenous heparin anticoagulation.
- The patient with intestinal necrosis after acute superior mesenteric artery embolization should, on the one hand, go through exploratory laparotomy for resection and anastomosis of necrotic intestines and, on the other, have their blood flow of the superior mesenteric artery recovered as soon as possible. Traditional therapy resorts to simultaneous revascularization of artificial vascular bypass, which is complicated with abdominal infection for patients with intestinal necrosis and high incidence of postoperative graft infection. However, mechanical aspiration thrombectomy can revascularize blood flow within the blood vessels, leaving no grafts, thus reducing the risk of postoperative graft infection.
- During mechanical aspiration thrombectomy, the risk that emboli breaking off leads to distal embolization exists.

Therefore, aspiration thrombectomy should be conducted gently and carefully. Selectively insert infusion catheter to conduct pulse thrombolysis before aspiration, which can ease the burden of embolic secondary distal thrombus, thus reducing the risk of distal embolization.

19.11 Case 11 Coil Embolization Technique for Treatment of Giant Splenic Artery Aneurysm

19.11.1 Patient Data

The male patient, aged 46, was found with splenic artery aneurysm after color Doppler imaging in a physical examination in April 2015, and subsequent reexamination also showed splenic artery aneurysm. The patient was admitted for splenic artery aneurysm in May.

19.11.2 Surgical Operation

As shown by the preoperative CTA findings, a 5-cm-diameter cystic aneurysm near the porta lienis of the splenic artery, the proximal splenic artery of the aneurysm, looked like a tortuous S, and it was assessed to adopt peripheral stent graft for aneurysm repair. However, the peripheral stent graft guide system is thick and poor in flexibility, which is hard to reach the lesion site. Even the peripheral stent graft could reach the lesion site, the aneurysm might not be completely excluded upon stent deployment, and instead, it would occlude the surgical approach for the embolization of the splenic artery aneurysm, thus losing the chance for minimally invasive endovascular therapy. After comprehensive consideration of the patient's all indexes, finally Interlock controllable spring coil and Cook spring coil were selected for combined embolization treatment of the splenic artery aneurysm. The subject gave informed consent for the procedure.

19.11.3 Device Preparation

Refer to Table 19.21.

19.11.4 Procedures and Intraoperative Coordination Process

Refer to Table 19.22.

Table 19.21 Device preparation

Name	Qty.	Name	Qty.
Puncture needle (Cook)	1	5F Cobra Catheter (AngioDynamics)	1
High-pressure connector (SCW Medicath)	2	5F common pigtail catheter (Optimed)	1
0.035 in. common hydrophilic wire 260 cm (Terumo)	1	5F short sheath (Terumo)	1
0.014 in. PT2 wire 300 cm (Boston Scientific)	1	6F Ansel long sheath 45 cm (Cook)	1
0.018 in. Embolization 8 mm × 140 mm (Cook)	4	Renegade STC 18 microcatheter (Boston Scientific)	1
Interlock-18 controllable embolization 10 mm × 300 mm (Boston Scientific)	2	Interlock-35 controllable embolization 10 mm × 400 mm (Boston Scientific)	1
Interlock-18 controllable embolization 12 mm × 300 mm (Boston Scientific)	1	Interlock-35 controllable embolization 8 mm × 200 mm (Boston Scientific)	2
Interlock-18 controllable embolization 14 mm × 300 mm (Boston Scientific)	4	Embolization (0.035 in.) 8 mm × 140 mm (Cook)	2
Complex Helical-18 free embolization 11 mm × 170 mm (Boston Scientific)	1	Embolization (0.035 in.) 5 mm × 500 mm (Cook)	1
6F ProGlide vascular closure device (Abbott)	1		

Note: The devices listed above (*A* mm × *B* mm), wherein *A* is the diameter of the device and *B* the length

Table 19.22 Procedures and intraoperative coordination process

Procedures	Intraoperative coordination process
1. Patient enters the operation room	(1) Mental nursing; (2) keep the patient warm; (3) help to lie at supine position, with two lower limbs slightly at abduction and extorsion position; (4) connect ECG to observe changes in blood pressure, heart rate, and oxygen saturation; (5) establish intravenous infusion
2. Routinely sterilize the bilateral groins from the umbilical down to the midthigh, exposing the groins	Prepare disinfectant (heated to 98.6 °F with incubator), and assist with draping; deliver iodixanol injection; prepare heparin diluent (1000 mL normal saline +100 mg heparin sodium injection)

Table 19.22 (continued)

Procedures	Intraoperative coordination process
3. Puncture the right common femoral artery with modified Seldinger technique under local anesthesia, implant a 5F short sheath and a 0.035 in. common hydrophilic wire 260 cm, implant a 5F common pigtail catheter to above the abdominal aortic splenic artery opening along the hydrophilic wire, withdraw the hydrophilic wire, and conduct angiography, showing tortuous proximal end of the splenic artery and aneurysm at its distal end (Fig. 19.27)	Deliver 1% lidocaine injection, puncture needle, high-pressure connector, 5F short sheath, 0.035 in. common hydrophilic wire 260 cm, and 5F common pigtail catheter; perform systematic heparinization; intraoperative endovascular devices should be flushed with the prepared heparin diluent
4. Withdraw the 5F common pigtail catheter and 5F short sheath, exchange to implant a 6F Ansel long sheath 45 cm and a 5F Cobra catheter, coordinate the hydrophilic wire with the 5F Cobra catheter to superselect access into the splenic artery	Deliver the 6F Ansel long sheath 45 cm and 5F Cobra catheter
5. Withdraw the 0.035 in. common hydrophilic wire 260 cm, exchange it with a 0.014 in. PT2 wire 300 cm, implant a Renegade STC 18 microcatheter to superselect access into the splenic aneurysm via the PT2 wire	Deliver the 0.014 in. PT2 wire 300 cm and Renegade STC 18 microcatheter
6. Implantation of 0.018 in. spring coil: withdraw the PT2 wire, and implant seven Interlock-18 controllable embolizations, four Cook embolizations (0.018 in.), and one complex Helical-18 free embolization into the aneurysm cavity along the Renegade STC 18 microcatheter	Deliver two Interlock-18 controllable embolization 10 mm × 300 mm, one Interlock-18 controllable embolization 12 mm × 300 mm, four Interlock-18 controllable embolization 14 mm × 300 mm, four 0.018 in. Cook embolizations 8mm × 140 mm, and one complex Helical-18 free embolization 11 mm × 170 mm
7. Implantation of 0.035 in. embolization: withdraw Renegade STC 18 microcatheter, and implant three Interlock-35 controllable spring coils and three Cook embolizations into the splenic aneurysm cavity and inflow tract along the 5F Cobra catheter	Deliver one Interlock-35 controllable embolization 10 mm × 400 mm, two Interlock-35 controllable embolization 8 mm × 200 mm, and one 0.035 in. Cook embolization 5 mm × 50 mm
8. Manually inject the iodixanol diluent via the 5F Cobra catheter, and conduct angiography, showing significantly reduced blood flow in the splenic aneurysm cavity and obvious embolization effect achieved (Fig. 19.28)	
9. Withdraw the 5F Cobra catheter and the 6F Ansel long sheath, coordinate the hydrophilic wire with the 6F ProGlide vascular closure device to suture the puncture site on the right common femoral artery	Deliver the 6F ProGlide vascular closure device
10. Compression dressing on puncture site	Deliver the gauze and elastic bandage, assist with dressing, escort the patient safely back to ward

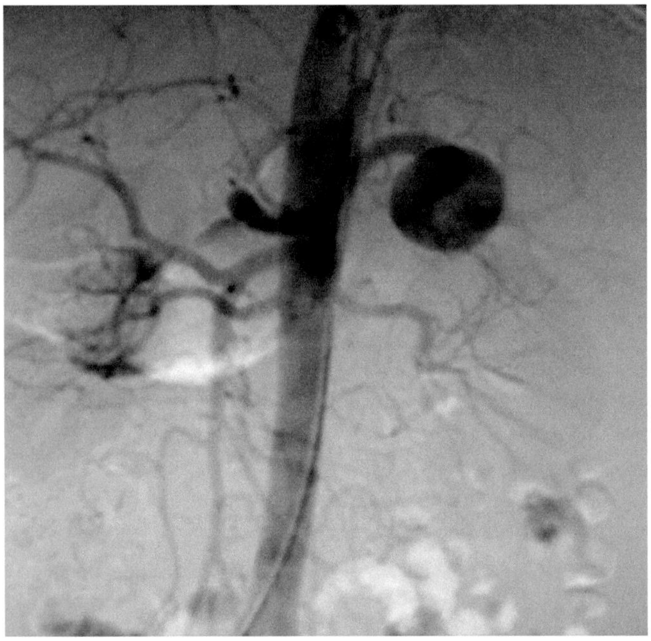

Fig. 19.27 Intraoperative angiography

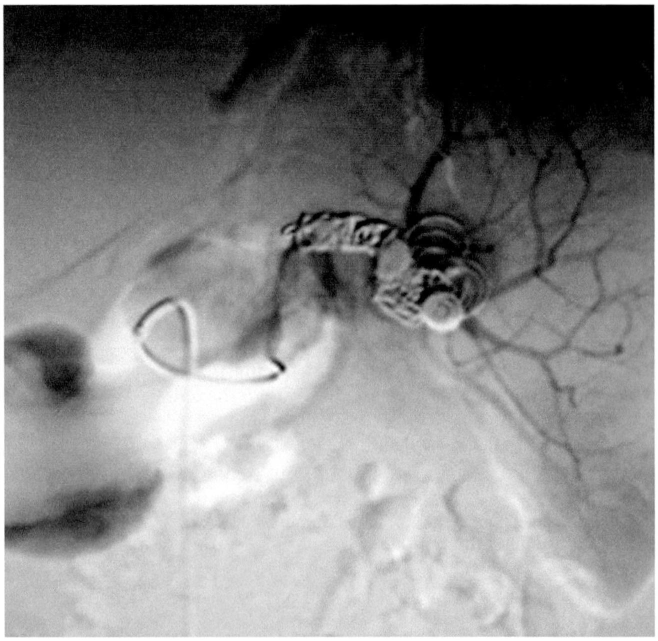

Fig. 19.28 Postoperative spring coil embolization angiography

19.11.5 Technical Essentials and Precautions

- Spring coil was used to fill the splenic artery aneurysm and inflow tract for the patient in this case, which has low technical requirements and is the main method for splenic artery aneurysm embolotherapy. Other endovascular therapies include aneurysm repair with peripheral stent graft, spring coil embolization assisted with self-expanding peripheral bare stent, etc. Aneurysm repair with peripheral stent graft requires smooth running of the guide approach and splenic artery, and this kind of lesions is mostly located at the beginning part of the splenic artery, which ensures the splenic blood flow is retained while conducting splenic artery aneurysm repair. However, due to thick delivery system, it is hard to introduce into the tortuous lesion. Therefore, the requirements for the anatomical site of this kind lesion are very high. The self-expanding peripheral bare stent is thinner than the stent graft system, easier to be advanced into the lesion site, which can retain the splenic blood supply and realize aneurysm embolization if assisted with spring coil embolization.
- Due to the tortuous splenic artery of the patient, the aneurysm is far from the abdominal trunk artery opening, and the aneurysm wall is thin. Therefore, operation must be carefully performed to avoid intraoperative rupture of the splenic artery aneurysm, and preparation should be made for open surgery. After operation, attention should be paid to the occurrence of the complications of spleen infarction. Spleen infarction is mostly focal infarction and often recovers after symptomatic treatment, which has no effect on the prognosis of the patient, but attention should be paid to the formation of abscess after spleen necrosis.

19.12 Case 12 Coil Embolization-Assisted Abdominal Aortoiliac Stent Technique for Endovascular Repair of Iliac Artery Aneurysm

19.12.1 Patient Data

The male patient, aged 49, presented himself with bilateral lower extremity numbness in March 2015, and DSA angiography showed right iliac artery aneurysm at another hospital. The patient was admitted to the hospital in April.

19.12.2 Surgical Operation

Intraoperative angiography showed the right iliac artery aneurysm was located at the bifurcation of the external and the internal iliac arteries. To completely exclude the aneurysm, it intended to use "spring coil embolization assisted with abdominal aorta iliac stent" technique, that is, to implant abdominal aortoiliac stent in the external iliac artery while using spring coil to embolize the internal iliac artery via the catheter retained in advance. The subject gave informed consent for the procedure.

19.12.3 Device Preparation

Refer to Table 19.23.

19.12.4 Procedures and Intraoperative Coordination Process

Refer to Table 19.24.

Table 19.23 Device preparation

Name	Qty.	Name	Qty.
Puncture needle (Cook)	1	4F Cobra catheter (AngioDynamics)	1
High-pressure connector (SCW Medicath)	2	5F common pigtail catheter (Optimed)	1
0.035 in. common hydrophilic wire 260 cm (Terumo)	2	5F short sheath (Terumo)	1
6F ProGlide vascular closure device (Abbott)	2	6F Balkin sheath 40 cm (Cook)	1
6F Angio-Seal vascular closure device (St. Jude)	1	5F Berenstein catheter (AngioDynamics)	1
5F super-slip catheter (Terumo)	1	0.035 in. Lunderquist super-stiff wire 260 cm (Cook)	1
Embolization 15 mm × 80 mm (Cook)	4	Endurant abdominal aortoiliac stent 16 mm × 13 mm × 95 mm (Medtronic)	1

Note: The devices listed above (A mm × B mm), wherein A is the diameter of the device and B the length; the abdominal aortic (aortoiliac) stent (A mm × B mm × C mm),
wherein A is the proximal diameter of the stent, B the distal diameter, and C the length

Table 19.24 Procedures and intraoperative coordination process

Procedures	Intraoperative coordination process
1. Patient enters the operation room	(1) Mental nursing; (2) keep the patient warm; (3) help to lie at supine position, with two lower limbs slightly at abduction and extorsion position; (4) connect ECG to observe changes in blood pressure, heart rate and oxygen saturation; (5) establish intravenous infusion
2. Routinely sterilize the bilateral groins from the umbilical down to the midthigh, exposing the groins	Prepare disinfectant (heated to 98.6 °F in incubator) and assist with draping; deliver iodixanol injection; prepare heparin diluent (1000 mL normal saline +100 mg heparin sodium injection)
3. Puncture the right common femoral artery with modified Seldinger technique under local anesthesia; implant a 5F short sheath, a 0.035 in. common hydrophilic wire 260 cm, and a 5F common pigtail catheter to the abdominal aorta; withdraw the hydrophilic wire; and conduct angiography, showing the right iliac artery lies at the bifurcation of the external and the internal iliac arteries (Fig. 19.29)	Deliver 1% lidocaine injection, puncture needle, high-pressure connector, 5Fshort sheath, 0.035 in. common hydrophilic wire 260 cm, and 5F common pigtail catheter; perform systematic heparinization; intraoperative endovascular devices should be flushed with the prepared heparin diluent
4. Puncture the left common femoral artery with modified Seldinger technique; implant 6F Balkin sheath 40 cm; sequentially use a 5F Berenstein catheter, a 4F Cobra catheter, and a 5F super-slip catheter to superselect access into the right internal iliac artery along the 0.035 in. common hydrophilic wire 260 cm; retain the 5F super-slip catheter in the right internal iliac artery; withdraw the 0.035 in. common hydrophilic wire 260 cm	Deliver the puncture needle, 6F Balkin sheath 40 cm, 0.035 in. common hydrophilic wire 260 cm, 5F Berenstein catheter, 4F Cobra catheter, and 5F super-slip catheter
5. Withdraw the 5F short sheath and 5F common pigtail catheter at the right common femoral artery, pre-implant two 6F ProGlide vascular closure devices	Deliver two 6F ProGlide vascular closure devices
6. Implant a 5F Berenstein catheter along the 0.035 in. common hydrophilic wire 260 cm on the right common femoral artery, exchange a 0.035 in. Lunderquist super-stiff wire 260 cm, withdraw the 5F Berenstein catheter, implant an Endurant abdominal aortoiliac stent 16 mm × 13 mm × 95 mm to external iliac artery via the super-stiff wire before deployment, withdraw the Endurant abdominal aortoiliac stent delivery system, implant the 5F common pigtail catheter, and conduct iliac artery angiography, showing endoleak with the right iliac aneurysm	Deliver the 0.035 in. Lunderquist super-stiff wire 260 cm and Endurant abdominal aortoiliac stent 16 mm × 13 mm × 95 mm
7. Implant four Cook embolizations 15 mm × 80 mm to the right internal iliac artery via the pre-implanted 5F super-slip catheter, and conduct iliac artery angiography again, showing right iliac aneurysm already excluded without obvious endoleak	Deliver four Cook embolizations 15 mm × 80 mm
8. Withdraw the catheter and vascular sheath, suture the right common femoral artery with the pre-implanted two 6F ProGlide vascular closure devices, and occlude the puncture site on the left common femoral artery with a 6F Angio-Seal vascular closure device	Deliver the 6F Angio-Seal vascular closure device
9. Compression dressing on puncture site	Deliver gauze and elastic bandage, assist with dressing

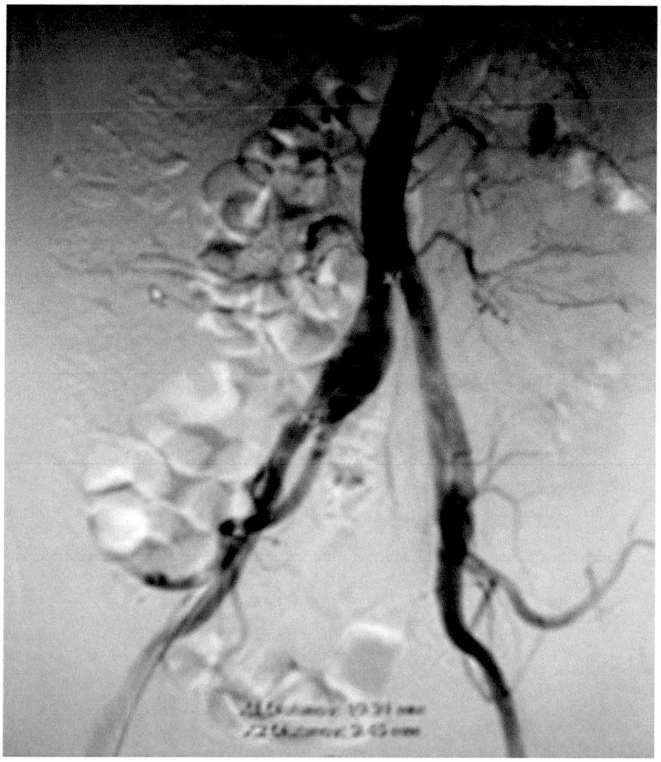

Fig. 19.29 Intraoperative angiography

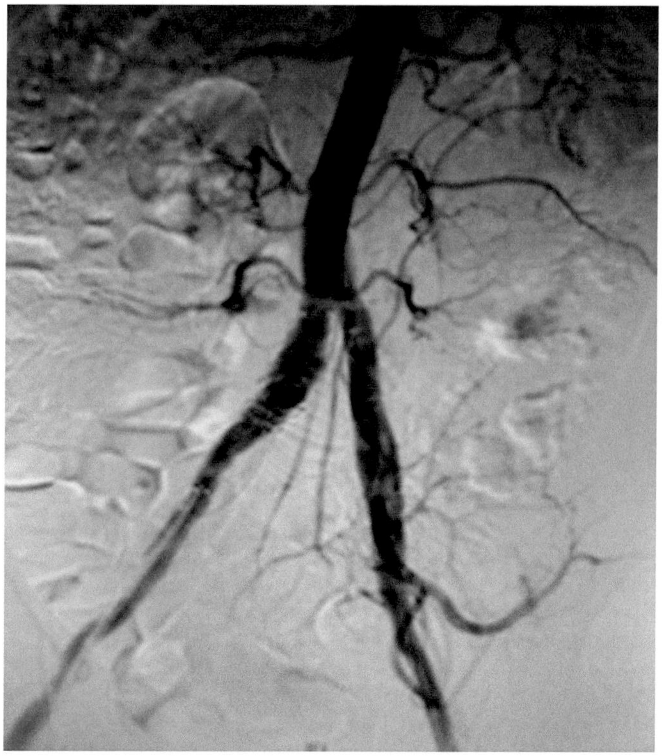

Fig. 19.30 Postoperative angiography

19.12.5 Technical Essentials and Precautions

- In order to avoid internal iliac artery reflux, the internal iliac artery often needs to be embolized, which may cause gluteal muscle limping, rectal ischemia, and other complications; the degree of ischemia depends on the collateral circulation after the internal iliac artery embolization. Generally, it is considered to retain at least unilateral internal iliac artery.
- There are many types of stent grafts, mainly depending on the position of the aneurysm. If necessary, integrated abdominal aortic stent can be selected to exclude the abdominal aorta and the iliac artery at the same time. Therefore, CTA should be carefully evaluated before operation, to understand the size of the tumor, the relationship between the internal iliac artery and the abdominal artery, the situation of the artery to be advanced, etc.

19.13 Case 13 Muff Coupling Technique for Lower Extremity Popliteal Aneurysm Repair

19.13.1 Patient Data

The male patient, aged 66, presented himself with sudden right limb soreness in May 2013, and a mass was palpated at the knee accompanied with strong throbbing. CT examination showed obvious enlargement of right popliteal artery, and the patient was admitted for "lower extremity popliteal aneurysm."

19.13.2 Surgical Operation

As shown by intraoperative angiography, the affected limb was tortuous from the inferior superficial femoral artery to the popliteal artery and accompanied with abnormal and uneven enlargement. According to DSA measurement, the diameter of the distal superficial femoral artery was enlarged to 30.8 mm and that of the popliteal artery to 42.7 mm (Fig. 19.31). The diameters of the superficial femoral artery and the popliteal artery of the patient were seven to eight times larger than normal, and once the aneurysm ruptured, massive hemorrhage would happen. Considering uneven and tortuous enlargement from the superficial femoral artery to the popliteal artery, where the proximal anchorage diameter reached 13 mm and distal 7.5 mm, it intended to con-

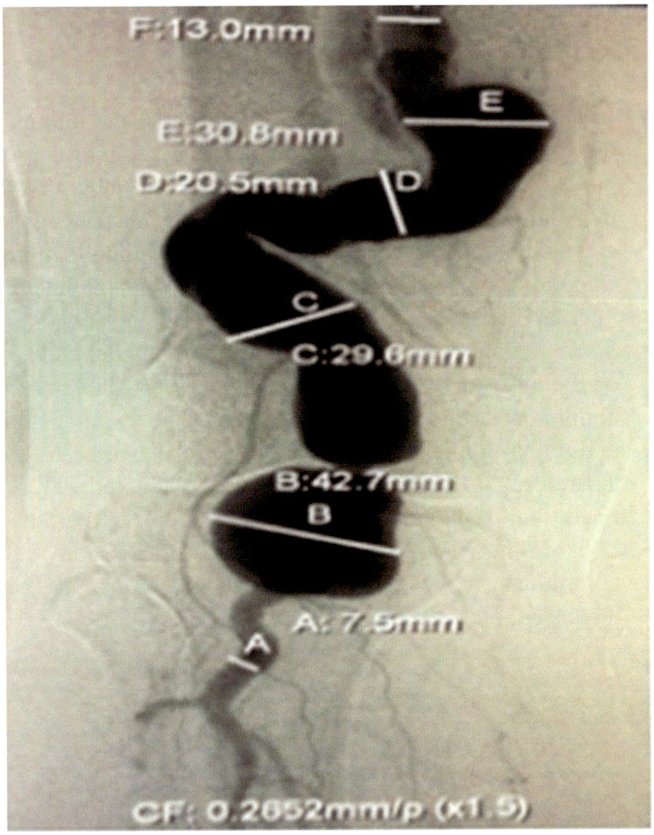

Fig. 19.31 Precision intraoperative measurement

duct aneurysm repair by "muff coupling" technique to deploy the peripheral stent graft from small to large and from far to near. The subject gave informed consent for the procedure.

19.13.3 Device Preparation

Refer to Table 19.25.

19.13.4 Procedures and Intraoperative Coordination Process

Refer to Table 19.26.

Table 19.25 Device preparation

Name	Qty.	Name	Qty.
Puncture needle (Cook)	1	4F Berenstein catheter (AngioDynamics)	1
High-pressure connector (SCW Medicath)	2	5F common pigtail catheter (Optimed)	1
0.035 in. common hydrophilic wire 260 cm (Terumo)	1	5F short sheath (Terumo)	1
Viabahn peripheral stent graft 8 mm × 100 mm (Gore)	1	12F short sheath (Cook)	1
Viabahn peripheral stent graft 10 mm × 100 mm (Gore)	1	0.035 in. hardened hydrophilic wire 260 cm (Terumo)	1
Viabahn peripheral stent graft 11 mm × 100 mm (Gore)	1	6F ProGlide vascular closure device (Abbott)	2
Viabahn peripheral stent graft 13 mm × 100 mm (Gore) 1	1		

Note: The devices listed above (*A* mm × *B* mm), wherein *A* is the diameter of the device and *B* the length

Table 19.26 Procedures and intraoperative coordination process

Procedures	Intraoperative coordination process
1. Patient enters the operation room	(1) Mental nursing; (2) keep the patient warm; (3) help to lie at supine position, with two lower limbs slightly at abduction and extorsion position; (4) connect ECG to observe changes in blood pressure, heart rate, and oxygen saturation; (5) establish intravenous infusion
2. Routinely sterilize bilateral groins up to the navel and down to the midthigh, exposing the groin	Prepare disinfectant (heated to 98.6 °F in incubator), and assist with draping; deliver iodixanol injection; prepare heparin diluent (1000 mL normal saline +100 mg heparin sodium injection)
3. Puncture the left common femoral artery with modified Seldinger technique under local anesthesia, implant a 5F short sheath and 0.035 in. common hydrophilic wire 260 cm, implant a 5F common pigtail catheter to the abdominal aorta along the hydrophilic wire, withdraw the hydrophilic wire, and conduct angiography for iliac artery, superficial femoral artery, popliteal artery, and infrapopliteal artery, showing tortuous lesion from the right distal superficial femoral artery to the popliteal artery, accompanied with abnormal dilatation	Deliver 1% lidocaine injection, puncture needle, high-pressure connector, 5F short sheath, 0.035 in. common hydrophilic wire 260 cm, and 5F common pigtail catheter; perform systematic heparinization; intraoperative endovascular devices should be flushed with the prepared heparin diluent

Table 19.26 (continued)

Procedures	Intraoperative coordination process
4. Implant a common hydrophilic wire via the 5F common pigtail catheter, and exchange to a 4F Berenstein catheter; coordinately advance the catheter and wire to the distal end of the lesion site	Deliver the 4F Berenstein catheter
5. Muff coupling technique: withdraw the 5F short sheath and 4F Berenstein catheter, exchange to implant a 12F short sheath and a 0.035 in. hardened hydrophilic wire 260 cm, and implant and deploy the Viabahn peripheral stent grafts 8 mm × 100 mm, 10 mm × 100 mm, 11 mm × 100 mm, and 13 × 100 mm in sequence from the right popliteal artery to the inferior superficial femoral lesion site along the hardened hydrophilic wire (Fig. 19.32)	Deliver the 12F short sheath, 0.035 in. hardened hydrophilic wire 260 cm, and Viabahn peripheral stent grafts 8 mm × 100 mm, 10 mm × 100 mm, 11 mm × 100 mm, and 13 mm × 100 mm
6. Withdraw the Viabahn peripheral stent graft delivery system, and conduct right lower extremity angiography, showing popliteal aneurysm already excluded with distal vascular patency (Fig. 19.33)	
7. Withdraw the wire and short sheath, use two 6F ProGlide vascular closure devices to suture the puncture site on the right common femoral artery	Deliver the two 6F ProGlide vascular closure devices
8. Compression dressing on puncture site	Deliver the gauze and elastic bandage, assist with dressing

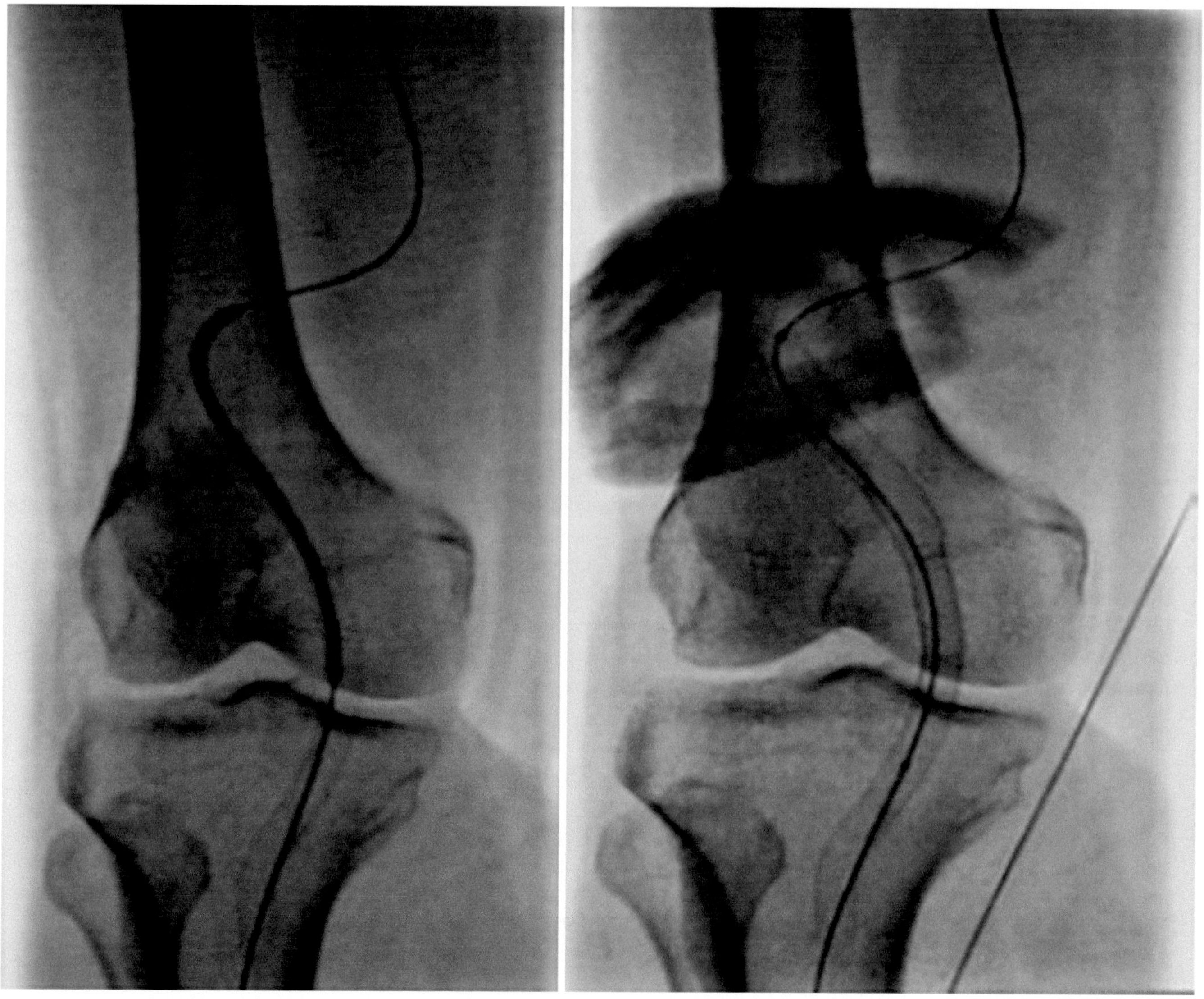

Fig. 19.32 Intraoperative stent graft deployment (right)

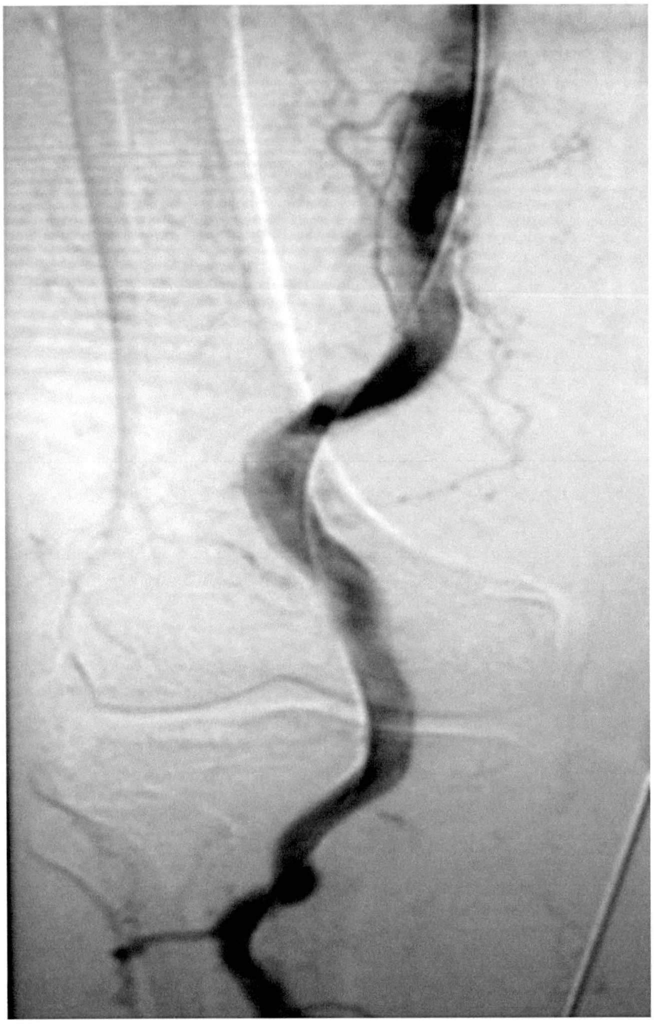

Fig. 19.33 Postoperative angiography

19.13.5 Technical Essentials and Precautions

- This case is very rare. Because the superficial femoral artery presented with full-range aneurysmal dilatation, traditional open bypass surgery may cause uncontrollable bleeding. Therefore, aneurysm repair technique by peripheral stent graft was selected. Moreover, because the patient's lesion was located at the popliteal artery and the long-term patency might decline after implantation of stent, so warfarin anticoagulation should be administered with the patient after operation.
- Considering different anchorage profiles between the popliteal artery and the superficial femoral artery, peripheral stent grafts with different profiles were selected for aneurysm repair by "muff coupling" technique. Furthermore, due to the severely tortuous artery lesion, it was difficult to advance the stent, and hardened wire with strong support should be used, and high-profile stent graft lacked matching long guide sheath in domestic market. Therefore, operation should be performed carefully when introducing the stent and using hardened or even super-stiff wire with strong support to enhance the supporting force and ensure smooth advancement of the stent system into the lesion site.

19.14 Case 14 Retrograde Approach with Stent Graft Technique for Treatment of Popliteal Arteriosclerosis Obliterans

19.14.1 Patient Data

The male patient, aged 73, presented himself with left lower extremity pelma ulcer in January 2013, and after conservative treatment in local hospital, ulcer area continually expanded with intermittent claudication. The patient was admitted for "left lower extremity arteriosclerosis obliterans."

19.14.2 Surgical Operation

Intraoperative angiography (Fig. 19.34) showed the left lower extremity popliteal artery segment occlusion. Firstly, puncture and cross via the right common femoral artery to revascularize the lower extremity artery. In case of severe atherosclerosis obliteration, it might be unavailable for the wire to revascularize the lesion site. It intended to conduct minimally invasive endovascular therapy for the left lower extremity popliteal artery occlusion by way of "retrograde approach revascularization" technique. The "retrograde approach revascularization" technique is to puncture the posterior tibial artery (also anterior, dorsalis pedis artery, etc.), reversely revascularize the occluded segment of the popliteal artery by wire and catheter so as to ensure docking of the wire and catheter tip with the catheter reversely crossing to the left superficial femoral artery via the right common femoral artery, and advance the wire out of the body via the right femoral artery catheter to establish the stretching wire. The subject gave informed consent for the procedure.

19.14.3 Device Preparation

Refer to Table 19.27.

19.14.4 Procedures and Intraoperative Coordination Process

Refer to Table 19.28.

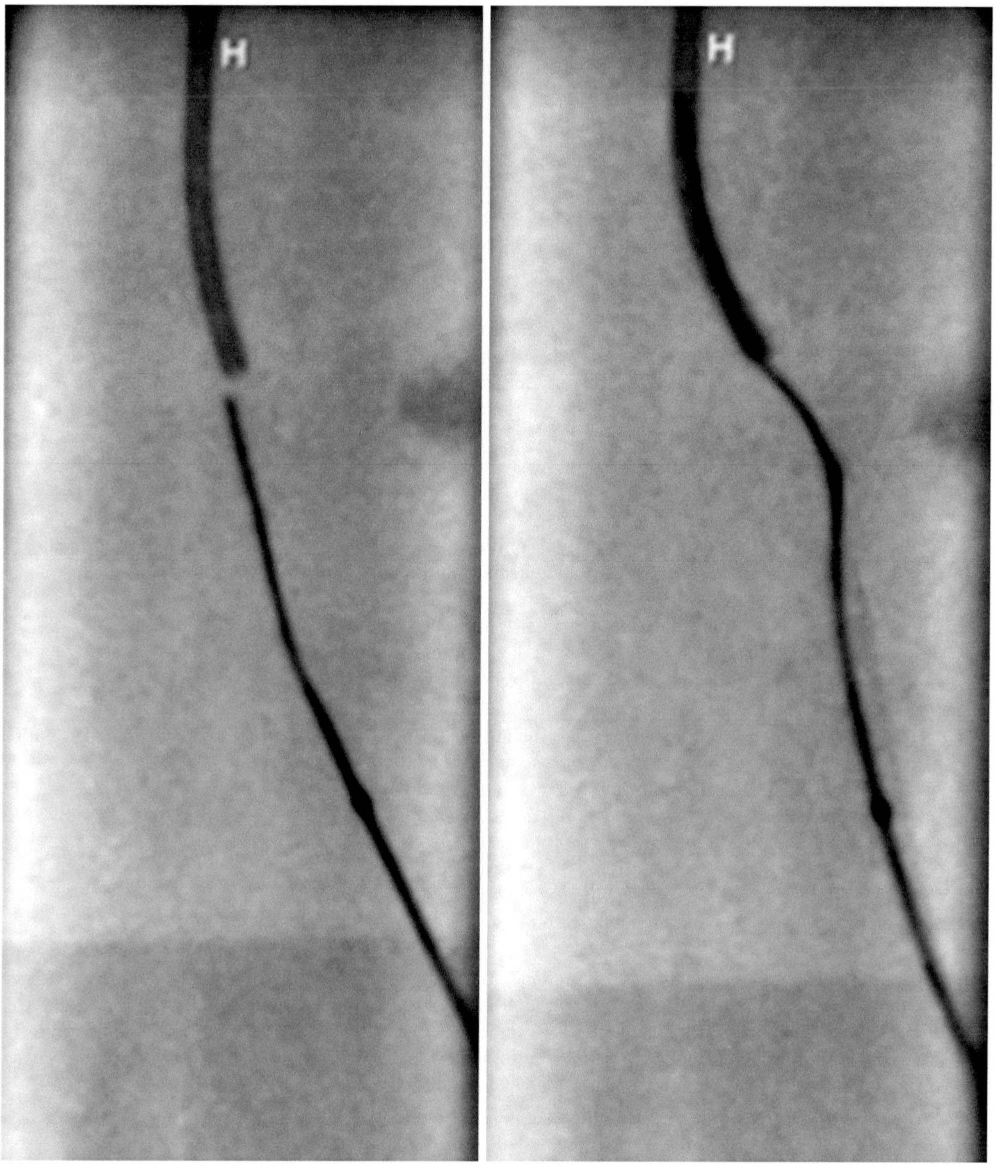

Fig. 19.34 "Docking" technique

Table 19.27 Device preparation

Name	Qty.	Name	Qty.
Puncture needle (Cook)	1	4F MPA catheter 125 cm (Cordis)	1
High-pressure connector (SCW Medicath)	2	5F common pigtail catheter (Optimed)	1
0.035 in. common hydrophilic wire 260 cm (Terumo)	1	5F short sheath (Terumo)	1
4F microsheath (Cook)	1	6F Balkin sheath 40 cm (Cook)	1
V-18 control wire 300 cm (Boston Scientific)	1	7F Balkin sheath 40 cm (Cook)	1
0.014 in. PT2 wire 300 cm (Boston Scientific)	1	6F ProGlide vascular closure device (Abbott)	1
Inflation device (Boston Scientific)	1	ReeKross18 balloon catheter 3 mm × 120 mm (Bard)	1
EverCross balloon catheter 5 mm × 100 mm (Medtronic)	1	Deep balloon catheter 2.5 mm × 120 mm (Medtronic)	1
Viabahn peripheral stent graft 5 mm × 100 mm (Gore)	1		

Note: The devices listed above (*A* mm × *B* mm), wherein *A* is the diameter of the device and *B* the length

Table 19.28 Procedures and intraoperative coordination process

Procedures	Intraoperative coordination process
1. Patient enters the operation room	(1) Mental nursing; (2) keep the patient warm; (3) help to lie at supine position, with two lower limbs slightly at abduction and extorsion position; (4) connect ECG to observe changes in blood pressure, heart rate, and oxygen saturation; (5) establish intravenous infusion
2. Sterilize the right groin up to the navel and down to the midthigh; sterilize left lower extremity up to the navel and down to the ankle	Prepare disinfectant (heated to 98.6 °F with incubator), and assist with draping; deliver iodixanol injection; prepare heparin diluent (1000 mL normal saline +100 mg heparin sodium injection)
3. Puncture the right common femoral artery with modified Seldinger technique under local anesthesia, implant a 5F short sheath and a 0.035 in. common hydrophilic wire 260 cm, implant a 5F common pigtail catheter to the abdominal aorta via the hydrophilic wire, and conduct left iliac artery, superficial femoral artery, popliteal artery, and infrapopliteal artery angiography, respectively, showing no imaging on the P2–P3 segments of the left lower extremity popliteal artery (Fig. 19.35)	Deliver 1% lidocaine injection, puncture needle, high-pressure connector, 5F short sheath, 0.035 in. common hydrophilic wire 260 cm, and 5F common pigtail catheter; perform systematic heparinization; intraoperative endovascular devices should be flushed with the prepared heparin diluent
4. Coordinately use the 0.035 in. common hydrophilic wire 260 cm with the 5F common pigtail catheter to cross and access into the left superficial femoral artery, withdraw the 5F common pigtail catheter, exchange to implant a 6F Balkin sheath and a 4F MPA catheter 125 cm along the hydrophilic wire, and revascularize the popliteal artery. Due to severe popliteal arteriosclerosis occlusion, lesion site is unable to be revascularized	Deliver the 6F Balkin sheath 40 cm and 4F MPA catheter 125 cm
5. "Retrograde puncture" technique: puncture the left posterior tibial artery with Seldinger technique under fluoroscopy; implant a 4F microsheath; implant a V-18 control wire 300 cm along the 4F microsheath to reversely perforate the popliteal artery occlusive segment till it reaches the superficial femoral artery; introduce the V-18 wire out of the body via the 4F MPA catheter by using docking technique to establish the stretching wire; access the 4F MPA catheter through the lesion segment along the stretching wire; and withdraw the V-18 wire	Deliver the 4F microsheath and V-18 control wire 300 cm
6. Infrapopliteal artery balloon dilatation: implant a 0.014 in. PT2 wire 300 cm into the infrapopliteal artery along the 4F MPA catheter 125 cm, and use a Deep balloon catheter 2.5 mm × 120 mm and a ReeKross18 balloon catheter 3 mm × 120 mm to dilate the infrapopliteal artery lesion site in sequence	Deliver the 0.014 in. PT2 wire 300 cm, Deep balloon catheter 2.5 mm × 120 mm, ReeKross 18 balloon catheter 2.5 mm × 120 mm, and inflation device
7. Withdraw the balloon catheter, and conduct angiography via the 6F Balkin sheath 40 cm, showing vascular patency of infrapopliteal artery	
8. Popliteal artery balloon dilatation: withdraw the 0.014 in. PT2 wire 300 cm and 6F Balkin sheath 40 cm, exchange to implant a 7F Balkin sheath and 0.035 in. common hydrophilic wire 260 cm, and implant an EverCross balloon catheter 5 mm × 100 mm to the popliteal artery lesion site for balloon dilatation via the hydrophilic wire	Deliver the 7F Balkin sheath 40 cm, 0.035 in. common hydrophilic wire 260 cm, and EverCross balloon catheter 5 mm × 100 mm
9. Implantation of peripheral stent graft: withdraw the EverCross balloon catheter, and implant a Viabahn peripheral stent graft 5 mm × 100 mm to popliteal artery lesion site along the 0.035 in. common hydrophilic wire 260 cm	Deliver the Viabahn peripheral stent graft 5 mm × 100 mm
10. Withdraw the Viabahn peripheral stent graft delivery system, and conduct angiography to the iliac artery, superficial femoral artery, and infrapopliteal artery in sequence via the 7F crossing sheath 40 cm, showing vascular patency of the left lower extremity artery (Fig. 19.36)	
11. Withdraw the wire and 7F Balkin sheath; suture the puncture site of the right common femoral artery with 6F ProGlide vascular closure device; withdraw the 4F microsheath; compress the left posterior tibial artery for 5–10 min till no bleeding is visible	Deliver the 6F ProGlide vascular closure device
12. Compression dressing on the puncture sites on the right common femoral artery and left posterior tibial artery	Deliver the gauze and elastic bandage, assist with dressing

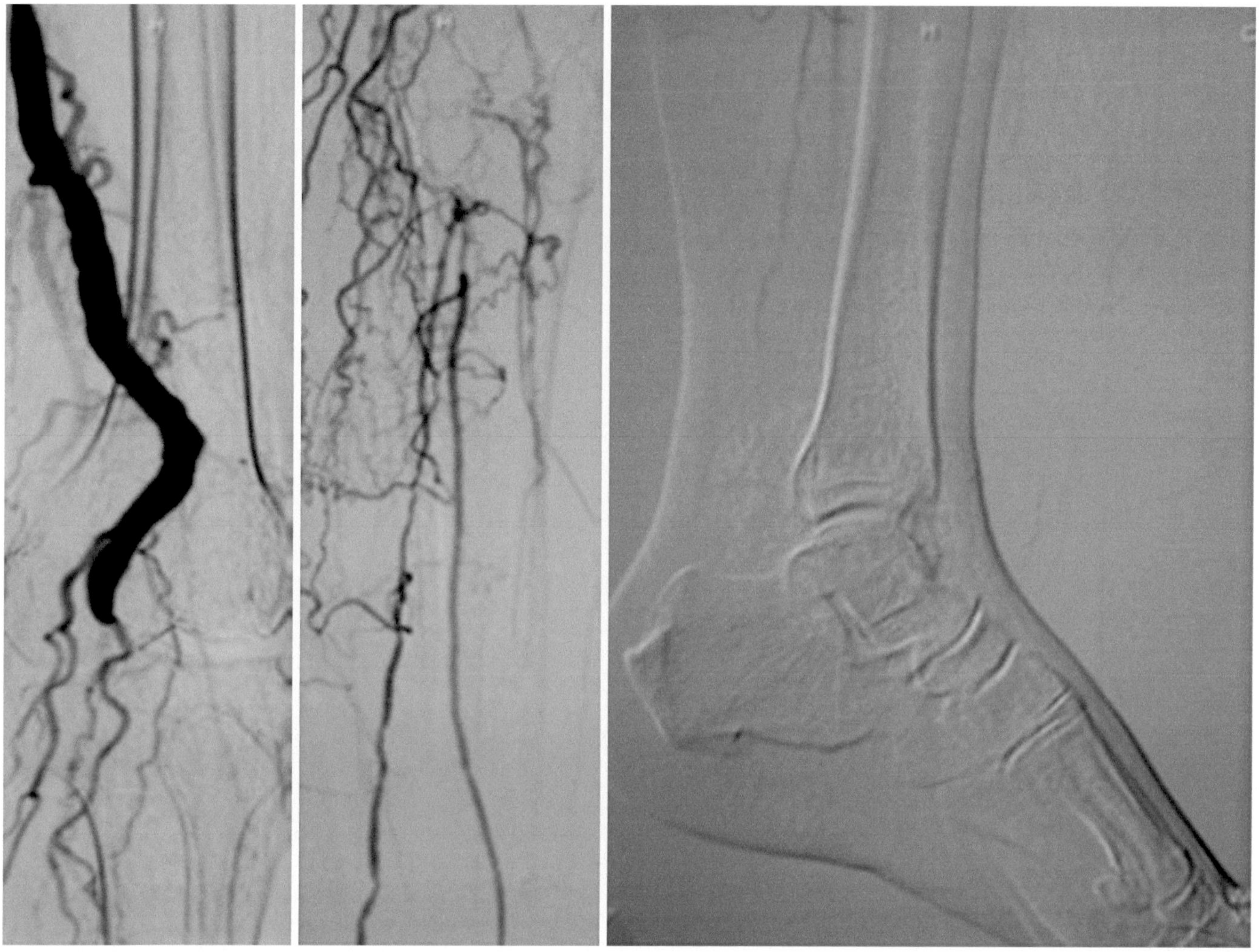

Fig. 19.35 Intraoperative angiography

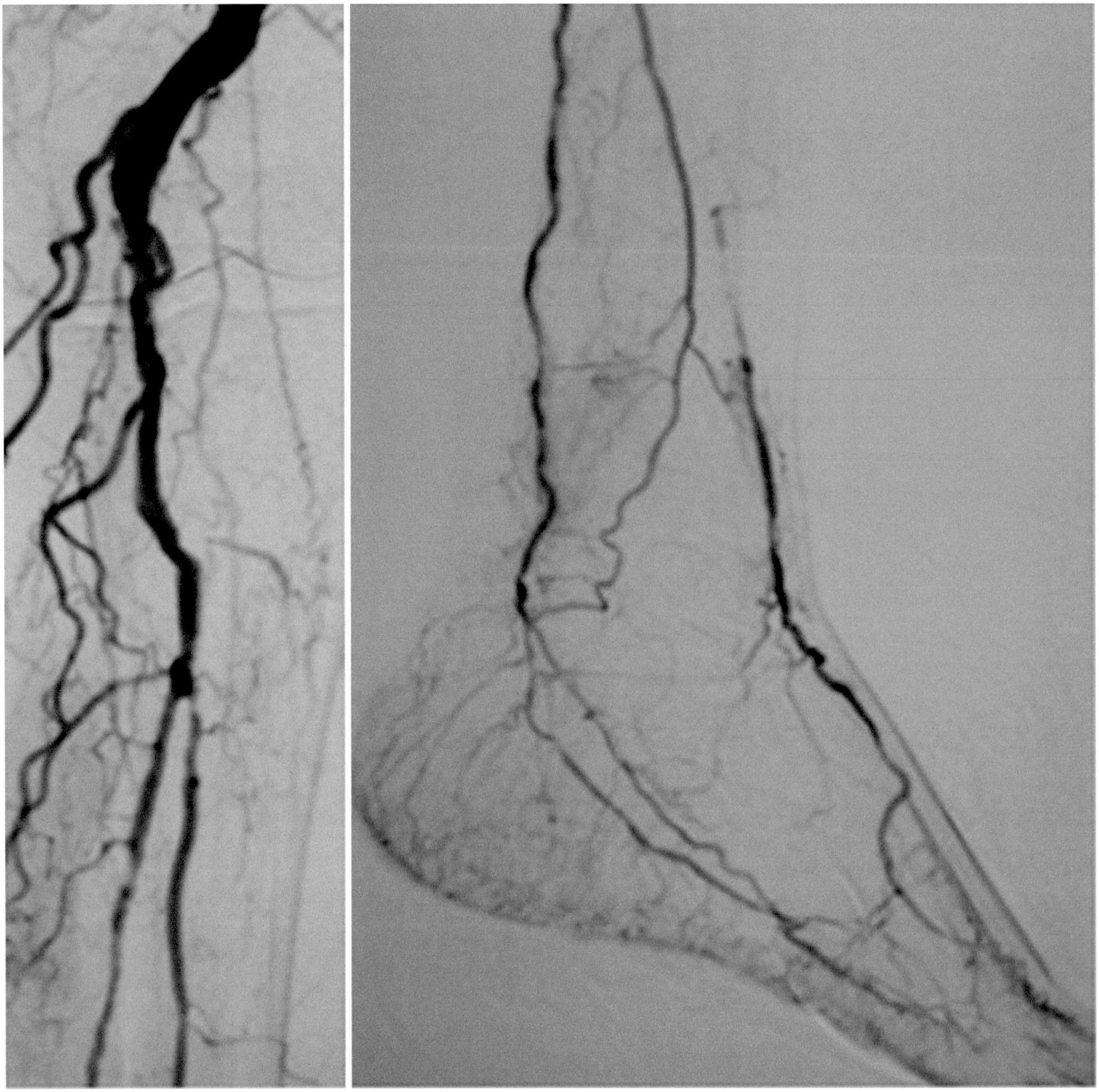

Fig. 19.36 Postoperative angiography

19.14.5 Technical Essentials and Precautions

- In anterograde revascularization of the distal occlusive segment of the popliteal artery in this case, the wire is liable of access into the subintima via the proximal end of the occlusive segment and hard to go back into the true lumen. Usually it can return to the true lumen only in the infrapopliteal artery. Otherwise, it is liable of damaging many normal blood vessels.
- Because of many collateral circulations around the popliteal artery, catheter and wire are liable of entering the downward collateral blood vessels at the proximal end of the occlusive segment, making further revascularization unavailable. If infrapopliteal artery retrograde puncture is used to implant catheter and wire for revascularization, it can not only avoid interference by bifurcated small arteries but also provide strong support for the catheter and wire because of the straight running of the infrapopliteal artery, which facilitates access through the occlusive segment of the popliteal artery.
- In most of the lower limb lesions, retrograde revascularization is often smoother, which may relate to the different pathological structures on the both ends of the occlusive vascular lesions. Proximal vascular occlusion presents with obvious atherosclerotic calcification and relatively hard plaque and fibrous cap texture; distal thrombosis is relatively fresh, with relatively soft fibrous cap texture. If infrapopliteal artery retrograde puncture is used, the retrograde wire first passes through the occlusive blood vessels of the soft segment, the blood vessel in the remaining hard occlusive segment is rather short, and therefore, success rate of revascularization is high.
- For the retrograde puncture of the infrapopliteal artery, ultrasound-guided puncture technique can be used, or puncture is conducted under real-time DSA imaging or road map. Before the retrograde puncture, first conduct angiography to determine the location, profile, and running direction of the infrapopliteal artery. In operation, blood vessel with large lumen, straight running, and no plaque is generally selected to facilitate puncture.

19.15 Case 15 Direct Stent Puncture Technique for Treatment of In-Stent Restenosis of Femoropopliteal Artery

19.15.1 Patient Data

The male patient, aged 61, suffered from lower extremity arteriosclerosis occlusion for years. In June 2011, the patient received "right lower extremity artery and left iliac artery stent angioplasty" at another hospital. In February 2013, the patient presented with right lower extremity intermittent claudication and was admitted for "in-stent restenosis of femoropopliteal artery."

19.15.2 Surgical Operation

Intraoperative angiography showed total occlusion from the superficial femoral artery opening to the inferior superficial femoral artery. If revascularization was conducted by crossing to the right lower extremity through puncturing the left common femoral artery, the catheter and wire might not be able to access the occlusive stent and through the lesion site. After assessment, it intended to use direct stent puncture technique (DSPT), that is, the retrograde puncture of the stent by the puncture needle under DSA fluoroscopy (Fig. 19.37). The subject gave informed consent for the procedure. This technique features simple puncture, safety and avoidance of the severe hyperplasia at both ends of the stent, and less complications.

19.15.3 Device Preparation

Refer to Table 19.29.

19.15.4 Procedures and Intraoperative Coordination Process

Refer to Table 19.30.

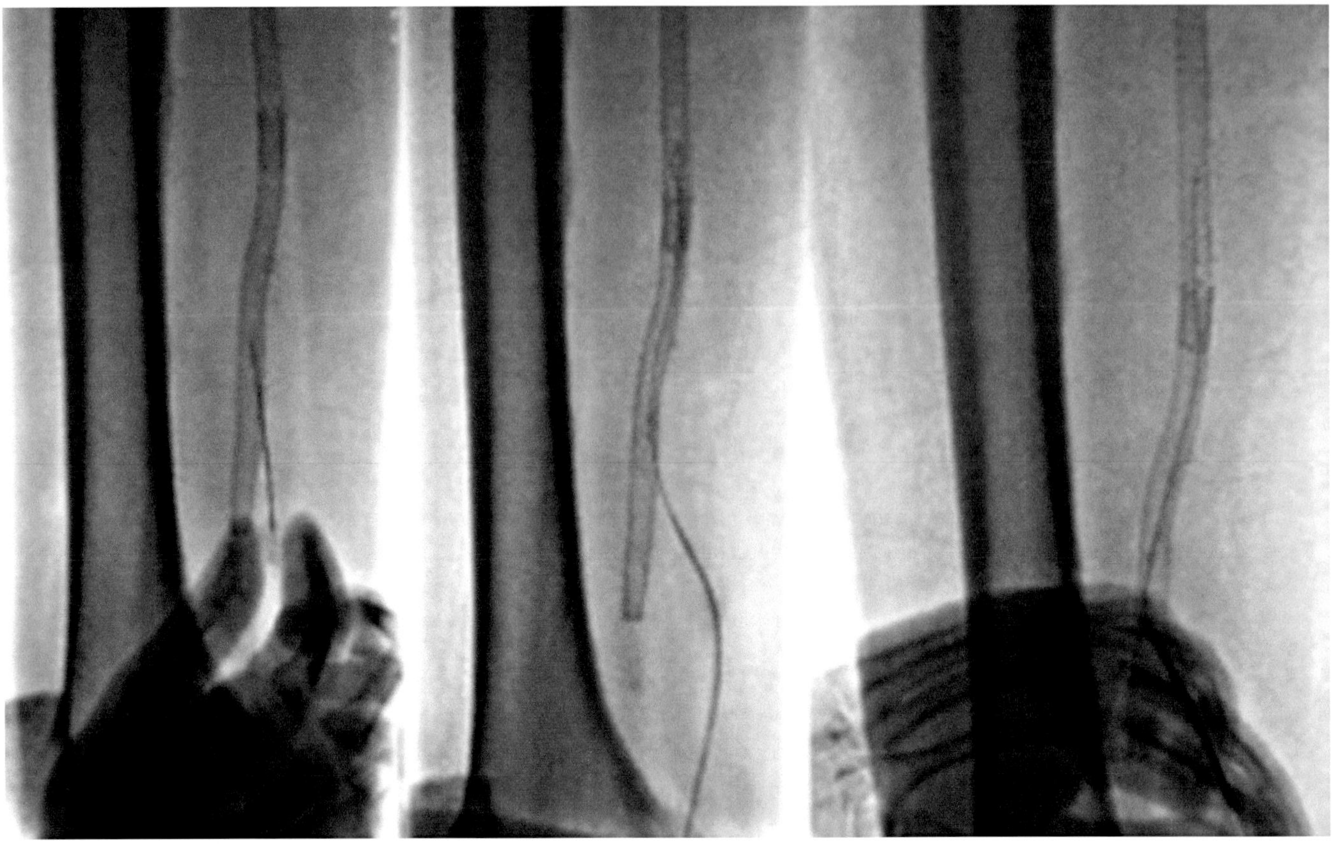

Fig. 19.37 Direct stent puncture technique

Table 19.29 Device preparation

Name	Qty.	Name	Qty.
Puncture needle (Cook)	1	4F MPA catheter 125 cm (Cordis)	1
High-pressure connector (SCW Medicath)	2	5F common pigtail catheter (Optimed)	1
0.035 in. common hydrophilic wire 260 cm (Terumo)	1	Inflation device (Boston Scientific)	1
0.035 in. hardened hydrophilic wire 260 cm (Terumo)	1	Admiral balloon catheter 6 mm × 120 mm (Medtronic)	1
5F short sheath (Terumo)	1	ReeKross18 balloon catheter 2.5 mm × 120 mm (Bard)	1
6F Balkin sheath 40 cm (Cook)	1	0.014 in. PT2 wire 300 cm (Boston Scientific)	1
Complete SE (self-expanding) peripheral bare stent 6 mm × 120 mm (Medtronic)	1	6F ProGlide vascular closure device (Abbott)	1
Omnilink balloon-expandable peripheral bare stent 8 mm × 29 mm (Abbott)	1		

Note: The devices listed above (*A* mm × *B* mm), wherein *A* is the diameter of the device and *B* the length

Table 19.30 Procedures and intraoperative coordination process

Procedures	Intraoperative coordination process
1. Patient enters the operation room	(1) Mental nursing; (2) keep the patient warm; (3) help to lie at supine position, with two lower limbs slightly at abduction and extorsion position; (4) connect ECG to observe changes in blood pressure, heart rate, and oxygen saturation; (5) establish intravenous infusion
2. Sterilize the left groin up to the navel and down to the midthigh; sterilize right lower limb up to the navel and down to the knee joint	Prepare disinfectant (heated to 98.6 °F with incubator), and assist with draping; deliver iodixanol injection; prepare heparin diluent (1000 mL normal saline +100 mg heparin sodium injection)
3. Conduct the retrograde puncture to the left common femoral artery with modified Seldinger technique under local anesthesia, implant a 5F short sheath and a 0.035 in. common hydrophilic wire 260 cm, implant a 5F common pigtail catheter to the abdominal aorta along the hydrophilic wire, and conduct angiography for iliac artery, superficial femoral artery, popliteal artery, and infrapopliteal artery, showing stenosis of the right iliac artery, total occlusion from the superficial femoral artery opening to its inferior segment, and stenosis of popliteal and infrapopliteal arteries (Fig. 19.38)	Deliver 1% lidocaine injection, puncture needle, high-pressure connector, 5F short sheath, 0.035 in. common hydrophilic wire 260 cm, and 5F common pigtail catheter; perform systematic heparinization; intraoperative endovascular devices should be flushed with the prepared heparin diluent
4. Coordinate 0.035 in. common hydrophilic wire 260 cm with 5F common pigtail catheter to cross to and access into the right lower limb, withdraw the 5F common pigtail catheter and 5F short sheath, and exchange and implant a 6F Balkin sheath and 4F MPA catheter 125 cm along the hydrophilic wire	Deliver the 6F Balkin sheath 40 cm and 4F MPA catheter 125 cm
5. Use the 0.035 in. common hydrophilic wire 260 cm and the 0.035 in. hardened hydrophilic wire 260 cm successively to coordinate with the 4F MPA catheter 125 cm to revascularize the right lower limb, and the wire fails to access through the occlusive segment due to severe in-stent occlusion	Deliver the 0.035 in. hardened hydrophilic wire 260 cm
6. Direct stent puncture technique: conduct retrograde puncture to the distal end of the stent of the inferior right superficial femoral artery by puncture needle, implant the 0.035 in. common hydrophilic wire 260 cm via the end of the puncture needle, implant the common hydrophilic wire reversely into the right common femoral artery, and docking with the tip of the 6F Balkin sheath 40cmon the left common femoral artery, introduce the hydrophilic wire out of the body via the 6F crossing sheath by "sheath penetrating" technique to establish a stretching wire; implant the 4F MPA catheter 125 cm through the occlusive segment of the stent along the stretching wire	Deliver the puncture needle and 0.035 in. common hydrophilic wire 260 cm
7. Withdraw the 4F MPA catheter 125 cm, implant an Admiral balloon catheter 6 mm × 120 mm along the common hydrophilic wire to the stent's occlusive segment, and dilate it	Deliver the Admiral balloon catheter 6 mm × 120 mm and inflation device
8. Implantation of superficial femoral artery stent: withdraw the Admiral balloon catheter, implant a Complete SE (self-expanding) peripheral bare stent 6 mm × 120 mm to the superficial femoral artery opening and the proximal end of the occlusive stent via the wire (the distal end of the Complete SE stent is overlapped with the proximal end of the occlusive stent for 10 mm), and deploy it	Deliver the Complete SE (self-expanding) peripheral bare stent 6 mm × 120 mm
9. Implantation of iliac artery stent: withdraw the Complete SE (self-expanding) peripheral bare stent delivery system, implant an Omnilink balloon-expandable peripheral bare stent 8 mm × 29 mm along the 0.035 in. common hydrophilic wire 260 cm to the right iliac artery lesion site, and deploy it	Deliver the Omnilink balloon-expandable peripheral bare stent 8 mm × 29 mm and inflation device
10. Balloon dilatation of infrapopliteal artery: withdraw the balloon-expandable peripheral bare stent delivery system; exchange to a 0.014 in. PT2 wire 300 cm, and advance it to the infrapopliteal artery; implant a ReeKross18 balloon catheter 2.5 mm × 120 mm along the PT2 wire; and dilate the infrapopliteal artery lesion sites successively	Deliver the 0.014 in. PT2 wire 300 cm and ReeKross18 balloon catheter 2.5 mm × 120 mm
11. Withdraw the balloon catheter, and conduct angiography for iliac, superficial femoral, popliteal, and infrapopliteal arteries via the 6F Balkin sheath, showing vascular patency of the right lower extremity artery (Fig. 19.39)	
12. Withdraw the wire and 6F Balkin sheath, suture the puncture site on the left common femoral artery with 6F ProGlide vascular closure device, compress the puncture site on the right superficial femoral artery for 5–10 min till no presence of bleeding	Deliver the 6F ProGlide vascular closure device
13. Compression dressing on puncture site	Deliver the gauze and elastic bandage; assist with dressing

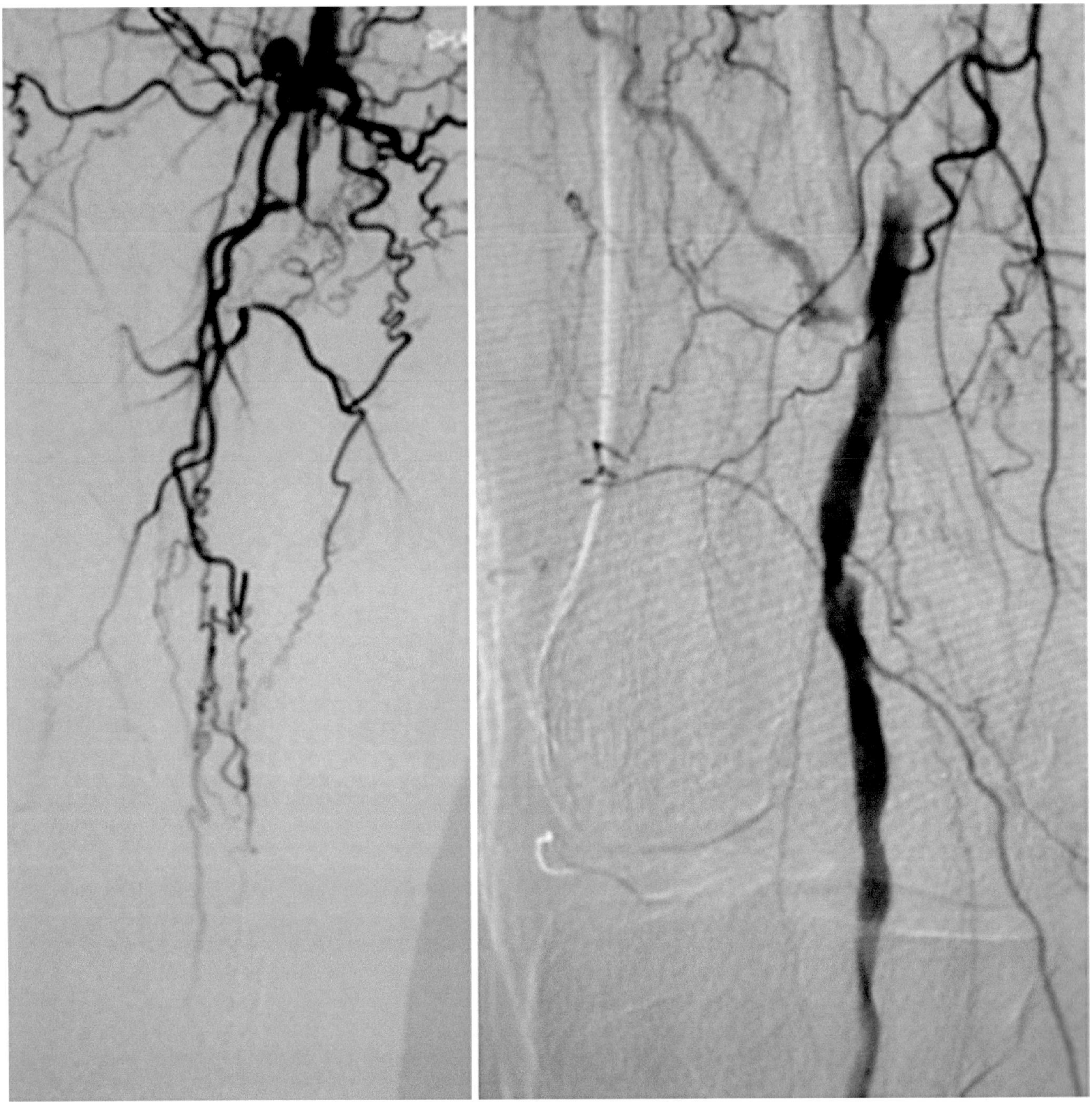

Fig. 19.38 Intraoperative angiography

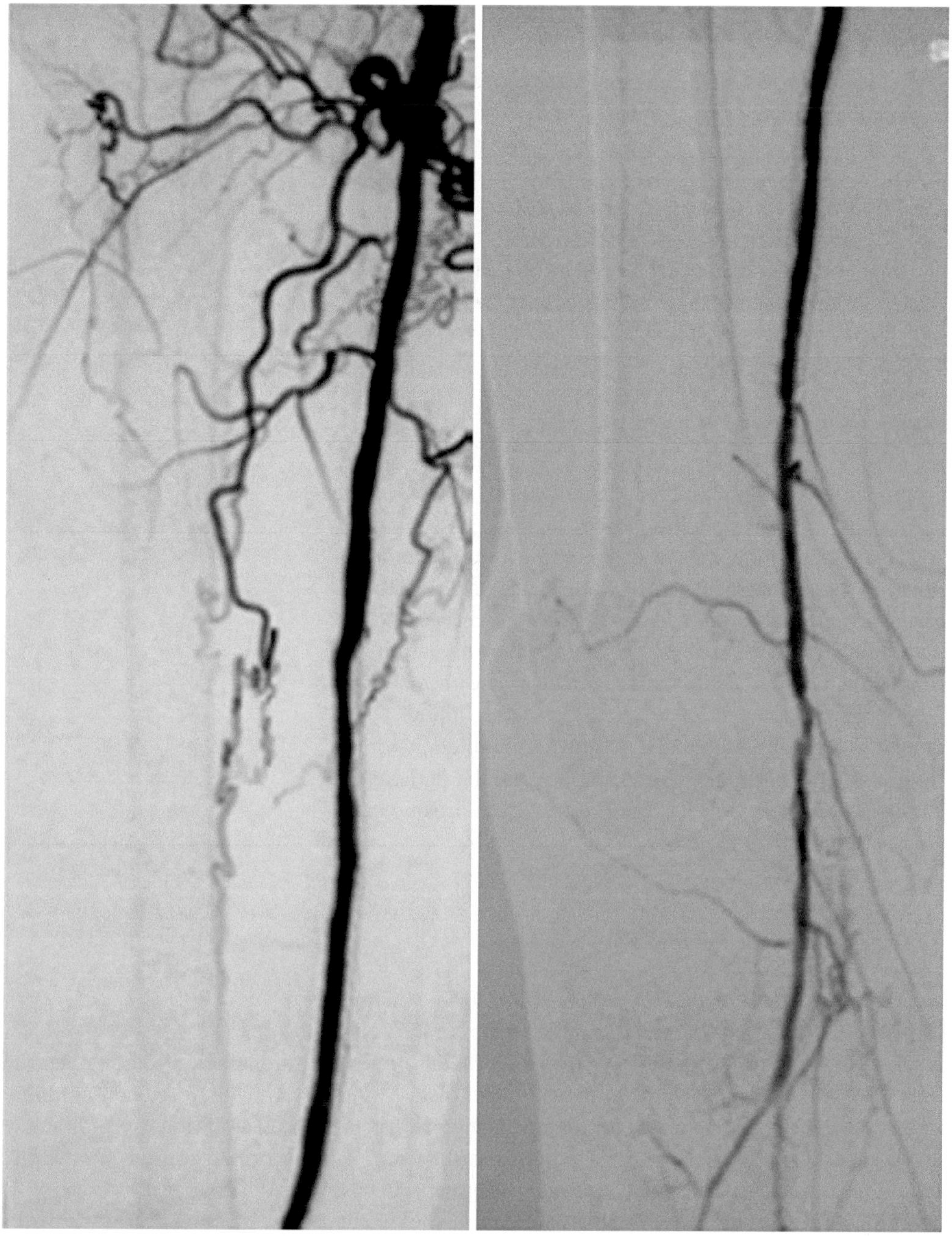

Fig. 19.39 Postoperative angiography

19.15.5 Technical Essentials and Precautions

- After understanding the lesion during operation through angiography, puncture the distal end of the stent under DSA fluoroscopy. The difficulty in puncture lies in that there is no return blood in the occlusive stent, and therefore it needs to repeatedly verify whether the wire is in the vascular lumen of the stent. After reverse access through the in-stent stenotic lesion by the wire, pull out the wire from the contralateral penetrating sheath by "sheath penetrating" technique to form the stretching wire before endovascular therapy.
- In-stent restenosis is one of the difficulties in the treatment of lower extremity arterial occlusive lesions. If the wire cannot access the proximal end of the occlusive stent and there is no normal blood vessel for retrograde puncture at the distal end of the occlusive blood vessel, then puncture stent will be the choice for endovascular therapy. Common balloon dilatation, cutting balloon dilatation, atherectomy, and other techniques can be chosen for the

treatment of in-stent restenosis. Drug-coated balloon and drug-eluting stent have a good therapeutic effect for in-stent stenosis treatment and are expected for early clinical practice in China.

19.16 Case 16 Retrograde Puncture and Bionic Stent Technique for Treatment of Seriously Calcified Femoral Artery Bifurcation Lesion

19.16.1 Patient Data

The male patient, aged 84, presented himself with cold feeling on the right lower extremity without obvious cause, accompanied with intermittent claudication, in 2016. The patient had CTA examination at our hospital on March 15, 2017, showing "bilateral lower extremities multiple arteriosclerosis occlusion, right femoral artery occlusion and bilateral anterior tibial artery occlusion." The patient was treated with "the left lower extremity artery balloon dilatation and stent implantation" technique under local anesthesia along with postoperative antiplatelet anticoagulant therapy. The patient was suggested to receive endovascular therapy for the right lower extremity. For further treatment, the patient was admitted for "right lower extremity arteriosclerosis occlusion" in April 2017.

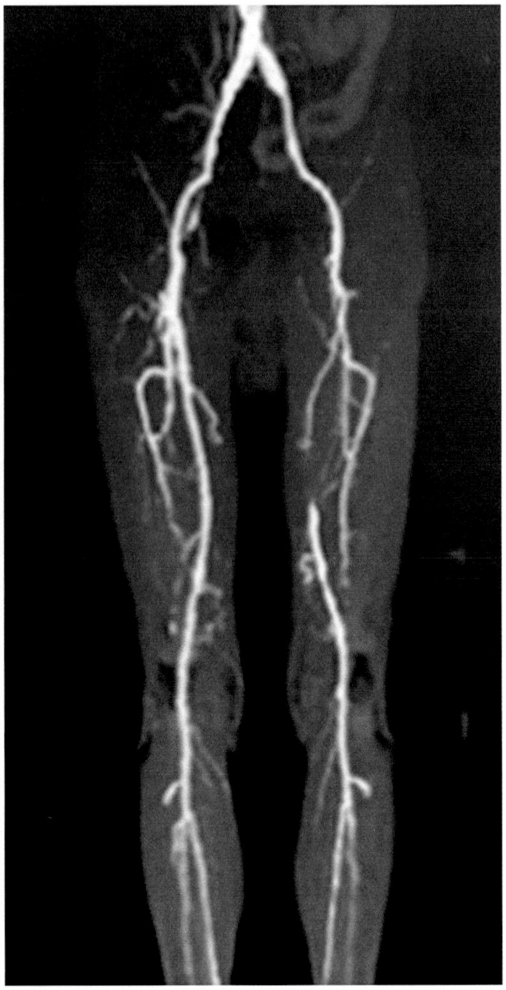

Fig. 19.40 Preoperative CTA

19.16.2 Surgical Operation

According to the patient's lower limb CTA findings (Fig. 19.40), it was considered to conduct anterograde revascularization by crossing to the right superficial femoral artery. In case of severe calcification that makes distal vascularization unavailable, conduct retrograde puncture for the distal superficial femoral artery or popliteal artery, and try bidirectional revascularization of the lesion segment. In case revascularization succeeds, first dilate the lesion site by cutting balloon with appropriate profile, and if post-dilatation effect is poor, implant self-expanding peripheral bionic bare stent, the reason for which is that the lesion segment is severely calcified and poses high requirement for stent support, while this stent not only has sound support but also can have its local compactness adjusted upon deployment to achieve the optimal therapeutic effect according to local lesion and calcification situation. However, in using this stent, it requires to pre-dilate the lesion site before stent implantation to come near to or even reach the stent diameter. Therefore, non-compliant high-pressure balloon larger than traditional pre-dilatation is required. The subject gave informed consent for the procedure.

19.16.3 Device Preparation

Refer to Table 19.31.

19.16.4 Procedures and Intraoperative Coordination Process

Refer to Table 19.32.

Table 19.31 Device preparation

Name	Qty.	Name	Qty.
Puncture needle (Cook)	1	V-18 control wire 300 cm (Boston Scientific)	1
High-pressure connector (SCW Medicath)	3	4F short sheath (Cordis)	1
0.035 in. common hydrophilic wire 260 cm (Terumo)	1	6F ProGlide vascular closure device (Abbott)	1
5F common pigtail catheter (Cordis)	1	Pacific balloon catheter 6 mm × 80 mm (Medtronic)	1
4F MPA catheter 125 cm (Cordis)	1	Admiral balloon catheter 6 mm × 40 mm (Medtronic)	1
7F Balkin sheath 40 cm (Cook)	1	Peripheral cutting balloon catheter 6 mm × 20 mm (Boston Scientific)	1
Inflation device (Boston Scientific)	1	Supera self-expanding peripheral bare stent 5.5 mm × 120 mm (Abbott)	1
0.018 in. Rubicon support catheter 150 cm (Boston Scientific)	1		

Note: The devices listed above (*A* mm × *B* mm), wherein *A* is the diameter of the device and *B* the length

Table 19.32 Procedures and intraoperative coordination process

Procedures	Intraoperative coordination process
1. Patient enters the operation room	(1) Mental nursing; (2) keep the patient warm; (3) help to lie at supine position, with two lower limbs slightly at abduction and extorsion position; (4) connect ECG to observe changes in blood pressure, heart rate, and oxygen saturation; (5) establish intravenous infusion
2. Sterilize the left groin up to the navel and down to the midthigh; sterilize right lower limb up to the navel and down to the middle calf	Prepare disinfectant (heated to 98.6 °F with incubator), and assist with draping; deliver iodixanol injection; prepare heparin diluent (1000 mL normal saline +100 mg heparin sodium injection)
3. Conduct retrograde puncture to the left common femoral artery with modified Seldinger technique under local anesthesia, implant a 7F Balkin sheath 40 cm and a 0.035 in. common hydrophilic wire 260 cm, implant a 5F common pigtail catheter to the abdominal aorta along the hydrophilic wire, and conduct angiography for right iliac artery, superficial femoral artery, popliteal artery, and infrapopliteal artery, respectively, showing lumen occlusion due to calcified plaque near the bifurcation of the right common femoral artery, with 5 cm occlusion length for the initial segment of the right superficial femoral artery and the superficial femoral artery at the lesion segment being calcified seriously, right anterior tibial artery occlusion, but normal patency of the right peroneal artery and posterior tibial artery (Fig. 19.41)	Deliver 1% lidocaine injection, puncture needle, high-pressure connector, 7F Balkin sheath, 0.035 in. common hydrophilic wire, and 5F common pigtail catheter 260 cm; perform systematic heparinization; intraoperative endovascular devices should be flushed with the prepared heparin diluent
4. Coordinate 0.035 in. common hydrophilic wire 260 cm with 5F common pigtail catheter to cross and to access into the right common femoral artery, withdraw the 5F common pigtail catheter, exchange to implant the a4F MPA catheter 125 cm along the hydrophilic wire to coordinate in revascularizing the right superficial femoral artery. After multiple trials, it is unable to revascularize from the proximal end. Then withdraw the 4F MPA catheter, and exchange to implant a V-18 control wire and 0.018 in. Rubicon support catheter, but it is still unable to revascularize from the proximal end (Fig. 19.42)	Deliver the 4F MPA catheter 125 cm, V-18 control wire 300 cm, and 0.018 in. Rubicon supporting catheter 150 cm
5. The "retrograde puncture" technique (Fig. 19.43): slightly bend the right knee joint, puncture the distal superficial femoral artery under proximal imaging guidance, implant a 4F short sheath, use the V-18 wire and support catheter to coordinate revascularization of the proximal occlusion of the superficial femoral artery, conduct subintimal revascularization of the occlusive segment, and return to the true lumen from the common femoral artery	Deliver the 4F short sheath
6. Lead the V-18 wire out of the body from inside the 7F Balkin sheath 40 cm; establish stretching wire; advance the 4F MPA catheter through the lesion segment via the stretching wire; forward implant the V-18 wire into the distal popliteal artery; withdraw the 4F short sheath; compress for 5–10 min till no presence of bleeding	
7. Withdraw the 4F MPA catheter, implant a Pacific balloon catheter 6 mm × 80 mm along the stretching wire, dilate the common femoral artery and proximal superficial femoral artery successively, withdraw the balloon catheter, and conduct angiography via the 6F Balkin sheath 40 cm, showing severe stenosis still exists with the distal end of the common femoral artery	Deliver the inflation device and Pacific balloon catheter 6 mm × 80 mm
8. Implant a peripheral cutting balloon 6 mm × 20 mm along the V-18 wire to dilate the stenotic segment	Deliver the peripheral cutting balloon catheter 6 mm × 20 mm
9. Withdraw balloon catheter, and conduct angiography again via the 7F Balkin sheath, showing poor dilatation effect by peripheral cutting balloon catheter	
10. Implantation of "bionic stent": implant a Supera peripheral self-expanding bare stent 5.5 mm × 120 mm to the distal stenotic segment of the superficial femoral artery along the V-18 wire, and deploy it	Deliver the Supera peripheral self-expanding bare stent 5.5 mm × 120 mm
11. Withdraw the "bionic stent" (Supera peripheral self-expanding bare stent) delivery system, implant an Admiral balloon catheter 6 mm × 40 mm along the wire to dilate the remaining stenotic segment	Deliver the Admiral balloon catheter 6 mm × 40 mm

Table 19.32 (continued)

Procedures	Intraoperative coordination process
12. Withdraw the balloon catheter, and conduct angiography via the 7F Balkin sheath, showing obvious removal of the stenotic lesion at the bifurcation of the right femoral artery and vascular patency in right common femoral artery, superficial femoral artery, deep femoral artery, popliteal artery, and infrapopliteal artery (Fig. 19.44)	
13. Withdraw the wire and 7F Balkin sheath, suture the puncture site on the left common femoral artery by 6F ProGlide vascular closure device	Deliver the 6F ProGlide vascular closure device
14. Compression dressing on the puncture site of the left common femoral artery	Deliver the gauze and elastic bandage; assist with dressing

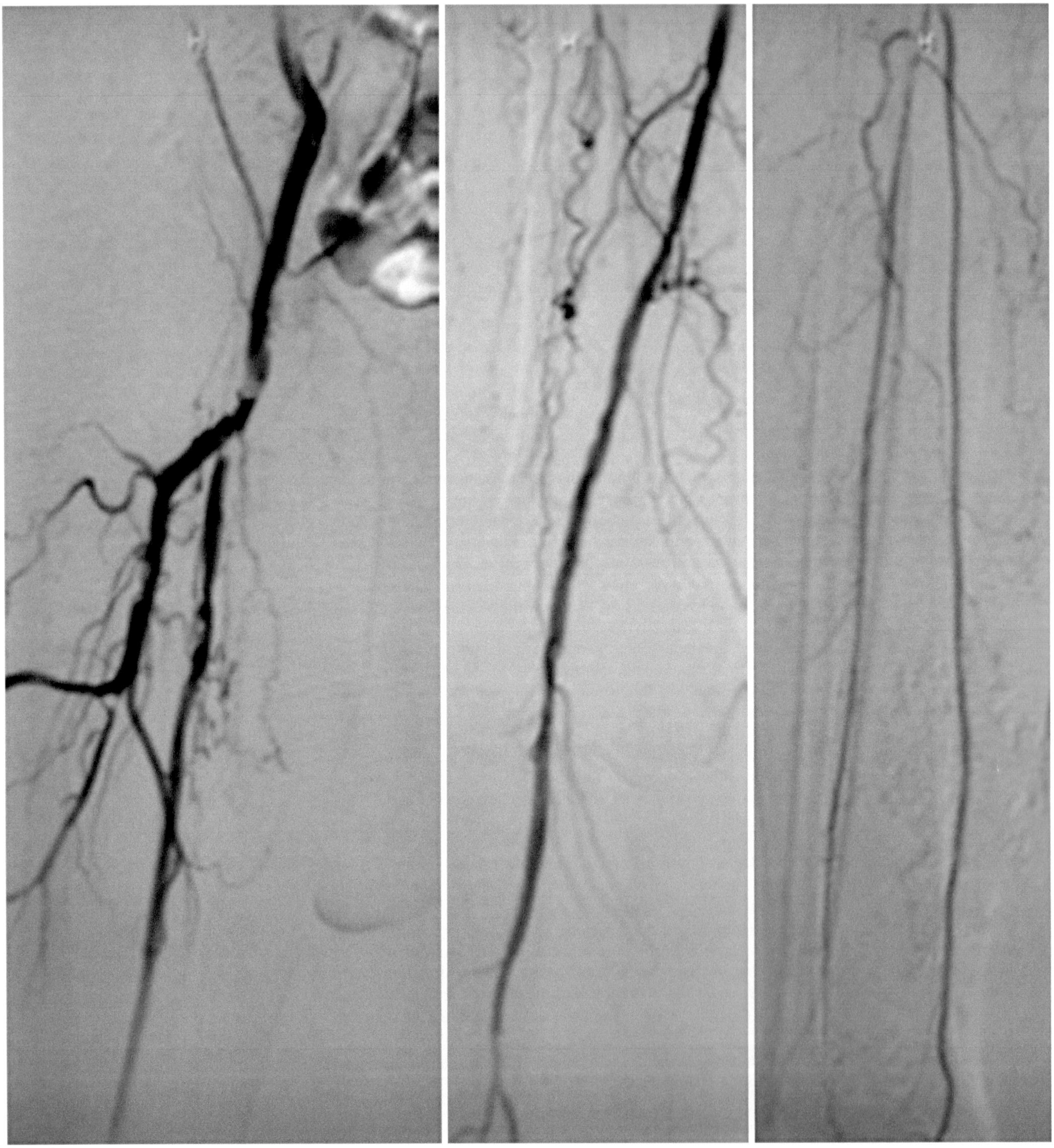

Fig. 19.41 Preoperative angiography

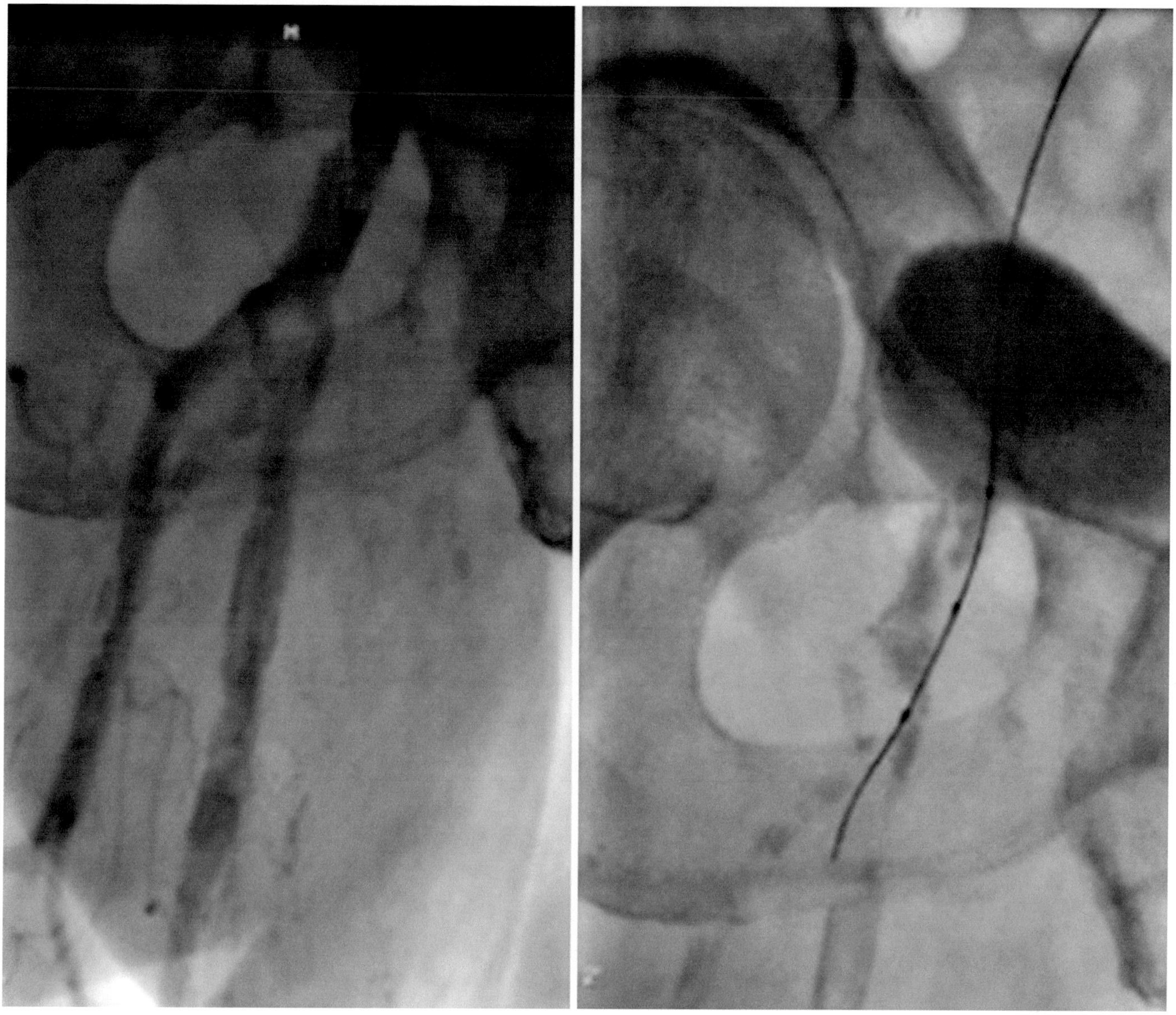

Fig. 19.42 Difficulty in proximal anterograde revascularization

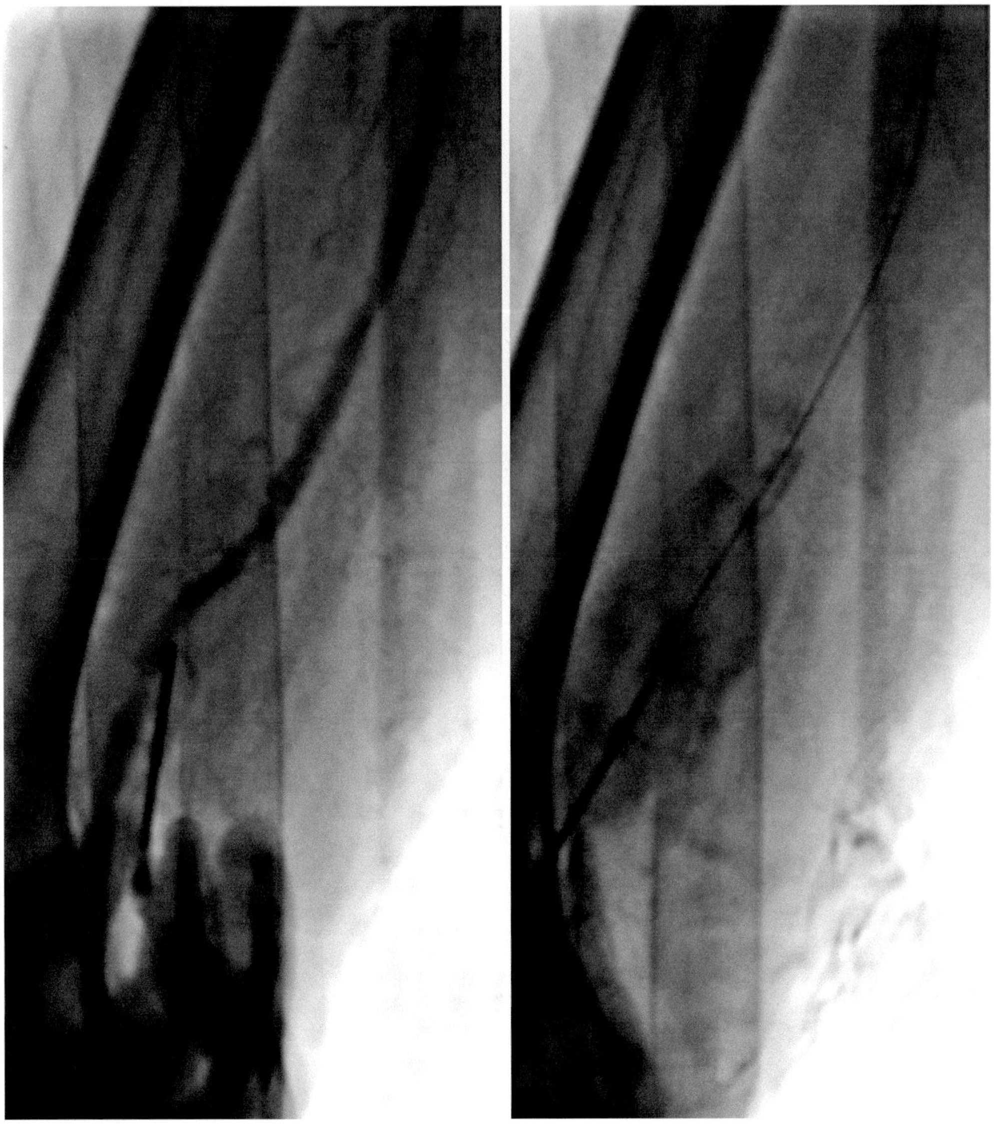

Fig. 19.43 "Retrograde puncture" technique

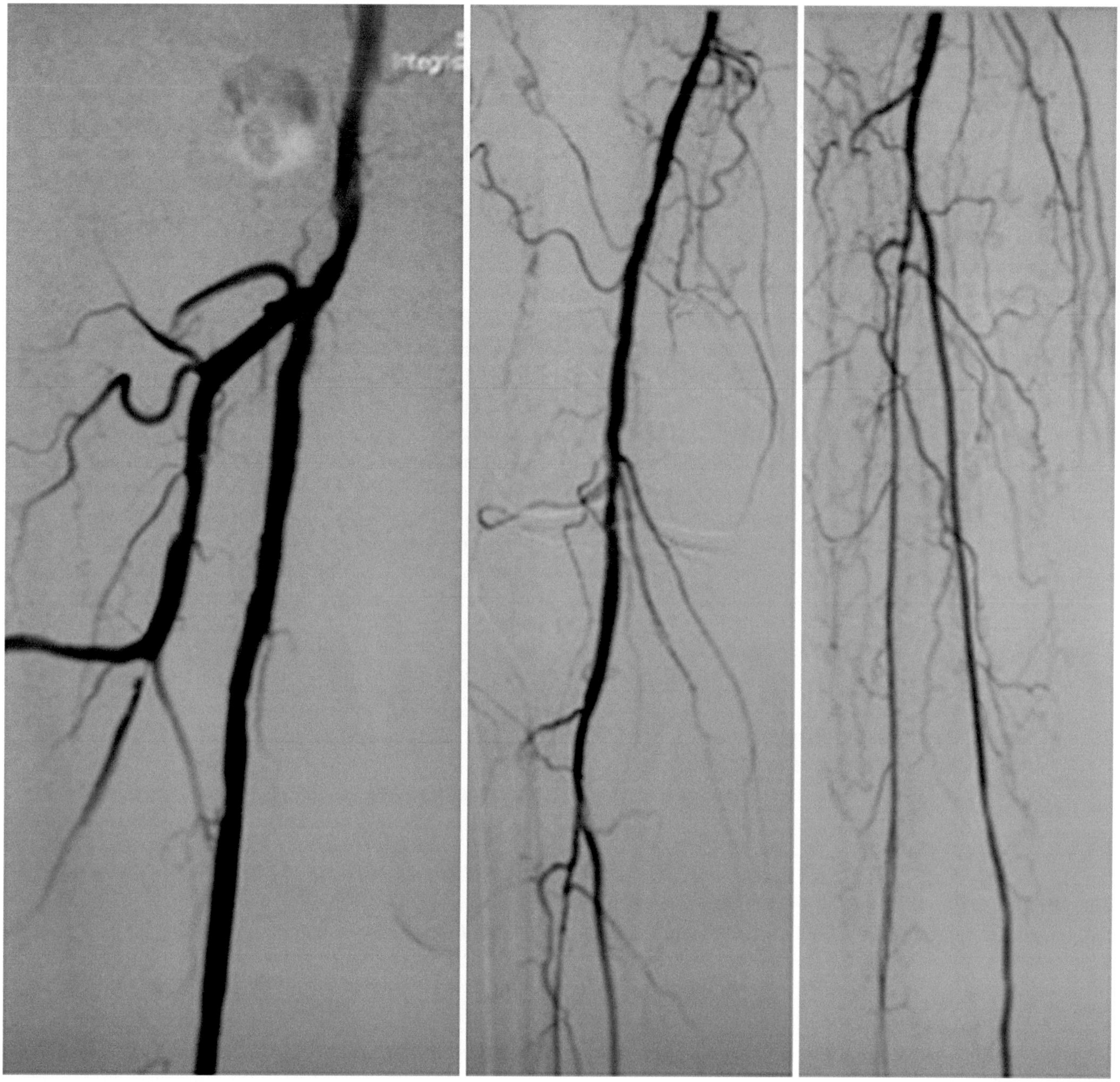

Fig. 19.44 Post-implantation of bionic stent

19.16.5 Technical Essentials and Precautions

- This patient presented with severely calcified lesion at the right femoral artery bifurcation. Although the distal femoral artery occlusion segment is only 1 cm long, it ca not be revascularized by forward puncture. Therefore, distal retrograde puncture technique is used to revascularize the lesion segment.
- In conducting retrograde puncture of the distal superficial femoral artery or popliteal artery, the knee joint should be bent appropriately. Inject radiocontrast from the proximal sheath, and use the collateral imaging as the reference for the artery puncture site. Select the puncture site at the upper medial of the calf and the posteromedial of the tibial plateau, and puncture forward, outward, and upward. Upon successful puncture, advance the 0.018 in. wire into

the vascular lumen to support the placement of the 4F short sheath.

- During retrograde revascularization, if the wire accesses through the lesion via the true lumen, directly draw out the wire from the proximal sheath to establish stretching wire. In case of subintimal access by the wire, place both the proximal and distal catheters under the intima of the occlusion segment, adjust the catheter tip frequently, zoom in the screen, and rotate the wire tip. If the wire can touch the catheter at a certain level, superselect to advance the wire into the catheter at this level and establish the stretching wire for femoral and popliteal arteries.
- Hemostatic operation for distal retrograde puncture site: upon completion of revascularizing proximal occlusion segment, retract the proximal wire into the puncture sheath, and superselect to the distal vascular true lumen of the puncture site. Taking the popliteal artery retrograde puncture in this case as an example, conduct low-pressure dilatation with 4-mm-diameter balloon at the puncture site so as to realize "endo-occlusion." Meanwhile, conduct in vitro hemostasis by compression for 5 min, and then cover the puncture site with aseptic bandage for compression hemostasis, thus facilitating subsequent operation.

19.17 Case 17 AngioJet Thrombus Aspiration Technique for Treatment of Acute Deep Vein Thrombosis

19.17.1 Patient Data

The female patient, aged 68, fell over and suffered from lumbar vertebra compression fracture in September 2015. The patient was treated with internal fracture fixation therapy at Changhai Hospital affiliated to the Naval Medical University and ordered for bed rest after operation. In October, the patient presented herself with obvious left lower limb swelling for 3 days, and color Doppler imaging showed left lower extremity deep vein thrombosis. The patient was consequently admitted for "left lower extremity deep vein thrombosis."

19.17.2 Surgical Operation

According to the case history of the patient, the case belongs to the lower extremity deep vein thrombosis, and according to conventional treatment, catheter-directed thrombolysis can be selected by puncturing the small saphenous vein or popliteal artery to implant the infusion catheter. Catheter-directed venous thrombolysis lasts longer time, during which the patient needs to stay in bed for a long time, and theoretically speaking, thrombolysis presents with certain risk of bleeding. In this case, it intends to use AngioJet aspiration thrombectomy for "one-stop" treatment. The subject gave informed consent for the procedure.

19.17.3 Device Preparation

Refer to Table 19.33.

19.17.4 Procedures and Coordination Process

Refer to Table 19.34.

Table 19.33 Device preparation

Name	Qty.	Name	Qty.
Puncture needle (Cook)	1	5F Berenstein catheter (AngioDynamics)	1
High-pressure connector (SCW Medicath)	2	6F Balkin sheath 40 cm (Cook)	1
0.035 in. common hydrophilic wire 260 cm (Terumo)	1	10F long sheath 65 cm (Arrow)	1
AngioJet Ultra console (Boston Scientific)	1	Inflation device (Boston Scientific)	1
6F AngioJet thrombectomy device (Boston Scientific)	1 set	Admiral balloon catheter 8 mm × 60 mm (Medtronic)	1
Wallstent self-expanding peripheral bare stent 12 mm × 60 mm (Boston Scientific)	1		

Note: The devices listed above (*A* mm × *B* mm), wherein *A* is the diameter of the device and *B* the length

Table 19.34 Procedures and intraoperative coordination process

Procedures	Intraoperative coordination process
1. Patient enters the operation room	(1) Mental nursing; (2) keep the patient warm; (3) help to lie at supine position, with two lower limbs slightly at abduction and extorsion position; (4) connect ECG to observe changes in blood pressure, heart rate, and oxygen saturation; (5) establish intravenous infusion
2. Routinely sterilize the bilateral groins from the umbilical down to the midthigh, exposing the groins	Prepare disinfectant (heated to 98.6°Fwith incubator) and assist with draping; deliver iodixanol injection; prepare heparin diluent (1000 mL normal saline +100 mg heparin sodium injection)
3. Puncture the right femoral vein with modified Seldinger technique under local anesthesia, implant a 6F Balkin sheath 40 cm and a 0.035 in. common hydrophilic wire 260 cm to cross over and revascularize the occlusive segment, implant a 5F Berenstein catheter via the common hydrophilic wire, withdraw the wire	Deliver 1% lidocaine injection, puncture needle, high-pressure connector, 6F Balkin sheath 40 cm, 0.035 in. common hydrophilic wire 260 cm, 5F Berenstein catheter; perform systematic heparinization; intraoperative endovascular devices should be flushed with the prepared heparin diluent
4. Conduct the left lower extremity vein angiography via the 5F Berenstein catheter, showing thrombosis from the left iliac vein to the long segment of the superior deep femoral vein (Fig. 19.45)	Connect the AngioJet Ultra console with power supply in advance. Prepare heparin diluent (500 mL normal saline + 50 mg heparin sodium injection), and hang it on the hook on one side of the console; prepare urokinase solution (100 mL normal saline +500,000 units of urokinase), and hang it on the hook on the other side of the console
5. Thrombus aspiration: withdraw the 5F Berenstein catheter, immerse the catheter tip of the 6F AngioJet thrombectomy system fully into the prepared heparin diluent, step on the foot pedal to exhaust air till AngioJet Ultra console displays 0; implant a 6F AngioJet thrombectomy device catheter into the lesion segment along the hydrophilic wire, control the foot pedal, and slowly advance the catheter for thrombus aspiration	Deliver the 6F AngioJet thrombectomy device; insert the pump of the AngioJet device into the AngioJet Ultra console; connect the syringe needle of the infusion bag inside the AngioJet device with the prepared heparin diluent hung on the AngioJet Ultra console
6. Thrombolysis: the same as thrombus aspiration	Set the system to thrombolysis mode; connect the syringe needle of the infusion bag inside the 6F AngioJet thrombectomy system with the prepared urokinase solution hung on the AngioJet Ultra console
7. Switch between aspiration and thrombolysis modes, withdraw the 6F AngioJet thrombectomy device catheter, implant the 5F Berenstein catheter along the hydrophilic wire, and conduct left lower extremity vein angiography via the 5F Berenstein catheter, showing vascular patency from the iliac to the deep femoral veins, but distal iliac artery stenosis	
8. Balloon dilatation technique: implant an Admiral balloon catheter 8 mm × 60 mm into the initial part of the left iliac vein via the 0.035 in. common hydrophilic wire 260 cm, inflate the balloon, and dilate the stenotic segment	Deliver the inflation device and Admiral balloon catheter 8 mm × 60 mm
9. Withdraw the Admiral balloon catheter and 6F Balkin sheath 40 cm, replace to implant a 10F long sheath 65 cm, implant a Wallstent self-expanding peripheral bare stent 12 mm × 60 mm to the left iliac vein stenotic segment along the common hydrophilic wire, and deploy it	Deliver the 10F long sheath 65 cm and Wallstent self-expanding peripheral bare stent 12 mm × 60 mm
10. Withdraw the Wallstent self-expanding peripheral bare stent delivery system, implant the 5F Berenstein catheter via the hydrophilic wire, and conduct left lower extremity vein angiography again, showing vascular patency from the left iliac vein to the deep femoral vein and disappeared stenosis at the initial part of the iliac vein (Fig. 19.46)	
11. Withdraw the common hydrophilic wire and 10F vascular sheath, compress the puncture site of the right femoral vein, apply compression dressing	Deliver the gauze and elastic bandage, assist with dressing

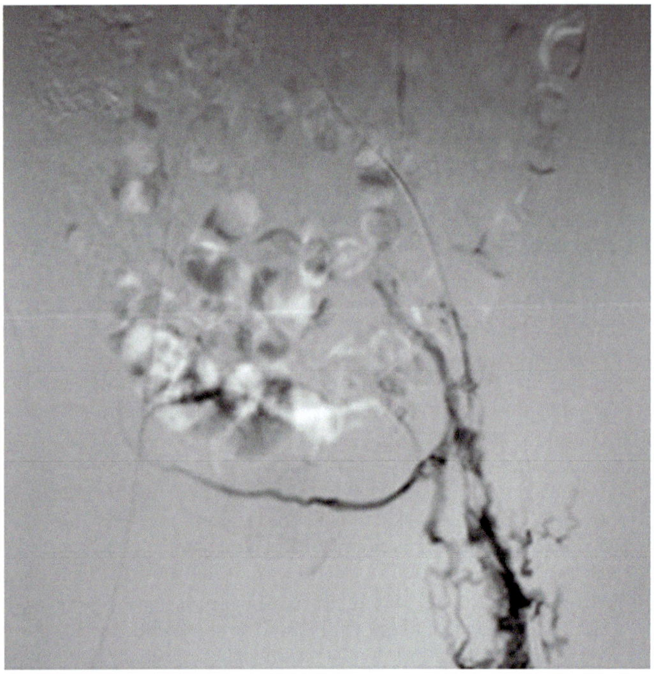

Fig. 19.45 Preoperative angiography

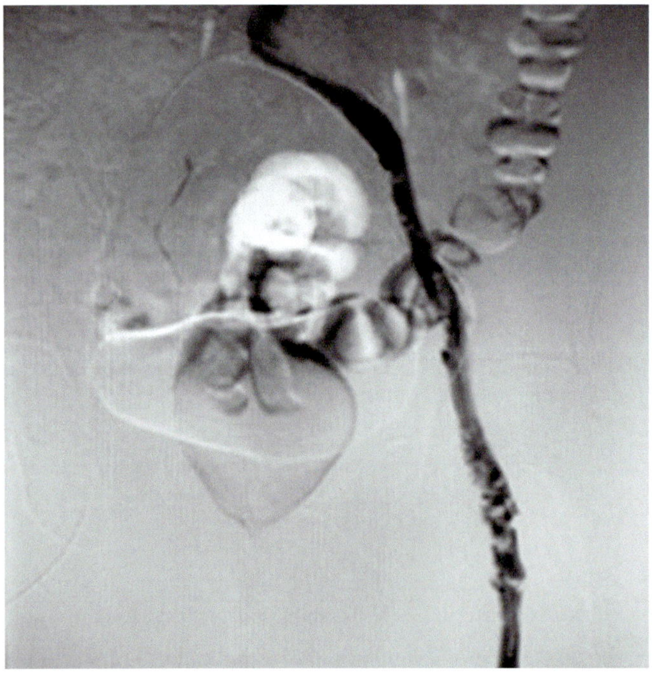

Fig. 19.46 Postoperative angiography

19.17.5 Technical Essentials and Precautions

- The approach in this case is anterograde puncture of the contralateral unaffected femoral vein. If revascularization by crossing is unavailable, conduct anterograde puncture of the affected popliteal, common femoral, small saphenous, and posterior tibial veins (depending on thrombus length and vascular conditions), and cross to the unaffected common femoral vein via the wire to establish operation path. Puncture can also be conducted via the affected popliteal vein, facilitating follow-up stent implantation and filter recovery.
- For the patient still with stenosis after iliac vein aspiration thrombectomy, "balloon dilatation and implantation of self-expanding peripheral bare stent" technique can be used. The stent available can be self-expanding peripheral bare stent of 10–16 mm diameter so as to dilate the vein stenotic site as far as possible.
- In the process of AngioJet aspiration thrombectomy, possible emboli breaking off may threaten the life of the patient. Therefore, operation should be performed under filter protection as far as possible, and recoverable filter is preferred.

19.18 Case 18 Coil Embolization and Peripheral Stent Graft Technique for Treatment of Left Subclavian Arteriovenous Fistula

19.18.1 Patient Data

The male patient, aged 38, was found by accident an egg-sized "unknown mass" on the left neck, without pain. Later, the mass was found to enlarge gradually, accompanied with obvious bouncing. Neck CT showed "arteriovenous fistula, AVF" (Fig. 19.47), and the patient was admitted for "left subclavian arteriovenous fistula" in April 2013.

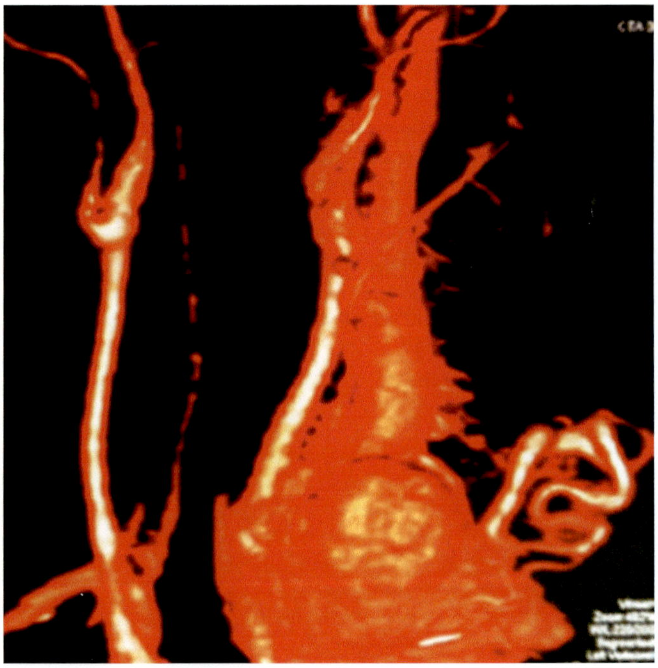

Fig. 19.47 Neck CT

19.18.2 Surgical Operation

MRI showed that the patient's arteriovenous fistula (AVF) involved multiple collateral branches. If only spring coil was used for treatment, embolization of all collateral branches would be impossible; in case of repair only of peripheral stent graft, it might lose the chance for any follow-up treatment. After multiple preoperative assessments, it intended to use "spring coil embolization and peripheral stent graft repair" technique to treat the left subclavian arteriovenous fistula. The subject gave informed consent for the procedure.

19.18.3 Device Preparation

Refer to Table 19.35.

19.18.4 Procedures and Intraoperative Coordination Process

Refer to Table 19.36.

Table 19.35 Device preparation

Name	Qty.	Name	Qty.
Puncture needle (Cook)	1	5F MPA catheter 125 cm (Cordis)	1
High-pressure connector (SCW Medicath)	2	5F common pigtail catheter (Optimed)	1
0.035 in. common hydrophilic wire 260 cm (Terumo)	1	5F short sheath (Terumo)	1
6F Raabe long sheath 90 cm (Cook)	1	10F Raabe long sheath 80 cm (Cook)	1
Fluency peripheral stent graft 10 mm × 100 mm (Bard)	1	Embolization 10 mm × 80 mm (Cook)	3
Viabahn peripheral stent graft 8 mm × 50 mm (Gore)	1	Embolization 8 mm × 50 mm (Cook)	11
Hemostatic patch	1	Embolization 5 mm × 50 mm (Cook)	11
6F ProGlide vascular closure device (Abbott)	1		

Note: The devices listed above (*A* mm × *B* mm), wherein *A* is the diameter of the device and *B* the length

Table 19.36 Procedures and intraoperative coordination process

Procedures	Intraoperative coordination process
1. Patient enters the operation room	(1) Mental nursing; (2) keep the patient warm; (3) help to lie at supine position, with two lower limbs slightly at abduction and extorsion position; (4) connect ECG to observe changes in blood pressure, heart rate, and oxygen saturation; (5) establish intravenous infusion
2. Routinely sterilize the bilateral groins from the umbilical down to the midthigh, exposing the groins	Prepare disinfectant (heated to 98.6 °F with incubator), and assist with draping; deliver iodixanol injection; prepare heparin diluent (1000 mL normal saline +100 mg heparin sodium injection)
3. Puncture the right common femoral artery with modified Seldinger technique under local anesthesia, implant a 5F short sheath and a 0.035 in. common hydrophilic wire 260 cm, implant a 5F common pigtail catheter to the ascending aorta via the hydrophilic wire, withdraw the hydrophilic wire, and conduct aortic arch angiography, showing left subclavian arteriovenous fistula (Fig. 19.48)	Deliver 1% lidocaine injection, puncture needle, high-pressure connector, 5F short sheath, 0.035 in. common hydrophilic wire 260 cm, and 5F common pigtail catheter; perform systematic heparinization; intraoperative endovascular devices should be flushed with the prepared heparin diluent
4. Withdraw the 5F common pigtail catheter and 5F short sheath, exchange to insert a 6F Raabe long sheath 90 cm and a 5F MPA catheter 125 cm, coordinate the hydrophilic wire with the 5F MPA catheter to superselect access to the left subclavian lesion site, withdraw the hydrophilic wire, and conduct embolization for all branch arteries in sequence	Deliver the 6F Raabe long sheath 90 cm and 5F MPA catheter 125 cm
5. Implantation of Cook embolization: implant 25 embolizations into the branch arteries of the left subclavian arteriovenous fistula in sequence via the 5F MPA catheter 125 cm	Deliver 11 embolizations 8 mm × 50 mm, 11 embolizations 5 mm × 50 mm, and three Cook embolizations 10 mm × 80 mm
6. Implantation of Viabahn peripheral stent graft: withdraw the 5F MPA catheter 125 cm and the 6F Raabe long sheath 90 cm, exchange to implant a 10F Raabe long sheath 80 cm, implant a Viabahn peripheral stent graft 8 mm × 50 mm to the left subclavian lesion site along the 0.035 in. common hydrophilic wire 260 cm before deployment	Deliver the 10F Raabe long sheath 80 cm and Viabahn peripheral stent graft 8 mm × 50 mm

Table 19.36 (continued)

Procedures	Intraoperative coordination process
7. Withdraw the Viabahn peripheral stent graft delivery system, and conduct left subclavian artery angiography via the 10F Raabe long sheath, showing significant decrease in blood flow of the collateral artery of the left subclavian arteriovenous fistula. To ensure perfect effect, implantation of another peripheral stent graft should be considered during operation	
8. Implantation of Fluency peripheral stent graft: implant a Fluency peripheral stent graft 10 mm × 100 mm to the left subclavian lesion site via the 0.035 in. common hydrophilic wire 260 cm before deployment	Deliver the Fluency peripheral stent graft 10 mm × 100 mm
9. Withdraw the Fluency peripheral stent graft delivery system, implant a 5F common pigtail catheter to the ascending aorta along the hydrophilic wire, withdraw the hydrophilic wire, and conduct angiography, showing the left subclavian arteriovenous fistula has been excluded (Fig. 19.49)	Deliver the 5F common pigtail catheter
10. Withdraw the 5F common pigtail catheter and the 10F Raabe long sheath 80 cm, suture the puncture site of the right common femoral artery with the 6F ProGlide vascular closure device	Deliver the 6F ProGlide vascular closure device
11. Cover the hemostatic patch on the puncture site of the right common femoral artery, compress for 5 min, and apply compression dressing on the puncture site	Deliver the hemostatic patch, gauze, and elastic bandage, assist with dressing

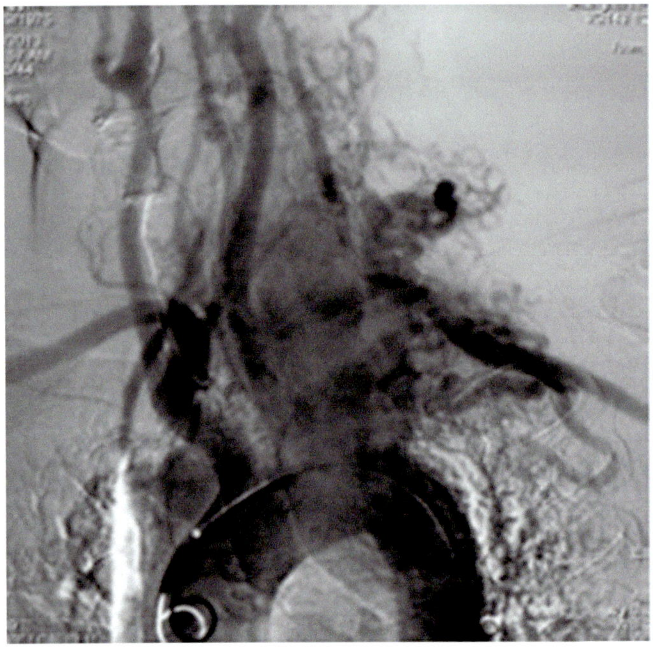

Fig. 19.48 Intraoperative angiography

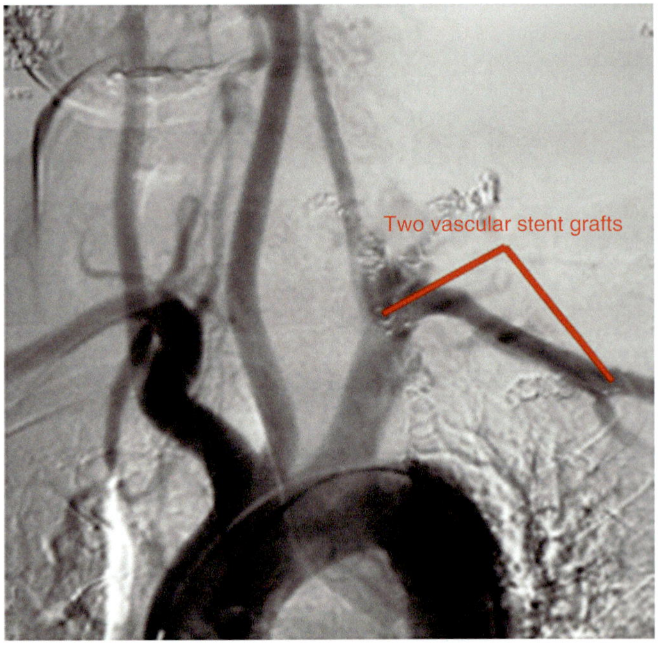

Fig. 19.49 Postoperative angiography

19.18.5 Technical Essentials and Precautions

- In using the spring coil for embolization therapy for this patient, the diameter of the spring coil should be greater than the diameter of the arteries where embolization is performed, and the spring coil should be coiled into shape so as to prevent the spring coil from accessing into the intracranial blood vessels along the blood flow and leading to malignant results. If necessary, controllable spring coil should be selected to improve treatment safety.
- The patient in this case cannot be completely cured if only embolization therapy is used. Therefore, in most times, peripheral stent graft is used to isolate the corresponding feeding arteries, and embolization should be as close to the fistula as possible in the treatment of arteriovenous

malformations. Due to numerous collateral branches of arteriovenous fistula, pay attention to using the stent grafts, and ensure complete coverage of the abnormal vascular networks as far as possible, and thus reduce AVF recurrence.

19.19 Case 19 Reinforced Bar and Concrete Technique for Treatment of Lower Extremity Arteriovenous Fistula

19.19.1 Patient Data

The female patient, aged 19, presented herself with left lower extremity swelling discomfort after long-time standing in August 2015, which was alleviated after taking a rest at supine position. In September, the patient's CTA showed "left lower extremity arteriovenous malformation" at another hospital, and in October, the patient was admitted to the hospital for "the left lower extremity arteriovenous fistula."

19.19.2 Surgical Operation

Intraoperative angiography suggested that the left lower extremity suffered from multiple arteriovenous fistulas. Due to numerous AVF collateral branches, using stent graft might make the patient lose the approach for subsequent treatment. Therefore, it intended to use "rebar (embolization) and concrete (Onyx liquid embolic agent)" technique to embolize the branch blood vessels of arteriovenous fistula. The subject gave informed consent for the procedure.

19.19.3 Device Preparation

Refer to Table 19.37.

19.19.4 Procedures and Intraoperative Coordination Process

Refer to Table 19.38.

Table 19.37 Device preparation

Name	Qty.	Name	Qty.
Puncture needle (Cook)	1	5F Berenstein catheter (AngioDynamics)	1
High-pressure connector (SCW Medicath)	2	5F short sheath (Terumo)	1
0.035 in. hydrophilic wire 260 cm (Terumo)	2	Echelon-10 microcatheter (Medtronic)	1
6F Balkin sheath 40 cm (Cook)	1	Onyx18 liquid embolic agent (Medtronic)	2
Interlock-35 controllable embolization 6 mm × 200 mm (Boston Scientific)	3	6F ProGlide vascular closure device (Abbott)	1
Onyx liquid embolic system (Medtronic)	1 set		

Note: The devices listed above (*A* mm × *B* mm), wherein *A* is the diameter of the device and *B* the length

Table 19.38 Procedures and intraoperative coordination process

Procedures	Intraoperative coordination process
1. Patient enters the operation room	(1) Mental nursing; (2) keep the patient warm; (3) help to lie at supine position, with two lower limbs slightly at abduction and extorsion position; (4) connect ECG to observe changes in blood pressure, heart rate, and oxygen saturation; (5) establish intravenous infusion
2. Routinely sterilize the bilateral groins from the umbilical down to the midthigh, exposing the groins	Prepare disinfectant (heated to 98.6°Fwith incubator), and assist with draping; deliver iodixanol injection; prepare heparin diluent (1000 mL normal saline +100 mg heparin sodium injection)
3. Puncture the right common femoral artery with modified Seldinger technique under local anesthesia; implant a 5F short sheath, 0.035 in. common hydrophilic wire 260 cm, and 5F Berenstein catheter to the left lower limb; withdraw the common hydrophilic wire; and conduct angiography, showing left lower extremity multiple arteriovenous fistula (different embolic methods for different fistulas)	Deliver 1% lidocaine injection, puncture needle, high-pressure connector, 5F short sheath, 0.035 in. common hydrophilic wire 260 cm, 5F Berenstein catheter; perform systematic heparinization; intraoperative endovascular devices should be flushed with the prepared heparin diluent

(continued)

Table 19.38 (continued)

Procedures	Intraoperative coordination process
4. Withdraw the 5F short sheath, exchange to insert a 6F Balkin sheath 40 cm, and implant an Echelon 10 microcatheter to the left lower extremity arteriovenous fistula via the 5F Berenstein catheter	Deliver the 6F Balkin sheath 40 cm and Ev3 Echelon 10 microcatheter, open the package box of the Onyx18 liquid embolic agent, and check supportive items in the box: 1.5 mL DMSO liquid, 1.5 mL Onyx18 liquid embolic agent, and three vials of 1 mL syringes (yellow syringe specially for DMSO liquid aspiration, white one for aspiration of Onyx18 liquid embolic agent); oscillate the Onyx18 liquid embolic agent on the liquid oscillator 20 min in advance (heated before oscillation in the event of low room temperature)
5. Embolization by Onyx18 liquid embolic agent: first suck up the DMSO liquid with the 1 mL yellow syringe, and inject it into the Echelon 10 microcatheter to flush the catheter (if several Onyx18 liquid embolic agents are used during operation, flush the catheter only once); then suck up the Onyx18 liquid embolic agent with the white syringe, and inject it into the fistula via the Echelon10 microcatheter; conduct angiography by manual push via the Echelon 10 microcatheter, showing significant decrease of branches at the fistula (Fig. 19.50)	Deliver three 1 mL syringe and 2 Onyx18 liquid embolic agents; coordinate with the physicians to suck up DMSO liquid and the oscillated Onyx18 liquid embolic agent
6. Embolization by Interlock-35 spring coil: retract the Echelon 10 microcatheter, use the 0.035 in. common hydrophilic wire 260 cm and 5F Berenstein catheter to superselect access into other fistulas, implant three Interlock-35 controllable spring coils 6 mm × 200 mm along the Berenstein catheter for embolization; conduct angiography by manual push along the 5F Berenstein catheter, showing significant decrease in the branches at the fistula	Deliver three Interlock-35 controllable spring coils 6 mm × 200 mm
7. Coordinate the Onyx18 liquid embolic agent with the Interlock-35 controllable spring coil till all fistulas are embolized	
8. Conduct left lower extremity artery angiography via the 5F Berenstein catheter, showing no obvious bypass at the lower extremity AVF and successful embolization (Fig. 19.51)	
9. Withdraw the catheter and short sheath, suture the puncture site on the right common femoral artery with 6F ProGlide vascular closure device	Deliver the 6F ProGlide vascular closure device
10. Compression dressing on puncture site	Deliver the gauze and elastic bandage, assist with dressing, escort the patient safely back to ward

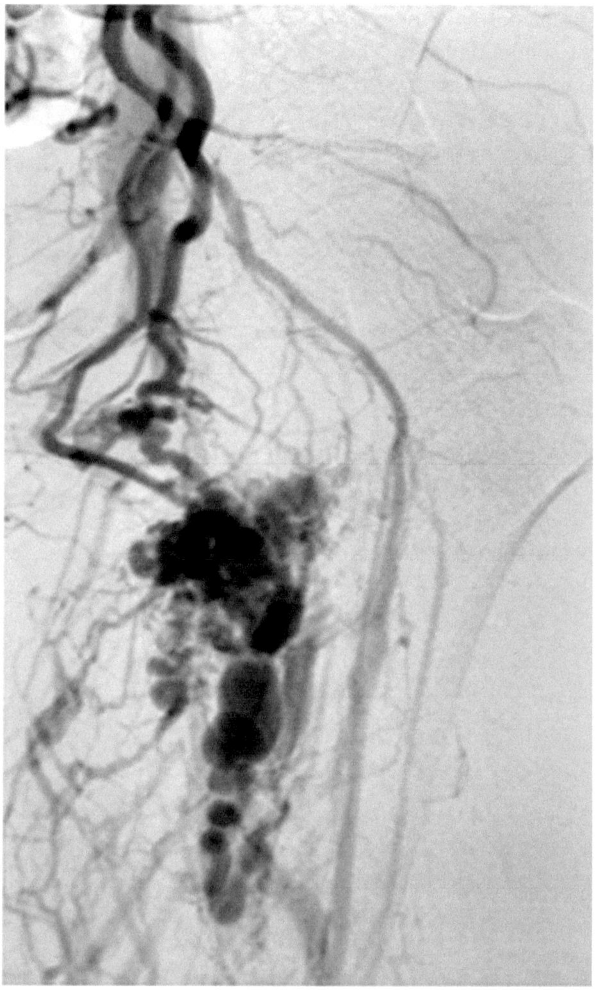

Fig. 19.50 Preoperative angiography

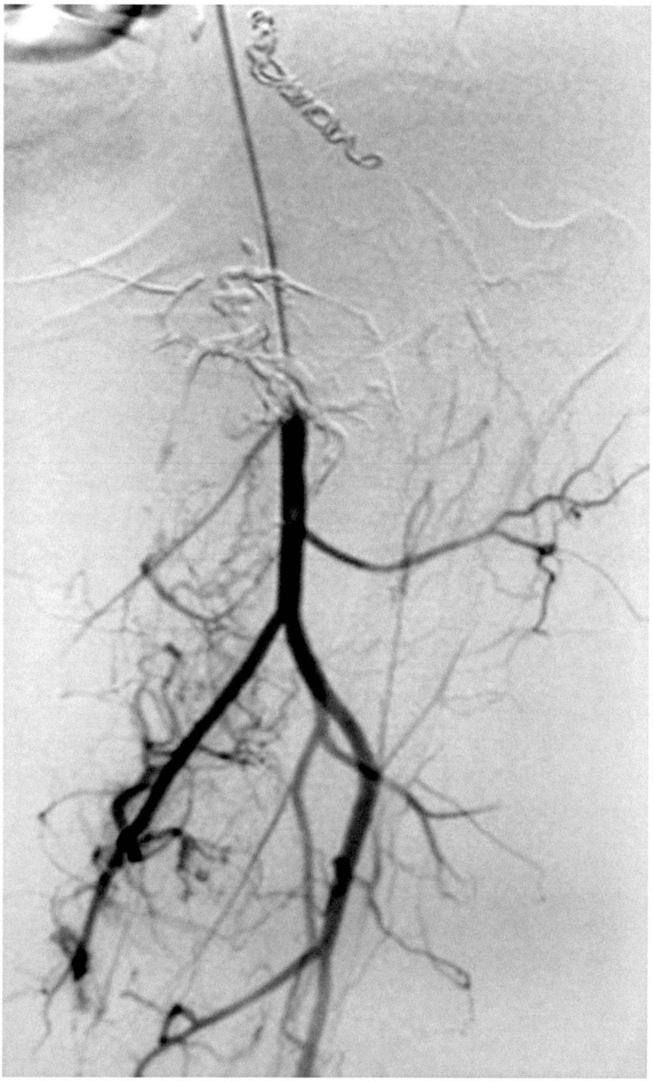

Fig. 19.51 Postoperative angiography

19.19.5 Technical Essentials and Precautions

- The treatment of arteriovenous malformations has always been a major challenge for vascular surgeons. In recent years, with the development of endovascular devices, the progress of technology, and the popularity of the concept, AVF endovascular repair has been proved to be an effective and reliable method.
- The Onyx liquid embolic agent used in this case has the advantages of long injection time, high controllability, and high embolization rate and has been widely used in clinical practice. Completely occluding or occluding as much as possible occlusive malformations can reduce remaining blood flow and the volume of the arteriovenous malformations and alleviate artery stealing, venous hypertension, and other symptoms.
- The slowdown of high-volume flow rate after spring embolization will lead to fading or disappeared imaging, but the original low-volume lesion will display imaging during angiography. In conducting embolization by Onyx liquid embolic agent, try to advance the embolic agent to the fistula location under the coordination of the microcatheter, which will increase the embolization rate.

19.20 Case 20 High Ligation + Punctate Stripping + Sclerotherapy for Treatment of Great Saphenous Varicose with Superficial Thrombophlebitis

19.20.1 Patient Data

The male patient, aged 53, presented himself with left lower extremity varicose veins for more than 20 years and had an about 5 cm × 7 cm mass on the left lower extremity 2 weeks ago, accompanied by pain and tenderness along the great saphenous vein running course. Duplex-ultrasonography examination showed great saphenous vein thrombosis and deep vein patency. The patient was admitted for "left lower extremity varicose veins with superficial thrombophlebitis" in August 2016.

19.20.2 Surgical Operation

Combined with the physical examination and duplex-ultrasonography findings, thrombosis concentrated in the trunk infrapopliteal great saphenous vein, forming a 5 cm × 7 cm mass at 10 cm of the infrapopliteal artery, and no thrombus was found in the femoral great saphenous vein, and scattered infrapopliteal venous branches with dolichoectasia were visible. According to the venous characteristics of different parts, it intended to conduct high ligation for the great saphenous vein under local anesthesia, sclerotherapy for supra-popliteal great saphenous vein, thrombectomy for infrapopliteal great saphenous vein, and sclerotherapy for thin collateral veins. The subject gave informed consent for the procedure.

19.20.3 Device Preparation

Refer to Table 19.39.

19.20.4 Procedures and Intraoperative Coordination Process

Refer to Table 19.40.

Table 19.39 Device preparation

Name	Qty.	Name	Qty.
Disposable operation kit	1	Suture scissors, tissue scissors	One each
5 mL, 2 mL, 1 mL empty needle	One each	Medium-curved forceps	2
Disposable gloves	2 pairs	Michel clips	1
Large gauze	10	Small-curved forceps	6 pairs
T valve	1	Mosquito pliers	6 pairs
1% lidocaine	2 vials	Handle, blade	One each
Silk suture (1#)	1 bag	1% polidocanol injection	1–2 vials
Traumatic suture	1	5F Berenstein catheter (Cook)	1
Toothed forceps	2 pairs	Histoacryl sealant (Braun)	1 tube
Muller hook	1 pair	Mepore self-adhesive sterile wound dressing (Molnlycke)	Several
Skin retractor	2	Therapeutic anti-varicose vein compression stockings (HSD)	1 pair
Needle holder	1	Elastic bandage (HSD)	2 tapes

Note: The devices listed above (*A* mm × *B* mm), wherein *A* is the diameter of the device and *B* the length

Table 19.40 Procedures and intraoperative coordination process

Procedures	Intraoperative coordination process
1. Guide the patient to enter the operation room and take a supine position, mark the varicose vein, and pre-mark the incision site (Fig. 19.52)	(1) Mental nursing; (2) keep the patient warm; (3) help to lie at supine position, with two lower limbs slightly at abduction and extorsion position; (4) connect ECG to observe changes in blood pressure, heart rate, and oxygen saturation
2. Routinely sterilize up to the navel and down to all affected limbs of the lower extremities and 1/3 upper part of the contralateral thigh	Prepare disinfectant (heated to 98.6 °F with incubator), and assist with draping; tidy up the operation table; and prepare surgical devices
3. Conduct local anesthesia at the root of the thigh where saphenofemoral junction is and along the superficial varicose veins	Deliver 1% lidocaine injection
4. Start from the pulsatile point of the left femoral artery, cut a 3 cm incision on the medial of the inguinal, cut open the skin, subcutaneous fat, and scape fascia, in turn, to dissociate the trunk of the great saphenous vein. Devascularize the root branches of the great saphenous vein, and conduct ligation, respectively. Dissociate to the oval fossa toward the proximal end, and devascularize the great saphenous vein at 0.5 cm from the point where the great saphenous vein converges with the femoral vein, conduct ligation, and clamp the distal end	Deliver the surgical devices

Table 19.40 (continued)

Procedures	Intraoperative coordination process
5. Cut open the skin marked on the knee, with longer incision for place having thrombus. Dissociate the adhesion between the thrombotic vein and the skin, and pay attention to reduce extrusion. Cut small incision at the thrombotic vessel, pull out the thrombus (Fig. 19.53), and strip out the blood vessel when the thrombi in the blood vessel are basically pulled out. Conduct punctated stripping for varicose veins on other sites of the calf	Deliver the surgical devices; closely observe the change in oxygen saturation
6. Insert a 5F Berenstein catheter from the proximal end to the root via the knee joint great saphenous vein, prepare sclerosing foam of 1% polidocanol injection and air at a proportion of 1:4, inject the foam via the 5F Berenstein catheter into the superior knee segment of the trunk of the great saphenous vein, withdraw the catheter while injecting. Ligate both ends of the great saphenous vein, find out the site with obvious great saphenous dilation at the mid-piece of the thigh, sever the great saphenous vein, strip off part of the vein and ligate (Fig. 19.53)	Deliver the 5F Berenstein catheter and 1% polidocanol injection
7. Close the inguinal incision, seal the incision and other small incisions with Histoacryl tissue glue, and wrap the wounds with Mepore self-adhesive sterile dressing wounds; apply compression dressing by elastic bandage after intraoperative use of therapeutic anti-varicose vein stockings	Deliver the Histoacryl tissue glue and Mepore self-adhesive sterile dressing; assist with dressing and wearing therapeutic anti-varicose vein stockings

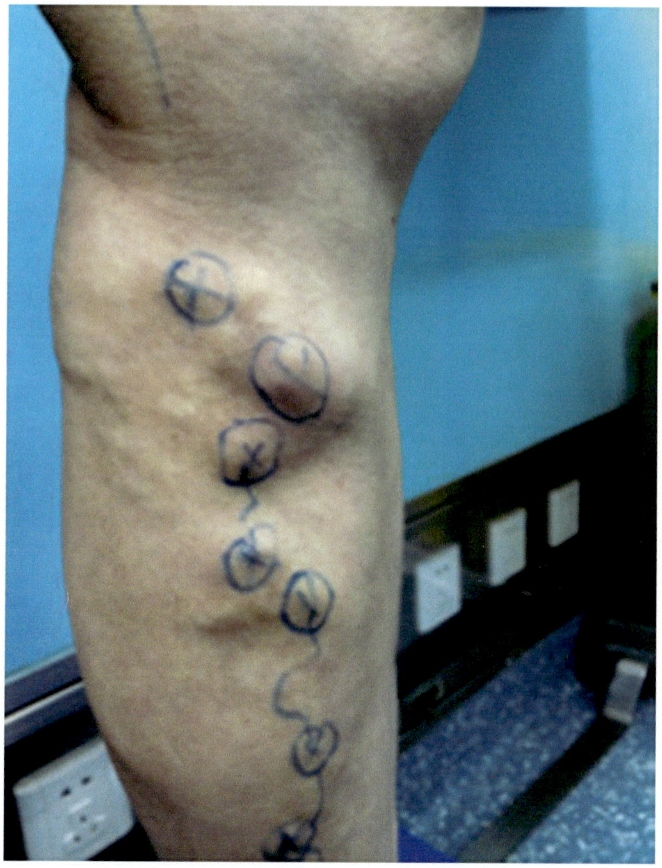

Fig. 19.52 Marking at varicose vein

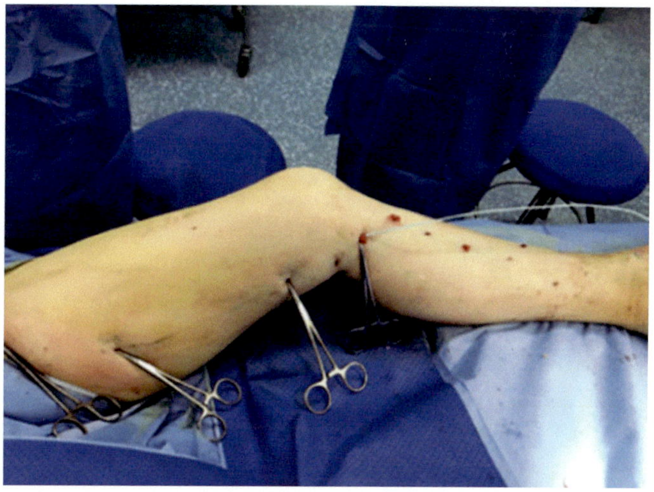

Fig. 19.53 High ligation + punctate stripping + sclerotherapy

19.20.5 Technical Essentials and Precautions

- The most important thing in conducting superficial thrombophlebitis therapy is to avoid excessive extrusion and pulling of the great saphenous vein and thus prevent the thrombi from being squeezed to the deep vein and causing pulmonary embolism. Therefore, before stripping, the great saphenous vein at the thrombus segment should be dissociated carefully. Small incisions are cut on the great saphenous vein segment by segment for decompression and providing access to thrombi so as to avoid access into perforating branches. Oxygen saturation should be closely monitored during operation.
- When the patient with superficial thrombophlebitis is treated with high ligation of the great saphenous vein, special attention should be paid to the presence of thrombosis at the root of the great saphenous vein. Sometimes duplex-ultrasonography cannot reflect the real-time situation. Therefore, the action must be gentle during the operation, to avoid excessive extrusion and stretching.
- The longer operation time for superficial thrombophlebitis does not necessarily mean that the thrombi do not easily break off. Sometimes, thrombi will appear liquefied 1–2 months later, resulting in chocolate-dipped thrombosis, which, under extrusion, are very liable of entering the deep vein via the perforating branches.

References

1. Mier J. Clinical vascular surgery. 3rd ed. Beijing: Science Press; 2011.
2. Guo W. Endovascular surgery. Beijing: People's Military Medical Press; 2011.
3. Wang S. Vascular surgery. Beijing: People's Medical Publishing House; 2011.
4. Cronenwett JL, Johnston KW. Rutherford's vascular surgery. 8th ed. American: Saunders; 2014.

Part III

Management Over Endovascular Devices

Management Theories and Methods

20

Weihui Dai and Huajuan Mao

Abstract

The management of endovascular devices consists of the internal management in clinical departments and the supply chain management from suppliers to clinical departments. Based on the objects of management, it can be classified into device management, supplier management, device technician or nurse management, and patient management. The internal management in clinical departments related to endovascular devices mainly involves the barcode information entry of various devices, warehousing and ex-warehouse registration, use traceability, classified placement, optimized layout, and other links; attentions must be paid to requirements on the period of validity and storage environment for devices in the principle of "first in, first out," so as to conveniently and precisely pick up and maximally avoid contamination, failure, loss, or wastage in other manners and properly conduct related management work. Based on the above-mentioned management requirements and characteristics, this chapter discusses the management theories and methods of endovascular devices from the perspective of the whole-process supply chain.

Keywords

Endovascular devices · Agile supply chain management · Autonomous intelligent decision-making

W. Dai (✉)
School of Management, Fudan University, Shanghai, China
e-mail: whdai@fudan.edu.cn

H. Mao
Department of Vascular Surgery, Changhai Hospital, Second Military Medical University, Shanghai, China

20.1 Agile Supply Chain Management of Endovascular Devices

The endovascular devices possibly used in clinical operations are diversified and multifarious, the storage, keeping, and use of which are subject to strict requirements [1–3]. Compared with general medical devices, the significant difference in management of the endovascular devices lies in that the endovascular devices, especially high-value consumables, are often subject to special distribution by suppliers according to the operation schedules in view of their high stocking cost and limited expiry date as well as the devices urgently and accidently required during operation are delivered urgently to the operation room directly by suppliers [1, 2]. With the development of endovascular devices and the increasing popularity of modern information network application, the management over endovascular devices must take into account the characteristics of following new demands in view of the delivery coordination for clinical surgery [1, 4–8].

20.1.1 Diversity, Complexity, and Professionalism

Many critical endovascular devices have become the important guarantee for the success of clinical surgery. They have highly added value and are the focus of research for relevant institutions and one of the fastest growing domains in technological development. As the products are increasingly updated and diversified, product design and application also tend to be subdivided, and professional development, and clinical surgery will face more complexities. Therefore, the latest knowledge and clinical application practice should be provided in this regard [9, 10].

Z. Jing et al. (eds.), *Endovascular Surgery and Devices*, https://doi.org/10.1007/978-981-10-8270-2_20

20.1.2 Dynamic Change and Emergency Delivery Demand

In the arrangement of clinical operation, although the requirements for the preparation and delivery of critical devices are given in advance, in actual operation, various complex situations will arise, and the arrangement of original operation should be changed accordingly, thus resulting in dynamic change in the device requirements. Emergency delivery measures should be taken for unprepared devices. Therefore, the demand for endovascular devices in clinical surgery is dynamic and changing according to actual situations.

20.1.3 Personalized Preference and Intelligent Recommendation

Considering the difference in knowledge, experience, and habits during clinical operation, different doctors show different preferences for device selection. To ensure smooth surgical operation, personalized preferences of the doctors should be satisfied as far as possible. Considering from the perspective of safety, effectiveness, and economy, the most appropriate devices should be recommended promptly via intelligent technology, providing tips on the important characteristics and use instructions of the devices [9].

20.1.4 Adverse Reaction Predication and Safety Precautions

For devices that may bring adverse reaction in clinical surgery, in particular, products that are not indicated for clinical use, predication and safety precautions should be given promptly [11, 12]. For the safety precautions, in addition to the notices from the health administration, big data mining and analysis must be carried out for the existing cases and Internet information, so as to obtain important information in a timely manner.

In view of the relevant management theories and methods for endovascular devices [13–22], S. E. Heinbuch proposed the idea of realizing precision management and cost reduction through JIT (just-in-time) model under the concept of applying advanced logistic technology and total quality management (TQM) [20]. L. Ritchie et al. pointed out that purchase and inventory system must consider the reverse logistics [21]. S. T. Young proposed a new model of supplier-based dynamic monitoring of the hospital inventory and inventory management [22], which is essentially the prototype of virtual inventory and "zero inventory" management model for hospitals [1].

With the increasing in-depth application of information technology and the continuous improvement at hospital information level, the application of digital barcode technology, radiofrequency identification technology, data-mining technology, intelligent monitoring technology, and ERP (enterprise resource planning) systems have provided powerful means for the full-range integrated management of the demand analysis, optimized purchase, inventory management, and use monitoring of the devices. The said device management has been transformed from inventory and use management to the management of the entire integrated supply chain so as to achieve the best overall economic benefits in a dynamically changing environment. Therefore, the research scholars put forward a new model of process optimization management based on information integration from the perspective of integrated supply chain management and use the theory of scenario analysis to perfectly design the supply chain management system, which, on the one hand, highlights the economical nature and, on the other, increasingly values the device safety and proposes a full-range new safety monitoring model pertinent to the safety characteristics of the said devices [1, 14, 16].

At the end of the 1990s, Stanford University proposed a new theory of agile supply chain (ASC) management in view of the dynamic changes in the market and the increasing complexity in personalized demands, providing systematic principles and mechanism to quickly respond to the dynamic demands and more effectively reduce the total cost of the entire supply chain in the context of uncertainty and increasingly changing environment. The management model of agile supply chain transforms the traditional supply chain structure from a serial structure to a parallel one centered on personalized demands of customers and uses information technology to build a new reactive mechanism integrating dynamic supply and demand network with collaborative operation, which can quickly respond to dynamic demands under uncertain environment and more effectively reduce the total cost of the whole supply chain. In particular, the development of mobile communication technology extends the supply chain terminal to customers under mobile environment. Therefore, the optimal matching and dynamic integration of the supply chain resources must be realized in view of the ever-changing demands of customers and location information [23–28]. T. Y. Eng believed that under the said mobile environment, the mobile communication technology, mobile devices, and Internet technology should be used to manage the specific key information resources of relevant enterprises providing certain common goods or services whenever and wherever possible. He also analyzed the technologies on how to effectively configure the goods and services coverage, meet customer needs in real time, guarantee the quality of customer service, and enhance customer satisfaction [26].

The coordinated delivery of clinical surgery-oriented endovascular devices is characteristic of agile custom-made service under mobile environment, and the management theory of agile supply chain provides important theoretical basis for the abovementioned coordinated delivery management [27, 28]. In the said management, the decision on the automatic device variety and quantity replenishment is the key link affecting system performance. In allusion to the aforesaid demand characteristics, the contradiction between the coordinative delivery service level and inventory cost control should be solved from the perspective of effectiveness, safety, and economy while satisfying the personalized preference of doctors and available with intelligent recommendation, adverse reaction predication, safety precautions, and other functions, so as to meet the satisfaction of the patients, doctors, suppliers, and all other stakeholders [1, 2, 14, 22]. Considering the complexity of the said management, multiple agent techniques must be applied to devise the supply chain management system. In recent years, along with the development in studying code mobility and agent autonomous intelligence, the application of mobile agent and autonomous intelligent agent in supply chain management has won extensive concern. The said agent can move freely among computers via the computer network and autonomously perform specific functions in line with the presence of relevant contextual information. This mobility and autonomous intelligence enable the agent programs of users to truly reside in others' computers and perform information processing on behalf of the users, which greatly improves the processing flexibility, intelligence and efficiency, hence playing a significant role in solving the massive dynamic negotiations and decision-making problems in agile supply. Supported by the National 863 Program of China, Yu Yue and Huang He conducted studies on the networked organization pattern, dynamic negotiation mechanism, and integrated technology of agile supply chain in the context of mobile environment based on the said agent technology, bringing forth brand-new supply chain system structure and its operation mechanism scheme [27, 28]. Meanwhile, technologies of virtual enterprise modeling, distributed computing, software reconfiguration, legacy system package, and various information safeties have also been extensively used for the management over agile supply chain [28]. In view of the current development trend, medical information system application is evolving from information management to big data-driven intelligent decision-making [19, 23, 24], from rational intelligence of the machine to smart healthcare combined with emotional intelligence, and from in-hospital management to patient-centered integrated ubiquitous services, which brings revolutionary change to the traditional medical management pattern [29–32]. The management over clinical surgery-oriented endovascular devices must start from the new requirements for optimal management of the whole supply chain and agile, precision, safe, and intelligent coordinated delivery service under mobile environment and build a fully new management model based on modern agile supply chain management theories and advanced intelligent technologies [1, 14, 31].

20.2 Autonomous Intelligent Decision-Making for Coordinated Delivery

The agile supply chain management over the endovascular devices involves massive decision-making issues. For example, in coordinated delivery decision (Fig. 20.1), first consideration should be given to various demands for clinical surgery, doctors' familiarity with relevant devices, and their

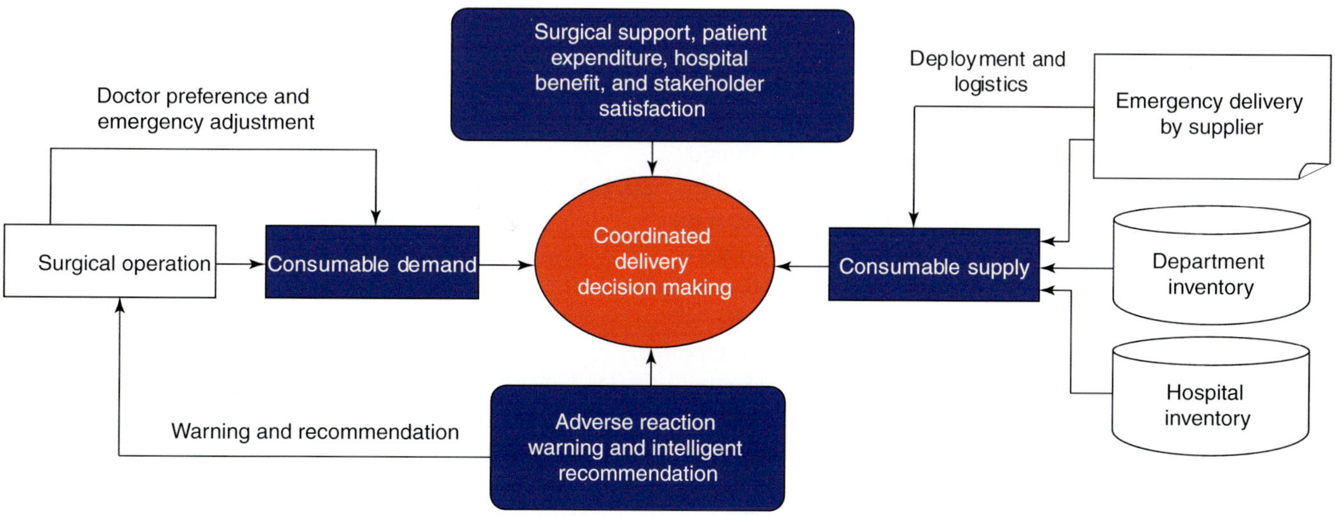

Fig. 20.1 Coordinated delivery decision for endovascular devices

use preference. Moreover, attention should also be paid to the demands for critical devices resulting from various complex situations occurring during operation and emergency programs enforced accordingly [1, 2].

In addition to the stocks provided by hospital and department inventory, many urgently needed devices are subject to emergency delivery by the suppliers, and the ability of suppliers in device allocation and logistics distribution plays a key role in the said service of emergency delivery. Among the decision-making objectives for the coordinated delivery service, surgical support, patient expenditure, hospital and supplier's benefits are all important objectives to be taken into consideration, which play a significant role in improving the synergic innovation ability in coordinated delivery, maintaining its sustainable development and making better use of social and economic benefits [1, 9, 14]. Meanwhile, in making the aforesaid decisions, prompt warning should be given to the adverse reaction already found in device use. Intelligent recommendation and references should also be provided for clinical surgery according to the latest trend of development and updated experience of the devices [11, 12].

Concerning the coordinated delivery mode for the said devices, both conventional and emergency coordinated delivery modes should be taken into consideration. Among them, conventional coordinated delivery refers to prompt and accurate supply of relevant devices according to the surgical scheme and device demand plans predefined by the clinical surgical group, while emergency coordinated delivery refers to delivery of devices urgently needed at the fastest time according to the changes occurred during the surgery. In particular, the waiting time for allocation and delivery of the said critical devices from different suppliers' inventories plays an extremely important role in rescuing the life of the seriously ill patients. The coordinated delivery service of the devices mainly involves decision-making in two aspects: device selection scheme and device delivery scheme. The decision objectives and constraint conditions involved in the above two aspects are somewhat different under conventional and emergency delivery modes.

In the actual selection of decision-making, supply constraints, warning of adverse events, hospital's cost should also be taken into account, in addition to paying attention to surgical support, doctors' use experience and preference, and patients' expenditure. On the one hand, the supplier's interests should also be considered, guaranteeing its reasonable income through data analysis and increasing the supplier's enthusiasm in coordinated delivery service and synergic surgical innovation. But, adequate competitive mechanism should be introduced to avoid falsely high price level. While under emergency coordinated delivery mode, its decision selection is not only subject to influence by the above factors, and furthermore, but also waiting time for the coordination and delivery of critical devices is the primary consideration. As the surgery progresses and delivery situations changed, the above decision should be in-depth analyzed from the angle of dynamic optimization, and in decision for delivery scheme, the major considerations should be real-time inventory distribution, transportation conditions, and time of the devices. In actual situations, the above decision may also involve in a series of random and dynamic decision-making problems.

For further analyzing the above decision-making issues, the decision-making model for the selection scheme and delivery scheme of the above devices is expressed as follows:

20.2.1 Device Selection Scheme Decision

$$\begin{cases} \max Z(C_i) = f_c(p_1, p_2 \ldots, p_m) \\ s.t. C_i \in C, i = 1, 2, 3 \ldots, n \end{cases}$$

wherein $Z(C_i)$ is the multipurpose function of the selection scheme decision; $p_1, p_2, \ldots, p_m$ are the device adaptability, surgical success rate, incidence of complications and other adverse events, total device cost, stakeholders' interests' appeal, and other subgroup objective variables; and C is the optional device scheme set, including all optional device schemes satisfying supply constrain conditions, doctors' use experience and preference, and exclusion of possibilities of adverse reaction under the same patient conditions. Considering the rapid updating of the devices and the fast accumulation of relevant use experience, the said optional device selection scheme set C should not be generated only by retrieving historical data, and rather, intelligent recommendations should also be provided based on the combination use rules and relevant knowledge of the devices.

20.2.2 Device Delivery Scheme Decision

$$\begin{cases} \max S(D_i) = f_s(t_i, c_i) \\ s.t. q(D_i) \le Q, l(D_i) \in L, i = 1, 2, 3 \ldots, n \end{cases}$$

wherein $S(D_i)$ is the multipurpose function of the delivery scheme decision; t_i and c_i are the subgroup objective variable of transportation time and transportation cost, respectively; q (D_i) is the demand quantity of the device; Q the real-time inventory number of the said devices; I (D_i) the transportation scheme; and L all the optional transportation scheme set satisfying the said transportation requirements, including special requirements for transportation conditions and tools. Because device demand generally involves in combined use of various devices and possibly involves in device allocation of suppliers' inventories at different places, the L set of the above transportation scheme is diversified, and complex and transportation time t_i and cost c_i are subject to the influence of the dynamic change of transportation conditions.

In the above decision, the calculation of the objective variables such as total device cost, balance of interests and transportation time and cost basically belongs to structural issues and can be solved by model optimization under certain environmental conditions or with stable random distribution properties. However, recommendation of device selection scheme, doctor's use experience and preference, and warning of adverse events are of nonstructural or semi-structural issues. Moreover, with the extensive use of new devices and continual updating of relevant knowledge, it must consider integrating model optimization with empirical knowledge guidance, case-based reasoning and data driving, and other nonstructural decision modes. In the above decisions, it also involves in acquiring relevant external information, in particular, random optimization and dynamic decision should be ensured under emergency delivery mode according to the ongoing surgical demands and dynamic change of transportation conditions. Among them, device selection and allocation may involve in combination optimization of the suppliers' inventories from different places to reduce transportation waiting time to the maximum extent, which is somewhat complicated.

Through the above analysis, it can be seen that the decision-making for the coordinated delivery of clinical surgical devices is different from the centralized purchase decision of the hospital. It should take into consideration of the multifaceted requirements for service level and quality for clinical surgery and its dynamic changes, involving in the influential factors for the dynamic changes to all external links of the full-range supply chain and having high complexity and high values for in-depth study. Meanwhile, the abovementioned devices include a large number of high-value consumables and special devices that are not subject to centralized purchase and inventory stock by the hospital, which poses significant impact to medical cost and all stakeholders. To properly solve the abovementioned decision-making issues can result in significant economic and social benefits for clinical surgical support, control of medical cost, reasonable interests distribution, improvement in patient's satisfaction, and promotion of experience exchange and learning among different surgical groups.

Viewing from the perspective of decision theory, the coordinated delivery decision-making for clinical surgery-oriented endovascular devices is a multi-objective dynamic decision-making. K. Yu, S. T. Young et al. analyzed in-depth the complexity in their interest relationship and pointed out that the selection and coordinated delivery of the abovementioned devices are not only related to the success of clinical surgery but also had close relationship with the patient's medical costs, hospital benefits, supplier's interests, and wishes for collaborative innovation [14, 22]. M.S. Pishvaee et al. expounded the complexity of the various influencing factors in clinical application and demand's dynamic characteristics [13]. W. Padula and other scholars proposed Markov dynamic prediction model by analyzing the changing characteristics of the abovementioned demands [14, 19]. Based on thorough analysis of the abovementioned issues, the above decision-making problems must be solved by building new intelligent decision-making model through machine learning, data mining, and various artificial intelligence means in combination with effective empirical knowledge [14, 17, 23].

In the above decision-making, the analysis of the existing cases and study on various stakeholders can be used to analyze the demand characteristics in coordinated device delivery; the main complains of the patients, hospital, suppliers, and all other stakeholders; as well as the index level parameters by comparing the current status with their expectations, and comprehensive analysis of the medical, economic, and social factors that influence the coordinated delivery and their decision-making objectives and principles is carried out to build influencing factor model and decision objective model. Based on this, big data-driven decision-making mechanism, methods, and models are studied according to the decision characteristics of the clinical surgical devices under the relevant big data-driven decision-making theories. Finally, build big data-driven decision model scheme oriented to clinical surgery and integrate it with empirical decision, forming intelligent solution. This is the development direction for the coordinated delivery decision of the endovascular devices.

In view of the nature and requirements of the abovementioned decision-making issues and starting from the perspective of combining data driving, empirical knowledge, and model optimization, we put forward a new hybrid decision-making solution based on analysis and systematic in-depth thinking over the coordinated device delivery cases accumulated in the past decade (Fig. 20.2).

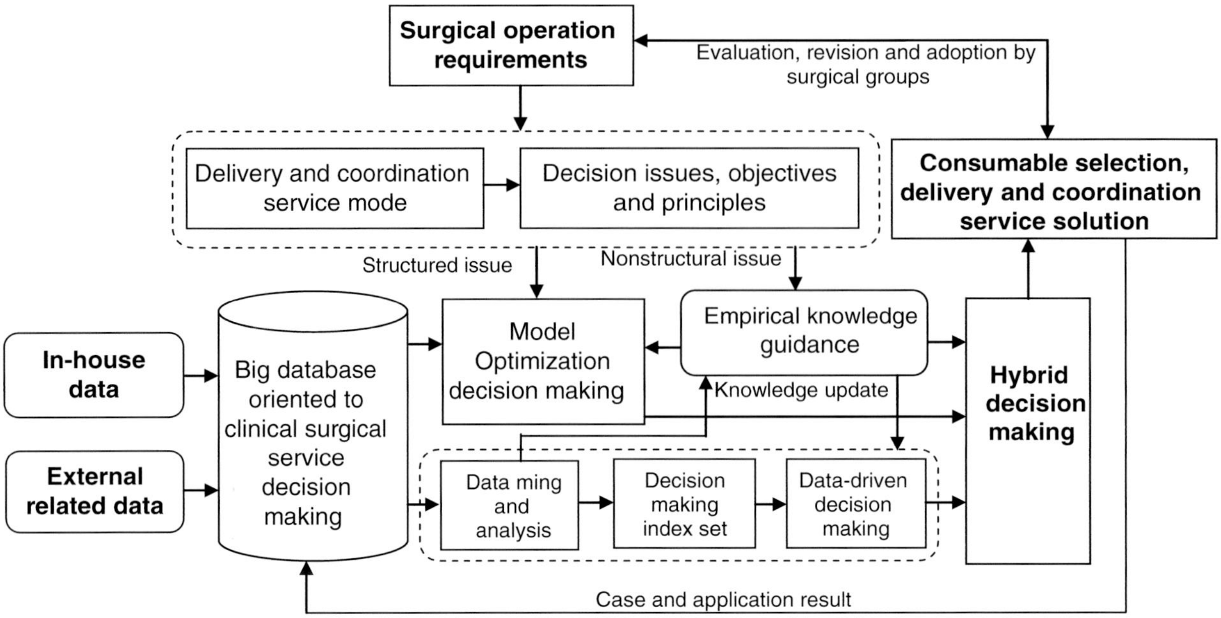

Fig. 20.2 Hybrid decision-making model concerning coordinated delivery service for clinical surgical devices

In the above decision-making model, we first collect in-house data and various related external data, such as supplier's product data, inventory data, transportation tools and conditions, polices and rules by health administration on device use, notices on adverse events, online comments on supplier's products, reports on relevant medical events, literature study and other information, and then establish big database oriented to clinical surgical service decision. Subsequently, data-driven decision-making index set is established by smart mining and analysis of the collected data. When data changes so that the said indexes reach certain level, relevant decision schemes are generated through the autonomous data-driven decision-making function. The said data-driven decision-making is specific to the overall strategy, basic support and common demands by all surgical groups of the coordinated device delivery service, such as use preference analysis for different surgical groups, surgical effect evaluation and stock level configuration based on statistical analysis of device use conditions and surgical effect, as well as device recommendations and overall purchase strategy made according to the foregoing analysis.

In the face of specific clinical surgery, first, select appropriate coordinated delivery service mode according to the analysis of surgical demands, and then, decompose the decision-making issues in line with relevant decision-making problems involved in the foregoing service mode and its decision-making objectives and principles. The structural issues will be solved by model optimization decision-making mode. To improve the efficiency in model optimization and the feasibility of the decision scheme, relevant empirical knowledge will be used to guide the optimization. Nonstructural issues will be solved via guidance by empirical knowledge and data mining and analysis technique based on the said guidance, such as case-based reasoning, and the existing empirical knowledge is updated according to the knowledge acquired from data mining and analysis and objective facts. Finally, the decision scheme generated from the foregoing decision-making mode is comprehensively analyzed and recommended to the surgical group, which is adopted after evaluation and amendment by the surgical group and satisfies the requirements for coordinated delivery of the foregoing clinical devices. The foregoing decision scheme and its actual results in use are sent back to the big database and used as reference for subsequent decision-making.

In general, the large number of complex decision-making and operation problems involved in the management of agile supply chain and the coordinated delivery of the endovascular devices are difficult to be solved on manual basis under limited time constraints and must be responded promptly by autonomous intelligent management of the machines to produce and autonomously carry out optimized decision-making schemes under certain rules [1, 14]. The autonomous intelligence technology differs from the general one mainly in (1) autonomously taking preset actions based on the dynamic monitoring of the target objects and relevant environment information, such as automatic initiating emergency order procedures to the suppliers according to the device changes and surgical knowledge base during clinical surgery, and (2) adopting mobile agent available for self-migration among

Table 20.1 Demand predication probability for some devices

Type	Specification	Demand probability (%)
Cook aneurysm body stent	TFFB-26-96	28.13
Cook aneurysm body stent	TFFB-30-125	2.44
Cook aneurysm iliac stent	TFLE-12-105	24.84
Cook aneurysm iliac stent	TFLE-22-54	1.12
Coda balloon catheter	Coda-10.0-35-120-40	74.58
Cook puncture needle (modified)	G00003 BSDN-18-7.0	100.00
Cook Lunderquist super-stiff wire	G31453 TSMG-35-260-LES	100.00
AngioDynamics angiography catheter	10722702	94.66
Optimed radiographic catheter	1080-4100 110 5	78.77
Optimed nitinol stent	6406-7060	9.84
Perclose AT suture closure system	12673 6F	49.18

different organizations in the service chain so as to solve the massive intelligent negotiation and decision problems in the service chain. Clinical surgery involves in diversified and multifarious surgical devices, and the abovementioned autonomous intelligence technology provides a powerful technological means for the agile, precision, safe, and intelligent coordinated device delivery.

For example, through the in-depth analysis of the previous surgical cases, the demand requirements for relevant devices are consolidated and summarized based on various surgical characteristics and doctor-specific preferences, and based on this, the dynamic demand predication model is built for the critical device as follows:

$$p_{i,j} = f\left(t,d,i,j\right)$$

wherein $p_{i,j}$ represents the demand predication probability of the device of Type i and specification of j, and t, d, i, j represents surgical name, doctor's name, device type, and specification, respectively. For example, Table 20.1 is the demand predication probability for some devices by certain surgeon in an abdominal aortic aneurysm repair operation [1].

Then, stock demand level is figured out according to the surgical schedules of the doctors. Based on this, the optimal model for automatic replenishment is built through the dynamic monitoring to the existing inventory change [1]:

$$s_{i,j} = \min\cos t\left(p_{i,j}, q_{t,d}, c_{i,j}, w_{i,j}\right) \mid l_{i,j} \le L_{i,j}$$

wherein $s_{i,j}$ is the automatic replenishment quantity of the device of Type i and specification j; cos $t()$ is the replenishment cost function of the above consumables, a variable related to demand predication probability $p_{i,j}$, doctor's surgical quantity $q_{t,d}$, device cost $c_{i,j}$, and existing inventory level $w_{i,j}$; and $l_{i,j}$ is the emergency delivery time of the above devices, $L_{i,j}$ the allowable waiting time from the time when the device is decided for use to the time when the device is delivered to the clinical surgery site. The optimized calculation results of the above model can reduce the total replenishment cost without compromising the specific coordinated device delivery service level. Autonomous intelligent agent can take into account the demands by the doctors, patients, hospital, suppliers, and all other stakeholders according to the automatic replenishment quantity calculated by the model, automatically work out replenishment decisions, issue replenishment orders to relevant suppliers, and monitor the distribution of the above devices. The above agent together with the demand information can be migrated to the interface area of the supplier's information system and, after information exchange and autonomous negotiation with the supplier's agent, work out new replenishment decision under certain constraint rules, providing a new model for autonomous intelligent management of coordinated endovascular device delivery.

References

1. Mao H, Jin S, Dai W, et al. Study of the agile supply chain on high-value consumables used in surgical operations. Chinese Journal of Hospital Administration. 2014;6(30):466–9.
2. Mao H, Chen Z, Dai W, et al. Informationization management of high-value interventional consumables to face the dynamic demand. Journal of Medical Informatics. 2014;8(27):57–8.
3. Mao Y. Interventional therapy nursing. Beijing: People's Military Medical Press; 2013.
4. Zhang Z. Operation room nursing technology manual. Beijing: People's Military Medical Press; 2000.
5. Wei K, Liu S. Operation Room Nursing. Beijing: People's Military Medical Press; 2003.
6. Ministry of Construction of the People's Republic of China, General Administration of Quality Supervision, Inspection and Quarantine of the People's Republic of China. Specifications of hospital clean operation room building. Beijing: Ministry of Construction of the People's Republic of China, General Administration of Quality Supervision, Inspection and Quarantine of the People's Republic of China; 2002.
7. Shou H, Xu X, Zhang X, et al. Effects of ambient temperature on core temperature of senile patients during operation in the operating room. J Pract Med. 2005;21(6):555–7.
8. Zhong C, Jiang X. Evaluation of application effect of hydrocolloid transparent paste in treatment of stage I bedsore of the elderly patient. Chin J Pract Nurs. 2014;30(16):42–3.
9. Wang Z, Lou H, Lou Y, et al. Application of use amount and effect analysis in medical consumables. Chin J Hosp Adm. 2012;18(1):54–6.
10. Wu J, Sun C, Liu H. Research report on income and expenditure of medical consumables. Money China. 2015;5:72.
11. Xie L, Xie H, Wei H. Medical instrument not good event risk guard and management. Chin Health Serv Manage. 2006;8:510–1.
12. Han Y, Wang X, Hu C, et al. Analysis of medical devices events in clinical nursing and management. Chin J Nurs. 2008;43(10):924–6.
13. Pishvaee MS, Razmi J, Torabi SA. An accelerated Benders decomposition algorithm for sustainable supply chain network design

under uncertainty: A case study of medical needle and syringe supply chain. Transport Res E-Log. 2014;67:14–38.
14. Yu K. Dynamic supplying management research of medical consumables for clinical surgery. Master dissertation of Fudan University; 2014.
15. Rosales CR, Magazine M, Rao U. The 2Bin system for controlling medical supplies at point-of-use. Eur J Oper Res. 2015;243(1):271–80.
16. Christopher M. Supply chain migration from lean and functional to agile and customized. Supply Chain Manag Int J. 2000;5:206–13.
17. Kong X, Feng M, Wang R. The current status and challenges of establishment and utilization of medical big data in China. Eur Geriatr Med. 2015;6(6):515–7.
18. Ramani KV. Managing hospital supplies. Health Organ Manag. 2006;20(3):218–26.
19. Padula W, Makic MB, Epstein Z, et al. Using machine learning to populate a Markov model by mining big data directly from hospital ehrs-An application to dynamically predict hospital-acquired pressure ulcers. Value Heal. 2015;18(7):PA694.
20. Heinbuch SE. Total quality materials management and just-in-time. Manag Med. 1995;9(2):48–56.
21. Ritchie L, Burnes B, Whittle P, et al. The benefits of reverse Logisties. Supply Chain Manag. 2000;5(3):226–33.
22. Young ST. Prime vendor and hospital purchasing relationships. Int J Phys Distrib Logist Manag. 2007;19(9):27–30.
23. Luo X, Liu Y. Medical big data research situation and its clinical application. J Med Inform. 2015;36(5):10–4.
24. Xu Z, Feng Z, Guo X, et al. Big data-driven management and decision frontier topics. Manage World. 2014;11:158–63.
25. Huajuan Mao, Research and realization of doctor's prescription behavior analysis system. master dissertation of Fudan University, 2010.
26. Eng TY. Mobile supply chain management: challenges for implementation. Technovation. 2006;26(5–6):682–6.
27. Yu Y. Study on grid model and dynamic negotiation mechanism for agile supply chain under mobile environment. Master dissertation of Fudan University; 2010.
28. Huang H. Study and realization of integrated technology for agile supply chain under mobile environment. Master dissertation of Fudan University; 2010.
29. Cacioppo JT, Berntson GG. Social psychological contributions to the decade of the brain: doctrine of multilevel analysis. Am Psychol. 1992;47:1019–28.
30. Ma Q, Wang X. From Neuroeconomics and Neuromarketing to Neuromanagement. J Ind Eng Eng Manag. 2006;20(3):129–32.
31. Dai W. Study on China's translational medicine development strategy: forward-looking medical information technology (1st draft). Major strategic advisory report of Chinese Academy of Engineering; 2014
32. Dai W. Context awareness and emotional intelligence: the gateway to smart city. Urban Manag. 2012;4:29–32.

Device Management

21

Huajuan Mao, Weihui Dai, and Yufeng Zhuang

Abstract

With the continuous progress in medical technology and the all-round improvement at hospital service level, the varieties and use of endovascular devices increase year by year. These devices set high requirements for safekeeping and use. How to store these devices in the limited operation room, realize precision in-out management, and ensure perfect registration and traceability of grafts according to the relevant requirements by National Health Commission of the People's Republic of China are a difficulty faced in actual work. The development of information technology has brought great convenience for the management mentioned above and also provided advanced management model. This chapter expounds the endovascular device management mainly from four aspects: storage management, information management, registration management, and management system.

Keywords

Endovascular devices · Storage management · Information management · Use management

21.1 Storage Management of Endovascular Devices

The development of endovascular minimally invasive techniques relies heavily on the innovation of endovascular devices. In recent years, various new endovascular devices, such as vascular sheath, wire, spring coil, etc., have been extensively used in minimally invasive endovascular surgery. These devices are of multifarious varieties, complex specifications, and different forms, occupying large operation room space and thus making the operation room appear crowded and messy. Moreover, ambiguous marking also leads to difficulties in identifying these devices or misusing them, resulting in malpractice. Therefore, storage management should be carried out strictly according to the structures and forms, use characteristics, and storage requirements of various devices, having the arrangement, purchase date, and use sequence of the devices carefully considered. To solve the problems mentioned above, Huajuan Mao at the Department of Vascular Surgery of Changhai Hospital affiliated to the Second Military Medical University designed special storage utilities for the storage management of the devices mentioned above, greatly facilitating the device management. Please refer to the following three patented products designed by Huajuan Mao for detail.

21.1.1 Medical Consumable Storage Unit

Medical consumable storage unit (Patent No. ZL201320560946.4) (Fig. 21.1) is made of organic glass, equipped with different frames and partitions according to the size, diameter, and dimension of the common consumables so that the consumables are arranged by category and identified clearly. The unit is characterized in that the first supporting frame passes through the first backplate, the first side plate, and the bracket and connects with the second supporting frame in a fixed manner or dismountable manner. The unit is not easy for deformation, durable and sturdy, available for storing consumables of different dimensions, and greatly reducing the space occupied by medical consumable storage devices and the increasing storage area. There are more than 40 kinds of standby wires used by the department of Vascular Surgery of Changhai Hospital affiliated to the Second Military Medical University, all of which can be readily arranged into the device mentioned above, with models, diameters, and lengths being clearly marked. This sig-

H. Mao (✉) · Y. Zhuang
Department of Vascular Surgery, Changhai Hospital, Second Military Medical University, Shanghai, China

W. Dai (✉)
School of Management, Fudan University, Shanghai, China
e-mail: whdai@fudan.edu.cn

Z. Jing et al. (eds.), *Endovascular Surgery and Devices*, https://doi.org/10.1007/978-981-10-8270-2_21

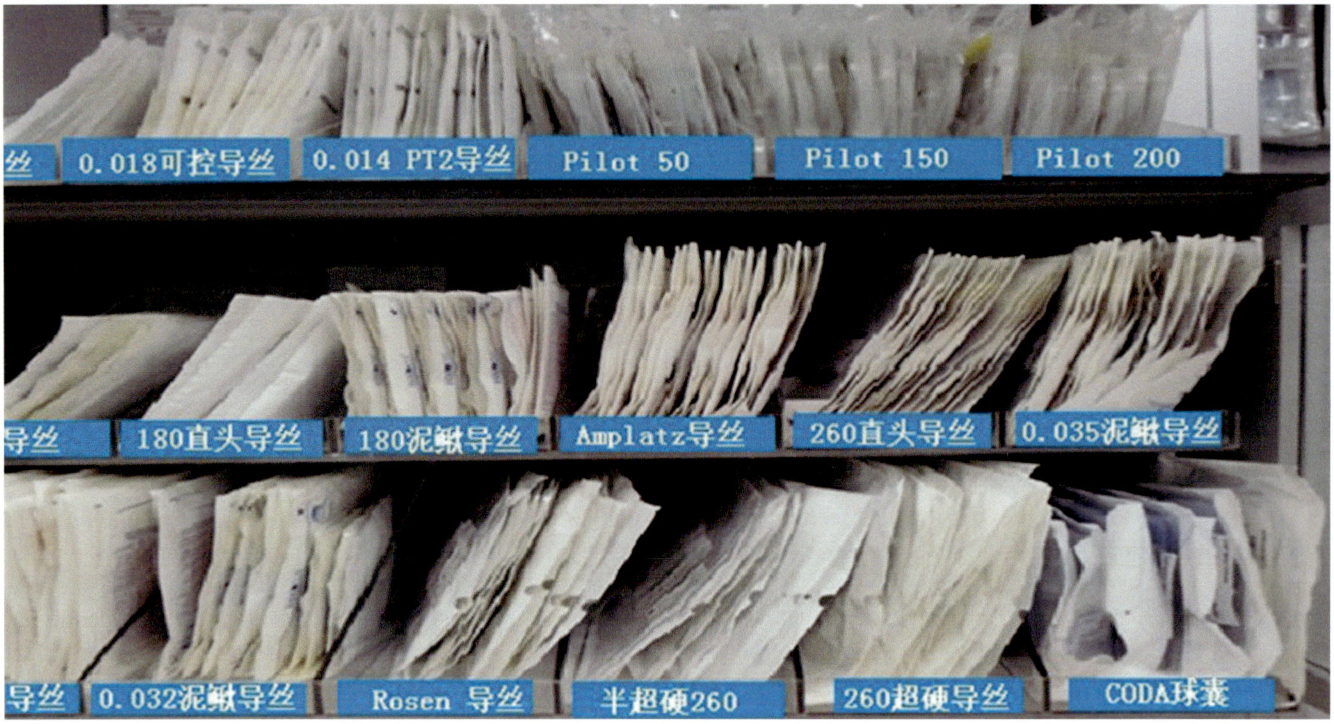

Fig. 21.1 Medical consumable storage unit

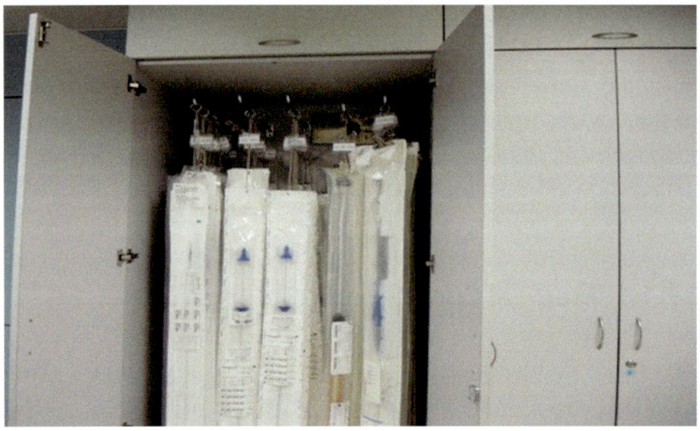

Fig. 21.2 Stent storage cabinet

nificantly reduces the occupied space of the operation room and also reduces the error rate in clinical surgical coordination. Since the use of the said unit, no errors in coordinated delivery have occurred to any consumables, having achieved safe and agile results in practical use.

21.1.2 Stent Storage Cabinet

Stent storage cabinet (Patent No.: ZL201320617605.6) (Fig. 21.2) is made of wooden boards, mainly used for storage of large artery stents in thoracic and abdominal aortic surgeries, by which the large artery stents of various lengths can not only be hung up vertically and are not liable of damage, but also the newly purchased stents are arranged at the back so as to use the stents according to their production date and avoid waste and invalid use upon expiration. The storage cabinet greatly increases the storage space. The original cabinet can accommodate only about 20 stents for large arteries, but now it can accommodate more than 100 stents. Meanwhile, the cabinet facilitates the nurses to quickly find and accurately obtain the required stents during operation, preventing them from working in a rush and greatly reducing surgical waiting time.

21.1.3 Aortic Stent Hanging Piece

Aortic stent hanging piece (Patent No. ZL201320585533.1) (Fig. 21.3) is made of organic glass, metal chains, coils, and hooks in a double-skin design, facilitating putting in and taking out of the transparent plates marked with different stent model labels. The stents are classified and displayed, avoiding the waste of time or mistakenly taking in a rush due to the printed small serial number on the stent package.

For the operation rooms with limited space, orderly and classified arrangement of surgical devices with clear identification and reasonable design of endovascular storage devices is of critical importance. In particular, during surgical coordination, various devices can be delivered quickly, accurately, and orderly according to the actual demands present at any time during the operation. The use of the storage devices mentioned

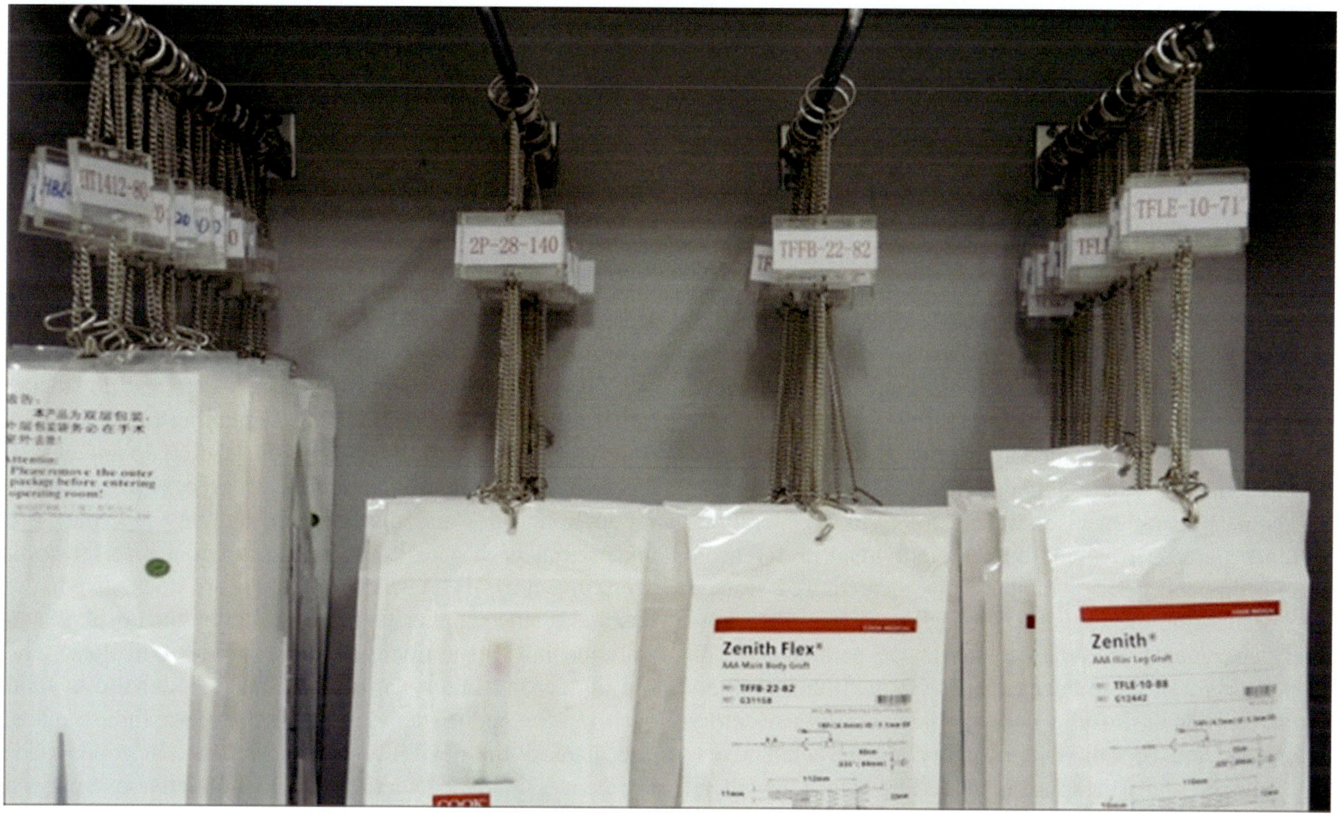

Fig. 21.3 Aortic stent hanging piece

above not only facilitates the coordination work of the nurses but also provides guarantee for the success in operation, reducing errors due to wrong surgical devices on the operation table and eliminating all medical errors. Using the device mentioned above also facilitates inventory taking, ensuring first-in and first-out, and avoiding device waste due to expiration. By network monitoring with information system, the device can also be used to optimize replenishment quantity and make up the inventory at any time, avoiding stock out and greatly reducing cost. Through years' practical use, the device can not only increase the work efficiency but also greatly improve the satisfaction of the doctors, suppliers, and patients.

21.2 Information-Based Management of Endovascular Devices

21.2.1 Current Status of Information-Based Management of Endovascular Devices

Endovascular devices can be classified as high-value and low-value endovascular devices, among which low-value endovascular devices are diversified in varieties, huge in quantities, vast in specifications, and frequently used. To ensure prompt and convenient supply, these devices are generally subject to high inventory. Numerous low-value endovascular devices have different shelf lives and negligence in noticing these shelf lives will result in huge waste. In addition, the market price for some low-value endovascular devices is tremendous, which poses high loss risks for inventory. But high-value endovascular devices feature expensive price and high requirements for storage; in particular, the effectiveness and safety of the grafts are subject to rigid control. Therefore, the management over high-value endovascular devices is an important part for hospital device management.

In the face of the above characteristics of the endovascular devices and the complexity of their management, the traditional management methods can no longer meet the requirements for lean coordinated management among clinical demands, planned procurement, and cost control [1, 2]. In particular, in current practice, the cost of the devices is collected after the use by the patient. If the above monies have been paid at the time of purchase and once product quality problems arise, it is often difficult to recover the cost. The abovementioned devices are usually kept directly by the department users, but the demands for endovascular devices often change in actual operation process, for example, the devices readily prepared before operation are not used in actual operation, or new devices are used for emergency purpose, easily leading to disagreement between the book entries and the actual inventory or even device loss, thus resulting in direct economic loss.

In the face of the management of the high-value endovascular devices mentioned above, we have adopted a new information-based management model for agile supply chain.

21.2.2 Information-Based Management Model for High-Value Endovascular Devices

High-value endovascular devices refer to the consumable medical devices directly acting on human bodies, having strict requirements for safety, strictly controlled in production and use, and having relatively high value. For vascular surgery, high-value endovascular devices mainly include balloons, stents, filters, spring coils, and other devices. In face with the management characteristics of the high-value endovascular devices, we have proposed a new model for the information-based management of the agile supply chain of endovascular devices (Fig. 21.4) [1].

In the management model mentioned above, dynamic device demand prediction model is provided first by analyzing the past operation cases and according to the operation-specific characteristics and doctor's individual preferences, establishing the basic parameters for the required storage level and asking the suppliers to meet the order for the hospital departments according to the above parameters. The property right of these devices still vests with the suppliers before use, and the hospital only establishes virtual inventory record and safekeeps the said inventory, and the actual inventory number of the hospital is zero. The virtual inventory information mentioned above is provided to the suppliers, and by dynamic monitoring of the virtual inventory and in comparison with the required stock level, replenishment order is automatically sent to the suppliers by short messages.

To meet the dynamic demands for different devices during operation and provide prompt services, the said system should provide on-demand services according to the rules of demands for the devices by different operations and doctors, and under special circumstances, the suppliers should provide emergency delivery to the operation room. Under the aforesaid management model, the hospital adopts "zero inventory" stock. It is worth noting that the said "zero inventory" does not necessarily mean no reserves and no stocks; rather, it means that the materials (including raw materials, semifinished products, finished products, etc.) do not exist in the form of warehouse storage in the process of purchase, production, sale, and distribution, and, instead, they are under circulation state. "Zero inventory" stock refers to book "zero inventory" stock where the stocks are stocked up in the hospital by the suppliers and safely kept by the hospital, and warehousing registration is conducted after surgical use. The use of "zero inventory" model can make better use of fund performance, reduce department cost, save warehouse space, and increase the flexibility and convenience in goods management. The management model mentioned above plays a significant role in standardizing department management procedures for the high-value endovascular devices and

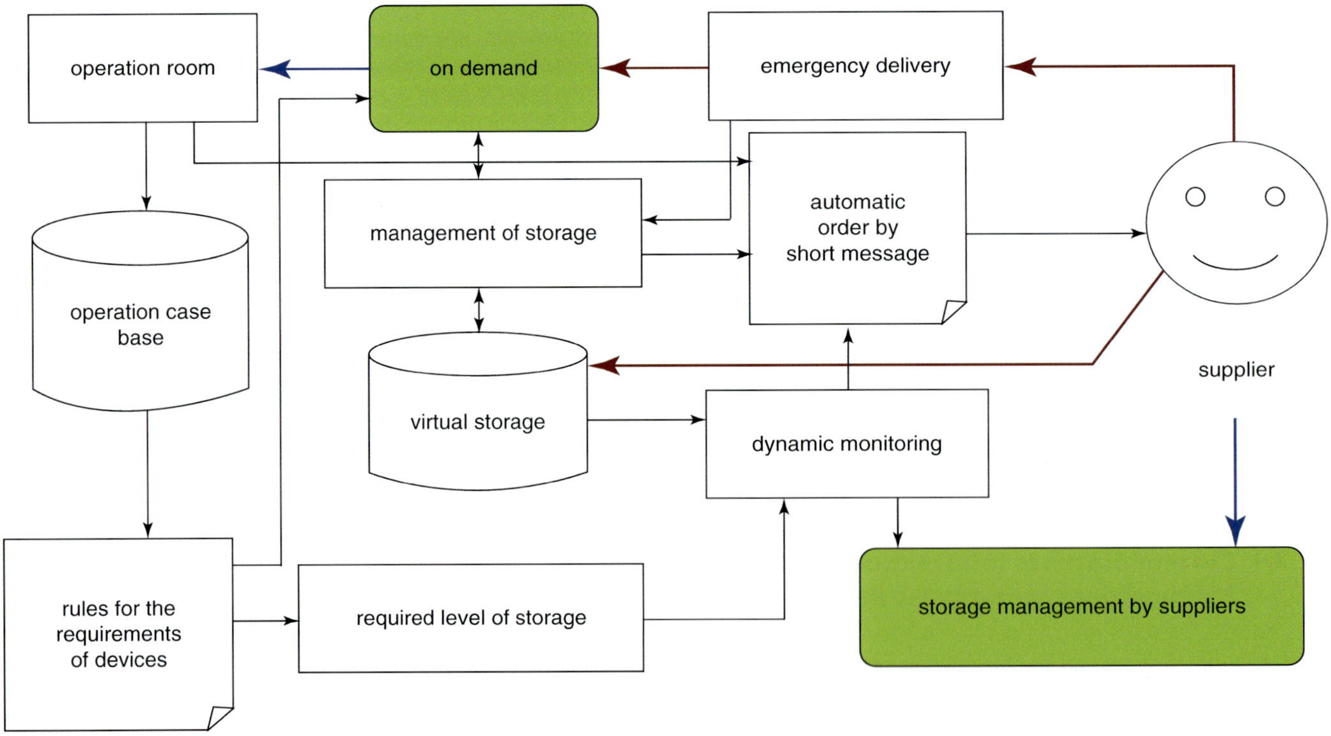

Fig. 21.4 Information-based management model for agile supply chain of endovascular devices

ensuring accurate pricing, effective tracking, and better risk avoidance.

In the "zero inventory" management, we adopt the following two order management methods:

1. Quantitative ordering method: An inventory management practice where replenishment order is placed at specified quantity when the virtual inventory declines to the preset minimum inventory level, the advantage of which is the prompt knowledge about the dynamic inventory because detailed inspection and inventory taking are carried out for high-value endovascular devices each time after use. However, frequent inspection and inventory taking take a lot of time and labor and thus increase the cost to maintain and safely keep the inventory.
2. Periodic ordering method: An inventory management method where replenishment order is placed at a preset fixed interval. A fixed interval is preset for order placement by the enterprise based on its past experience or business objectives, and order is placed at each preset time interval with different order quantity each time. For periodic ordering, the order cycle and maximum inventory level must be defined, and the order quantity each time is the maximum inventory level minus current inventory minus floating order minus delayed purchase by the customer. In using periodic ordering method, multiple goods are purchased at the same time, which reduces order processing cost and transportation cost. Moreover, this method requires no frequent inspection and inventory taking, thus reducing inventory maintenance cost.

After a 9-year practice, the "zero inventory" management model has achieved significant results, saving both the waiting time for the doctors and the patients and the stock cost for the suppliers and providing a whole information-based supply chain management model for the endovascular devices [1, 2].

21.2.3 Information-Based Management System for High-Value Endovascular Devices

In information-based management for the endovascular devices, first, use the barcode to label all devices. Each device has its unique barcode, similar to the ID card number. Products of the same specifications have different ID card numbers due to different lot numbers. Relevant information, inventory quantity, and settlement charges of the devices can be input just by scanning the barcode. When the endovascular devices are warehoused, the supplier should complete the endovascular device delivery note as required, clearly indicating the model, quantity, production lot number, expiry date, and other information of the devices. The hospital should verify and accept the product package, quantity, barcode, expiry date, lot number, and other information. Finally, the endovascular devices are warehoused by scanning the barcode by the information system. When the endovascular devices are used by the patients, fees are charged via the above system, and when the patient's admission number is entered, the information on the use of the endovascular devices is associated with patients. The labels of the devices used during operation should be attached onto the Department Implant Registration Book as required for traceability purpose. Meanwhile, the warehouse-out list of the supplier's surgical materials can be generated by entering the patient's admission number and the supplier's Pinyin code.

21.2.4 System Functions and Operation Procedures

The main functions and operation procedures of the information-based management system mentioned above are as follows [1]:

- Personnel responsible for device management should consult with the supplier and prepare routinely used balloons, stents, filters, and other devices according to the demands by clinical operation departments and rooms. The quantity for each model can be prepared according to the surgical quantity and the characteristics of each doctor. Supplier's inventory stock information on high-value endovascular devices is established in the information-based management software used by the departments or rooms (Fig. 21.5).
- Replenish and prepare high-value endovascular devices 1 day before the operation according to the surgical quantity under appointment. During the operation, if the patient presents with different situations and the surgical procedures need to be changed, some high-value endovascular devices that have not been prepared may be temporarily required. In this case, the demand can be satisfied by agile supply chain and on-demand coordination service.
- The traceability information and barcode of the patient's implants should be registered promptly during operation, marking clearly the surgical site and used implants on the surgical map (Fig. 21.6).

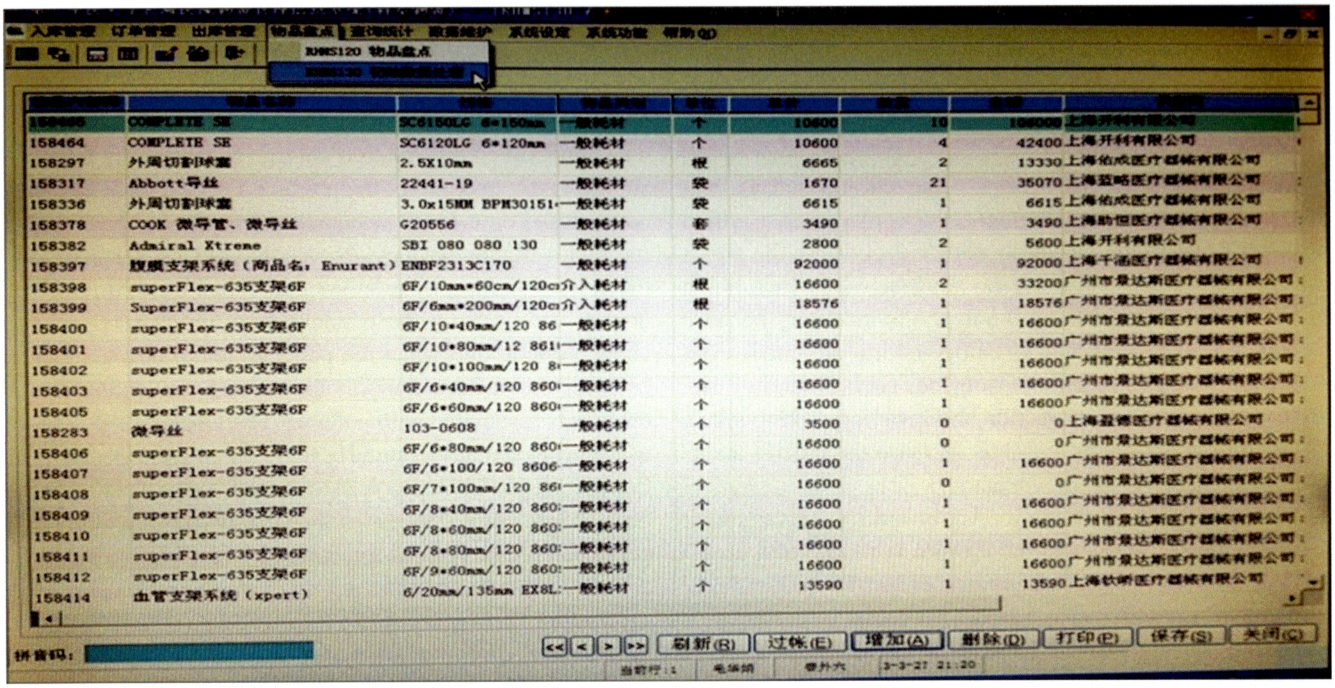

Fig. 21.5 Inventory information

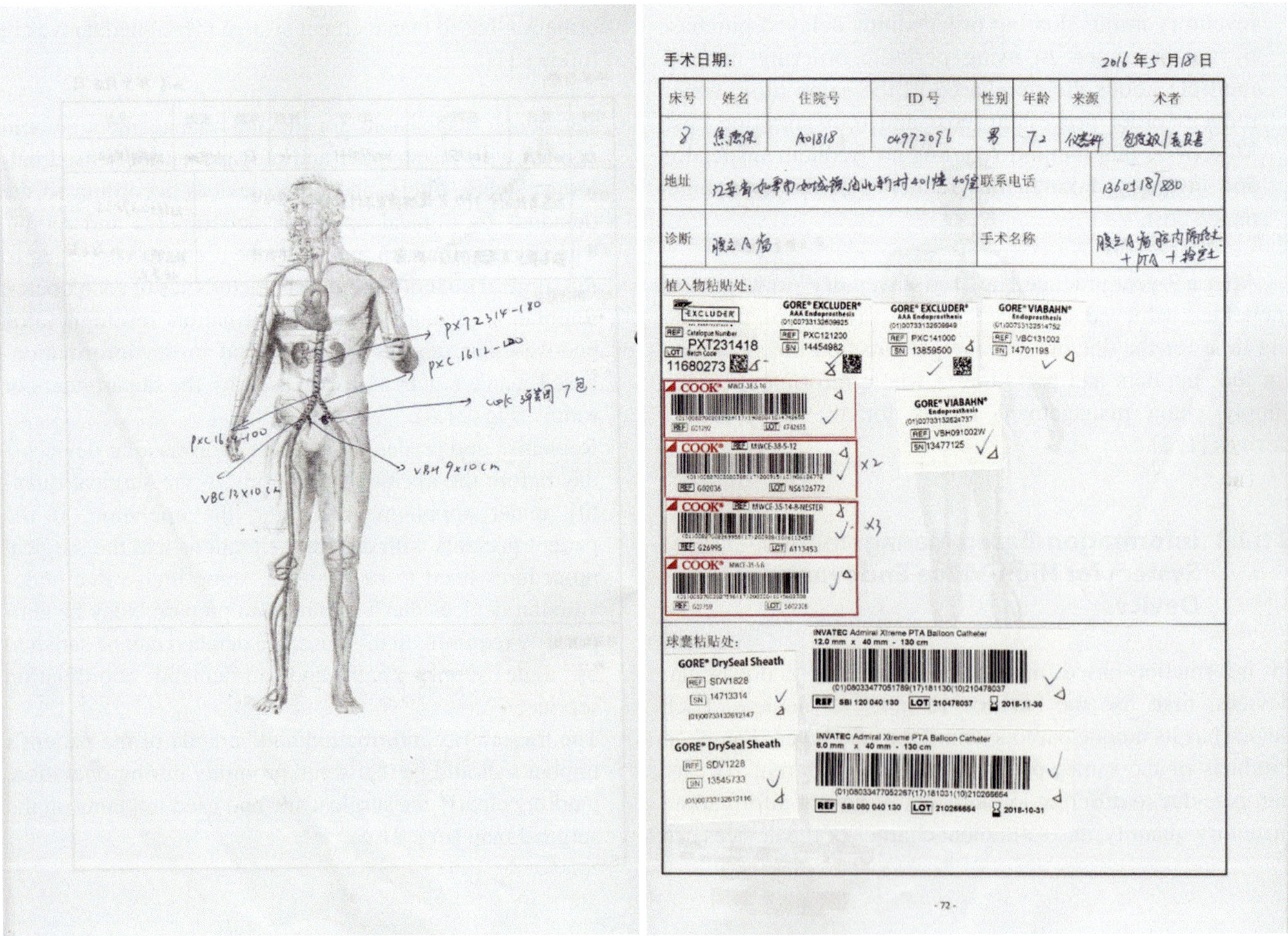

Fig. 21.6 Implant information registration and traceability record

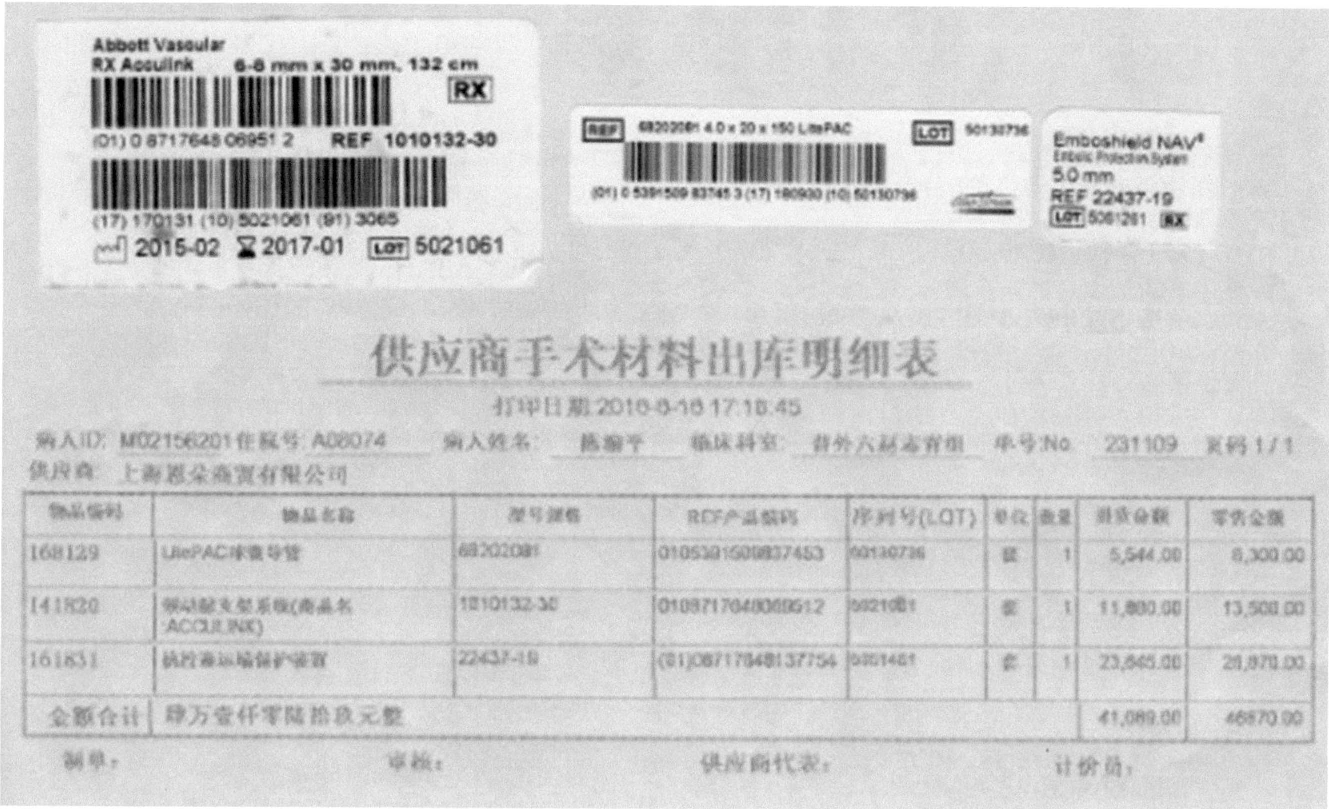

Fig. 21.7 Warehouse-out list of supplier's surgical materials

- Fees are collected promptly and accurately after operation; the warehouse-out list of supplier's surgical materials (Fig. 21.7) is printed in four copies.
- Enter the used high-value endovascular devices into the direct log-on page of the purchase application form of the hospital material management system, and open the notice of purchase arrival.
- Send the name, model, quantity, and unit price of the supplier's high-value endovascular devices used on the current day to the supplier-specific mobile phones (Fig. 21.8). The device for sending the message consists of the SMS package and the SIM card of the mobile phone, directly connected with the computer by USB interface.
- Upon successful message transmission, establish and review warehouse-out inventory.
- The supplier makes up the order at 9:30–10:30 the next morning according to the message received, which is the best time for replenishment based on years' experience. The supplier signs on the warehouse-out list of supplier's surgical materials (Fig. 21.7) and leaves one copy, and the other three copies are taken back to the company for selling, sealing, and invoicing and handed over directly to hospital device section for accounting upon completion of invoicing.
- Enter all the delivery notes of suppliers (Fig. 21.9) onto the review page of the notice of purchase arrival according to the entries on the warehouse-in list.

In the implementation of the above process, SMS notice not only meets the intraoperative demands of the patients and the surgeons but also saves the nurse's time in notifying the suppliers, reduces the occurrence of various accidents, improves the timeliness and accuracy in delivery by the salespersons, and alleviates the messy and busy work of the nurses and the salespersons. Moreover, it enables quick inquiry into the patient's past case history, providing the clinical doctors with accurate guidance in looking up and comparing the intraoperative materials and selecting appropriate operation procedures. The doctors and the nurses need not spend a lot of time and efforts to look up the original registrations or perform manual statistics so as to obtain all these data information and materials. For example, for the patient with endovascular therapy again due to in-stent restenosis, the specifications of the previously implanted stent must be known so as to guide the selection of stent used in the current operation. In the past, such information could only be looked up by reading over the registration books, but after the use of information management system, the past surgical history of the patient can be looked up immediately only by entering the initials of the patient's name, greatly reducing the waiting time for intraoperative inquiry and comprehensively improving the medical nursing quality. The phenomenon of being in disorder, overdue, lost, charged less, omitted charge of the high-value endovascular devices

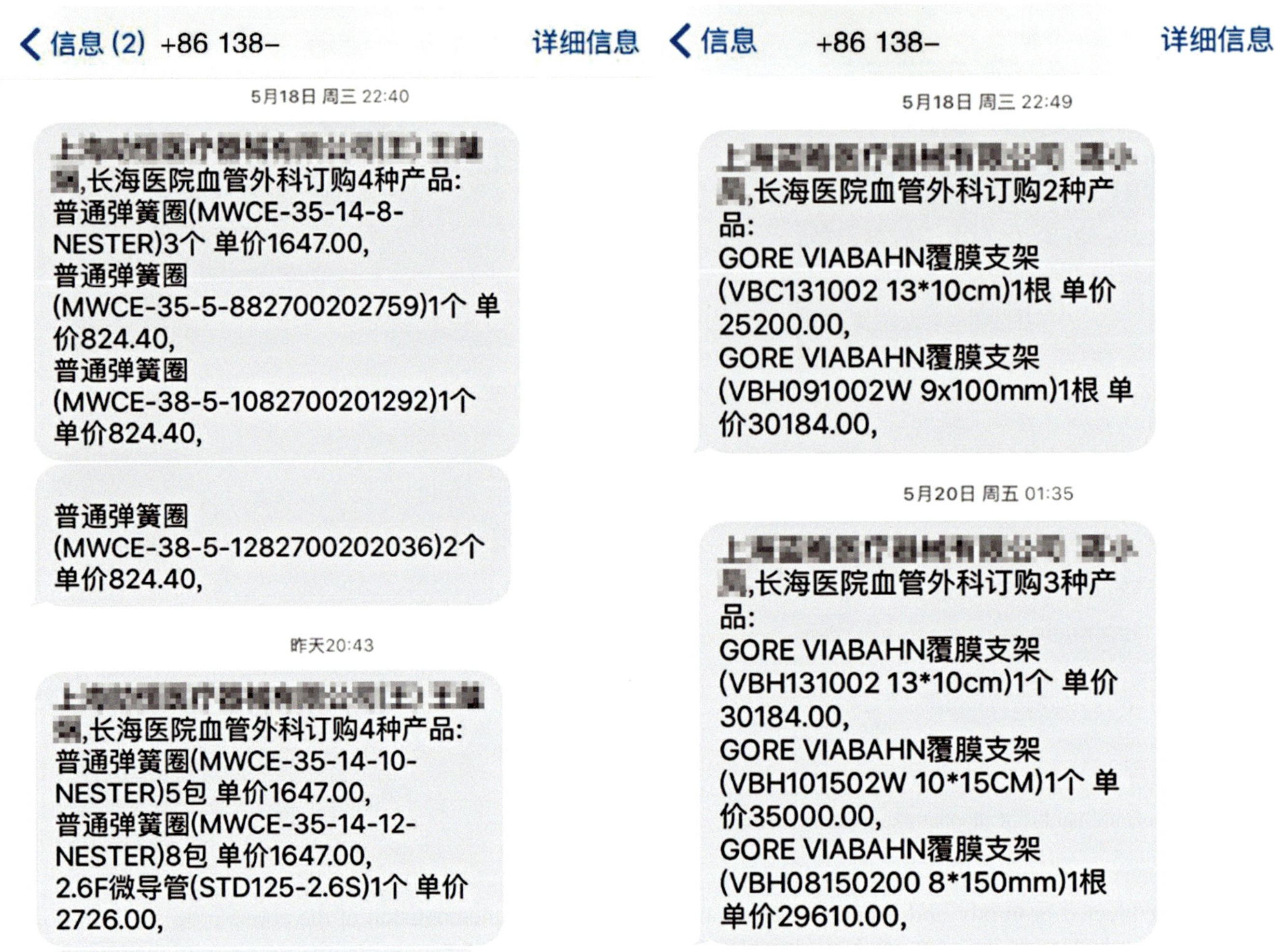

Fig. 21.8 Mobile phone SMS page

is eliminated by standardized management, which not only enables convenient and effective work by the special management personnel but also enhances the sense of responsibility of nurses and improves their service quality for mutual benefits. The research results of the medical consumable information management system have been published on the *Journal of Chinese Hospital Administration* (6th Issue, 2014) [1] and obtained a national invention patent (Patent No.: ZL201310488851.0).

With the application of the autonomous intelligent technology, massive complex decision-making tasks and the whole supply chain management in the above system will be completed by intelligent agent and interfaced with information system of suppliers, thus providing agile, precision, safe, and intelligent coordinated delivery service for clinical surgeries.

21.3 Registration Management of Endovascular Devices

Registration management over endovascular devices is a basic work for device management. Among the endovascular devices, implants refer to the implantable endovascular devices that can be placed in vivo during operation, such as vascular stent, spring coil, heart valve, etc. During each operation, the implants used by the patient should be registered for filing. On the implant registration form, medical workers should record the name and quantity of the implants used and sign off upon multiple examinations so as to avoid errors in pricing the implants and consequentially any medical disputes due to the negligence of medical workers. However, this simple registration form cannot clearly record the barcode information and implantation

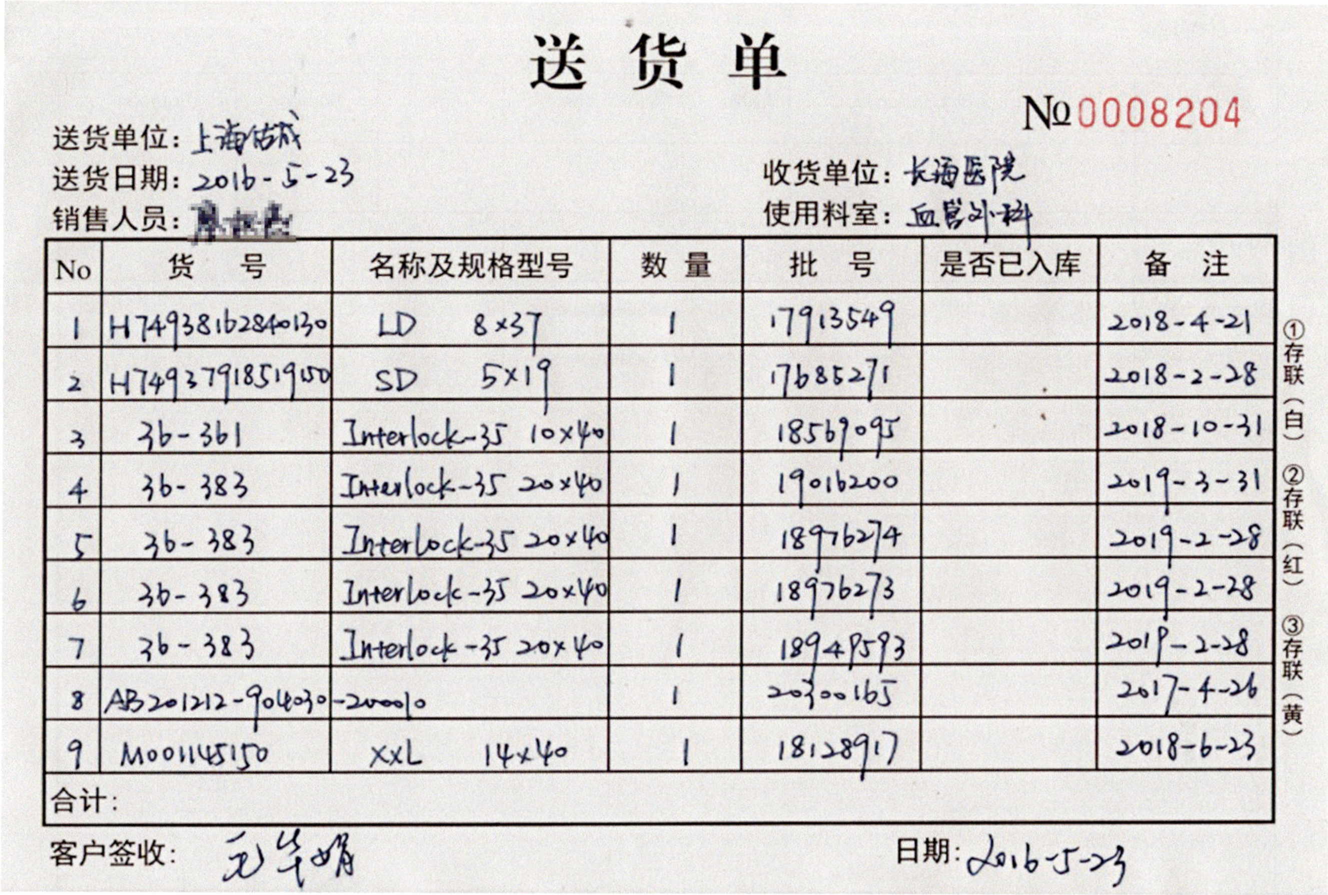

送 货 单

№0008204

送货单位：上海佑成
送货日期：2016-5-23
销售人员：[redacted]

收货单位：长海医院
使用料室：血管外科

No	货 号	名称及规格型号	数 量	批 号	是否已入库	备 注
1	H74938162840130	LD 8×37	1	17913549		2018-4-21
2	H74937918519150	SD 5×19	1	17685271		2018-2-28
3	36-361	Interlock-35 10×40	1	18569095		2018-10-31
4	36-383	Interlock-35 20×40	1	19016200		2019-3-31
5	36-383	Interlock-35 20×40	1	18976274		2019-2-28
6	36-383	Interlock-35 20×40	1	18976273		2019-2-28
7	36-383	Interlock-35 20×40	1	18948593		2019-2-28
8	AB201212-904030-200010		1	20300165		2017-4-26
9	M001145150	XXL 14×40	1	18128917		2018-6-23
合计：						

①存联（白） ②存联（红） ③存联（黄）

客户签收：[illegible]　　日期：2016-5-23

Fig. 21.9 Delivery note

location of the in vivo implants and, as a result, cannot track and inquire about the implants implanted in the patient's body.

To ensure better registration management for the implants mentioned above, Huajuan Mao designed a special implant information registration and traceability record (Patent No. ZL201530303843.4) based on clinical demands, as shown in Fig. 21.10.

This record is the original record maintained strictly in accordance with the barcode traceability requirements by National Health Commission of the People's Republic of China. The bottom of the registration front page is printed with the implant information column used for attaching the implant barcode, available for recording the barcode information of the implants used during operation. The back is printed with a human body structure diagram, available for marking the implantation location(s) of the implant(s) recorded on the next page, thus enabling tracking and inquiry of the implants. The use of the implant information registration and traceability record eliminates the situations of unclear models or quantities in the supplier's inventory management, reduces the situations of less or omission in fee collection in department inventory management, provides precious first-line surgical information for the follow-up patients, and, for the doctors, provides them with scientific research information. Ultimately, all implant information registration and traceability records are arranged and filed in chronological sequence (Fig. 21.11).

21.4 Management System for Using Endovascular Devices

Use management of endovascular devices should have special management system according to the types, characteristics, and use requirements of the devices. The following management system has been worked out for the device use management by Changhai Hospital affiliated to the Second Military Medical University for reference only.

<table>
<tr><td colspan="8">Date of Operation: day month year</td></tr>
<tr><td>Bed No.</td><td>Name</td><td>Admission No.</td><td>ID No.</td><td>Gender</td><td>Age</td><td>Source</td><td>Surgeon</td></tr>
<tr><td></td><td></td><td></td><td></td><td></td><td></td><td></td><td></td></tr>
<tr><td>Add ress</td><td colspan="3"></td><td>Contact Tel.</td><td colspan="3"></td></tr>
<tr><td>Diagnosis</td><td colspan="3"></td><td>Nomenclature
of Operation</td><td colspan="3"></td></tr>
<tr><td colspan="8">Attach implant (s) here</td></tr>
<tr><td colspan="8">Attach balloon (s) here</td></tr>
</table>

Fig. 21.10 Implant information registration and traceability record

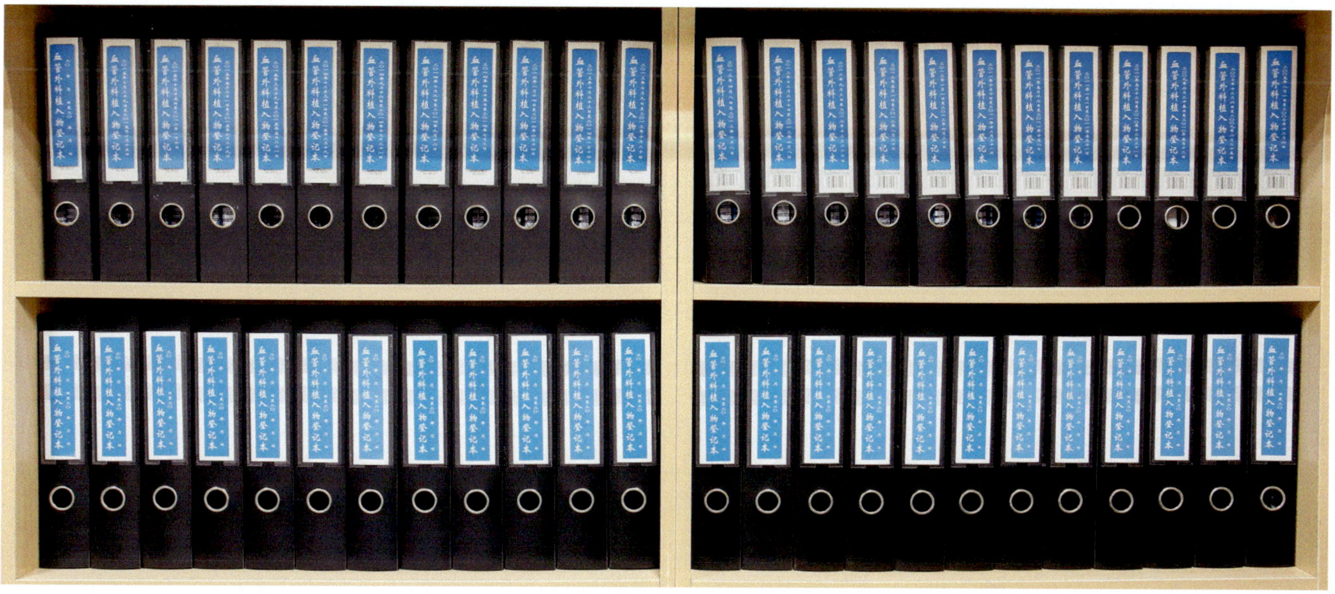

Fig. 21.11 Consolidated and filed implant information registration and traceability records

21.4.1 Management System for Using Low-Value Endovascular Devices

- All endovascular devices are subject to barcode management.
- Engineers of special device management are responsible for requisition application, use, bookkeeping, payment collection, and other formalities of the consumables.
- Inventory taking is carried out at the end of each month, periodically checking the shelf life of the devices to see if the packages are damaged or invalid before use.
- All disposable endovascular devices are subject to centralized purchase by the hospital and should not be purchased by departments without permission.
- Disposable endovascular devices must be conforming products turned out by manufacturers obtaining medical device manufacturing license, industrial product manufacturing license, and medical device registration certificate issued by provincial drug regulatory authorities or higher and health license issued by health administration or distributed by dealers obtaining medical device operation license; imported disposable catheter and other endovascular devices must have medical device registration certificate issued by the National Drug Administration.
- For each procurement, the purchase department must carry out quality inspection; confirm the order contract, place of departure, and payment account are consistent with the manufacturer/dealer; and verify the inspection certificate, production date, date of sterilization, product logo, and shelf life of each package of products. Imported disposable catheter and other interventional consumables must have date of sterilization, shelf life, and other contents in Chinese.
- Products are arranged in cool and dry storage cabinets according to their shelf lives, kept at ≥20 cm over the ground and ≥5 cm from the wall.
- Engineers of special device management should establish endovascular device registration forms (Fig. 21.12), recording the supplier unit, delivery date, product name, specifications, unit price, quantity, product lot number, shelf life, sign-off date, sender, recipient, invoice price, invoicing date, invoice number, and others.

21.4.2 Management System for Implantable High-Value Endovascular Devices

- Forbid using implantable medical devices and high-value endovascular devices not purchased by the hospital through public bidding.
- Medical Device Section should ensure the used implantable medical devices and high-value endovascular devices conform to product quality requirements according to relevant national laws and regulations and carry out authentication procedures as specified to confirm the legal qualifications of manufacturers.
- Preoperative doctor-patient communication must be performed for all high-value endovascular devices to be used during the operation (such as spring coil, filter, stent, etc.), explaining the type, purpose, price, and adverse reaction of the high-value endovascular devices to be used and signing the Informed Consent for Using Medical Implants (Fig. 21.13) upon consent by the patient or his/her family members.
- The barcode of the high-value endovascular devices implanted into the patient's body must be attached on the

Company:														
Date	Product Name (Specifications and models)	Unit Price	Qty.	Lot No.	Useful Life	Sign-off date	Sender	Receiver	Invoice Price	Invoice Date	Invoice No.	Total Price	Signature on Invoice

Fig. 21.12 Registration Form for Low-Value Endovascular Devices

Registration Form for Using Medical Implant (Fig. 21.14) and registered. The surgeon must also register the brand, model, and quantity of the high-value endovascular devices used during the operation on the Operation Record.

- All departments should establish registration systems for warehousing, use, and delivery for all high-value endovascular devices, and all registration information should be kept for over 30 years for product quality traceability.
- Device Section should be responsible for the purchase and quality inspection of the high-value endovascular devices and carry out relevant registration accordingly for the filing. Medical Service Management Section should be responsible for checking if the patient's records are filled with the product qualification certificate and barcode as completed in the Informed Consent for Using Medical Implants and the Registration Form for Using Medical Implant.
- In using high-value endovascular devices, in case of any problems with product quality, the devices involved should be kept properly, and further product quality authentication should be carried out, with Report on the Suspected Medical Device Adverse Event (Fig. 21.15) being completed and delivered to Medical Device Section for reporting.
- Forbid purchasing and using high-value endovascular devices without permission. Once any unauthorized purchase or use is found, the same will be handed over to and treated by the hospital Discipline Inspection Commission.

Shanghai Changhai Hospital

Informed Consent for Using Medical Implants

Patients name: Gender: Age: Department: Bed No.: Admission No.:

Representative (Guardian)Name: Relationship with the Patient:

Minutes of talks:

1. Preoperative diagnosis:
2. Intended operation:
3. Name of medical implant(s) to be used:
4. Purpose of using the medical implant (s):
5. Possible major complications, accidents and intended countermeasures:

Patients opinion: (the patient to fill in Agree or Disagree)

I have been informed of my state of illness, the surgical program, the treatment purpose, benefits, possibility of success, possible risks, and possible problems occurringduring rehabilitation and alternative therapeutic regime. I have understood and given full consideration to the aforesaid information, I hereby decide and am willing to acceptthe useof the medical implant(s) mentioned herein above and bearall risks incurred therewith and related thereto.

The foregoing minutes of talks shall be signed by the patient (the representativeor guardian) if being consistent with the facts and shall come into effect upon signatures by both parties.

Signature of the patient (or agent, or guardian): Date:

Signature of the attending doctor: Date:

Fig. 21.13 Informed Consent for Using Medical Implants

Registration Form for Using Medical Implants			
Patient's Name	Admission No.	Operation Time	Surgeon's Signature
Product Name	Specifications & Models	Product Tracking No./Production Lot No.	
Manufacturer	Manufacturer's Address	Manufacturer's Contact Tel.	
Attach product information here:			
Remarks:			
Instructions for Filling in the Form: 1. The form is to be filled by the surgeon. 2. Attach the barcode related to the product serial number at the "Attach product information here" column. 3. The form must be filled at the same day as the operation. 4. The form shall be attached to medical records of the patient.			

Fig. 21.14 Registration Form for Using Medical Implants

Appendix 1:

Report on the Suspected Medical Device Adverse Event

Report Date: Code □□□□□□□□□□□

Source of Report: □ Manufacturer □ Distributor □ User Name:

Mailing Address.: Post Code: Contact Tel.:

A. Information on the Patient		
1. Name:	2. Age:	3. Gender: □ Male □ Female
4. Intended use:		
B. Adverse Event		
5. Main Event Manifestations:		
6. Date of Occurrence: 7. Discovery or Informed Date:		
8. Place of Use □ Medical establishment □ Home □ Others (please specify):		
9. Consequences of Event □ Death_________________(time) □ Threat to life □ Permanent damage to organic structure □ Possible permanent damage to organic structure □ Internal and surgical treatment required to avoid permanent damage to organic structure □ Others (Please specify in the Event Statement):		
10. Event statement: (at least include the time of using the device, purpose of use, basis for use, conditions in use, adverse event occurring, impact on the victim, therapeutic measures taken and combined use of devices)		

C. Information on Medical Device
11. Product Name:
12. Trade Name:
13. Registration Certificate No.:
14. Manufacturer'sName: Manufacturer's Address: Contact Tel.:
15. Specifications and models: Product S/N: Product Lot No.:
16. Operator: □ Professional □ Non-professional □ Patient □ Others (please specify):
17. Expiry Date: 18. Production Date: 19. Stop Using Time: 20. Date of Implantation:
21. Initial Analysis of Event
22.Initial Measures Taken Against the Event:
23. Reporting State of Event: □ Notified the user □ Notified the manufacturer □ Notified the distributor □ Notified drug authorities
D. Evaluation of Adverse Event
24. Opinions by Shanghai Municipal Supervision Institution (additional pages available):

Reported by: Doctor □ Technician □ Nurse □ Others □

Signature of the reporter: **Prepared by State Food and Drug Administration**

Fig. 21.15 Report on the Suspected Medical Device Adverse Event

References

1. Mao H, Jin S, Dai W, et al. Study of the agile supply chain on high-value consumables used in surgical operations. Chin J Hospital Administration. 2014;6(30):466–9.
2. Mao H, Chen Z, Dai W, et al. Informationization management of high-value interventional consumables to face the dynamic demand. J Med Informatics. 2014;8(27):57–8.

22 Personnel Management

Huajuan Mao, Weihui Dai, and Haiyan Li

Abstract

Personnel management constitutes an important part of endovascular device management and consists of three aspects, i.e., supplier management, device technician or nurse management, and patient management. It aims to ensure that the delivery, safekeeping, and use of devices can meet relevant requirements on safety and specialization; with the aid of information systems and intelligent technology, it also aims to enhance management efficiency, reduce losses and errors, provide more precise guarantee for clinical departments, and ultimately improve patient experience and satisfaction with medical services. This chapter provides a comprehensive elaboration on parties related to endovascular devices, i.e., supplier management, patient management, device platform and device technician management, and radiological safety management. To be specific, in the section of patient management, it introduces how to use neuromanagement to improve patient experience with medical services and promote the new concept of smart medical services. In the section of device platform and device technician management, it puts forward the construction of professional management platforms for endovascular devices and relevant requirements on device technician.

Keywords

Endovascular devices · Personnel management · Device platform · Neuromanagement · Smart medical services

H. Mao · H. Li
Department of Vascular Surgery, Changhai Hospital, Second Military Medical University, Shanghai, China

W. Dai (✉)
School of Management, Fudan University, Shanghai, China
e-mail: whdai@fudan.edu.cn

22.1 Supplier Management

In the management of personnel related to endovascular devices, the ability of suppliers to cooperate and professional quality function as the most critical elements. The device stock should be updated in line with the personalized demands by the clinical surgeons, and each product has its unique characteristics, advantages, and disadvantages. The suppliers for the devices mentioned above should provide sufficient guidance and suggestions for the clinical doctors according to product structure, performance, model, applicable object, and use method. In the management of the supplier team, we have worked out the following regulations based on our practical experience for years.

- Regularly evaluate the supplier's products, services, and goodwill, classify the suppliers, employ different management strategies and incentive measures accordingly, and cancel the qualification of the non-compliant suppliers.
- All ordered devices must be within the scope of the device catalog, and all new devices can be ordered and stocked up only after approval by the hospital administration.
- For the service conditions and problems found with each device, device-specific service condition list is prepared based on statistical analysis, and the supplier should analyze, explain, and provide opinions on product service conditions, thus providing evaluation reference for the follow-up orders.
- From 9:00 a.m. to 10:30 a.m. each day, the supplier should complete the normal delivery, understand the service conditions and problems with his products, and provide relevant guidance.
- The supplier should guarantee sufficient stocks for and verify the stocktaking data of the high-value endovascular devices and commonly used critical devices in line with the operation arrangement and the requirements for the stock level.

Z. Jing et al. (eds.), *Endovascular Surgery and Devices*, https://doi.org/10.1007/978-981-10-8270-2_22

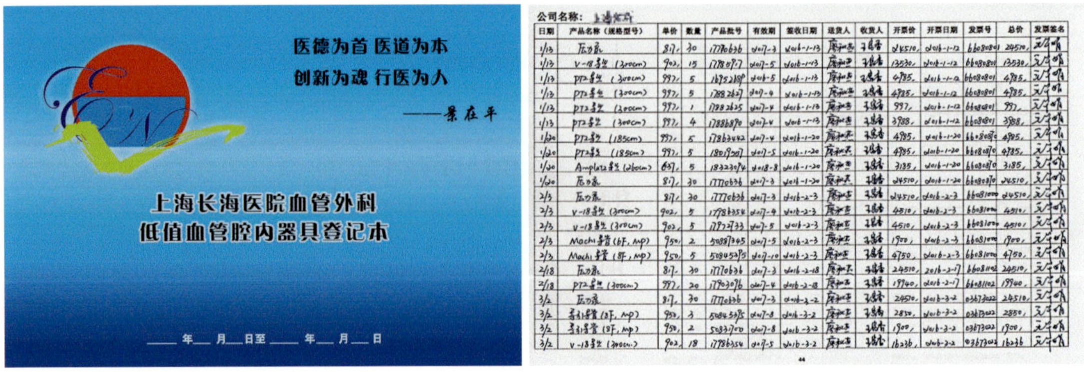

Fig. 22.1 Low-value endovascular device register

- Special device register (Fig. 22.1) is designed for the diversified low-value endovascular devices by Huajuan Mao, facilitating looking up and verifying these devices at any time.

The management of suppliers needs not only to establish a necessary guarantee system and the survival-of-the-fittest mechanism but also to build a favorable symbiotic ecosystem through effective incentive measures to achieve sustainable development under an all-win and cooperative relationship.

22.2 Patient Management

An important idea for modern medical service is patient-centered. The demands of patients are reflected not only in efficient, safe, and economical service, and also the perception, cognition, and experience of the patient exert significant influence on service satisfaction. With the development in medical technology, the time for endovascular therapy is shortened significantly; most patients receive their surgeries under local anesthesia and are fully aware of their situations. Intraoperative and postoperative care to the patients is an issue to be meticulously considered in patient management. In line with the characteristics of the patients under endovascular therapy, we have taken the following measures in the management of patients mentioned above.

22.2.1 Emotion Management

In the emotion management over the patients, the environmental atmosphere has an important impact, in addition to the care by the medical workers. In 1997, Zaiping Jing put forward the idea of installing musical equipment in the wards.

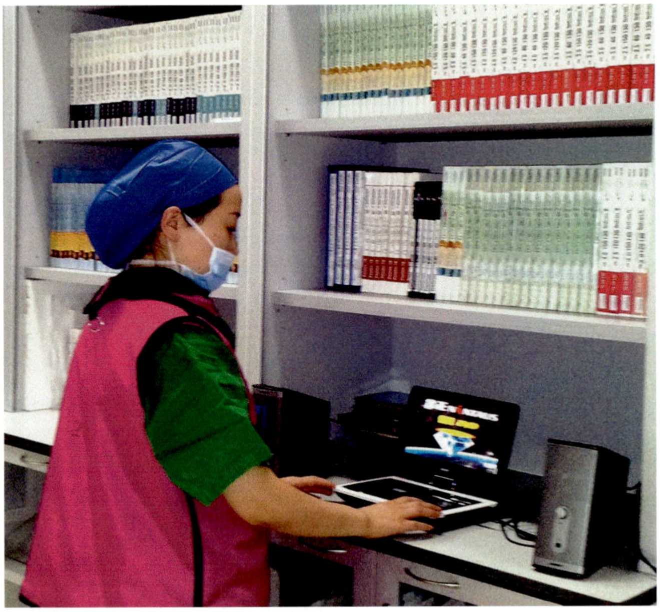

Fig. 22.2 Music playback devices

Relaxed and cheerful music can improve the function of the brain and the entire nervous system, rhythmic music makes people refreshed and eliminates depression and tension, and melodious music can make people at ease, distract the patient's nervous mood, and be conducive to the restoration of the patient's physical and mental health. The patients have been highly appreciative of our SRS musical equipments installed in our wards since 2000. In 2009, at the suggestion of Zaiping Jing, we also installed light music playback devices in the catheter rooms of the vascular surgery (Fig. 22.2). The music installations mentioned above not only alleviate and reduce the mental stress and pain of the anxious and nervous patients but also bring good experience to the surgeons, improving both the surgical efficiency and quality.

22.2.2 Temperature Management

As pointed out in the *Operation Room Nursing Technical Manual*, the temperature in the operation room is very important, and the operation room should be equipped with temperature-regulating devices to keep room temperature at 24–26 °C and humidity of about 50% [1]. According to Operation Room Nursing and Building Specifications of Hospital Clean Operation Room, the operation room temperature should be maintained at 22–25 °C with relative humidity of 50–60%. Each operation room should be equipped with thermometer, humidometer, and temperature-regulating switch [2, 3]. Related studies have shown that during operation for the elderly people, the operation room temperature should be kept at about 22 °C, which can both effectively prevent the core body temperature of the elderly patient from excessively declining during operation and also prevent or reduce microbial reproduction while satisfying the requirements for comfort [4]. Therefore, in the management over patients, the ambient temperature should be properly regulated, which will have an important impact on the patient's physiology, psychology, and prevention of reproduction of microorganisms.

22.2.3 Skin Management

Surgical patients will be subject to postural restriction and other factors and become the high-risk group for bedsores. Among them, bedsores due to body position rank No.4 among the operation room safety risks [5]. Therefore, before the patient is arranged to lie at any position, the status of the force-bearing point of the patient body should be taken into account, and appropriate position mattress should be cushioned. In case of high-risk surgical patient, bedsore paste or transparent paste can be used to protect the related area of the skin. The said bedsore paste can improve the friction and shear force, alleviate the vertical pressure and skin pressure, ease hemodynamic disorder, prevent the infiltration of external moisture, keep skin dryness and better permeability, and better prevent the occurrence of bedsores. In order to prevent the occurrence of acute bedsores during operation, when the patient is moved by two persons, the bedsheet must be lifted up, avoiding the formation of shear force by pulling and dragging the patient. In addition, the operation sheet should be kept clean and dry, avoiding skin irritation and occurrence of other accidents. For example, the gauze for skin disinfection needs to be moderately dry and wet to prevent excessive disinfectant from flowing to other parts of the patient body and wetting the bedsheets. Operation sheets and position constraint tapes should be kept dry, smooth, and soft without wrinkles, trying to eliminate all risks of bedsores as far as possible. Position constraint tapes should also be padded with adequate tightness to prevent the tissue damage to the related area of the skin and reduce its bedsore incidence.

22.2.4 Safety Management

For patients accommodated in the catheter room, the nurses of the nursing station should check whether various tubes of the patient are in place and smooth so as to ensure the normal use during operation. For patients without indwelling venous needles or with obstructed venous needles, prompt placement and treatment should be ensured, thus reducing preoperative preparation time, accelerating operation process, and improving hand-and-taking-over system. When the patient enters the catheter room, the nurse of the catheter room should verify the patient identity according to the case history and, upon confirmation, help the patient to move to the waiting area, conduct health propaganda, and reassure the patient. When the patient receives operation, the technician takes the patient case history and verifies his/her information according to the wrist identification tape, and after careful confirmation, the patient is moved to the operation room. When the patient lies on the operation table, the patient information should be reverified together by the surgeon, nurse, and anesthetist or technician in the operation room to ensure surgical safety.

22.3 Neuromanagement and Smart Medical Services

The psychologies and behaviors in medical service are marked by strong situational characteristics and are affected by the complexity of disease diagnosis and treatment, the asymmetry of information, and the confidence mechanism between doctors and patients. The above services pose differences and uncertainty in personalized demands, asymmetry of knowledge between doctors and patients, and other aspects of the particularity. The above services not only need professional knowledge on medical technology but also take into account the influence in social, economic, psychological, and other factors [6, 7]. A large number of empirical studies have shown that how to form a good understanding, comprehension, and cooperation through effective communication between doctors and patients is the key to guarantee the success of these services and to improve service satisfaction [6]. With the development of modern neuroscience and artificial intelligence technology, how to study the perception, cognition, and affective characteristics of patients in the course of medical service from the neurological mechanism and use the intelligent context awareness and analysis technology to provide the patients with better medical care service has become a hot topic in related fields and a new trend in application development [7, 8].

In the 1970s, the combination of neuroscience, brain science, and psychology, especially the development of cognitive neuroscience, enabled people to make breakthrough progress in researches on neurological mechanisms of brain functions, such as learning, memory, thinking, language, and feeling, from molecular and cellular level to overall and behavioral level. In the 1990s, the emergence of fMRI (functional magnetic resonance imaging) provided new technical means for direct noninvasive observation of brain functional activities and promoted the fast development of neurological science and cognitive neuroscience. The development does not only provide a new basis for brain-like and brain-inspired design in the interdisciplinary research areas of computational neuroscience, artificial intelligence science, and other engineering disciplines but also gives rise to many emerging disciplines in interdisciplinary social and human sciences. In 1992, Cacioppo and Berntson proposed a new field of research in "social neuroscience," which takes the social processes of normal people and the neurobiological mechanisms of social behavior as the object of study [9]. In 2002, Vernon Smith, Nobel Prize winner in economics, proposed the new development trend of using brain imaging technique to explore neuroeconomics issues. In 2004, International Society of Mind, Brain, and Education was established, cultivating a new area for research in educational neuroscience. In 2006, Prof. Qingguo Ma gave in-depth analysis of the foregoing development trends, proposed the new concept of neuromanagement, and expounded the difference and connection of the foregoing disciplines with other relevant disciplines [10].

Neuromanagement is an emerging interdisciplinary system exploring into management issues and its inherent mechanism, finding new management rules, and proposing new management theories by using the theories, methods, and techniques of neuroscience [11]. The development of neuromanagement provides new theoretical basis and techniques in studying relevant management issues from the perspective of brain cognitive characteristics and neurological mechanism of management activities, provides empirical knowledge on the inherent mechanism of human psychology and behavior for big data analysis, and provides new support for brain-like and brain-inspired artificial intelligence design oriented to advanced brain functions. Meanwhile, the development in brain science and neuroscience is also exerting significant influence to modern psychology, pedagogy, linguistics, sociology, economics, law, military science, and other social science and humanities and arts disciplines, giving rise to cognitive neuroscience, educational neuroscience, language neuroscience, social neuroscience, cultural neuroscience, neuroeconomics, neurolaw, military neuroscience, and other interdisciplinary sciences and disciplines [11]. On December 13, 2015, Neuromanagement and Neuroengineering Research Committee, Society of Management Science and Engineering of China was founded at Zhejiang University. In May 2016, the first academic annual meeting was convened at Ningbo University. In July 2017, the second academic annual meeting was convened at Guangdong University of Technology. In August 2017, Neuromanagement and Intelligent Computing Forum was held at Fudan University chaired by Prof. Weihui Dai, under the joint sponsorship by Shanghai Charter of China Computer Federation (CCF), Neuromanagement and Neuroengineering Research Committee, and Department of Information Management and Information Systems of School of Management at Fudan University. After a decade's development, neuromanagement has aroused worldwide attentions, given rise to a vigorous research team in China and exerted significant influence to the creative development of relevant disciplines.

The research results in the field of neuromanagement provide important theoretical guidance for us to understand the psychological and behavioral characteristics of medical services and their law of change, avoid the contradiction, and build a harmonious relationship between doctors and patients.

By employing various experimental imaging techniques such as fMRI (functional magnetic resonance imaging), EPRs (event-related potentials), and the use of various wearable devices, the neurological activity characteristics and their brain mechanism for emotional experience of the patients in the process of medical service are studied, achieving many important results. Viewing from the emotional brain mechanism, the abovementioned emotions are first generated by the stimulus signals resulting from specific outside or in vivo situations, which are transmitted to cerebral limbic system and center systems via various sensory organs and paths and excite the brainstem reticular formation along the transmitted collateral branches, causing extensive brain arousal state and stimulating relevant brain functional activities. The emotions generated by the above stimulus signals are divided into two categories: the first category is the rapid instinctive response produced under external stimuli, which are the advanced cognitive process mainly produced by the cerebral limbic system rather than through the cerebral cortex, known as "primary emotion." The second category refers to those emotions that occur slowly after cognitive censorship through the cerebral cortex, known as "secondary emotion." The primary emotion often forms intuitive emotional response, based on which, the secondary emotion forms through the interactive activities between the cerebral limbic system and the cerebral cortex after the advanced cognitive process of the brain, thus forming rather rational cognitive response.

The emotional changes mentioned above will also induce a series of physiological reactions through neural regulation mechanism, in addition to producing corresponding active signals in the specific cerebral functional area, leading to changes in both of various human peripheral physiological signals (such as EEG, skin conductance, ECG, breathing, body temperature, and others) and external manifestations, such as the voice, face expression, posture, action, etc., and even resulting in further follow-up behaviors. On the other hand, human peripheral and external behavioral activities aggregate in the cerebral structure through the feedback from the neural sensory path, forming subjective experience to emotional changes. Therefore, the identification methods of human emotions can be classified into four categories [8, 11]: (1) description and identification of subjective experience of emotions by self-reports, (2) direct observations of activities in the brain functional area closely related to emotional changes through fMRI (functional magnetic resonance imaging), (3) identification by collecting and analyzing various human peripheral physiological signals, and (4) analysis and identification based on-site observations of external expressions and follow-up behaviors through various audio, video, infrared imaging, and other observation technologies in combination with specific situations and relevant empirical knowledge. Based on the work mentioned above, the generation, expression mechanism, and identification methods of human emotions are consolidated and summarized as follows (Fig. 22.3) [8, 11].

By observing the neural activities of emotions and analyzing its relations with peripheral reactions, external expressions, and follow-up behaviors, we can use affective computing technology to realize intelligent monitoring and analysis of the patient's emotional state by collecting relevant physiological signals or on-site observations under a noninterventional and on-contact site environment, thus providing better care service. Moreover, the sound, lighting, color, temperature, humidity, smell, and other conditions of wards and operation rooms are specially designed, by using ultrathin wall-adhesive screen, temperature, and humidity control devices, olfactory odor generation devices, and other intelligent devices to create a natural landscape atmosphere and provide various sensory stimulation signals helpful for emotional regulation. Prof. Weihui Dai in the School of Management at Fudan University pointed out: viewing from the intelligence trend of the medical service, the services mentioned above will not only provide the best clinical path and treatment decision for the patients through the rational intelligence of the machines but should also integrate with emotional intelligence, providing the patients with the best human-centered services according to their physiological state and emotional experience throughout all links of the medical service and defining the "smart service" as a service integrated with the emotional and rational intelligence [8]. In view of the definition above, having emotional intelligence distinguishes the "smart service" significantly from general intelligent services. Meanwhile, the meaning of "smart" in such concepts as smart city, smart healthcare, and smart government can also be understood as the combination of both rational and emotional intelligence [8].

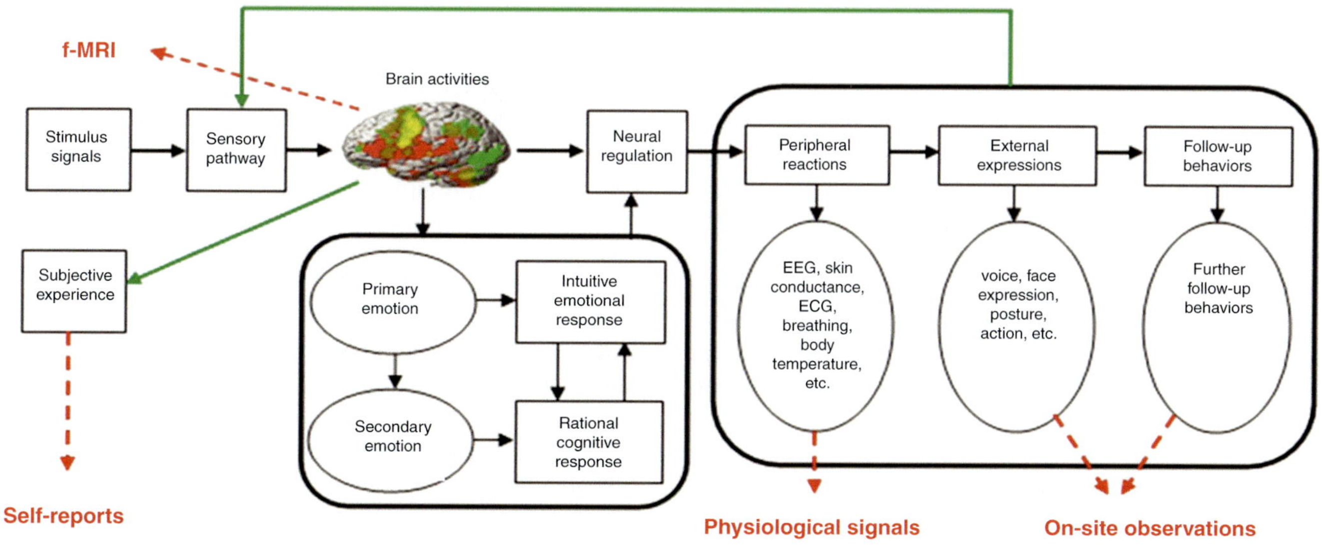

Fig. 22.3 Emotion's generation, expression mechanism, and identification method

22.4 Management of Device Platforms and Device Management Engineers

With the development of and the ever-increasing professional requirements for endovascular devices, a new management mode has come into being by establishing special device platforms equipped with corresponding device management engineers. The said-device platforms refer to the comprehensive platforms providing endovascular surgical devices as well as management, coordination, and research of associated services. Device management engineers function as the leading role for the platforms and are professional technicians among surgeons and nurses. The said-device platforms have been listed as one of the nine platforms for department development as proposed by Professor Zaiping Jing.

22.4.1 Establishing Endovascular Device Platform

As a new platform that comes with the minimally invasive endovascular surgery, device platform is performed by nurses of catheter, clinical, or operation rooms at many Chinese large class 3 grade-A hospitals. As endovascular devices develop rapidly in terms of types, models, and brands, different types of stocking also become increasingly multifarious. Many nurses feel unable to do as they would wish, hence failing to keep pace with the surgeons because they have to take on both intraoperative nursing and intraoperative coordination. Furthermore, for lack of frontier knowledge and the trend of development as well as no comprehensive consideration for intraoperative stocking, technological progress for the surgeons is hindered and surgical result of the patients affected. To this end, device platform is established and developed.

At present, devices used by large class 3 grade-A hospitals in first-tier cities are no longer distributed directly by the suppliers but delivered to the operation rooms through logistics, where the operations are coordinated mainly by catheter room nurses, reemployed staff after retirement, department doctors, and operation room nurses. For class 3 grade-A hospitals in second- and third-tier cities, salespersons of suppliers shall take on distribution as well as intraoperative coordination. After analyzing the aforesaid persons involved, we have to think over the following issues.

22.4.1.1 Poor Professionalism

Some hospitals practice surgical coordination with nurses of catheter and operation rooms, but basically they do not work on fixed shifts or work on rotation with other departments. Therefore, such job mobility often leads to poor professionalism and short-term learning. Many problems also exist with surgical coordination with suppliers. Most salespersons of suppliers are not graduates from specialized medical schools and often lack knowledge of aseptic operation and infection control, thus increasing the risk of post-operation infection on the part of the patients. Meanwhile, several salespersons from various suppliers are allowed access to the operation rooms by some hospitals, resulting in artificially mutual competition and seriously affecting the overall quality and effect of surgical operations.

22.4.1.2 Lack of Frontier Knowledge

To reduce the cost of labor, some hospitals or departments employ retired medical staff to manage the endovascular devices. They are devoted and responsible, but when facing the multifarious and quickly developing devices, they are often late in acquiring the latest knowledge and situations. Nurses are asked to monitor these devices together with these people at some hospitals, but they are not fixed professionals and unable to understand the adaptability and particularity of each brand and each device, which, however, requires continuous accumulation of clinical experience.

22.4.1.3 Failure to Meet Dynamic Demands

Complex and changing situations often happen during minimally invasive endovascular operations. Therefore, surgical procedures often change while the types and models of devices also change accordingly. In case of too many intermediate links, delivery time will be delayed or messages sent wrong after retelling, thus delaying the operation or rescue time for patients.

22.4.1.4 Delayed Information Exchange with Suppliers

Any adverse reactions or problems happening in using the devices shall be promptly communicated to the manufacturers by professionals for consultancy, guidance, and treatment, and any adverse reactions with the devices shall be reported and registered.

22.4.1.5 Chaotic Device Management

Lack of specialized management, manual operation, irregular or delayed charges, wrong or missing accounts, and other issues often exist with device management.

Therefore, establishing a unified device platform can ensure professional management and improve management efficiency for endovascular devices.

22.4.2 Managing Professional Skills of Device Management Engineers

Device management engineers of endovascular devices shall, at first, have the following qualities:

- Being correct in thinking, highly responsible, and quick-witted.
- A strong team spirit: Patients undergoing vascular surgery involve extensive operations and diversified anesthesia as well as various medical staffs from related departments. For example, in aortic valve replacement via transfemoral balloon dilation, it involves multifarious surgical devices and complex operations as well as coordination with multidisciplinary departments and rooms such as anesthesia, ultrasonography, cardiovascular medicine, thoracic surgery, operation room, and others. Therefore, the proficiency and mutual understanding of the device management engineers are of paramount importance throughout operations.
- High professional requirements: As new minimally invasive endovascular techniques and therapies evolve continuously, device management engineers have to understand the performance and use of radiographic wire, the catheter, the puncture kit, and endovascular devices and deliver the devices quickly as required at each operation step to shorten the operation time to ensure successful completion of the operation.

22.4.3 Professional Requirements for Device Management Engineers

22.4.3.1 Size of Devices

Patients undergoing vascular surgery have complex conditions, suffering from an extensive range of lesion and involving the use of thousands of catheters, wires, vascular sheath, balloons, and stents of various sizes throughout their bodies. For example, there are more than 30 kinds of stent grafts just in terms of diameter, ranging from max. 46 mm to min. 5 mm, let alone their different lengths. There are nearly 100 kinds of stent grafts just for one brand. In operation, stent grafts of different sizes are required according to different conditions, surgical procedures, and vascular diameters.

22.4.3.2 Models of Devices

Devices of each brand have different models. Conventional models shall be clearly understood, especially the special models of each brand, so that we can make the best of each brand in preparing stocking. For example, Bard self-expanding stent has a minimum diameter of 6 mm and a maximum length of 17 mm. However, in clinical practice, most patients are fit for 5 mm or 4 mm. Therefore, models of Biotronik self-expanding stent below 6 mm diameter shall be stocked up excessively. As a result, models of each brand shall be clearly understood in stocking and use.

22.4.3.3 Types of Devices

Devices are diversified, for example, there are various types of stents: balloon-expandable stent, self-expanding bare stent, stent graft, drug-eluting stent, etc. Catheter and wire can also be classified into several dozens according to their tip and hardness. Therefore, different balloons and stents should be configured according to the actual models of the wire and vascular sheaths.

22.4.3.4 Features of Devices

Devices of different brands have different characteristics. Taking peripheral self-expanding bare stent as an example, some are flexible and some rather rigid. Rigid stent is indicated for venous lesions. It must be understood which characteristics match with which spectrum of diseases. This must not be used wrongly.

22.4.3.5 Use of Devices

The use of devices is very important; each vascular sheath, wire, catheter, balloon, and stent has its own indications and use and should not be wrongly used during operation. For example, using peripheral self-expanding bare stent with the carotid artery may lead to stent rupture due to longtime neck movement. Therefore, the carotid artery requires special carotid artery stent.

22.4.3.6 Development and Frontier Knowledge of Devices

In recent years, centering on the problems found in clinical surgery, medical device companies have made great progress in the development of new materials. Hi-tech devices become more and more popular, such as drug-eluting balloon, drug-eluting stent, absorbable stent, etc. A professional engineer of device management must have expert mastery of the devices so as to successfully coordinate with the surgeons during operation.

22.4.4 Essentials for Intraoperative Coordination by Device Management Engineers

22.4.4.1 Planning

Understand and communicate with the surgeons about the patient's operative program 1 day before the operation, and prepare devices to be used the next day according to the communication results. Any special devices, if required, should be ordered as early as possible, and generally device order is placed before 12 o'clock at noon so as to leave sufficient time for suppliers to prepare goods.

22.4.4.2 Flexibility

In the clinical operation program, although the preparation and delivery requirements for critical devices are given in advance, the actual operation process often encounters various complicated situations so that the original operation program has to be changed, thus resulting in dynamic change in the device demands, and emergency delivery must be carried out for unprepared devices.

22.4.4.3 Professionalism

Many high-value endovascular devices have become the key to the success of clinical surgery, having high added value and becoming the focus of research and development by related institutions and one of the fastest growing areas. With the continually updating and ever-enriching devices, segmentation of device use also shows a rapid trend of development, and clinical surgery will face more diversified, complex, and professional choices. Therefore, it is necessary to learn and master relevant knowledge and accumulate critical experience in clinical application.

22.4.4.4 Adaptability

In clinical surgery, due to the difference in knowledge, experience, and habits, different doctors have different preference in the selection of devices. To ensure smooth operation, personalized preference of doctors should be satisfied as far as possible. Moreover, in line with the ever-changing operation situations and considered from the prospective of safety, efficiency, and economy, the most appropriate endovascular devices should be recommended by intelligent methods, providing their important characteristics and operation instructions.

22.4.4.5 Creativity

In developing new technologies and therapies, device management engineers must learn together with the surgeons and cooperate for innovation. For example, when the doctor flushes the thoracic aortic stent graft delivery system with the prepared heparin diluent, the entire system is about 155 cm long, but common operation device table is only 90–100 cm long, and thus this kind of devices cannot be operated on the table. In particular, for surgeons with different heights, the fixed height of the operation device table also causes inconvenience to them. To solve the problems mentioned above, the department of Vascular Surgery of Changhai Hospital affiliated to the Second Military Medical University has specially designed a national invention patent of the operation device table (Patent No.: ZL201310468529.1) (Fig. 22.4).

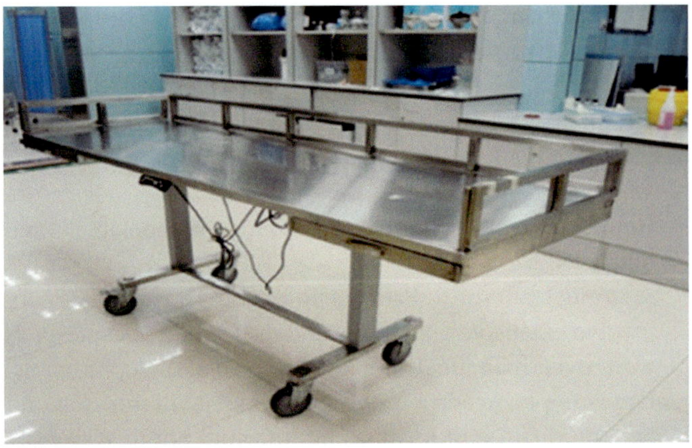

Fig. 22.4 Operation device table

The operation device table is 250 cm long, preventing personnel from bumping into the operation device on the table when they pass by the table, hence playing a positive role in preventing infection. Meanwhile, the telescopic structure of the table enables the surgeons to adjust the table to the appropriate height according to the corresponding data between body height and table height, thus achieving optimal operation state.

22.4.4.6 Economy

The rapid development of the doctor's technique and the endovascular devices has led to the accelerated pace of operation, the shortening of the hospitalization time, and faster turnover rate of the bed. Upon completion of each operation, device management engineers should promptly follow through on fee charging.

With continuous development of various minimally invasive endovascular therapies, more and more endovascular device brands and models emerge, and more professionals are required to understand their performance and operations. These professionals are highly valued by relevant hospital and department authorities, but for the entire layout and personnel arrangement of a hospital, there is still much room for improvement. This profession poses broad demands and prospects of development. What follows is how to train and cultivate professional device management engineers in a more standard manner and promote the implementation of access qualification, which is worthy of our further thinking.

22.5 Radiological Safety Management

22.5.1 Basic Requirements for Interventional Radiological Protective Articles

Personal interventional radiological protective articles should conform to the nature of the interventional operation, delicate, convenient, durable, and harmless to the human body. Protective tube should be designed according to the difference in the lower and the upper-tube X-ray machines so that radiation exposure to the workers of interventional therapy is as low as possible, while normal work is not affected. The design of these articles is subject to the following requirements [12].

- Conveniently applicable: The aim is that under the prerequisite of not affecting the operations, the designed protective devices and personal protective articles are flexible and convenient in use, without affecting surgical operation.
- Safely shielded: The doctor's operation area should be adequately shielded from the patient's irradiation area. The better the area is separated, that is, the better the radioactive source is shielded, the better the protective effect will be.
- Extensively available: In design protective devices, the compatibility with single type C-arm, double type C-arm, and common X-ray machines should be considered, which can have extensive application value.
- Easily disinfected: Interventional devices are often polluted by blood and should be sterilized regularly. Therefore, protective devices and articles should be acid and oxidant resistant so as to reduce pollution and the spread of diseases. In the use of lead collars, it is not suitable for washing and direct contact with the skin, and after using for some time, it is liable of cross infection among the medical workers. To solve this problem, Huajuan Mao has specially designed a national patented of the lead collar jacket (Patent No.: ZL201520114715.X) (Fig. 22.5).

The lead collar jacket easily absorbs sweat and is convenient in use. In using the lead collar, cover the jacket over the lead collar to avoid direct contact with the skin. Upon completion of operation, remove the jacket and leave the lead collar unpolluted. In addition, lead collar jacket is easy to be washed and carried and used just by one person, thus reducing the probability of cross infection.

- Shapely and durable: Material selection and structure design weigh whether it is durable, for example, not easy of failure to the mechanical parts, no deformation after long use, no surface corrosion, etc. Exquisite workmanship and pleasant appearance are required to match with the advanced X-ray machines (Fig. 22.6).
- Optimal cost performance: Take into account the best integration of the protective effect, applicability, and economic cost, that is, to optimize the design scheme. According to the actual measurement and scientific calculation, 0.6 mm, 0.7 mm, 1.0 mm, and 1.4 mm lead equivalent protection thickness is chosen for different protective articles, which achieves over 90% shielding efficiency while reducing the weight and cost at the same time.

22.5.2 Use and Management of Interventional Radiological Protective Articles

The protective article brands currently available on market include Lite Tech (US), InFab (US), Medical Index (German), YOUMYOU (China), Kolida (China), etc., covering a variety of products, like radiation-proof clothes, collars, hats,

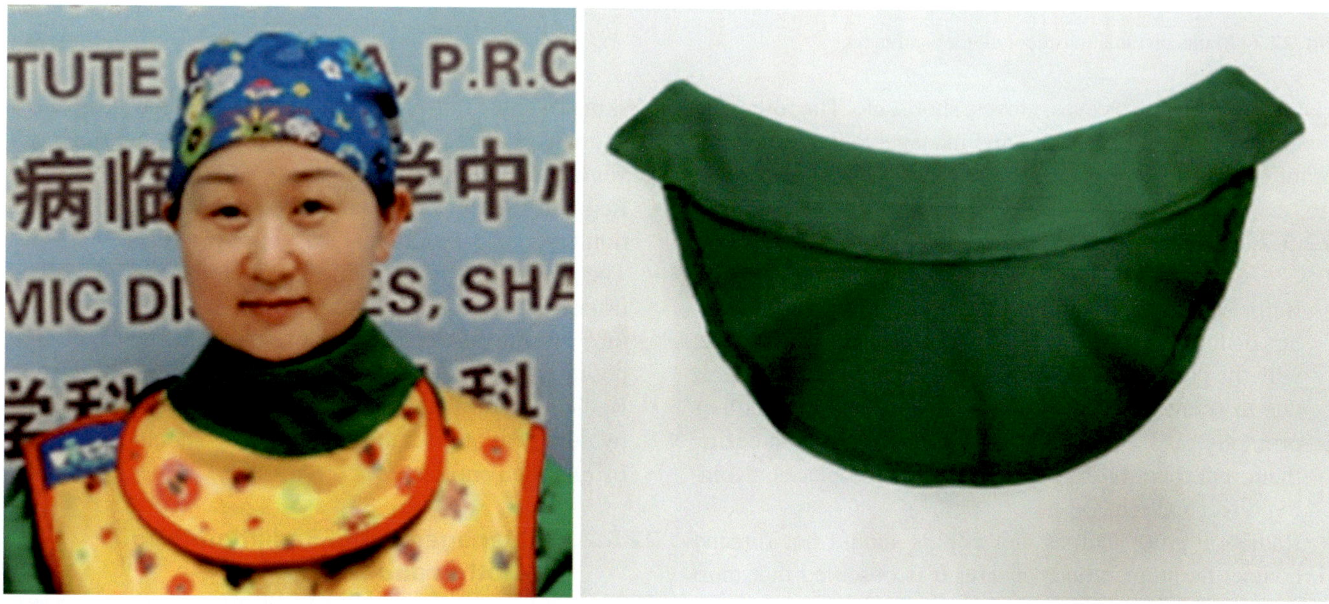

Fig. 22.5 Lead collar jacket

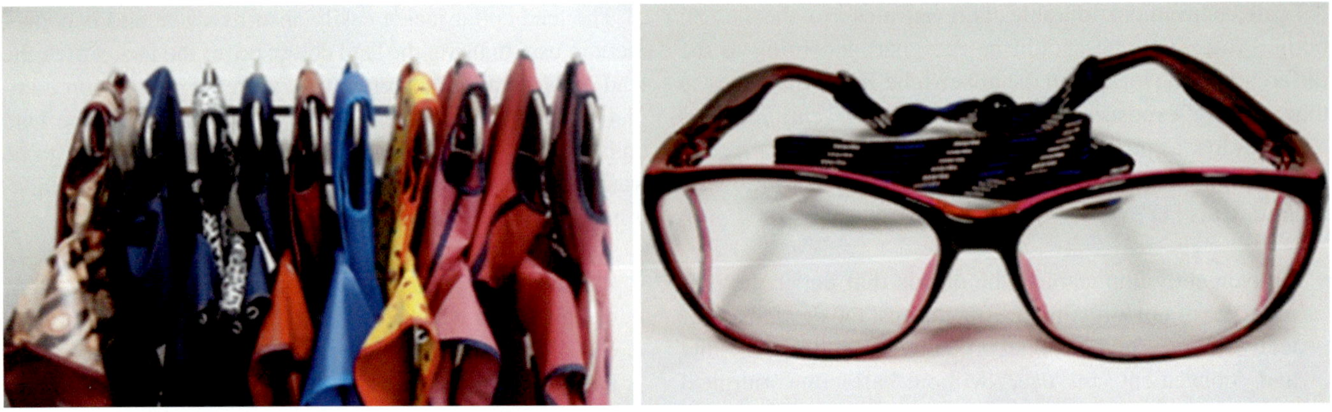

Fig. 22.6 Materials and structures for protective articles

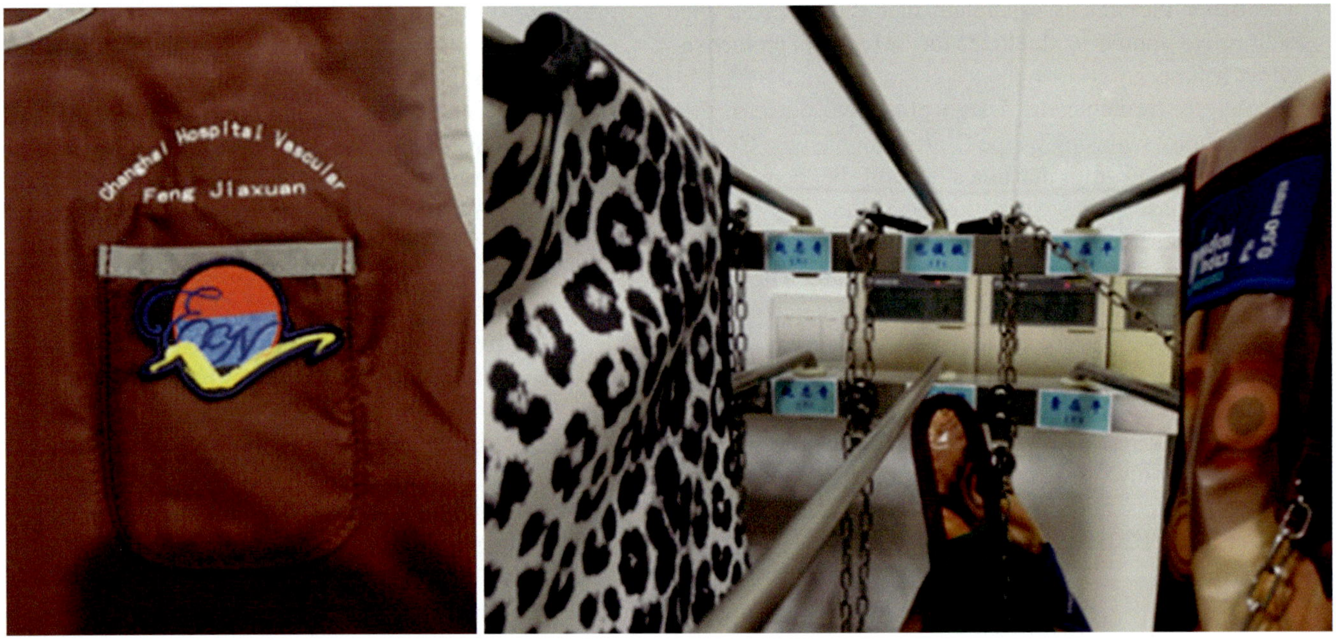

Fig. 22.7 Marks on radiation-proof clothes and racks

glasses, hoods, arm sleeves, gloves, shorts, etc. The following text mainly introduces the use and management of radiation-proof clothes and collars [12].

22.5.2.1 Principles in Using Radiation-Proof Clothes and Collars

- Before use, check if the radiation-proof clothes and collars dislocate, fall off, or loosen; during use, avoid contact with the pointed article as this affects the protective effect due to scratches. After use, hang the clothes and collars promptly on special racks, without folding or squeezing them; put them in dry and well-ventilated places, avoiding direct sunlight.
- Radiation-proof clothes and collars should not directly contact the human body in use. It is observed that most doctors directly wear the collars on the necks or cushion the collars with paper, gauze, towel, etc. near the neck skin. To solve this problem, Huajuan Mao has designed a national patented of the lead collar jacket, featuring convenient use and washing.
- Regularly inspect by imaging or send to special inspection units for inspection at least once per year.
- The service life of radiation-proof clothes and collars is usually 3–5 years, and those with cracks or damage (rupture >5 mm) under imaging examination should be disposed promptly.
- Radiation-proof clothes and collars should not be washed by detergent at discretion; rather, they should be cleaned by qualified entities.

22.5.2.2 Management of Radiation-Proof Clothes and Collars

- Clearly labeled (Fig. 22.7): Each suit of radiation-proof clothes should be labeled with serial number or have the unit name and name of doctor embroidered on the clothes. The name and serial number of each doctor should be attached on the clothes racks, and each suit of radiation-proof clothes, collars, and hats should be hung on corresponding racks and hooks, locked and chained.

- Use by just one person (Fig. 22.8): Lead clothes should be assigned to concrete person for self-management under the support by each hospital and department.
- Safekeeping by specially assigned person (Fig. 22.9): The radiation-proof clothes and collars for public use should be managed by specially assigned persons. After use, the doctors are urged to put them on the racks and lock them promptly.
- Suggestions: For the manufacturers and suppliers, the radiation-proof articles need corresponding supporting services in clinical use, such as follow-up maintenance, annual inspection, establishing data library, etc.

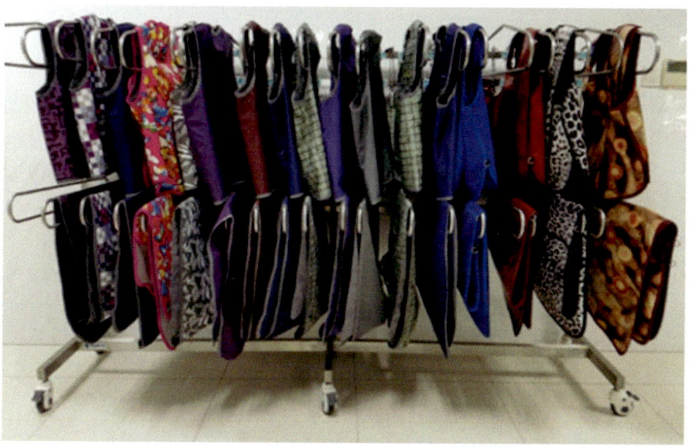

Fig. 22.8 Radiation-proof clothes and racks assigned to concrete person

22.5.3 Common Protective Measures

22.5.3.1 General Protection

Inherent Protection of X-Ray Machine

The inherent safety protection performance of X-ray machine is the most important part of X-ray protection. Tube sleeve and lighttight shutter should be X-ray leakproof, with aluminum filter plate mounted at the window. The air exposure rate at the place where the useful beam accesses into the patient skin should be less than 6R /min. Especially with the bed tube for imaging purpose, in case of radiation leakage happening to the X-ray tube and its accessories, the staffs and the patient will be subject to direct radiation.

Time Protection

Try to shorten X-ray radiation time. The cumulative exposure time in operation should not exceed 30 min. Optimize the best exposure conditions and avoid repeated exposure.

Distance Protection

By enlarging the distance of the operator with the radioactive source (tube focus) and the patient, reduce the exposure dosage to the operator. If the distance doubles, the exposure dosage will be reduced by 3/4.

Shielding Protection

Shield is equipped between the radioactive source and the staff to reduce or eliminate exposure (such as lead barrier).

22.5.3.2 Patient Protection

Reducing exposure dosage to the patient is the key for patient protection. ICRP report published in 2000 classifies the interventional operation according to the maximum cumulative exposure dosage on the patient's skin: high-dose operation is defined as operation resulting in hundreds of mGy dosage, medium dosage as in dozens of mGy dosage, and

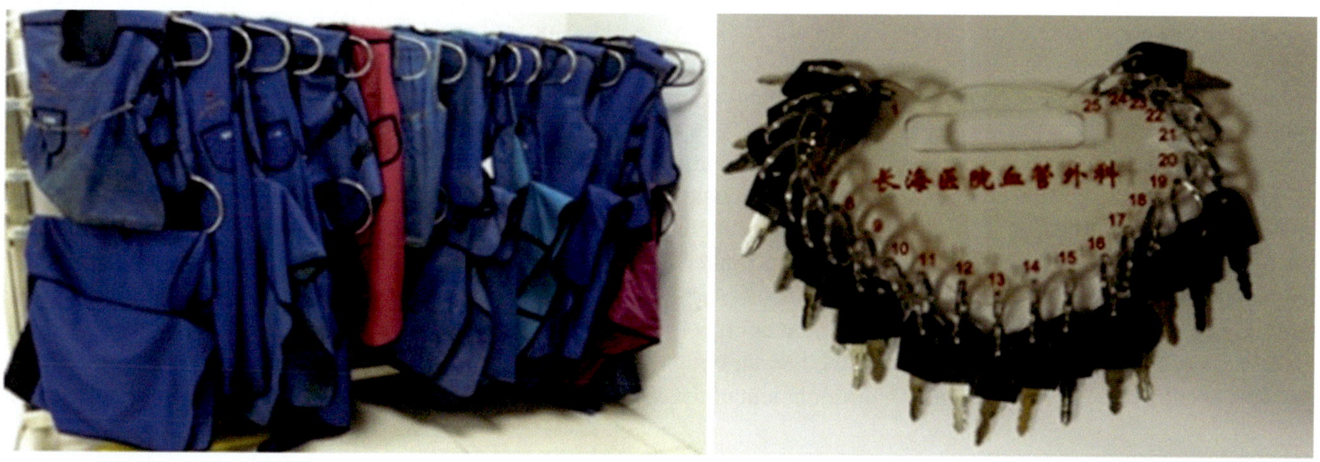

Fig. 22.9 Radiation-proof clothes and racks managed by specially assigned person

low dosage as in less than 10 mGy dosage. Therefore, the staff must be skillful, select the best conditions, reasonably use light-shield device and X-ray filter, adopt shielding protection and position protection, and use lead product to cover the non-irradiation field (especially the genitals and fetuses) to reduce the exposure dosage to patients. The aim is to achieve the best diagnostic and therapeutic effect with the minimum exposure dosage.

22.5.3.3 Staff Protection

Wear Dose Detector

Report personal exposure dosage once every month. The dosage exposed to interventional worker each year should not exceed 5%. To limit X-ray exposure dosage, the number of operations can be adequately limited according to the device and protective conditions of the catheter room.

Observe Protective Regulations

Wear lead clothes, lead collars, and protective goggles. Adjust the ray shield at any time, try to reduce the irradiation field, and forbid access into the irradiation field by any part of the staff's body. Pay attention to protection of critical organs. Tissues highly susceptible to X-ray radiation include the hematopoietic tissue, lymphoid tissue, gonad, intestinal epithelium, and fetus. Tissues moderately and highly susceptible to X-ray radiation include oral mucosa, salivary glands, hair, sweat glands, skin, capillaries, and eye lens.

Regularly Inspect Protection

Conduct blood routine test for staff once every month and systematic physical examination once every year.

Others

Adequately increase nutrition and outdoor activities and avoid overfatigue. Arrange work-shift reasonably and strictly control leave.

22.5.3.4 Protection of DSA Room

The workplace for interventional operation should conform to the stipulations in the Medical Diagnostic X-Ray Health Protection Standards. The indoor area of the interventional operation room relates to the rated tube current of the X-ray machine. The indoor area for X-ray machine of over 200 mA should not be less than 36m^2; indoor wall should have adequate thickness to prevent infiltration of X-ray. Indoor arrangement should be reasonable, without storing matters unrelated to this operation so as to reduce occurrence of scattered rays. Effective ventilation devices should be equipped inside the building, so as to reduce harm to the human body by harmless air. Viewing from the current development of the interventional radiology, X-ray machine equipped with TV imaging device is the minimum requirement for interventional operation. X-ray machine with type C-arm, bipolar imaging, and digital subtraction is more convenient for operation, shortens treatment and diagnosis time, reduces X-ray exposure dosage to both the operators and the patients, and is the preferred interventional fluoroscopic device. X-ray machine without TV monitor should be restricted from the protection safety point of view.

22.5.4 Healthcare System for Interventional Radiotherapy Personnel

22.5.4.1 Health Management

- Personnel involved in radiation-exposed work must receive physical examination, and those unqualified should not be assigned with radiation work.
- Regular physical examination: Those with exposure dosage close to allowable annual maximum exposure level should go through physical examination once every year; those lower than 3/10 once every 2–3 years. Those with onetime exposure dosage exceeding allowable maximum level under special situations should go through physical examination and receive necessary treatment promptly.
- Establish health archives for radiation-exposed workers, which are transferred as their job transfers.
- Forbid radiation contact during radiological healthcare.
- Labor protection measures for radiation-exposed workers should conform to the existing regulations by labor protection authorities and relevant departments.

22.5.4.2 Items for Regular Physical Examination

- Hemogram test: White cell count and classification, blood platelet count, and bone marrow examination, if necessary
- Lens examination
- Hepatic and renal functions
- Skin, hair, fingernail, and blood capillary examination

22.5.4.3 Nutrition Healthcare for Interventional Radiotherapy Personnel

Purposeful adjustment of the nutrition and diets of the medical staffs engaged in the work of interventional radiotherapy can change the body's sensitivity to ionizing radiation to certain extent, and the body's ability to resist radiation damage and repair damage can be improved somewhat. The main principle is to first meet the normal physiological needs of the body, based on which, special nutritional supplements are provided according to the special role by radiological damage. Its ultimate goal is to meet the reasonable nutritional needs of the body to improve the body resistance against external factors.

Special Nutritional Requirements for Interventional Radiotherapy Workers

- Protein: Nutritional requirement is qualitatively higher than that of the normal people.
- Vitamins: Requirements for riboflavin (vitamin B2), vitamin B_{12}, vitamin A, vitamin C, and vitamin D must be first satisfied.
- Excessive supplements for sugar, fat, minerals, trace elements, and water are not necessary.
- Cooked food and diet planning should be reasonable.
- Maintain dietary balance and diversified foods.

Drugs and Healthcare Products Conducive to Reducing Radiation Damage

- Yeast autolysate and yeast ribonucleic acid and hydrolysate can protect against radiation damage to certain extent.
- Herbal drugs: Such as *Astragalus membranaceus*, herba cistanche, etc.
- Polysaccharides: Such as *Trionyx sinensis* Wiegmann crude polysaccharides, mushroom polysaccharides, etc.
- Vitamins.
- Free radical scavenger.
- Others: It is found that mushrooms have a certain anti-radiation effect. Animal experiments confirmed that cabbages have certain protective effect against radioactive damage, the active ingredient of which is not yet clear. Carrots have a certain effect on radiation-induced leukopenia. Honey, almonds, ginseng, etc. also have a certain protective effect against radioactive damage.

22.5.4.4 Health Standard for Interventional Radiotherapy Personnel

In case the following situations happen to the interventional radiotherapy personnel, it is suggested to reduce exposure, suspend work for a short time, and recuperate or transfer to other job.

- Hemoglobin: Male, <120 g/L or > 160 g/L; female, <110 g/L or > 150 g/L
- Red blood cell count: Male, $<4 \times 10^{12}$/L or $> 5.5 \times 10^{12}$/L; female, $<3.5 \times 10^{12}$/L or $> 5 \times 10^{12}$/L
- Total white blood cell continually (over 6 months) $< 4 \times 10^{9}$/L or $> 1.1 \times 10^{9}$/L
- Platelet continually $<100 \times 10^{9}$/L
- Patients suffering from cardiovascular, liver, renal, respiratory, and endocrine disorders, blood diseases, skin disorders, severe lens opacity or high myopia, and severe neurosis or mental illness
- Other organic or functional disorders, which are comprehensively determined by the health sector based on the state of disease or actual exposure to radioactive damage (including radioactive work types, level), ability to work, and professional and technical needs

22.5.5 Regulations on Catheter Room X-Ray Protection Management

- Catheter room X-ray protection work should be the responsibility of the special personnel or coordinated with assigned part-time workers.
- Catheter room workers should have awareness of and sense of responsibility for radiological protection, observe the principle of justification of medical exposure and optimization of radiological protection during work, and organize periodic inspection to radiological protection against working areas, equipment, and personnel.
- DSA devices must have work permit for large medical radiation unit; workers must have relevant qualifications; various personnel at various levels must be familiar with the main structure and safety performance of the DSA device to ensure equipment safety and prevent occurrence of radiation accidents.
- The radiation protection of all examination and control rooms of the catheter room of the Radiology Department should conform to relevant national requirements; all examination rooms should be equipped with ionizing radiation warning signs and work indicators; radiation protection articles should be equipped for working personnel and the persons under examination.
- Before examination, notify the patient of radiation influence on health, and set up notice board at conspicuous places. If not particularly necessary, radiation examination should be avoided for pregnant women, especially for those with 8–15 weeks gestation. The patient's sensitive organs and tissues adjacent to the irradiation field should be shielded.
- Before the DSA examination, close the door of the examination room, and forbid access into the examination room by unrelated personnel. Necessary protective articles should be ensured for the personnel accompanying the patient, if necessary, and the accompanying personnel should stay away from the X-ray tube as far as possible.
- Technical personnel should strictly observe the operation procedures of the DSA device to ensure imaging quality and avoid repeated irradiation.

- Catheter room staff must wear personal dosimeter during their work, receive professional and radiological protection training, and receive regular health examination. The hospital should establish files about personal dose, occupational health management, and educational training.

References

1. Zhang Z. Operation room nursing technology manual. Beijing: People's Military Medical Press; 2000.
2. Wei K, Liu S. Operation Room Nursing. Beijing: People's Military Medical Press; 2003.
3. Ministry of Construction of the People's Republic of China, General Administration of Quality Supervision, Inspection and Quarantine of the People's Republic of China. Specifications of hospital clean operation room building. Beijing: Ministry of Construction of the People's Republic of China, General Administration of Quality Supervision, Inspection and Quarantine of the People's Republic of China; 2002.
4. Shou H, Xu X, Zhang X, et al. Effects of ambient temperature on core temperature of senile patients during operation in the operating room. J Pract Med. 2005;21(6):555–7.
5. Zhong C, Jiang X. Evaluation of application effect of hydrocolloid transparent paste in treatment of stage I bedsore of the elderly patient. Chin J Pract Nurs. 2014;30(16):42–3.
6. Mao H. Research and realization of doctor's prescription behavior analysis system. In: master dissertation of Fudan University; 2010.
7. Dai W. Study on China's translational medicine development strategy: forward-looking medical information technology (1st draft). Major strategic advisory report of Chinese Academy of Engineering; 2014
8. Dai W. Context awareness and emotional intelligence: the gateway to smart city. Urban Manag. 2012;4:29–32.
9. Cacioppo JT, Berntson GG. Social psychological contributions to the decade of the brain: doctrine of multilevel analysis. Am Psychol. 1992;47:1019–28.
10. Ma Q, Wang X. From Neuroeconomics and Neuromarketing to Neuromanagement. J Ind Eng Eng Manag. 2006;20(3):129–32.
11. Dai W. Neuromanagement: disciplinary development and research paradigm [J]. Journal of Beijing Technology and Business University (social science edition). 2017;32(4):1–10.
12. Mao Y. Interventional therapy nursing. Beijing: People's Military Medical Press; 2013.

MIX
Papier aus verantwortungsvollen Quellen
Paper from responsible sources
FSC® C105338

If you have any concerns about our products,
you can contact us on
ProductSafety@springernature.com

In case Publisher is established outside the EU,
the EU authorized representative is:
Springer Nature Customer Service Center GmbH
Europaplatz 3, 69115 Heidelberg, Germany

Printed by Libri Plureos GmbH
in Hamburg, Germany